Springer-Verlag Italia Srl.

A. Gullo (Ed.)

Anaesthesia, Pain, Intensive Care and Emergency Medicine - A.P.I.C.E.

Proceedings of the

14th Postgraduate Course in Critical Care Medicine
Trieste, Italy - November 16-19, 1999

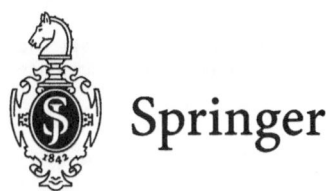 Springer

Prof. ANTONINO GULLO, M.D.
Head, Department of Anaesthesiology and Intensive Care
Trieste University School of Medicine
Trieste, Italy

Library of Congress Cataloging-in-Publication Data: Applied for

© Springer-Verlag Italia 2000
Originally published by Springer-Verlag Italia, Milano in 2000
ISBN 978-88-470-0095-7   ISBN 978-88-470-2286-7 (eBook)
DOI 10.1007/978-88-470-2286-7

SPIN 10753419

Table of Contents

RESPIRATORY CARE

Principles of Laboratory Research on Respiratory Mechanics
W.A. ZIN.. 23

RESPIRATORY MONITORING AT BEDSIDE AND TECHNIQUES

Static and Dynamic Pressure - Volume Curves
G. SERVILLO, M. COPPOLA, AND R. TUFANO... 37

Lung Function Evaluation by Capnography
U. LUCANGELO, G. BERLOT, AND A. GULLO 43

Clinical Implications of the Mechanical Effects of Heat and Moisture Exchangers
A. BRASCHI, M.C. OLIVEI, AND M.A. VILLANI 57

FOCUS ON PULMONARY HYPERTENSION

Pulmonary Hypertension in ARDS: Management Strategies
A. BRIENZA, AND N. BRIENZA.. 65

Focus on Pathophysiology, Diagnosis and Management of Chronic Thromboembolic Disease
I. LANG, AND M. KNEUSSL... 69

EVIDENCE-BASED MEDICINE - PULMONARY SURFACTANT

Rationale for Exogenous Surfactant in Acute Respiratory Distress Syndrome
J.J. HAITSMA, AND B. LACHMANN... 79

Surfactant in the Airways: Function and Relevance in Asthma
J.M. HOHLFELD 85

Alveolar Surfactant and Inflammatory Mediators
M. HALLMAN 91

Role of Surfactant in Ventilation-Induced Lung Injury
S.J.C. VERBRUGGE, J.J. HAITSMA, AND B. LACHMANN.. 101

UPDATE ON ARDS

Has ARDS Epidemiology Changed in the Last 30 Years?
A. ARTIGAS.. 109

Mechanism of ARDS
L. BRAZZI, P. PELOSI, AND L. GATTINONI... 113

Dynamics of Recruitment and Collapse of the Lung in Models of ARDS
P. NEUMANN, AND G. HEDENSTIERNA... 121

Regional Lung Blood Flow and Inhalation of Nitric Oxide
G. HEDENSTIERNA, K. HAMBRAEUS JONZON, AND F. FREDÉN 125

AIRFLOW LIMITATION

Mechanisms and Detection of Tidal Expiratory Flow Limitation
J. MILIC-EMILI.. 133

Clinical Consequences of the Airflow Limitation
C. TANTUCCI, A. FERRETTI, AND V. GRASSI 139

Mechanisms of Intrinsic PEEP
W.A. ZIN.. 147

Static and Dynamic Intrinsic PEEP and Respiratory Mechanics in Mechanically Ventilated COPD Patients
V. ANTONAGLIA, A. PERATONER, AND L. DE SIMONI................................. 153

Respiratory Rehabilitation
R. BRANDOLESE, AND U. ANDREOSE 161

PERIOPERATIVE MEDICINE

EVOLUTION OF THE USE OF ANAESTHETIC DRUGS

Clinical Biochemistry of N_2O: Recent Advances
J. RUPREHT... 173

Anticholinergics: Towards Selective Antimuscarinic Agents?
J. RUPREHT... 179

Evolution of the Use of Anaesthetic Drugs: Neuromuscular Blocking Agents
A. D'HOLLANDER, AND M. BAURAIN... 185

Working Mechanisms of Anaesthetic Agents
M. DZOLJIC 191

FAST-TRACK ANAESTHESIA AND POSTOPERATIVE CARE

Fast-Track Anaesthesia in Cardiac Surgery and Postoperative Care
J.O.C. AULER JR, AND M.J.C. CARMONA 201

Fast-Track Program for Abdominal Surgery
F. CARLI 211

Fast-Track Anaesthesia and Postoperative Care: Orthopaedic Surgery
N.E. SHARROCK 219

Failure to Regain Consciousness After Anaesthesia
D.F. ZANDSTRA, AND M. KUIPER 225

FOCUS ON PERIOPERATIVE MANAGEMENT IN PAEDIATRICS

New Insights into Mechanical Ventilation During Paediatric Anaesthesia
J.O.C. AULER JR, D. FANTONI, AND M.H.C. PEREIRA 235

Perioperative Management Strategy for Cardiac Surgery in Paediatrics
J.O.C. AULER JR, S. COPPOLA GIMENEZ, AND D. MONTEIRO ABBELAN 251

MANAGEMENT OF ANAESTHESIA IN OBSTETRIC PATIENTS

Anaesthetic Management of Obstetric Emergencies
G. LYONS.. 265

Neonatal Resuscitation
D. TREVISANUTO, AND F. ZACCHELLO 271

CHALLENGES IN CARDIOVASCULAR ASSESSMENT, MONITORING
AND MANAGEMENT

Preoperative Cardiovascular Assessment
B. ALLARIA, M. FAVARO, AND M. DEI POLI 281

Perioperative Haemodynamic Monitoring: Invasive Vs. Non-Invasive
B. ALLARIA, M. DEI POLI, AND D. CULOTTA 291

Extracorporeal Circulation: Prevention and Management of Complications
J.O.C. AULER JR 301

Beta Blockers and General Anaesthesia: Prevention of Myocardial Ischaemia
R. MUCHADA.. 311

Heart and Electrolytes
F. SCHIRALDI, P. FERRARO, AND B. MAGLIONE 317

RECOMMENDATIONS ON PERIOPERATIVE MANAGEMENT

Patient-Assessment in the Postanaesthesia Care Unit (PACU)
H.V. SCHALK.. 327

HOW TO SET UP AN ACUTE PAIN SERVICE

How to Set Up Acute Pain Services
N. RAWAL, R. ALLVIN, AND C. ZETTERBERG 333

CENTRAL NERVOUS SYSTEM

DEVELOPMENT, DAMAGE AND REPAIR IN THE CENTRAL NERVOUS SYSTEM

Neural Development in the CNS: Biochemical Mechanisms of Cell Fate Determination
A. CESTELLI, G. SAVETTIERI, AND I. DI LIEGRO 349

Cellular Mechanisms of Brain Damage
G. SAVETTIERI, I. DI LIEGRO, AND A. CESTELLI 369

Repair Mechanisms in the CNS
D.A. SIEGEL, M. HUANG, AND S. WALKLEY 377

STROKE IN THE YOUNG

Stroke in the Young: Epidemiology
G. SAVETTIERI, G. CUCCIA, AND G. SALEMI 389

Pathogenesis of Stroke in Young Adults
A. ANZINI, M. RASURA, AND C. FIESCHI 401

TRAUMA OPERATIVE PROCEDURES

Update on Trauma Scoring
A.J. SUTCLIFFE 411

Trauma Management: From the Field to the Emergency Department
G. NARDI, S. DI BARTOLOMEO, V. MICHELUTTO 417

Intensive Care for Trauma Patients: The First 24 Hours
M.J.A. PARR, AND J.P. NOLAN 427

Intensive Treatment of the Patient with Hepatic Trauma
B. KREMŽAR, AND A. ŠPEC-MARN 439

Mistakes in the Management of Trauma Patients
M. FISHER 449

FOCUS ON NEUROTRAUMA

Integrated Intensive Care Management of Severe Head Injury
N. STOCCHETTI, L. LONGHI, AND S. MAGNONI 457

METABOLISM, ARTIFICIAL NUTRITION, CRRT

Organ Transplantation and Metabolism
G. Sganga, and M. Castagneto 469

Clinical Aspects of Nutrition in Acute Renal Failure
H.P. Kierdorf 477

The Tricks and Traps of Enteral Nutrition
G.J. Dobb 489

Update on CRRT Therapy
P. Rogiers 499

Haemofiltration in Neonates
G. Zobel, S. Rödl, and B. Urlesberger 507

DRUGS IN ICU - USE, ABUSE AND MISUSE

Use, Abuse and Misuse of Drugs in ICU: Muscle Relaxants
G. Conti, R. Marella, and M.C. Marini 517

Use of Corticosteroids in the Severely Ill Patient
M. Antonelli, and M. Passariello 523

ADVANCES IN CPR

On Field Resuscitation
M.A. Baubin 535

The Chain of Survival: Focus on Early Defibrillation
F. Kette 543

EVIDENCE-BASED MEDICINE AND POLICY IN THE ICU

Evidence-Based Medicine in the ICU
J.-L. Vincent 551

The Performance of an ICU
G.J. Dobb 557

Care of Dying Patients in ICU
M. Fisher 567

Cost-Effectiveness in the ICU
D. Reis Miranda, and M. Jegers 573

Index 579

Authors Index

Allaria B.
Dept. of Intensive Care National Institute for Cancer Research, Milan (Italy)

Allvin R.
Dept. of Anaesthesiology and Intensive Care, Örebro Medical Centre Hospital, Örebro (Sweden)

Andreose U.
Rehabilitation Centre, Intensive Care Unit, Padua City Hospital, Conselve (Italy)

Antonaglia V.
Dept. of Anaesthesiology and Intensive Care, Trieste University School of Medicine, Trieste (Italy)

Antonelli M.
Dept. of Anaesthesia and Intensive Care, La Sapienza University, Umberto I Hospital, Roma (Italy)

A. Anzini
Dept. of Neurological Sciences, La Sapienza University, Rome (Italy)

Artigas A.
Intensive Care Unit, Sabadell Hospital, and Dept. of Cellular Biology and Physiology, Medical Physiology Unit, Autonomous University of Barcelona (Spain)

Auler J.O.C. Jr
Dept. of Anaesthesia and Intensive Care, Heart Institute, Hospital das Clínicas, São Pãulo University, São Paulo (Brazil)

Baubin M.A.
Dept. of Anaesthesia and Intensive Care Medicine, University of Innsbruck, Innsbruck (Austria)

Baurain M.
Dept. of Anaesthesiology and Resuscitation, Erasme Hospital, University of Bruxelles, Bruxelles (Belgium)

Berlot G.
Dept. of Anaesthesiology and Intensive Care, Trieste University School of Medicine, Trieste (Italy)

Brandolese R.
Rehabilitation Centre, Intensive Care Unit, Padua City Hospital, Conselve (Italy)

Braschi A.
1st Dept. of Anaesthesia and Intensive Care, S. Matteo University Hospital - IRCCS, Pavia (Italy)

Brazzi L.
Dept. of Anaesthesia and Intensive Care, Maggiore University Hospital - IRCCS, Milan (Italy)

Brienza A.
Dept. of Emergency Medicine and Organ Transplantation, Anaesthesia and Intensive Care Unit, Bari University, Bari (Italy)

Brienza N.
Dept. of Emergency Medicine and Organ Transplantation, Anaesthesia and Intensive Care Unit, Bari University, Bari (Italy)

Carli F.
Dept. of Anaesthesia, McGill University, Montreal, Quebec (Canada)

Carmona M.J.C.
Dept. of Anaesthesia and Intensive Care, Heart Institute, Hospital das Clínicas, São Pãulo University, São Paulo (Brazil)

Castagneto M.
Dept. of Surgery, Division of Organ Transplantation, Catholic University, and CNR, Centre for the Pathophysiology of Shock, Rome (Italy)

Cestelli A.
Dept. of Cellular Biology and of Development, Palermo University School of Medicine, Palermo (Italy)

Conti G.
Dept. of Anaesthesia and Intensive Care, La Sapienza University, Umberto I Hospital, Roma (Italy)

Coppola Gimenez S.
Dept. of Paediatric Critical Care, Heart Institute, Hospital das Clínicas, São Pãulo University, São Paulo (Brazil)

Coppola M.
Dept. of Surgery, Anaesthesiology, Intensive Care and Emergency Medicine, Federico II University, Naples (Italy)

Cuccia G.
Dept. of Neuropsychiatry, Palermo University School of Medicine, Palermo (Italy)

Culotta D.
Dept. of Intensive Care National Institute for Cancer Research, Milan (Italy)

De Simoni L.
Dept. of Anaesthesiology and Intensive Care, Trieste University School of Medicine, Trieste (Italy)

Dei Poli M.
Dept. of Intensive Care National Institute for Cancer Research, Milan (Italy)

Di Liegro I.
Dept. of Cellular Biology and of Development, Palermo University School of Medicine, Palermo (Italy)

D' Hollander A.
Dept. of Anaesthesiology and Resuscitation, Erasme Hospital, University of Bruxelles, Bruxelles (Belgium)

Di Bartolomeo S.
Friuli-Venezia Giulia Emergency Helicopter Service (Italy)

Dobb. G.J.
Intensive Care Unit, Royal Perth Hospital, Perth (Australia)

Dzoljic M.
Dept. of Anaesthesiology, Academic Medical Centre, Amsterdam (The Netherlands)

Fantoni D.
Dept. of Veterinary Medicine, Heart Institute, Hospital das Clínicas, São Pãulo University, São Paulo (Brazil)

Favaro M.
Dept. of Intensive Care National Institute for Cancer Research, Milan (Italy)

Ferraro P.
Dept. of Emergency Medicine, San Paolo Hospital, Naples (Italy)

Ferretti A.
Dept. of Pneumology, Sant'Orsola-Malpighi Hospital, Bologna (Italy)

Fieschi C.
Dept. of Neurological Sciences, La Sapienza University, Rome (Italy)

Fisher M.
Dept. of Anaesthesia and Intensive Care, University of Sydney (Australia)

Fredén F.
Dept. of Thoracic Anaesthesia, Uppsala University Hospital, Uppsala (Sweden)

Gattinoni L.
Dept. of Anaesthesia and Intensive Care, Maggiore University Hospital - IRCCS, Milan (Italy)

Grassi V.
Institute of Internal Medicine I, University of Brescia, Brescia (Italy)

Gullo A.
Dept. of Anaesthesiology and Intensive Care, Trieste University School of Medicine, Trieste (Italy)

Haitsma J.J.
Dept. of Anaesthesiology, Erasmus University, Rotterdam (The Netherlands)

Hallman M.
Dept. of Paediatrics, University of Oulu, Oulu (Finland)

Hambraeus Jonzon K.
Dept. of Anaesthesiology and Intensive Care, Karolinska Hospital, Stockohlm (Sweden)

Hedenstierna G.
Dept. of Clinical Physiology, Uppsala University Hospital, Uppsala (Sweden)

Hohlfeld J.M.
Dept. of Respiratory Medicine, Hannover Medical School, Hannover (Germany)

Huang M.
Dept. of Neuroscience, Albert Einstein College of Medicine, Bronx, New York (U.S.A.)

Jegers M.
Center for Financial Analysis and Policy, Free University of Brussels, Brussels (Belgium)

Kette F.
Dept. of Anaesthesia and Intensive Care Unit, Udine University Hospital, Udine (Italy)

Kierdorf H.P.
Dept. of Nephrology, Clinic Braunschweig, Braunschweig (Germany)

Kneussl M.
Dept. of Internal Medicine IV - Pulmonary Medicine, Vienna General Hospital, University of Vienna, Vienna (Austria)

Kremžar B.
Dept. of Anaesthesiology and Intensive Therapy, University Medical Centre, Ljubljana (Slovenia)

Kuiper M.
Dept. of Intensive Care, Onze Lieve Vrouwe Hospital, Amsterdam (The Netherlands)

Lachmann B.
Dept. of Anaesthesiology, Erasmus University, Rotterdam (The Netherlands)

Lang I.
Dept. of Internal Medicine II - Cardiology, Vienna General Hospital, University of Vienna, Vienna (Austria)

Longhi L.
Dept. of Neurosurgical Intensive Care, Anaesthesia and Intensive Care Unit, Maggiore University Hospital - IRCCS, Milan (Italy)

Lucangelo U.
Dept. of Anaesthesiology and Intensive Care, Trieste University School of Medicine, Trieste (Italy)

Lyons G.
Dept. of Obstetric Anaesthesia, St. James University Hospital, Leeds (U.K.)

Maglione B.
Dept. of Emergency Medicine, San Paolo Hospital, Naples (Italy)

Magnoni S.
Dept. of Neurosurgical Intensive Care, Anaesthesia and Intensive Care Unit, Maggiore University Hospital - IRCCS, Milan (Italy)

Marella R.
Dept. of Anaesthesia and Intensive Care, La Sapienza University, Umberto I Hospital, Roma (Italy)

Marini M.C.
Dept. of Anaesthesia and Intensive Care, La Sapienza University, Umberto I University Hospital, Roma (Italy)

Michelutto V.
Friuli-Venezia Giulia Emergency Helicopter Service (Italy)

Milic-Emili J.
Meakins-Christie Laboratories, McGill University, Montreal, Quebec (Canada)

Monteiro Abbelan D.
Dept. of Paediatric Critical Care, Heart Institute, Hospital das Clínicas, São Pãulo University, São Paulo (Brazil)

Muchada R.
Dept. of Anaesthesia and Intensive Care, E. André Hospital, Lyon (France)

Nardi G.
Intensive Care Unit, S. Camillo Hospital, Rome (Italy)

Neumann P.
Dept. of Anaesthesiology, Emergency and Intensive Care Medicine, University Hospital, Göttingen (Germany)

Nolan J.P.
Royal United Hospital, Bath (U.K.)

Olivei M.C.
Laboratory of Biotechnology and Biomedical Technologies, IRCCS, S. Matteo University Hospital, Pavia (Italy)

Parr M.J.A.
Dept. of Intensive Care and Anaesthesia, Liverpool Hospital, University of New South Wales, Sydney (Australia)

Passariello M.
Dept. of Anaesthesia and Intensive Care, La Sapienza University, Umberto I Hospital, Roma (Italy)

Peratoner A.
Dept. of Anaesthesiology and Intensive Care, Trieste University School of Medicine, Trieste (Italy)

Pelosi P.
Dept. of Anaesthesia and Intensive Care, Maggiore University Hospital - IRCCS, Milan (Italy)

Pereira M.H.C.
Dept. of Anaesthesia and Intensive Care, Heart Institute, Hospital das Clínicas, São Pãulo University, São Paulo (Brazil)

Rasura M.
Dept. of Neurological Sciences, La Sapienza University, Rome (Italy)

Rawal N.
Dept. of Anaesthesiology and Intensive Care, Örebro Medical Centre Hospital, Örebro (Sweden)

Reis Miranda D.
Health Services Research Unit, University Hospital, Groningen (The Netherlands)

Rodl S.
Dept. of Paediatrics University of Graz, Graz (Austria)

Dept. of Intensive Care, Middelheim General Hospital, Antwerp (Belgium)

Rupreht J.
Dept. of Anaesthesiology, Erasmus University Hospital (The Netherlands) and University of Ljubljana, Ljubljana (Slovenia)

Salemi G.
Dept. of Neuropsychiatry, Palermo University School of Medicine, Palermo (Italy)

Savettieri G.
Dept. of Neuropsychiatry, Palermo University School of Medicine, Palermo (Italy)

Schalk H.V.
Dept. of Anaesthesiology and Intensive Care Medicine, Klagenfurt (Austria)

Schiraldi F.
Dept. of Emergency Medicine, San Paolo Hospital, Naples (Italy)

Servillo G.
Dept. of Surgery, Anaesthesiology, Intensive Care and Emergency Medicine, Federico II University, Naples (Italy)

Sganga G.
Dept. of Surgery, Division of Organ Transplantation, Catholic University, and CNR, Centre for the Pathophysiology of Shock, Rome (Italy)

Sharrock N.E.
Dept. of Anaesthesiology, The Hospital for Special Surgery, New York, New York (U.S.A.)

Siegel D.A.
Dept. of Neuroscience, Albert Einstein College of Medicine, Bronx, New York (U.S.A.)

Špec-Marn A.
Dept. of Anaesthesiology and Intensive Therapy, University Medical Centre, Ljubljana (Slovenia)

Stocchetti N.
Dept. of Neurosurgical Intensive Care, Anaesthesia and Intensive Care Unit, Maggiore University Hospital - IRCCS, Milan (Italy)

Sutcliffe A.J.
Neurosciences Critical Care Unit, Queen Elizabeth Hospital, Birmingham (U.K.)

Tantucci C.
Dept. of Semeiotics and Medical Methodology, University of Ancona, Ancona (Italy)

Trevisanuto D.
Dept. of Paediatrics, Padua University, Padua (Italy)

Tufano R.
Dept. of Surgery, Anaesthesiology, Intensive Care and Emergency Medicine, Federico II University, Naples (Italy)

Urlesberger B.
Dept. of Neonatology, University of Graz, Graz (Austria)

Verbrugge S.J.C.
Dept. of Anaesthesiology, Erasmus University, Rotterdam (The Netherlands)

Villani M.A.
1st Dept. of Anaesthesia and Intensive Care, S.Matteo University Hospital - IRCCS, Pavia (Italy)

Vincent J.-L.
Dept. of Intensive Care, Erasme University Hospital, Free University of Brussels, Brussels (Belgium)

Walkley S.
Dept. of Neuroscience, Albert Einstein College of Medicine, Bronx, New York (USA)

Zacchello F.
Dept. of Paediatrics, Padua University, Padua (Italy)

Zandstra D.F.
Dept. of Intensive Care, Onze Lieve Vrouwe Hospital, Amsterdam (The Netherlands)

Zetterberg C.
Dept. of Obstetrics and Gynecology, Örebro Medical Centre Hospital, Örebro (Sweden)

Zin W.A.
Laboratory of Respiratory Physiology, Carlos Chagas Filho Institute of Biophysics, Rio de Janeiro Federal University, Rio de Janeiro (Brazil)

Zobel G.
Dept. of Paediatrics, University of Graz, Graz (Austria)

Abbreviations

AA, amino acid

ACD, active compression decompression

ACh, acetylcholine

ACLA, anticardiolipin antibodies

ACLS, advanced cardiac life support

AED, automated and semi-automated external defibrillator

AHME, active heat and moisture exchanger

ALI, acute lung injury

ALS, amyotrophic lateral sclerosis

AMI, acute myocardial infarction

AMP, adenosine-5-monophosphate

AP, arterial pressure

APC, activated protein C

ARDS, acute respiratory distress syndrome

ARF, acute respiratory failure

ASA, atrial septal aneurysm

ATP, adenosine-triphosphate

AVB, atrio-ventricular block

BAL, bronchoalveolar lavage

BALF, bronchoalveolar lavage fluid

BCAA, branched chain amino acid

BDNF, brain derived neurotrophic factor

BFCNs, basal forebrain cholinergic neurons

BIA, body impedance analysis

BLS, basic life support

BMP, bone morphogenetic protein

BMT, bone marrow transplantation

BPD, bronchopulmonary dysplasia

CA, cardiac arrest

CADASIL, cerebral autosomal dominant subcortical arteriopathy with ischaemic leukencephalopathy

CAO, chronic airway obstruction

CAS, central anticholinergic syndrome

CAVH, continuous arterio-venous haemofiltration

CHDF, continuous haemodiafiltration

CHF, chronic heart failure

CI, cardiac index

CLD, chronic lung disease

CNS, central nervous system

CO, cardiac output

COPD, chronic obstructive pulmonary disease

CPP, cerebral perfusion pressure

CPR, cardiopulmonary resuscitation

CRRT, continuous renal replacement therapy

CSF, cerebrospinal fluid

CT, computed tomography

CTEPH, chronic thromboembolic pulmonary hypertension

CVP, central venous pressure

CVVH, continuous veno-venous haemofiltration

DAD, delayed after depolarization

DAP, diastolic arterial blood pressure

DH, dynamic hyperinflation

DO_2, oxygen delivery

DPL, diagnostic peritoneal lavage

DPPC, dipalmitoyl phosphatidylcholine

DVT, deep vein thrombosis

EAA, essential amino acid

EAD, early after depolarization

ECC, external chest compression

ECG/EKG, electrocardiogram

ECM, external cardiac massage

ECM, extracellular matrix

EE, epicardial echocardiography

EELV, end-expiratory lung volume

EFL, expiratory flow limitation

EGF, epidermal growth factor

EMS, emergency medical service

EMT, emergency medical technician

ERC, European Resuscitation Council

ERV, expiratory reserve volume

ESFR, end-stage renal failure

FRC, functional residual capacity

GIT, gastrointestinal tract

GM-CSF, granulocyte-macrophage colony-stimulating factor

GPB, glossopharyngeal breathing

HD, Huntington's disease

HEA, hypotensive epidural anaesthesia

HME, heat and moisture exchanger

HPV, hypoxic pulmonary vasoconstriction

HR, heart rate

IC, inspiratory capacity

ICP, intracranial pressure

IgG, immunoglobulin G

IH, intracerebral haemorrhage

IL-1, interleukin-1

ILCOR, International Liaison Committee on Resuscitation

INF-γ, interferon-γ

IUI, intrauterine infection

KGF, keratinocyte growth factor

LAC, lupus anticoagulant

LICAM, low invasivity cardiovascular monitor

LMA, laryngeal mask airway

LMWH, low molecular weight heparin

LVET, left ventricular ejection time

MAP, mean arterial pressure

MELAS, mitochondrial encephalopathy, lactate acidosis and strokelike episodes

MI, myocardial infarction

MOF, multiple organ failure

MOFS, multiple organ failure syndrome

mPAP, mean pulmonary arterial pressure

MS, methionine-synthase

MSUD, maple syrup urine disease

MTHFR, methylentetrahydrofolate reductase

MVO$_2$, myocardial consumption of O_2

MVP, mitral valve prolapse

MVV, maximal voluntary ventilation

N$_2$O, nitrous oxide

NDNMBA, nondepolarizing neuromuscular blocking agent

NEAA, non essential amino acid

NEP, negative expiratory pressure

NGF, nerve growth factor

NIBP, non invasive blood pressure

NICO, non invasive cardiac output

NIPPV, non invasive positive pressure ventilation

NO, nitric oxide

NTF, neurotrophic factor

PAC, pulmonary artery catheter

PAF, platelet activating factor

PAN, polyacrylonitrile

PCBF, pulmonary capillary blood flow

PCEA, patient-controlled epidural analgesia

PCV, pressure-controlled ventilation

PEA, pulseless electrical activity

PEEP, positive end expiratory pressure

PEEPi, intrinsic positive end expiratory pressure

PEF, peak expiratory flow

PEP, pre-ejection period

PFO, patent foramen ovale

PGI$_2$, prostacyclin

PH, pulmonary hypertension

PMMA, polymethylmethacrylate

PMX-F, polymyxin

POCD, postoperative consciousness disorders

POD, postoperative delirium

Poes, oesophageal pressure

PPH, primary pulmonary hypertension

PTC, post-tetanic count

PTE, pulmonary thromboendarterectomy

PTT, partial thromboplastin time

PVR, pulmonary vascular resistance

RES, reticuloendothelial system

ROSC, return of spontaneous circulation

RV, right ventricular

RVEDP, right ventricular end diastolic pressure

SH, subarachnoid haemorrhage

ShvO$_2$, hepatic venous O$_2$ saturation

SOD, superoxide dismutase

STI, systolic time interval

STR, systolic time ratio

SV, stroke volume

SvO$_2$, mixed venous O$_2$ saturation

SVR, systemic vascular resistance

Te, expiratory time

TEE, transesoephageal echocardiography

TGF, transforming growth factor

TH, thyroid hormones

THR, total hip replacement

TKR, total knee replacement

TNF, tumour necrosis factor

TOF, train of four

TTE, transthoracic echocardiography

VF, ventricular fibrillation

$\dot{V}O_2$, oxygen consumption

Vr, relaxation volume

VT, ventricular tachycardia

WP, wedge pressure

ZEEP, zero end expiratory pressure

RESPIRATORY CARE

Principles of Laboratory Research on Respiratory Mechanics

W.A. ZIN

In treating a patient presenting respiratory functional impairment, the physician is left with the task of running tests to determine whether there is a mechanical component to the illness. At this point he must be qualified to extract the desired information from a given measurement. Although not difficult to accomplish, the precise interpretation of the results demands awareness of exact methodological and theoretical concepts.

Fundamental aspects of measurements

Physical characteristics of measuring instruments

Dynamic characteristics of measuring instruments are partially described by their frequency response [1]. Consider a signal represented by a square wave. An overdamped recording device smoothes out the sharp corners and delays the rise and fall of the input wave, providing a somewhat rounded output signal. On the other hand, for the same input signal an underdamped apparatus generates an output wave that oscillates after each transient [2]. Of course, the ideally damped apparatus would provide a true "copy" of the original curve (Fig. 1).

One should also bear in mind that the measuring assembly must not delay the signal. For instance, if two simultaenously occurring pressure changes are recorded, one should not lag behind the other when finally displayed or recorded, as shown in Figure 2. When adequately dealt with, this phase lag can be eliminated.

Another very important aspect of a pressure measuring device is represented by its common mode-rejection profile. Briefly, when a differential pressure transducer has both its chambers equally pressurized to a certain degree, the resulting signal should be nil. Furthermore, the ideal transducer should not present pressure transients when its chambers are compressed or decompressed simultaneously to the same degree.

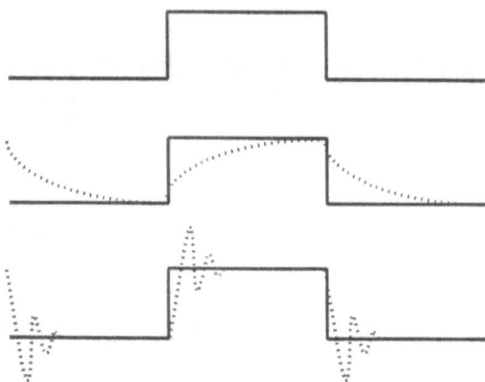

Fig. 1. Frequency response of measuring assembly. The true signal is represented by the solid lines, whereas the dotted lines depict the output provided by the equipment. From top to bottom: in an ideal system, the input and the output signals should be identical, hence the two lines are superimposed. In an overdamped assembly, the sharp corners are rounded and the input signal's rise and fall are delayed. An underdamped system generates an output signal that oscillates after transient changes in the input wave

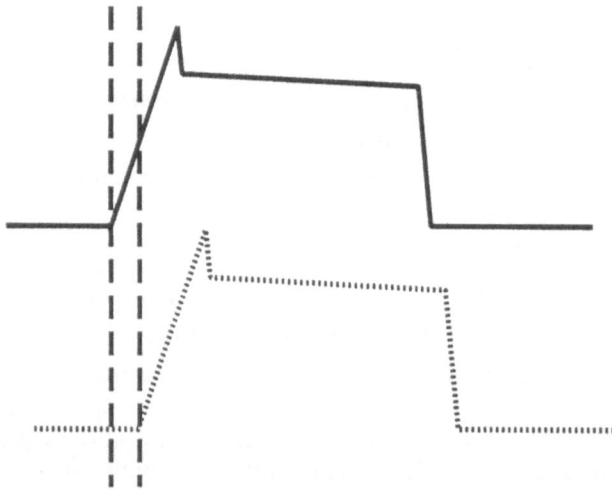

Fig. 2. Phase lag. The pressure variation was simultaneously measured by two different assemblies, as represented by the solid and dotted lines. Note that the pressure changes recorded lag a certain amount of time behind the other, which is the distance between the two vertical broken lines

Compliance and resistance of the experimental circuit

Not considering the frequency response aspect, compliance and resistance of the experimental circuit may distort the measurements to a great extent. For example, a very compliant piece of rubber tubing added in series will reduce the amount of gas injected into the lungs by retaining part of the tidal volume delivered by the ventilator. If the resistance of the circuit (Req) is not subtracted from the total resistance measured, the patient's real resistance will be overestimated. Furthermore, if turbulence occurs, the relationship between equipment resistive pressure (Pres,eq) and flow ($\dot{V}$):

$$Pres,eq = Req \cdot \dot{V} \tag{1}$$

will be adequately expressed either by Rohrer's Equation:

$$Pres,eq = K_1 \cdot \dot{V} + K_2 \cdot \dot{V}^2 \tag{2}$$

where K_1 and K_2 are constants, or by the power function:

$$Pres,eq = a \cdot \dot{V}^b \tag{3}$$

where *a* representes the pressure when $\dot{V}$ equals 1 L/s, and *b* is a dimensionless index of the shape of the curve.

Tracheal tubes

Within the physiological range of airflows, tracheal tubes always add a flow-dependent resistance (Equations 2 and 3) to the system [3]. As a consequence, for the same driving pressure, the tidal volume achieved will be smaller than in the non-intubated condition. Naturally, the lost volume augments disproportionately with diminishing tube diameter and increasing flow or driving pressure [4].

Analogue-to-digital conversion

Analogue information is data that correspond to a physical measurement, which is usually provided electronically as a change in either voltage or current. With the aid of an analogue-to-digital (A-D) converter the continuous electrical signal can be converted to discrete digital format in order to be processed by a computer. Ideally, the interval between each sample should be as small as possible so that the digital data points closely approximate the analogue signal. Therefore the faster the changes in the input signal, the higher the sampling frequency should be [5]. Similarly, the better the resolution of the A-D converter the closer the points will be spaced on the Y-axis (Fig. 3). Basically, the resolution improves as the number of bits of the A-D converter increases.

A-D Sampling Rate

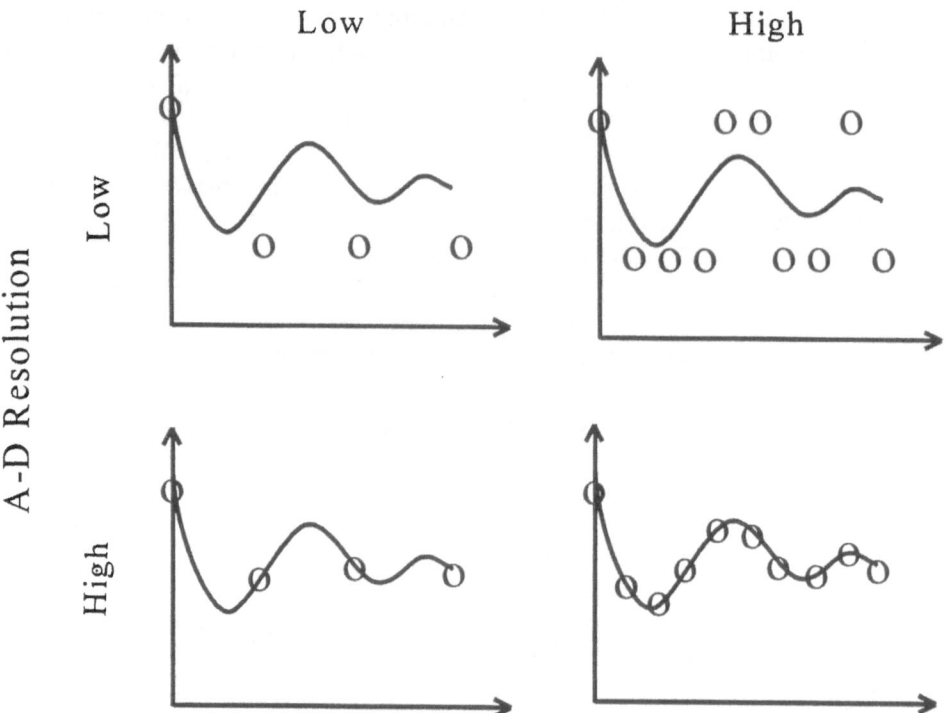

Fig. 3. Different A-D resolutions and sampling rates of the digitalized data points. With a high resolution the points are more closely spaced on the ordinate, whereas with a high sampling rate the spaces are more closely spaced on the abscissa

Oesophageal pressure measurement

Pleural pressure measurement is essential for splitting respiratory system mechanical properties into their pulmonary and chest wall components. Because of the risks involved in direct pleural pressure determination, oesophageal pressure (Poes) is registered instead. The most widely used method for recording Poes employs air-containing latex balloons sealed over catheters which in turn transmit balloon pressures to transducers. Although this approach was proposed more than a century ago by Luciani, its precise standardization occurred not earlier than 1964 [6]. Poes measurements should be validated in all instances. For such purpose, static Valsalva and Mueller manoeuvres or the dynamic "occlusion test" can be used [7].

In neonates and small animals a liquid-filled catheter has been used since 1957 [8]; it substitutes for the oesaphageal balloon. Because of hydrostatic factors, it can be difficult to obtain absolute values of Poes with the liquid-filled catheter. But there is an advantage because its frequency response is inherently high, due to the fact that pressure transmission occurs through a noncompressible fluid.

A comprehensive description of oesophageal pressure measurement has recently been published [9].

Mechanical models of the respiratory system

The respiratory system, as well as its pulmonary and chest wall components, is comprised of a multitude of elements. The undisputed necessity to interpret the meaning of measurable varibles such as volume, airflow, and pressure under both physiological and pathological conditions has imposed the need for relatively simple models that should be able to describe as accurately as possible the mechanical behaviour of the system. The components of such models and their associated parametres should have reasonable physiological counterparts.

Linear one-compartment model

The simplest model of the respiratory system, which is still the most commonly used, incorporates two lumped elements [10]: one resistance (associated with the pipe) and one elasticity (balloon), as depicted in Figure 4a. The "equation of motion of the respiratory system" describes its behaviour:

$$P(t) = R\dot{V}(t) + EV(t) \qquad (4)$$

where P is the driving pressure, R is the resistance of the pipe to airflow ($\dot{V}$), E is the balloon elasticity, V represents the change in volume of the balloon above its relaxed configuration, and t is time. This single-compartment linear model assumes that R and E are independent of $\dot{V}$ and V, respectively, and that inertial forces are negligible. The latter postulate is probably acceptable within the physiological breathing frequencies up to 2 Hz [11].

Figure 4b also illustrates that from the mechanical standpoint the deformation of the respiratory system (i.e., volume change V) results from the movement of a Voigt body (one dashpot R, and a spring E, arranged in parallel constitute a Voigt body). One should always bear in mind that dashpots dissipate energy as heat, whereas springs store potential energy that will be returned to the system.

The values of E and R can be determined during continuous breathing by fitting Eq. 4 to P, V, and $\dot{V}$ using multiple linear regression [12, 13] or by the electrical subtraction method [14]. Alternatively, E and R can be obtained during relaxed expiration [15].

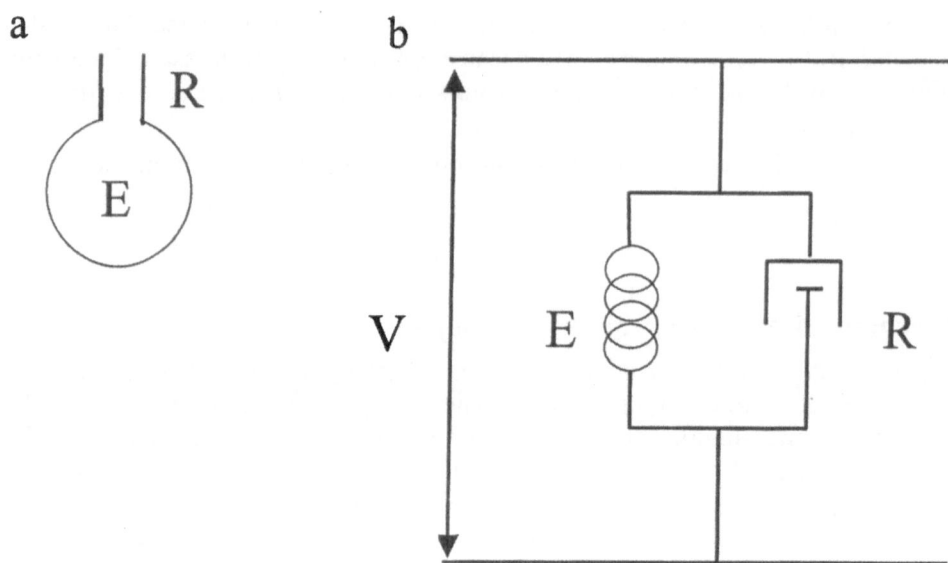

Fig. 4a, b. Linear one-compartment model. a) Anatomic representation; b) rheological representation by a Voigt body. R, respiratory system resistance; E, respiratory elastance; V, changes in lung volume

However, the linear one-compartment model cannot describe a few mechanical phenomena presented by the respiratory system, such as: 1) the slow decay in pressure observed after sustained airway occlusion at end inspiration [16-18]; 2) the frequency dependence of elasticity and resistance [13, 19-21]; and 3) the quasi-static pressure-volume hysteresis in isolated lungs. Therefore, in order to better describe the respiratory system mechanical profile more complex approaches are required.

Two-compartment models

Linear two-compartment models increase the mechanical degrees of freedom of the system, and explain the frequency dependence of respiratory parametres, stress adaptation, and the two-exponential decay of expired volume under relaxed conditions. They are divided into two main types: gas redistribution and rheologic models.

Gas redistribution models

These models describe the mechanical properties of the respiratory system based on the inhomogeneity of gas distribution within the lungs. In this context, they can be divided into two sub-types: parallel and series redistribution.

The *parallel gas redistribution model* [22] consists of two alveolar compartments with elasticity E_1 and E_2 served by parallel airways with fixed resistances R_1 and R_2. Additionaly, a resistance common to the two compartments can be added to the model, to represent central airways resistance [23]. Mechanically, the model serially associates two Voigt bodies characterized by their respective springs (E_1 and E_2) and dashpots (R_1 and R_2). The total deformation (i.e., volume V) is the sum of each of their respective deformations. This model associates stress adaptation to parallel Pendelluft, which consists of alveolar pressure equilibrium during airflow interruption, and depends on the difference between the two peripheral time constants (τ = R/E), and on volume history.

In the *serial gas redistribution model* [24], homogeneous lungs (represented by an alveolar compartment with elasticity E_2 and distal airways with resistance R_2) are served by central airways with an elasticity E_1 and a resistance R_1. E_1 behaves as a buffer between alveolar and driving pressures. Hence, a given fraction of the inspired volume remains in the central airways, depending on central and peripheral time constants (τ_1 and τ_2, respectively), thus decreasing the volume available for gas exchange. This kind of model is particularly useful in the interpretation of pathological conditions, such as chronic obstructive pulmonary disease. When elastic and resistive data of normal individuals are considered, the serial gas distribution model can not explain frequency dependence of resistance and elasticity in the normal range of breathing frequencies. However, when the peripheral resitance R_2 increases, the model confers a time dependence to R and E compatible with the real behaviour of COPD lungs. Finally, there are alternative anatomical interpretations for E_1, associated with either an alveolar gas compliance or a lung region with negligible resistance [25, 26]. However, the original association of E_1 with central airways elasticity still prevails [25, 27].

As also displayed by the parallel two-compartment model, there is gas redistribution between the compartments after flow interruption. In fact, the behaviour of both models may be identical, depending on the values chosen for the four parameters, since they are described by the same differential equation [28]:

$$P(t) + a\dot{P}(t) = bV(t) + c\dot{V}(t) + d\ddot{V}(t) \qquad (5)$$

where $\dot{P}(t)$ is the first time derivative of $P(t)$ and $\ddot{V}(t)$ corresponds to second time derivative of $V(t)$.

Rheological models

The *viscoelastic model* is a rheological two-compartment model that explains the frequency dependence of respiratory parameters, and stress adaptation. In fact, this approach extends the one-compartment model by incorporating a viscoelastic element in parallel [29, 30]. Furthermore, it does not consider the existence of uneven distribution of ventilation. Indeed, supporting this postulate inhomogeneous gas distribution could be detected under normal conditions [31, 32].

The viscoelastic model of the respiratory system considers that stress adaptation originates from lung/chest wall tissues and surfactant (E_2 and R_2, Fig. 5a). The deformation of the Maxwell body (E_2, R_2) shown in Figure 5b is the sum of the individual distortions of its elastic and resistive components, and its slow time constant ($\tau_2 = R_2/E_2$) might account for tissue stress adaptation. It should be pointed out that currently the precise structural basis of the viscoelastic parameters in Figure 5 is poorly understood.

As a result of viscoelastic pressure dissipation, the effective resistance of the respiratory system (pulmonary and chest wall components) is higher at low respiratory frequencies, f (or long inspiratory durations), than during elevated f [22, 33-35]. Indeed, at high f spring E_2 (Fig. 5b) will oscillate so quickly that no time will be allowed for the dissipation of its energy through dashpot R_2, Conversely, at low f R_2 will be given time to move and dissipate the applied energy and/or the energy stored in E_2. Therefore, it can be easily foreseen that according to the values of E_2, R_2, and f the respiratory system will display a broad range of lumped elasticity and resistance values, as originally proposed by Mount [29]. Finally, this model is also governed by a differential equation like Equation 5.

The *plastoelastic model* differs from the viscoelastic one by the substitution of a dry friction (Coulomb) element for the viscous element (R_2) in the Maxwell body, thus forming the Prandtl body [36]. The Coulomb element will only start moving after a pressure threshold has been reached. Henceforth, energy is continuously dissipated independent of the rate of displacement. This model could account for the quasi-static pressure volume hysteresis in isolated lungs. However, the plastoelastic model is rarely used in vivo under small volume excursions, where its parameter values are sometimes difficult to interpret mechanically [37, 38].

Multi-compartment models

An attempt to more accurately describe a set of experimental data can be performed by means of multi-compartment models. Hence, a varying number of Voigt, Kelvin, or Maxwell bodies could be added in parallel to the aforementioned models. In this line, a model has been proposed in which P(t) decreases linearly as a function of the logarithm of the time subsequent to a step change in volume (V), according to the equation [39-41]:

$$P(t)/V = A - B \times \ln t \tag{6}$$

Naturally, the existence of a multitude of time constants is implicit in this particular model. Nevertheless, the multi-compartment models yield a great deal of parameters, whose direct assigment to mechanical elements is unwarranted.

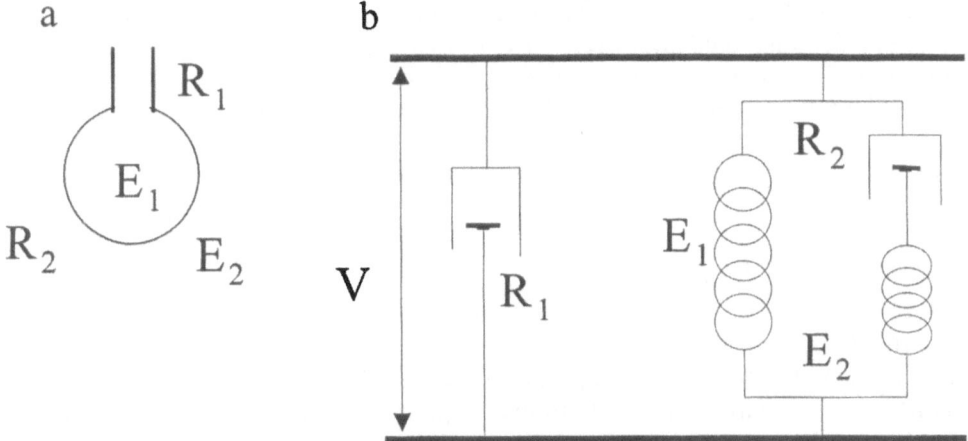

Fig. 5a, b. Rheological two-compartment model. a) Anatomic representation; b) rheological representation by a dashpot (R_1) associated in parallel with a spring (E_1) coupled in parallel with a Maxwell body (R_2, E_2); V, changes in lung volume

Non-linear models

Another way of increasing the complexity of the mechanical models of the respiratory system is to make the existing elements nonlinear. The simplest one consists in adding a flow-dependent (turbulent) term to the parametre representing airway resistance:

$$P(t) = K_1 \dot{V}(t) + K_2 \dot{V}(t)^2 + EV(t) \qquad (7)$$

where K_1 and K_2 are Rohrer's constants [42].

A non-linear viscoelastic model, where both tissue resistance and elasticity depend upon squared breathing frequency, is capable of quantitatively account for the known amplitude and frequency-dependent properties of lung tissue [43]. The non-linear viscoelastic model can be used instead of a plastoelastic one [44], which is also able to explain the same phenomena.

Another non-linear model states that the decay of P(t) after the volume increment V can be represented by:

$$P(t)/V = A \times t^{-k} \qquad (8)$$

where A and k are constants [45, 46]. Conversely, it can be concluded that tissue and lung impedances are inversely related to a given power of the breathing frequency.

Studies dealing with nonlinearities have provided interesting conclusions. It has been demonstrated that even an extremely inhomogeneous lung structure can produce virtually homogeneous mechanical behavior [45]. Furthermore, because of nonlinearities, it is feasible to measure respiratory system and pulmonary impedances during conventional mechanical ventilation only at and above normal breathing frequency [47].

Choosing the appropriate model

Naturally, the choice of the model will depend upon the intended physiological or pathophysiological goal. In other words, the most adequate model is that one in which the elements closely reproduce the actual system under study [28, 47]. Thence, it is virtually impossible to use a "perfect" model. However, the use of simple models that satisfactorily represent the general mechanical behaviour of the respiratory system and its lung and chest wall components is of paramount importance to the respirologist.

The models are to be chosen according to the scientific questioning, techniques and methods used, and, of course, experimental conditions. Furthermore, the easy gathering of parameters of a given model should never thwart the purpose of the most appropriate physiological interpretation of the data.

References

1. Fry DL (1960) Physiologic recording by modern instruments with particular reference to pressure recording. Physiol Rev 40:753-788
2. Butler JP, Leith DE, Jackson AC (1986) Principles of measurement: applications to pressure, volume, and flow. In: Macklem PT, Mead J (eds) Handbook of physiology. The respiratory system. Mechanics of breathing. American Physiological Society, Bethesda, sect 3, vol III, pp 15-33
3. Behrakis PK, Higgs BD, Baydur A et al (1983) Respiratory mechanics during halothane anesthesia and anesthesia-paralysis in humans. J Appl Physiol 55:1085-1092
4. Rocco PRM, Zin WA (1985) Modelling the mechanical effects of tracheal tubes on normal subjects. Eur Respir J 8:121-126
5. Beauchamp K, Yuen C (1979) Digital methods for signal analysis. George Allen & Unwin, London
6. Milic-Emili J, Mead J, Turner JM et al (1964) Improved technique for estimating pleural pressure from esophageal balloons. J Appl Physiol 19:207-211
7. Baydur A, Behrakis PK, Zin WA et al (1982) A simple method for assessing the validity of the esophageal balloon technique. Am Rev Respir Dis 126:788-791
8. Cook CD, Sutherland JM, Segal S et al (1957) Studies of respiratory physiology in the newborn infant: III. Measurements of mechanics of respiration. J Clin Invest 36:440-448
9. Zin WA, Milic-Emili J (1997) Esophageal pressure measurement. In: Tobin MJ (ed) Principles and practice of intensive care monitoring. McGraw-Hill, New York, pp 545-552
10. Otis AB, Fenn WO, Rahn H (1950) The mechanics of breathing in man. J Appl Physiol 2:592-607
11. Sharp JT, Henry JP, Sweany SK et al (1964) Total respiratory inertance and its gas and tissue components in normal and obese men. J Appl Physiol 43:503-509

12. Hantos Z, Daróczy B, Klebniczki J et al (1982) Parameter estimation of transpulmonary mechanics by a nonlinear inertive model. J Appl Physiol 52:955-963
13. Bates JHT, Shardonofsky F, Stewart DE (1989) The low-frequency dependence of respiratory system resistance and elastance in normal dogs. Respir Physiol 78:369-382
14. Mead J, Whittenberger JL (1953) Physical properties of human lungs measured during spontaneous respiration. J Appl Physiol 5:779-796
15. Zin WA, Pengelly LD, Milic-Emili J (1982) Single-breath method for measurement of respiratory mechanics in anesthetized animals. J Appl Physiol 52:1266-1271
16. Hughes R, May AJ, Widdicombe JG (1959) Stress relaxation in rabbits' lungs. J Physiol (Lond) 146:85-97
17. Don HF, Robson JG (1965) The mechanics of the respiratory system during anesthesia. Anesthesiol 26:168-178
18. Bates JHT, Rossi A, Milic-Emili J (1985) Analysis of the behavior of the respiratory system with constant inspiratory flow. J Appl Physiol 58:1840-1848
19. Barnas GM, Yoshino K, Loring SH et al (1987) Impedance and relative displacements of relaxed chest wall up to 4 Hz. J Appl Physiol 62:71-81
20. Brusasco V, Warner DO, Beck KC et al (1989) Partitioning of pulmonary resistance in dogs: effects of tidal volume and frequency. J Appl Physiol 66:1190-1197
21. Hantos Z, Daróczy B, Suki B et al (1986) Forced oscillatory impedance of the respiratory system at low frequencies. J Appl Physiol 60:123-132
22. Otis AB, McKerrow CB, Bartlett RA et al (1956) Mechanical factors in the distribution of pulmonary ventilation. J Appl Physiol 8:427-443
23. Bates JHT, Baconnier P, Milic-Emili J (1988) A theoretical analysis of interrupter technique for measuring respiratory mechanics. J Appl Physiol 64:2204-2214
24. Mead J (1969) Contribution of compliance of airways to frequency-dependent behavior of lungs. J Appl Physiol 26:670-673
25. Eyles JG, Pimmel RL (1981) Estimating respiratory mechanical parameters in parallel compartment models. IEEE Trans Biomed Eng 28:313-317
26. Peslin R (1986) Methods for measuring total respiratory impedance by forced oscillations. Bull Eur Physiopathol Respir 22:621-631
27. Michaelson ED, Grassman ED, Peters WR (1975) Pulmonary mechanics by spectral analysis of forced random noise. J Clin Invest 56:1210-1230
28. Lorino AM, Lorino H, Harf A (1994) A synthesis of the Otis, Mead, and Mount mechanical respiratory models. Respir Physiol 97:123-133
29. Mount LE (1955) The ventilation flow-resistance and compliance of rat lungs. J Physiol (Lond) 127:157-167
30. Bates JHT, Brown KA, Kochi T (1989) Respiratory mechanics in the normal dog determined by expiratory flow interruption. J Appl Physiol 67:2276-2285
31. Bates JHT, Ludwig MS, Sly PD et al (1988) Interrupter resistance elucidated by alveolar pressure measurements in open-chest normal dogs. J Appl Physiol 65:408-414
32. Saldiva PHN, Zin WA, Santos RLB et al (1992) Alveolar pressure measurement in open-chest rats. J Appl Physiol 72:302-306
33. Kochi T, Okubo S, Zin WA et al (1988) Flow and volume dependence of pulmonary mechanics in anesthetized cats. J Appl Physiol 64:441-450
34. Similovski T, Levy P, Corbeil C et al (1989) Viscoelastic behavior of lung and chest wall in dogs determined by flow interruption. J Appl Physiol 67:2219-2229
35. D'Angelo E, Calderini E, Torri G et al (1989) Respiratory mechanics in anesthetized-paralyzed humans: effects of flow, volume, and time. J Appl Physiol 67:2556-2564
36. Similowski T, Bates JHT (1991) Two-compartment modelling of respiratory system mechanics at low frequencies: gas redistribution of tissue rheology? Eur Respir J 4:353-358
37. Navajas D, Farré R, Cannet J et al (1990) Respiratory input impedance in anesthetized paralyzed patients. J Appl Physiol 69:1372-1379
38. Shardonofsky F, Sato J, Bates JHT (1990) Quasi-static pressure-volume hysteresis in the canine respiratory system in vivo. J Appl Physiol 68:2230-2236

39. Hildebrandt J (1969) Dynamic properties of air-filled excised cat lung determined by liquid plethysmography. J Appl Physiol 27:246-250
40. Hildebrandt J (1969) Comparison of mathematical models for cat lung and viscoelastic balloon derived by Laplace transform methods from pressure-volume data. Bull Math Biophys 31:651-667
41. Hildebrandt J (1970) Pressure-volume data of cat lung interpreted by a plastoelastic, linear viscoelastic model. J Appl Physiol 28:365-372
42. Rohrer F (1915) Der Strömungswiderstand in den menschlichen Atemwegen und der Einfluss der unregelmässigen Verzweigung des Bronchialsystems auf den Atmungsverlauf in verschiedenen Lungenbezirken. Arch Ges Physiol 162:225-300
43. Suki B, Bates JHT (1991) A nonlinear viscoelastic model of lung tissue mechanics. J Appl Physiol 71:826-833
44. Fredberg JJ, Stamenovic D (1989) On the imperfect elasticity of lung tissue. J Appl Physiol 67:2408-2419
45. Hantos Z, Daróczy B, Suki B et al (1992) Input impedance and peripheral inhomogeneity of dog lungs. J Appl Physiol 72:168-178
46. Lutchen KR, Suki B, Zhang Q et al (1994) Airway and tissue mechanics during physiological breathing and bronchoconstriction in dogs. J Appl Physiol 77:373-385
47. Rotger M, Peslin R, Navajas D et al (1995) Lung and respiratory impedance at low frequency during mechanical ventilation in rabbits. J Appl Physiol 78:2153-2160

RESPIRATORY MONITORING AT BEDSIDE AND TECHNIQUES

Static and Dynamic Pressure - Volume Curves

G. SERVILLO, M. COPPOLA, R. TUFANO

The pressure volume (P/V) curve of the respiratory system has been used for many years to describe the mechanical characteristics of the lungs in the acute respiratory distress syndrome (ARDS) [1-3] and more recently as a guide to modify the ventilatory settings at the bedside and limit lung damage related to mechanical ventilation [4-8].

Indeed, parameters used to titrate ventilatory settings can be identified on the shape of the P/V curve described, in ARDS, as having three main segments. A non-linear lower segment characterised by low compliance, separated by a lower inflection point (LIP) from a linear intermediate segment at higher compliance, and finally an upper non-linear segment over which compliance tends to fall with increasing volume [1, 2, 9, 10], these last two segments being separated by an upper inflection point (UIP).

In 1972, Lemaire et al. described the first measurement method of the P/V curve [11]. Using a super-syringe, the authors measured the visco-elastic properties of the respiratory system in ARDS patients. To measure the P/V curve from the resting volume of the respiratory system to the estimated total lung capacity, it appeared attractive to use a calibrated syringe of known volume, ranging from 1.5 to 2 L. The inflated gas volume from the syringe is electronically measured from the displacement of the plunger, while airway pressure is recorded with a transducer referenced to atmospheric pressure. The measurements are performed after the patient has been ventilated without positive end-expiratory pressure (PEEP) a few minutes before the study and oxygenated with a fractional inspired oxygen concentration (FiO_2) of 1. Disconnection from the ventilator to allow complete exhalation to the resting volume of the respiratory system is necessary before connection to the syringe.

After the initial enthusiasm following the description of the technique, essentially among European centres, some of the technical aspects and causes of errors or artifacts were examined more deeply. This manoeuvre is relatively long and the results can, therefore, be markedly affected by continuing gas exchange on lung volume. In paralysed subjects, the rate of decrease in thoracic lung volume due to continuing gas exchange should involve a 50% over estimation of the area of the hysteresis loop of the respiratory system using this method. In addition it requires the disconnection of the patient from the ventilator and could be harmful to a severely hypoxic ARDS patient.

Subsequently Levy et al. described a technique based on analysis of the behaviour of the respiratory system after constant inspiratory flow occlusion [12]. The measurements were performed rapidly to avoid gas-exchange problems and without disconnecting the patient from the ventilator. After ensuring the absence of leaks in the system, the authors used controlled ventilation with a constant inspiratory flow and standard ventilator settings. They measured auto-intrinsic PEEP using an end-expiratory pause manoeuvre before each studied insufflation to ensure the stability of end-expiratory volume and pressure. They then delivered different tidal volumes, starting from the same lung volume with the same constant inspiratory flow (achieved by altering inspiratory time) and performed an occlusion at the end of inspiration. After performing the occlusion, the pressure obtained after a pause of a few seconds was read; then, after release of the occlusion, the exhaled volume was read on the ventilator monitor. To change inspiratory time, frequency had to be changed during the end-expiratory occlusion immediately before the study breath. Using the same technique, a deflation static P/V curve was obtained by changing the frequency during the end-inspiratory occlusion, thereby changing expiratory time. The curve was constructed by plotting volume against the corresponding static pressure.

Today this is the most used method to define the static characteristics of the respiratory system, the procedure being possible with commercial ventilators, but it is complex, necessitating the manipulation of the two hold buttons on the ventilator and the frequency setting and monitoring of both pressure and volume at the same time. Moreover the technique is difficult to perform, time consuming, necessitating some training and the presence of at least two experimenters doing the study and it cannot be recommended for routine use at the bedside.

Recently, we used an automated method based upon constant flow, avoiding the limitations of previous methods [13]. The influence of resistance was minimised by reduction of flow rate, and calculation of the pressure in the distal lung by subtracting the resistive pressure in the connecting tubes and in the airways. The new automated low flow inflation (ALFI) technique was compared with a further developed version of the recognised static occlusion technique.

ALFI was recorded using the flow and pressure transducers of the Servo Ventilator. This was routinely calibrated with the calibration system of the ventilator, which was checked against a water manometer and a 1-L super-syringe. The signals of the pressure in the expiratory line and of combined inspiratory and expiratory flow were fed into an IBM compatible computer and A/D converted at 50 Hz. Application of an analogue signal to the external control socket of the ventilator allowed the computer to take over control of respiration rate, level of PEEP, and minute volume. ALFI was performed at a Ti/Ttot of 0.5. After a standard breath and another ordinary inspiration, the computer brought the PEEP to 0 and the frequency of the ventilator to five breath/min. At 50% expiratory time this gives a duration of expiration of 6 s. Thereby, we attempted to approach functional residual capacity (FRC) at zero end-expiratory pressure (ZEEP) and during the following inspiration the same frequency was maintained to prolong inspiration to 6 s. In order to insufflate a predetermined volume, the flow rate during the inspiration was controlled to a level equal to Vinsuff (ml)/6 in ml/s. This relatively low flow rate reduced the resistive pressure component during the insufflation. About 300 data points were recorded during insufflation. During the following prolonged expiration lung volume was allowed to return to ordinary levels.

In 19 patients with acute respiratory failure or ARDS we compared the curves obtained with an automated low flow inflation technique using the Servo 900C ventilator with static intermittent measurements. Very good agreement was obtained between the two methods. Slight differences existed at high lung volumes in some patients, but usually above the tidal range and thus having little practical relevance.

Interpretation and clinical applications

The lower inflection point on the P/V curve was considered in very early studies to be the minimal pressure above which mechanical ventilation should take place in ARDS patients [10, 14, 15] and thus was proposed as a means of titrating the level of PEEP. Setting PEEP above the inflection point was considered to be one of the optimal titration methods from a physiologic and clinical point of view, at least in the early phase of ARDS.

In clinical settings the level of best PEEP chosen is in the range of 8-15 cm H_2O. Ranieri et al. considered this point to be lower than the opening pressure of 20 cm H_2O described by Radford as the level of transpulmonary pressure needed to open collapsed alveolar units [16, 17]. This situation is different in many aspects from human ARDS lung where the chest/wall prevents the lung from collapsing fully.

This concept is also studied in a series of papers by Gattinoni and coworkers [10, 15]. These authors showed that, in an early phase of ARDS, there are alterations in the ventilation/perfusion ratio and a "healthy" non-dependent lung zone leans on an atelectasic region and an intervening poorly inflated region. This non-homogeneous ventilation/perfusion ratio is substantially caused by an increase of pulmonary water, that is why the opening pressure in the dependent zones could be much higher than suggested by the inflection point on the P/V curve.

Several authors considered the lower inflection point as a setting to be used in clinical practice to establish the "best PEEP", but no outcome study has substantiated this proposition until recently.

Amato et al. reported the beneficial effects of an "open-lung approach" to ventilator management in ARDS patients [8]. The mortality in the treated group was 38% and in the control group it was 71%. This was imputed to the different strategy of choosing mechanical ventilation, based on the analysis of the P/V curve. Because several important settings between the two treatment groups differed, i.e. not only the level of PEEP used, but also the tidal volume and ventilator mode, it is difficult to establish which of these settings influenced the improvement in outcome most of all. Although two multicentre randomised studies looking only at the effects of reducing tidal volume did not find any significant difference in outcome mortality, indirectly they suggested that the individual titration of the level of PEEP in the Amato study may have been the key factor.

Moreover it must be remembered that the lower inflection point can be influenced by chest wall compliance, particularly in patients with abdominal distension and it is therefore useful, in subsequent clinical studies, to measure this value.

However, there is no clear standard method of selecting the lower inflection point on the P/V curve because of the risk of subjective interpretation and individual observer variability.

In one of their first investigations, Lemaire et al. reported the values of the lower inflection points measured "visually" in 16 patients. No inflection point was found in four patients, but one patient had an inflection bend that ranged from 6 to 12 cm H_2O which demonstrates the difficulty in picking up a single number [11].

We have proposed that the curves be analysed with a moving regression curve and that the linear part can be defined as the segment of the curve consecutive subsegment with compliance above 80% of the steepest subsegments. This has the advantage of providing a mathematical description, and the inflection points are defined as the points at which compliance starts to fall below 80% of the large value. This can be calculated for both the lower and the upper inflection points [7].

Many authors have proposed the measurement of the compliance of the respiratory system on the limb part of the P/V curve in order to evaluate the nature and degree of parenchymal abnormalities in various types of lung diseases and to assess the severity of the lung disease. The compliance is influenced by aerated lung volume and a low compliance value more often reflects a "baby lung" than a fibrotic process.

Many authors reported conflicting results regarding the ability to predict alveolar recruitment from the measurement of the compliance [18, 19].

Many experimental animal studies suggested that ventilation with high-volume and high-pressure settings can cause acute lung damage; therefore many authors proposed the adoption of a ventilation reducing the volume and the pressure and suggested the utilisation of the P/V curve and its upper inflection point as a limit which should not be exceeded during tidal ventilation. In normal subjects, the upper inflection point on the P/V curve is observed at a lung volume of approximately 85 to 90 percent of total lung capacity. In 42 patients with ARF or ARDS, Roupie et al. identified an upper inflection point only in the group of patients with ARDS in the range of volumes studied, with a mean pressure of 26 cm H_2O. The authors determined a controlled reduced ventilation with following hypercapnia in these patients whose tidal ventilation exceeded the upper inflection point on the P/V curve [4].

Conclusion

Finally we consider it very important to adapt ventilator settings according to respiratory mechanics, gas exchange, and hemodynamics of ARDS patients, but it is also necessary, as suggested by Hubmayr et al., to have a better understanding of the pulmonary damage in ARDS and its effects on respiratory structure and function.

It is equally important to make the different flow techniques easier and faster in the future since these have several potential advantages over the measurement of the P/V curve at the bedside.

References

1. Falke KJ, Pontoppidan H, Kumar A et al (1972) Ventilation with positive end-expiratory pressure in acute lung disease. J Clin Invest 5:2315-2317
2. Suter PM, Fairley HB, Isenberg MD (1975) Optimum end-expiratory airway pressure in patients with acute pulmonary failure. N Engl J Med 292:284-289
3. Lemaire F, Harf A, Rivara D et al (1979) Pression pulmonaire de fin d'expiration et compliance pulmonaire au cours de l'insuffisance respiratoire aigue (lettre). Nouv Presse Med 8:47
4. Roupie E, Dambrosio M, Servillo G et al (1995) Titration of tidal volume and induced hypercapnia in acute respiratory distress syndrome. Am J Resp Crit Care Med 152:121-128
5. Ranieri VM, Mascia L, Fiore T et al (1995) Cardiorespiratory effects of positive end-expiratory pressure during progressive tidal volume reduction (permissive hypercapnia) in patients with acute respiratory distress syndrome. Anesthesiology 83:710-720
6. Amato MBP, Barbas CSV, Medeiros DM et al (1995) Beneficial effects of the "Open lung approach" with low distending pressures in acute respiratory distress syndrome: a prospective randomized study on mechanical ventilation. Am J Resp Crit Care Med 152:1835-1846
7. Servillo G, Svantesson C, Beydon L et al (1997) Pressure-volume curves in acute respiratory failure. "Automated low flow inflation" vs "occlusion". Am J Resp Crit Care Med 155:1629-1636
8. Amato MBP, Barbas CSV, Medeiros DM et al (1998) Effect of a protective-ventilation strategy on mortality in the acute respiratory distress syndrome. N Engl J Med 338:347-354
9. Matamis D, Lemaire F, Harf A et al (1984) Total respiratory pressure-volume curves in the adult respiratory distress syndrome. Chest 86:58-66
10. Gattinoni L, Pesenti A, Avalli L et al (1987) Pressure-volume curve of total respiratory system in acute respiratory failure: computed tomographic scan study. Am J Resp Crit Care Med 136:730-736
11. Lemaire F, Harf A, Simonneau G et al (1981) Echanges gazeux, courbe statique pression-volume et ventilation en pression positive de fin d'expiration. Ann Anesth Franç 5:435-441

12. Levy P, Similowski T, Corbeil C et al (1989) A method for studying the static volume-pressure curves of the respiratory system during mechanical ventilation. J Crit Care 4:83-89
13. Servillo G, De Robertis E, Coppola M et al (1999) Application of a computerised method to measure static pressure volume curve in acute respiratory distress syndrome. Intensive Care Med (in press)
14. Dall'Ava-Santucci J, Armaganidis A, Brunet F et al (1990) Mechanical effects of PEEP in patients with adult respiratory distress syndrome. J Appl Physiol 68:843-848
15. Gattinoni L, Pesenti A, Bombino M et al (1988) Relationships between lung computed tomographic density, gas exchange, and PEEP in acute respiratory failure. Anesthesiology 69: 824-832
16. Ranieri VM, Giuliani R (1994) PEEP, ARDS and alveolar recruitment. The physiologist's point of view. Intens Care Med 20:82-84
17. Radford E Jr (1964) Static mechanical properties of mammalian lungs. In: Fenn WO, Rahn H (eds) Handbook of physiology: sec 3, vol I. Washington, DC: American Physiological Society 429-449
18. Ranieri VM, Eisa NT, Corbeil C et al (1991) Effects of positive end-expiratory pressure on alveolar recruitment and gas exchange in patients with the adult respiratory distress syndrome. Am Rev Respir Dis 144:544-551
19. Mancebo J, Bak E, Fernandez RR et al (1995) Pressure volume curves in ARDS patients: curve morphology predicts lung recruitment and overdistension. Am J Respir Crit Care Med 151:A78

Lung Function Evaluation by Capnography

U. LUCANGELO, G. BERLOT, A. GULLO

Continuous monitoring of the expired concentration of carbon dioxide (CO_2) is routine practice universally accepted as a standard of safety in the operating theatre during anaesthesia [1, 2]. Thanks to recent technological innovations which have led to the development of portable equipment which is easy to use at the patient's bedside, breath-by-breath analysis of expired CO_2 is ever more frequently being carried out in intensive care [3-5]. Furthermore the use of "combined" pneumotachographic-capnographic sensors has meant that information on respiratory mechanics and alveolar CO_2 exchange can be gained from a single non-invasive monitoring session, thus allowing a more accurate and complete evaluation of the respiratory system.

Technical aspects

Capnometry is the technique which supplies digital, that is numerical, values of the carbon dioxide partial pressure throughout the respiratory cycle. Capnography, on the other hand, is the continuous graphical representation of the CO_2 concentration (ordinate axis) expressed as a function of time (abscissa). If values of expired volume are expressed on the abscissa, the result is volumetric capnography.

A capnograph is the instrument which provides the measurement of the concentrations of CO_2 in digital form and allows their contemporaneous graphic (analogic) visualization in real time.

The concentration of CO_2 can be expressed in terms of a fractional concentration (FCO_2) and thus as a percentage, or as a partial pressure (PCO_2) in mmHg.

Capnometry

The most widely used method for measuring CO_2 concentration in expired gas is based on the principle of infrared spectrophotometry [6-8].

There are two types of capnometer which exploit this principle; they differ from each other substantially only in the placement of the sensor and thus in the way in which the gas that reaches the measurement chamber or "cuvette" of the capnograph is sampled.

Mainstream (non diverting)

In the mainstream analyser the sensor is in series between the endotracheal tube and the "Y" of the ventilator. The measurement chamber in this case is crossed by the entire flow volume and thus its diameter must be the same as that of the endotracheal tube in order not to change the airway resistance. This type of analyser does, however, cause a substantial increase in both dead space and flow-dependent resistance.

The mainstream analyser produces a capnogram in real time because the values of the CO_2 concentration are calculated during the passage of the respiratory gases through the measurement chamber (cuvette). In order to prevent any condensation of water vapour, which would invalidate the capnographic reading, the sensor must be warmed to a temperature higher than that of the body (about 39°C). These strategies make the sensor heavy and bulky and therefore in need of a support system to avoid displacement of the endotracheal tube and the risk of causing burns by prolonged contact of the cuvette with the patient's skin [8, 9].

Sidestream (diverting)

In the sidestream analyser the sensor is located within the monitor and thus there is a delay in the capnographic reading caused by the longer time required by the gas sample to reach the measurement chamber. The gas is aspirated by a narrow tube which is between the endotracheal tube and the "Y" of the ventilator. For correct sampling this narrow tube must have the following characteristics: low compliance in order to avoid collapse during aspiration; impermeability to CO_2 (polyvinylchloride); internal diameter of at least 1-2 mm and a length not exceeding 183 cm if the readings are to be reliable.

The volume of gas sampled varies from 50 to 500 ml/min according to the type of equipment used. A sampling flow of at least 150 ml/min is considered optimal. This flow should be less in neonates in order not to change the capnogram. This is because the aspiration pump affects the low flow volumes supplied by ventilators for neonates [8, 9].

One of the major drawbacks of sidestream analysers is obstruction of the catheter by respiratory secretions or condensation which can lead to a complete loss of the signal reading.

Physiological aspects

The word capnograph derives from the Greek "capnos" (smoke) and "graphein" (to write). The "smoke" (CO_2) can be interpreted as the product of cell metabolism, from which the CO_2 diffuses into the capillaries to be carried to the right heart through the venous circulation.

The heart pump shunts the CO_2 rich blood into the pulmonary circulation where diffusion across the alveolar-capillary membrane takes place.

The PCO_2 of mixed venous blood ($PvCO_2$) is 46 mmHg, while that of alveolar air ($PACO_2$) is 40 mmHg, so the CO_2 diffuses from the blood to the alveoli following the pressure gradient which creates a reflux $PACO_2$ of 40 mmHg.

The clearance of the $PACO_2$ is associated with alveolar ventilation efficiency which is described by the following formula:

$$VA = f \times (Vt - Vd) \tag{1}$$

where f is the respiratory rate, and Vt and Vd are respectively, the flow volume and the volume of the dead space.

The fractional concentration of CO_2 in the alveolar space ($FACO_2$) is the dynamic result of the velocity of the production of carbon dioxide by the tissues (VCO_2) and the extent of the alveolar ventilation (VA):

$$FACO_2 - \frac{VCO_2}{VA} \tag{2}$$

In clinical practice it is easier to think in terms of partial pressure of CO_2 than in fractional concentration. The relationship between the two is based on the following presupposition: if $FACO_2$ exercises a partial pressure relative to barometric pressure (Pb), it can be stated that:

$$\frac{PACO_2}{Pb} = \frac{VCO_2}{VA} \tag{3}$$

where $PACO_2$ is the alveolar pressure of carbon dioxide expressed in mmHg, VA in L/min (BTPS) and VCO_2 in ml/min (STPD), then

$$PACO_2 = \frac{VCO_2 \times 0.863}{VA} \tag{4}$$

The constant 0.863 is a correction factor which takes into account the Pb, the different units of measurement of VA (l/min) and VCO_2 (ml/min) and of the convention of expressing $PACO_2$ in STPB.

Carbon dioxide elimination (V_ECO_2) on the other hand depends on F_ACO_2 and on alveolar ventilation, respecting the following relationship:

$$V_ECO_2 = F_ACO_2 \times VA \tag{5}$$

It can be seen from formulae (4) and (5) that any variation in alveolar ventilation will affect both CO_2 elimination and its alveolar concentration.

In healthy subjects with a normal distribution of ventilation/perfusion (V/Q) ratio, at the moment at which the blood leaves the alveolus there is a state of equilibrium between alveolar and end-capillary CO_2. The blood that leaves the alveolar unit is arterial blood whose carbon dioxide partial pressure ($PaCO_2$) depends on the same variables as those that regulate P_ACO_2:

$$P_ACO_2 = \frac{VCO_2 \times 0.863}{VA} \tag{6}$$

In the normal individual the $PaCO_2$ value is approximately the same as that of the P_ACO_2 ($PaCO_2 \approx P_ACO_2$) without however, ever equalling it, because of the mixing of the unoxygenated blood coming from the bronchial vessels and the part of the blood which perfuses the poorly or completely unventilated alveoli. This explains the alveolar-arterial CO_2 ($aADCO_2$) difference.

$$PaCO_2 = (aADCO_2) + P_ACO_2 \tag{7}$$

The physiological range of $aADCO_2$ is 2-5 mmHg, but its value can rise much higher in pathological conditions and indeed act as a quantitative index of the extent of alveolar dead space.

Thus in physiological conditions we can assume the approximation:

$$(PaCO_2 \approx P_ACO_2) \tag{8}$$

In healthy subjects the measurement of the carbon dioxide curve at the mouth during the end-expiratory phase allows a common part of the hypothetical $PaCO_2$ curve to be recorded. In particular, the value of PCO_2 at the mouth at the end of expiration ($PetCO_2$) is that which is closest to the real value of P_ACO_2. We can, therefore, state:

$$(PetCO_2 \approx P_ACO_2) \tag{9}$$

At this point the similarity between (8) and (9) is evident and we can reasonably suppose that in normal conditions, the $PetCO_2$ gives a good approximation of the value of $PaCO_2$ [7, 16-19].

$$(PetCO_2 \approx PaCO_2) \tag{10}$$

From this derives the simple view that the "smoke" exhaled via the airways is a sensitive representation of variations associated with metabolic changes, tissue perfusion abnormalities and changes in the pulmonary ventilation/perfusion ratio.

Analysis of variations in PetCO$_2$

Based on what was written in the previous paragraph we can say that the value of PetCO$_2$ is approximately the same as that of PaCO$_2$ in the absence of marked alterations in the V/Q ratio. In the face of a decrease in the V/Q ratio there is a longer equilibrium time between PaCO$_2$ and PvCO$_2$ with the result that the value of PaCO$_2$ and therefore of PetCO$_2$ approaches that of PvCO$_2$. Vice versa, if the V/Q ratio increases, the PaCO$_2$ and thus also the PetCO$_2$ approximates the value of PCO$_2$ in inhaled air, which is equal to zero. Thus the PetCO$_2$ can be as low as the PCO$_2$ in inspired air or as high as the PvCO$_2$ without, of course, ever exceeding it [11-15]. Table 1 lists the situations in which either increased or decreased alveolar ventilation, production of CO$_2$ or perfusion can cause changes in the PetCO$_2$ [9, 11, 12, 16-21].

Analysis of the relationship between PetCO$_2$ and PaCO$_2$

The PaCO$_2$ – PetCO$_2$ gradient in healthy subjects is 1 mmHg but can increase up to 4-5 mmHg during anaesthesia or mechanical ventilation. In patients with lung disorders that affect the V/Q ratio, the PaCO$_2$ – PetCO$_2$ gradient can be as high as 10-20 mmHg because of the effect of reduced alveolar ventilation. In this case the PetCO$_2$ no longer reflects the PaCO$_2$ [9]. As a general rule a gradient near to zero reflects a physiological condition, while an increase in the gradient may be the sign of one or more of the numerous events listed in Table 2.

The capnogram

The capnograph wave (Fig. 1) is characterized by four phases which are the indicators of distinct respiratory compartments:

In phase I (A-B) at the beginning of expiration the concentration of CO$_2$ is almost zero because the air being sampled has come from the anatomical dead space and the dead space of the instrument.

This is followed by phase II (B-C) in which there is a sharp rise in the concentration of CO$_2$ caused by the mixing of the gas, rich in CO$_2$, from the alveoli with that of the dead space.

Table 1. Different causes and situations which can affect PetCO$_2$

Increase in PetCO$_2$
Decrease in alveolar ventilation
Depression of respiratory centres
Muscle paralysis
Hypoventilation
Chronic obstructive airways disease
Increased production of CO$_2$
Pyrexia
Sepsis
Increased metabolism
Administration of bicarbonates
Convulsions
Increase in cardiac output
Technical problems
Re-inhalation
Used up CO$_2$ adsorbing filters
Losses in the ventilatory circuit
Decrease in PetCO$_2$
Increase in alveolar ventilation
Hyperventilation (voluntary or forced)
Decreased production of CO$_2$
Hypothermia
Cardiac arrest
Pulmonary embolism
Haemorrhage
Hypotension
Coma
Decrease in cardiac output
Technical problems
Detachment of ventilator
Intubation of the oesophagus
Airway obstruction
Endotracheal tube obstruction
Hyperventilation from ventilator autocycling
Obstruction of the sidestream aspiration catheter
Poor adherence of the endotracheal cuff

Table 2. Causes of an increase in the PaCO$_2$ – PetCO$_2$ gradient [12]

Increase in the PaCO$_2$ – PetCO$_2$ gradient
Ventilation of underperfused lung regions with consequent decrease of the PetCO$_2$
Increase in pulmonary shunt with relative increase in PaCO$_2$
Pulmonary embolism
Cardiac arrest
Positive end-expiratory pressure (PEEP)
Ventilation with low flow volumes and high respiratory rates

The third phase (C-D) or "alveolar plateau" represents expiration of the gas coming exclusively from the alveoli. Point D is the highest value of the CO_2 concentration which is also called the end-expiratory CO_2 concentration ($PetCO_2$).

With the beginning of the successive inspiratory phase the CO_2 concentration falls rapidly until it reaches point E (phase IV). Figure 1 represents the trend of CO_2 concentration in relation to flow and volume in a healthy subject undergoing mechanical ventilation. The four phases of the capnogram are clearly identifiable. The relative lack of slope of the alveolar plateau reflects alveolar homogeneity.

Figure 2 shows a pathological situation, for example chronic obstructive pulmonary disease (COPD) or adult respiratory distress syndrome (ARDS). Both these diseases are characterised by notable alveolar dishomogeneity. In this case the typical alveolar plateau is not found even in conditions of optimal gas exchange because of the different time constants which regulate the emptying of the alveoli [6, 8, 13]. The same pattern can be recorded during an attack of bronchial asthma or when there are mechanical problems such as kinking of the endotracheal tube or herniation of the cuff [4, 6, 8, 10, 22].

Volumetric capnography

Although the analysis of CO_2 expressed as a function of time is clinically useful, more accurate information can be gained from the CO_2 single breath test (SBT-CO_2), in which the changes in CO_2 are recorded as a function of the volume of expired gas instead of as a function of time. The advanced technology combination of airway flow monitoring and mainstream capnography allows the pulmonary dead space and CO_2 production ($V'CO_2$) to be calculated. The SBT-CO_2 system allows breath-by-breath calculation of this and other important parameters of ventilatory monitoring.

A typical SBT-CO2 is shown in Fig. 3 in which the threes phases which characterise it can be clearly distinguished [23].

Phase I represents the gas without CO_2 arriving from the airways (anatomical and instrument dead space).

The following phase II consists of a rapid S-shaped rise (the result of mixing of dead space gas and alveolar gas).

Finally, phase III or the alveolar plateau represents the CO_2 rich gas coming from the alveoli.

The variations in the phase III slope can be ascribed to the following physiological phenomena [23]:

1. Cyclic variation in alveolar CO_2 during ventilation (greater during expiration than during inspiration).

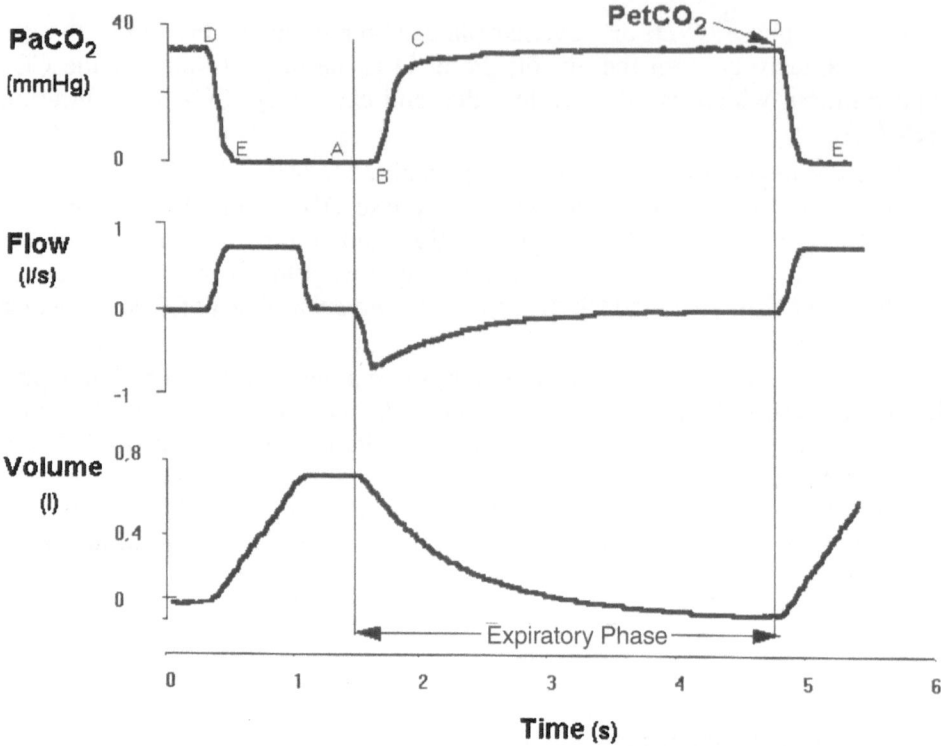

Fig. 1. Representative example of the capnographic wave related to flow, volume and the phases of the respiratory cycle

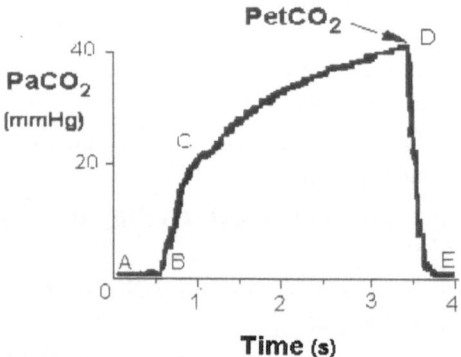

Fig. 2. Besides being difficult to identify, the slope of the alveolar plateau (C-D) is markedly increased as a result of alveolar dishomogeneity

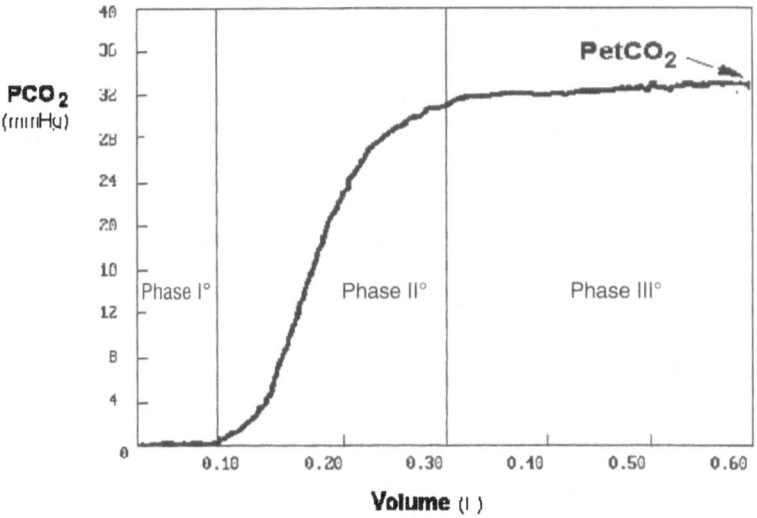

Fig. 3. The three phases of the volumetric capnogram

2. Late emptying of the alveoli with the lowest ventilation-perfusion (V/Q) ratio and, thus, with relatively higher PCO_2. If all the alveoli had the same PCO_2, phase III would be almost horizontal. In reality this "ideal" situation does not occur even in normal lungs which have a wide range of V/Q. Some alveoli have a higher V/Q ratio (overventilated) than that of "ideal" alveoli and, therefore, have a relatively lower PCO_2. Others have a lower V/Q ratio (underventilated) than that of ideal alveoli resulting in a relatively higher PCO_2. Delayed emptying of the alveoli with a low V/Q (high PCO_2) contributes to the increase in the slope of phase III. The mechanisms by which this effect can be produced are the following:

a) *Within the terminal respiratory units.* The difference in the V/Q between units can be caused by both incomplete mixing of the gases (alveolar mixing defect), and by the fact that the maximum ventilation and the maximum perfusion of that unit are out of phase (temporal mismatching - the perfusion is greater during the last part of expiration when the ventilation is less).

b) *Between the terminal respiratory units.* This can be the consequence of regional variations in the ventilation per unit of perfusion which produces a range of V/Q ratios (spatial mismatching). In this case the phase III slope is determined by the nature of the alveolar emptying: synchronous or asynchronous. If the alveolar units empty synchronously, the gas from well perfused and poorly perfused alveoli is exhaled simultaneously, resulting in a horizontal or only slightly inclined phase III slope. If the units empty in an asynchronous manner the units with a higher time constant, and thus a higher PCO_2, empty later (sequential emptying), resulting in a steeper phase III slope.

Other factors such as changes in cardiac output, the production of CO_2, airway resistance and functional residual capacity (FRC) can further influence the V/Q ratio of the various lung units affecting the height or slope of the phase III curve.

In the last analysis, the study of the phase III slope of the volumetric capnogram gives a more accurate picture of the state of pulmonary V/Q ratio than the corresponding CO_2 versus time trace.

Finally, a different approach to volumetric capnography is that of using the CO_2 elimination curve versus volume ($V'CO_2(V)$ curve). This curve has been used with success to measure the anatomical dead space, by retrograde linear extrapolation of the increase in $V'CO_2$ with volume [24, 25].

Furthermore, using the $V'CO_2(V)$ curve the fraction of the volume flow corresponding to alveolar gas exhalation (Vae) can be calculated [26, 27].

Alveolar ejection volume (Vae) can be defined as the fraction of tidal volume (Vt) with minimal dead space (Vd) contamination. According to the classical paradigm:

$$\lim {}_{vd \to 0} = [FACO_2 \ V'CO_2/Vt,]$$

VCO_2 versus Vt relationships tends asyntotically to a constant slope as it approaches endtidal volume. We have defined Vae as the volume that defines this relationship until a limit of 5% variation [27].

The method of Vae determination is presented in a normal subject and in an ARDS patient in Figure 4 where $V'CO_2(V)$ curves as a function of expired volume in a representative breath are recorded. After a given volume has been exhaled, $V'CO_2$ increases progressively to reach a total amount of CO_2 elimination in a single expiration ($V'CO_2$ tot). The increase in $V'CO_2$ is slightly nonlinear because of alveolar nonhomogeneity, i.e. the presence of a certain amount of alveolar gas contaminated by parrallel dead space. At the very end of expiration, exhaled gas comes only from alveoli, thus being pure alveolar gas.

Assuming a fixed amount of dead space contamination (dead space allowance (DSA)), we can obtain a point on the $V'CO_2(V)$ curve representing the beginning of the alveolar gas ejection volume (Vae). The Vae was then measured from the $V'CO_2(V)$ curve as follows.

First, the slope of the last 50 points of every cycle was obtained by linear fitting, using the least squares method. Then Vae was obtained as the value of the volume at the intersection between the $V'CO_2(V)$ curve and a straight line, having a maximal value at end-expiration and a slope equal to 0.95 (1-DSA) times the calculated slope (Fig. 4). Vae is expressed as a fraction of tidal volume (Vae/Vt) [29].

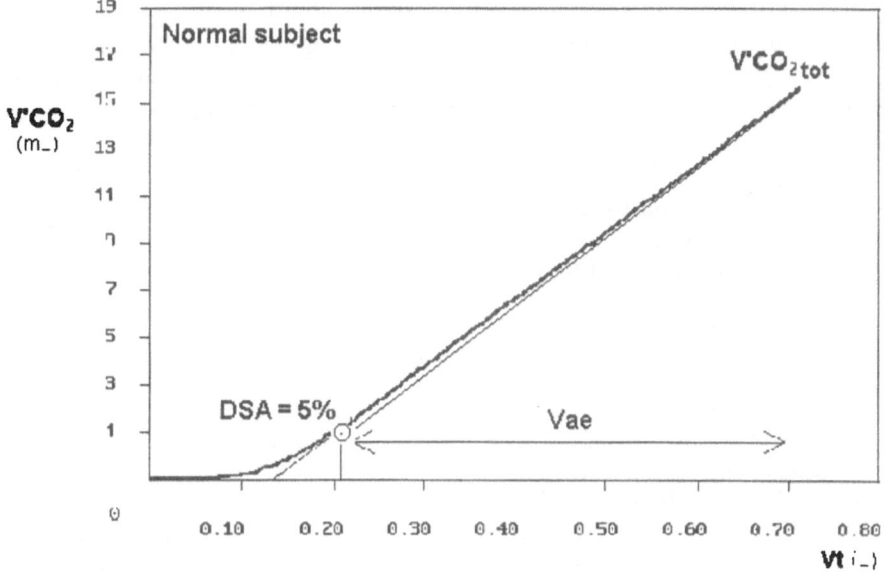

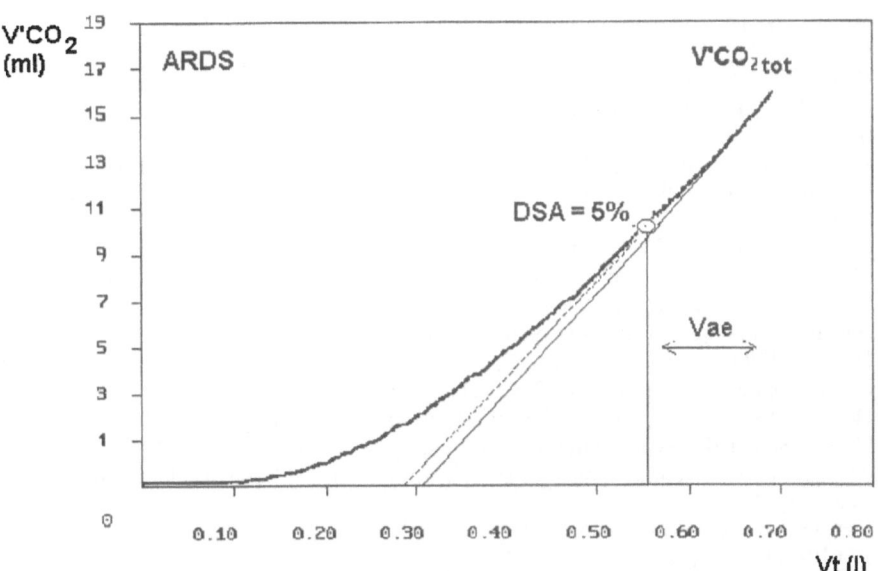

Fig. 4. Measurement of alveolar ejection to tidal volume (Vae/Vt) in a normal subject studied during anaesthesia for minor surgery and a patient with acute respiratory distress syndrome (ARDS). Curves represent CO_2 elimination versus volume $V'CO_2(V)$ curve as a function of expired volume: a first order polynomial is fitted to the last 50 points of the curve, and the equation of this line is represented. A second line is calculated by multiplying the slope by 0.95 (dead space allowance (DSA) of 5%). Vae is defined as the cross-point between this second line and the experimental $V'CO_2(V)$ curve. ($V'CO_2$ tot): total amount of CO_2 elimination in a single expiration [29]

Vae/vt has been shown to be a good index in that besides evidencing different behaviours between healthy subjects undergoing general anaesthesia and patients with ARDS, it retains this discriminative capacity independently of the flow volume and PEEP applied. Finally, apart from the phase III slope which bears no relation to any index of respiratory mechanics, Vae/Vt is inversely correlated with resistances and directly correlated with compliance of the respiratory system. It follows on from, and indeed this has already begun to be published in the literature [26-30], that Vae/Vt can have clinical applications in all those lung disorders characterised by marked alveolar dishomogeneity.

References

1. Swedlow DB (1986) Capnometry and capnography: the anesthesia disaster earlywarning system. Seminars in Anesthesia, vol V, 3:194-205
2. Eichorn JH, Cooper JB, Cullen DJ et al (1986) Standards for patient monitoring during anesthesia at Harvard Medical School. JAMA 256:1017-1020
3. Marini JJ (1988) Monitoring during mechanical ventilation. Clin Chest Med, vol 9, 1:73-99
4. Morley TF (1990) Capnography in the intensive care unit. Intensive Care Med 5:209-223
5. Tobin MJ (1988) Respiratory monitoring in the intensive care unit. Am Rev Respir Dis 138:1625-1642
6. Gravenstein JS, Paulus DA, Hayes TJ (1989) Capnography in clinical practice. Boston, Butterworth
7. Blanch Ll (1989) Capnography pulmonary function studies in mechanically ventilated patients. In: Net A, Benito S (eds) Update in intensive care and emergency medicine. Vol 13. Springer, Berlin, pp 251-266
8. Kesten S, Chapmann KR (1991) Capnometry and transcutaneous carbon dioxide monitoring. In: Tobin MJ, Grenvik A (eds) Contemporary management in critical care. Churchill Livingstone, pp 119-135
9. Jubran A, Tobin MJ (1994) Monitoring gas exchange during mechanical ventilation. In: Tobin MJ (ed) Principles and practice of mechanical ventilation. Mac Grow Hill, pp 919-943
10. Mangalaboyi J, Chopin C, Chambrin MC (1992) Utilisation de la capnographie en réanimation. In: Monitorage non invasive en réanimation. Masson, Paris
11. Hess D (1990) Capnometry and capnography: technical aspects, physiologic aspects, and clinical applications. Respiratory Care, vol 35, 6:557-576
12. Hess D (1993) Capnography: technical aspects and clinical applications. In: Kakmarek RM, Hess D, Stoller JK (eds) Monitoring in respiratory care. St Louis, Mosby 375-406
13. Nunn JF (1993) Nunn's applied respiratory physiology. 4th edn. Butterworth Heinemann, Cambridge
14. Fletcher R (1985) Relationship between arterial and end-tidal CO_2 tensions. Crit Care Med 13:610-611
15. Scheid P, Piiper J (1980) Blood/gas equilibrium of carbon dioxide in lungs. A critical review. Respir Physiol 39:1-31
16. Boysen PG, Broome JA (1988) Noninvasive monitoring of lung function during mechanical ventilation. Crit Care Clin 4:527-541
17. Good ML (1991) Clinical applications of capnography. American Society of Anesthesiologists, San Francisco Annual Refresher Course Lectures
18. Carlon GC, Ray C, Klein R et al (1988) Capnography in mechanically ventilated patients. Crit Care Med 16:550-556

19. Clark JS, Votteri B, Ariano RL et al (1992) Noninvasive assessment of blood gases. Am Rev Respir Dis 145:220-232
20. Gudipati CV, Weil MH, Bisera J et al (1988) Expired carbon dioxide: a noninvasive monitor of cardiopulmonary resuscitation. Circulation 77:234-239
21. Hatle L, Rokseth R (1974) The arterial to end-expiratory carbon dioxide tension gradient in acute pulmonary embolism and other cardiopulmonary diseases. Chest 66:352-357
22. Blanch L, Fernandez R, Lucangelo U, Artigas A (1994) Practical uses of capnography in intensive care medicine. In: Gullo A (ed) Anaesthesia Pain Intensive Care and Emergency Medicine. Fogliazza Editore, Trieste
23. Bhavani-Shankar K, Kumar AY (1992) Capnometry and anaesthesia. Can J Anaesth 39: 617-632
24. Ream RS, Screiner MS, Neff JD et al (1995) Volumetric capnography in children: influence of growth on the alveolar plateau slope. Anesthesiology 82:64-73
25. Fletcher R, Jonson B, Cumming G, Brew J (1981) The concept of dead space with special reference to the single-breath test for carbon dioxide. Br J Anaesth 53:77-88
26. Blanch L, Lucangelo U, Lopez Aguillar J et al (1995) Physiologic determinants of CO_2 elimination in mechanically ventilated patients. Int Care Med 21:S45
27. Romero P, Lucangelo U, Lopez Aguillar J et al (1995) Alveolar ejection ratio elucidated from VCO_2 versus Vt curves. Care Med 21:S45
28. Lucangelo U, Lopez Aguillar J, Fernandez R et al (1995) Capnographic indexes and lung mechanics in patients with acute lung injury receiving mechanical ventilation. Effect of PEEP. Int Care Med 21:S45
29. Romero P, Lucangelo U, Lopez Aguillar J et al (1997) Physiologically based indices of volumetric capnography in patients receiving mechanical ventilation. Eur Respir J 10:1309-1315
30. Blanch L, Lucangelo U, Lopez Aguillar J et al (1999) Volumetric capnography and respiratory system mechanics in patients with acute lung injury: effects of positive end expiratory pressure. Eur Resp J (in press)

Clinical Implications of the Mechanical Effects of Heat and Moisture Exchangers

A. BRASCHI, M.C. OLIVEI, M.A. VILLANI

Humidification of inspired gases during mechanical ventilation is a standard of care. The detrimental effects of inadequate humidity are well known [1-3], and include damage to the ciliary mucosa, thickening of secretions, and lung damage (atelectasis, shunt effect, and infection).

Heated humidifiers represent the current standard humidification technique in the ICU setting. In recent years, "passive" humidifiers, which are currently known as heat and moisture exchangers (HMEs), have been increasingly used on ICU patients submitted to long-term mechanical ventilation. The HMEs offer significant advantages over heated humidifiers, such as lower cost, simpler maintenance of the ventilator circuit, and the lack of need for electrical power. Moreover, the most recent HMEs, the combined HME and filter, combine humidification and antimicrobial filtering properties. Presently, the market offers a wide array of HMEs to the clinician, making the choice difficult. Indeed, the choice of an HME requires consideration of different parameters, which often have conflicting merits.

Several studies have evaluated the humidification efficiency and the antimicrobial properties of HMEs during long-term mechanical ventilation.

Only in recent years has attention been paid to the mechanical effects of the HMEs. The present paper examines the practical implications of the mechanical effects of the artificial noses.

The HMEs, being placed distally to the Y-piece in the circuit, are not just part of the ventilation circuit, but also part of the artificial airway. If we remove a heated humidifier and add an artificial nose, we can expect the following mechanical changes in the entire ventilation circuit:

1. an increase in the apparatus deadspace;
2. no relevant change in the inspiratory resistance;
3. an increase in the expiratory resistance, with potential generation of intrinsic positive end expiratory pressure (PEEPi);
4. a decrease in the compressible volume.

The extent of these mechanical effects is different, depending on the design and on the functions of the HMEs. In general, HMEs with a pure humidifying function have the lowest volume and lowest resistance, while combined HMEs and filters have the highest volume and highest resistance.

Increase in apparatus deadspace

HMEs increase the deadspace by an amount equal to their internal volume. The values for internal volume of HMEs range rather widely, and are mainly dependent on the design, and on the addition or not of a filtering function. The increase in volume of the HME is much less with electrostatic filtration than with mechanical filtration.

The HME volume does not affect the humidification performance of the device, except in those that have very low values [4]. In this case, the humidification performance is lower, remaining, however, acceptable if low tidal volumes (not higher than 0.5 l) are used [4].

The increase in deadspace is the most unfavourable mechanical effect of HMEs. Any increase in deadspace results in an increase in deadspace ventilation.

For a given minute ventilation level, an increase in deadspace ventilation implies a decrease in alveolar ventilation, and, hence, an increase in $PaCO_2$. To prevent this latter effect, the increase in deadspace ventilation due to the HMEs must be compensated by an increase in minute ventilation, which can be higher than 1 l/min in case of use of a HME combined with a filter [5-8].

Increase in the apparatus inspiratory resistance

Generally, the increase in the inspiratory resistance imposed by HMEs is mild. Indeed, the HMEs are for the major part low-resistive devices, although their resistance values are in a large range, going from 0.7 to 3.8 cm H_2O/l per second at an airflow of 60 l/min in dry state.

In vivo the resistance of artificial noses does not increase significantly after 24 h of clinical use, except in rare cases in which the filter membrane is exposed to particularly abundant secretions [9].

Increase in apparatus expiratory resistance and potential generation of PEEPi

The increase in the expiratory resistance imposed by HMEs does not affect the expiratory work, except when exhalation is active, when it invariably results in a decrease in the speed of exhalation, a condition which increases the risk of dynamic pulmonary hyperinflation. The increase in PEEPi due to HMEs is generally mild, and may be absent in COPD patients with dynamic bronchial collapse [10].

Increase in total work of breathing

All the above described mechanical effects of HMEs (i.e. increase in apparatus deadspace, increase in inspiratory resistance, and possible increase in PEEPi), lead to an increase in the inspiratory work, which should be compensated by an increase either in ventilator output, or in patient work. Although both approaches can be tolerated by most patients, some exceptions should be considered. The increased pressure and volume that are required to compensate for the artificial nose application increase the risk of barotrauma and volutrauma in the patients with the most severe alterations in respiratory mechanics, such as those observed in severe asthma, ARDS and lung fibrosis. Moreover, patients with very limited respiratory reserve may not be able to compensate for the inspiratory work imposed by an artificial nose. This latter aspect should be taken into account when the ability of a patient to be weaned from mechanical ventilation is evaluated.

Possible approaches for minimising the unfavourable mechanical effects of HMEs

When clinicians choose the artificial nose to be used in the ICU context, they should take into account the volume and resistance of the available devices.

The pure humidifying function is compatible with just a moderate increase in apparatus deadspace and resistance. In recent years, much effort has been done in the field of humidification, in order to maximise the humidification efficiency of HMEs, and to minimise the volume and resistance of these devices. A promising solution is represented by the active HME (AHME) (Humid-Heat, Gibeck, Upplands Väsby, Sweden). The AHME combines an HME with a unit which adds humidity and heat to the patient-side of the HME. The AHME is designed to achieve 100% humidity of inspired gases at 37°C. Of the two components of AHME, the HME provides 80% of the humidity and temperature outputs, while the remaining 20% is provided by the active unit. The principle of operation of AHME represents a way to optimise the performance of the HME, without substantial increases in the volume and the resistance of the device. Indeed, the AHME requires the use of an HME which has a low volume (73 ml, including the connector to the endotracheal tube), and a low resistance (2 cm H_2O/l per second at an airflow of 60 l/min). AHME has been shown to be an interesting alternative to heated humidifiers for humidification during long-term mechanical ventilation [11]. Indeed, AHME, besides being as efficient as heated humidi-fiers, maintains over these latter the same advantages that are typical of HMEs. In particular, AHME reduces the time-expenditure for handling, and eliminates the risk caused by water condensation in the ventilator tubings.

By contrast, combining the filtration function with the humidifying function appears more questionable. This combination may critically increase the volume and the resistance of the artificial nose, especially when a mechanical filter is used. On the other hand, there is not yet clear evidence that either simple artifi-cial noses or noses combined with filters decrease the incidence of ventilator-as-sociated pneumonia, especially when we consider that, in the ICU patient, colonisation and infection of the airways follow very complex pathways [12-14]. The possible anti-infective action of artificial noses might simply depend on the fact that these devices considerably reduce condensation accumulation in the ventilator circuit. Therefore, a reasonable compromise could be to forego the filtering function, a choice that enables a reduction in the volume and resistance of the device, and hence a reduction in its unfavourable mechanical effects.

References

1. Chalon J, Loew Day, Malebranche J (1972) Effects of dry anesthetic gases on tracheo-bronchial ciliated epithelium. Anesthesiology 37:338-343
2. Burton IDK (1962) Effects of dry anaesthetic gases on the respiratory mucous membrane. Lancet 1:235-238
3. Knudsen J, Lomholt N, Wisborg N (1973) Postoperative pulmonary complications using dry humidified anaesthetic gases. Br J Anaesth 45:363-368
4. Eckerbom B, Lindholm CE (1990) Laboratory evaluation of heat and moisture ment of draft International Standard (ISO/DIS 96330) in practice. Acta Anaesthesiol Scand 34:404-409
5. Natalini G, Bardini P, Latronico N et al (1994) Impact of heat and moisture exchangers on ventilatory pattern and respiratory mechanics in spontaneously breathing patients. Monaldi Arch Chest Dis 49:561-564
6. Le Bourdellès G, Mier L, Fiquet B et al (1996) Comparison of the effects of heat and mois-ture exchangers and heated humidifiers on ventilation and gas exchange during weaning trials from mechanical ventilation. Chest 110:1294-1298
7. Pelosi P, Solca M, Ravagnan I et al (1996) Effects of heat and moisture exchangers on minute ventilation, ventilatory drive, and work of breathing during pressure-support ventilation in acute respiratory failure. Crit Care Med 24:1184-1188
8. Iotti G, Olivei M, Palo A et al (1997) Unfavorable mechanical effects of heat and moisture ex-changers in ventilated patients. Intensive Care Med 23:399-405
9. Chiaranda M, Verona L, Pinamonti O et al (1993) Use of heat and moisture exchanging (HME) filters in mechanically ventilated ICU patients: influence on airway flow-resistance. Intensive Care Med 19:462-466
10. Conti G, De Blasi RA, Rocco M et al (1990) Effects of the heat-moisture exchangers on dynamic hyperinflation of mechanically ventilated COPD patients. Intensive Care Med 16: 441-443
11. Olivei M, Via G, Palo A et al (1999) A clinical evaluation of a new humidifier in long-term mechanical ventilation. Crit Care Forum 3:16

12. Branson RD, Davis K, Campbell RS et al (1993) Humidification in the intensive care unit. Prospective study of a new protocol utilizing heated humidification and a hygroscopic condenser humidifier. Chest 104:1800-1805
13. Dreyfuss D, Djedaïnin K, Gros I et al (1995) Mechanical ventilation with heated humidifiers or heat and moisture exchangers: effects on patient colonization and incidence of nosocomial pneumonia. J Respir Crit Care Med 151:986-992
14. Kirton O, DeHaven B, Morgan J et al (1997) A prospective, randomized comparison of an in-line heat moisture exchange filter and heated wire humidifiers: rates of ventilator-associated early-onset (community-acquired) or late-onset (hospital acquired) pneumonia, and incidence of endotracheal tube occlusion. Chest 112:1055-1059

FOCUS ON PULMONARY HYPERTENSION

Pulmonary Hypertension in ARDS: Management Strategies

A. Brienza, N. Brienza

Pulmonary hypertension (PH) is the consequence of either acute or chronic diseases resulting in the loss of the low pressure-high flow characteristics of pulmonary circulation. In 1977, Zapol and Snider demonstrated that PH is a physiological hallmark of ARDS as shown by the occurrence of a mean pulmonary arterial pressure (mPAP) > 25 mmHg in 58% of patients with severe ARF in the early phase [1]. In over 100 patients with ARDS, studied from 1-30 days after onset of symptoms, Zapol et al. observed mPAP to be around 22-28 mmHg in absence of severe hypoxemia, and in the range of 28-35 mmHg or more in presence of severe hypoxemia [2].

The causes of pulmonary hypertension in ARDS are multifactorial [3]. Vasoconstriction due to alveolar hypoxia or other vasoactive mediators like thromboxane and endothelin, and intravascular obstruction from platelet thrombi or perivascular edema, probably dominate in the early phase. In the late phase, sustained or worsening PH reflects the degree to which fibrosis is responsible for the obliteration of the vascular bed.

Acute PH was recognized as a negative prognostic factor in the late '70s [1] and its negative prognostic role has been recently confirmed. The European Collaborative ARDS Working Group has collected 2758 series of data from 586 severe ARDS patients admitted in 38 European Intensive Care Units [4]. Mean PAP was 26.1 + 8.5 mmHg at inclusion in the study and 26.7 + 8.1 mmHg after 48 hours. The study has shown that in addition to the cause of ARDS and the early time-course of lung function, a high systolic pulmonary arterial pressure and a low diastolic systemic arterial pressure were strong independent indicators of survival.

Although pulmonary blood pressure is usually only mildly to moderately elevated in ARDS patients, some patients develop right ventricular (RV) failure. While under physiological conditions, right heart role seems minimal, the development of acute PH may induce RV abnormalities and dysfunction. These abnormalities include increased RV end diastolic volume, decreased RV ejection fraction [5] or rightward shift of the right ventricle pressure-volume loop, and represent the RV response to overload. An increased RV end-diastolic volume with decreased ejection fraction is not in itself suggestive of RV failure. Dambrosio et al. [6] have shown that an acute increase in Positive End Expiratory Pressure (PEEP), considered as an acute afterload challenge for the right heart, while shifting RV pressure-volume loop to the right (i.e., higher RV volumes) does not affect the slope of the relationship (i.e., contractility does not change). The unchanged contractility with an increase in RV volumes suggests that the decreased RV performance is likely related to an increase in afterload causing a change in RV geometry, and, hence, alterations in the ejection pattern.

However, if RV afterload increases further and/or right ventricular contractile function is depressed, such as in sepsis [7], RV failure may occur, influencing systemic circulation (by reducing left ventricular preload), and even limiting survival. Therefore, when RV failure may be a major problem, the acute benefits of treating acute PH and reducing RV afterload are considered extremely useful in ARDS patients.

A pathophysiologic approach to the treatment of acute PH in ARDS includes:

a) identification and treatment of the underlying ARDS cause;
b) decreasing resistance to pulmonary blood flow by using oxygen and other pulmonary arterial vasodilators;
c) management of right heart failure.

Oxygen is a safe vasodilator and relieves pulmonary hypoxic vasoconstriction in ARF [8] as well as in COPD and primary PH patients.

The ideal pulmonary vasodilator has still yet not been found, although many have been. Most vasodilating substances systemically administered in order to treat acute PH, for example, nitroglycerin, nitroprusside, and, more recently, prostaglandin E_1 and prostacyclin are able to reduce pulmonary arterial pressure and capillary leakage, and to improve right ventricular function [9, 10]. Initial enthusiasm was based on a clinical study by Holcroft et al [11] suggesting reduced mortality in patients with ARDS treated with prostaglandin E_1. However, Bone et al. [12] while confirming the ability to reduce pulmonary vascular resistance showed no effect on mortality. Moreover, intravenously administered vasodilators cause a non selective pulmonary and systemic vasodilation; and by acting on pulmonary vessels perfusing non ventilated lung units, through the loss of hypoxic pulmonary vasoconstriction, contribute to worsen shunting of blood, Va/Q mismatch and severe hypoxemia. This lack of selectivity becomes critical when treating acute PH secondary to ARDS, in which hypoxemia is a major problem.

A vasodilator may become selective if administered through the "right route". When administered through the transbronchial route, the vasodilating action might be restricted only to pulmonary vessels perfusing well-ventilated areas (i.e., the lung areas the drug can effectively reach) causing a selective reduction of pulmonary vascular resistance with no change in systemic pressure and no increase in venous admixture [13].

Nitric oxide. Inhaled nitric oxide (NO) relaxes smooth muscles in arteries and veins in a similar way to endogenous NO by activating soluble guanylate cyclase and increasing cyclic guanosine 3'-5'-monophosphate. NO is rapidly inactivated by hemoglobin binding and does not reach systemic circulation. Therefore, delivered to ventilated lung units, it selectively dilates vessels in ventilated areas resulting in increasing flow to these areas. A recent meta-analysis has focused on administration of NO in ARDS [14]. Several short-term noncomparative and small noncomparative prospective trials concluded that NO improves oxygenation and decreases pulmonary vasoconstriction and pulmonary artery pressure in a dose-dependent way without effects on systemic hemodynamics; however, the minimal effective dose varied and evidence that NO improves outcome in ARDS patients is still insufficient because mortality remained high, and the number of subjects in each study was low [14]. Moreover, the complex and expensive technology, the potential occurrence of toxic metabolites and methemoglobinemia, the lack of benefit in non-responder patients, and the difficulty of weaning some patients from the gas, make its use not entirely safe and effective.

Prostacyclin. Prostacyclin (PGI_2) may represent an alternative to NO. It is a powerful physiological vasodilator with a short half-life, released by endothelial cells. Under physiological conditions it has a critical role in modulating pulmonary vascular tone. At physiological pH values, its half-life is 2-3 minutes because it is spontaneously hydrolyzed into an inactive metabolite, 6-keto-prostaglandin F1a. It binds to vessel smooth muscle cells receptors and increases the intracellular level of cyclic adenosine monophosphate (cAMP) by activating adenylate cyclase. cAMP activates the protein kinase A and decreases free intracellular calcium inducing vasorelaxation of the vascular smooth muscle.

Both inhaled NO and PGI_2 improve oxygenation by redistributing flow from shunt to well ventilated lung units, and pulmonary vasodilation seems more pronounced with inhaled PGI_2 than with NO in primary and secondary PH [15]. In severe ARDS, PGI_2 causes consistent and predictable effects on oxygenation and hemodynamics. Mean PAP decrease by about 4-5 mmHg [16, 17] and the effects on PH are more marked with PGI_2 than with NO. Moreover, due to the redistribution of flow from non ventilated to ventilated lung units, an increase in PaO_2/FiO_2 ratio is obtained with PGI_2 as well as with NO, although NO-related improvement seems slightly greater than PGI_2-related improvement [16, 17]. However, when PGI_2 is administered for a longer time period (24 hours) the improvement in oxygenation becomes significant [18].

In this setting both inhaled NO [19] and PGI_2 [20] show beneficial effects on RV performance, and prostacyclin can directly affect RV function through a positive inotropic effect.

In summary, PH management in ARDS is focused on the reduction in pulmonary arterial pressure and the prevention of right ventricular dysfunction/failure. The mainstay of treatment consists of ameliorating the underlying disease; however, pharmacological manipulation of pulmonary vascular tone is feasible in ARDS, and is better accomplished by the inhaled route of administration with NO and PGI_2. Although until now there is no clear proof that decreasing PH can affect prognosis of ARDS, inhaled substances through the combined effects of reducing mPAP, improving oxygenation and preventing/treating right ventricular dysfunction play a key role in ARDS treatment.

References

1. Zapol WM, Snider MT (1977) Pulmonary hypertension in severe acute respiratory failure. N Engl J Med 296:476-480
2. Zapol WM, Snider MT, Rie MA et al (1986) Pulmonary circulation during adult pulmonary distress syndrome. In: Zapol WM, Falke KJ (eds) Acute respiratory failure. New York, Marcel Dekker, vol 24, pp 241-273
3. Jones R, Reid LM, Zapol WM et al (1992) Pulmonary vascular pathology: Human and experimental studies. In: Zapol WM, Falke KJ (eds) Lung biology in health and diseases. New York, Marcel Dekker, pp 23-160
4. Squara P, Dhainaut JF, Artigas A et al (1998) Hemodynamic profile in severe ARDS: results of the European Collaborative ARDS study. Int Care Med 24:1018-1028
5. Brienza A, Cinnella G, Dambrosio M et al (1991) Incidence of pulmonary arterial hypertension and right ventricular impairment in moderate and severe acute respiratory failure. Acta Anaesthesiologica Italica 42[Suppl 1]:45-55
6. Dambrosio M, Fiore G, Brienza N et al (1996) Right ventricular myocardial function in ARF patients. Int Care Med 22:772-780
7. Brunet F, Dhainaut JF, Devaux JY et al (1988) Right ventricular performance in patients with acute respiratory failure. Int Care Med 14:474-477
8. Abraham AS, Cole RB, Greene ID et al (1969) Factors contributing to the reversible pulmonary hypertension in patients with acute respiratory failure studied by serial observation during recovery. Circ Res 24:51-60
9. Melot CP, Lejeune M, Leeman JJ et al (1989) Prostaglandin E_1 in the ARDS. Benefit for pulmonary hypertension and cost for pulmonary gas exchange. Am Rev Respir Dis 139:106-116
10. Radermacher P, Santak B, Wust J et al (1990) Prostacyclin and right ventricular function in patients with pulmonary hypertension associated with ARDS. Int Care Med 16:227-232
11. Holcroft JW, Vossar MJ, Weber CJ (1986) Prostaglandin E_1 and survival in patients with the adult distress syndrome. Ann Surg 203:371-380
12. Bone RC, Slotman G, Maunder R et al (1989) Randomized double-blind multi-centre study of prostaglandin E_1 in patients with the adult respiratory distress syndrome. Chest 96:114-119
13. Brienza N (1998) Inhaled prostacylin: from pulmonary hypertension to splanchnic hypoperfusion. Int Care Med 24:1228-1230
14. Ferreira E, Shalansky SJ (1999) Nitric oxide for ARDS - what is the evidence? Pharmacotherapy 19:60-69
15. Mikhail G, Gibbs JSR, Richardson M et al (1997) An evaluation of nebulized prostacyclin in patients with primary and secondary pulmonary hypertension. Eur Heart J 18:1499-1504
16. Zwissler B, Kemming G, Habler O et al (1996) Inhaled prostacyclin (PGI_2) versus inhaled nitric oxide in Adult Respiratory Distress Syndrome. Am J Respir Crit Care Med 154:1671-1677
17. Walmrath D, Schneider T, Schermuly R et al (1996) Direct comparison of inhaled nitric oxide and aerosolized prostacyclin in Acute Respiratory Distress Syndrome. Am J Respir Crit Care Med 153:991-996
18. Brienza N, Grasso S, Bruno F et al (1996) Effects of continuous administration of aerosolized prostacyclin on hemodynamics and gas exchange in ARDS. Int Care Med 22(3):S427
19. Rossaint R, Slama K, Steudel W et al (1995) Effects of inhaled nitric oxide on right ventricular function in severe acute respiratory distress syndrome. Int Care Med 21:197-203
20. Zwissler B, Welte M, Messmer K (1995) Effects of inhaled prostacyclin as compared with inhaled nitric oxide on right ventricular performance in hypoxic pulmonary vasoconstriction. J Cardiothor Vasc Anesth 9(3):283-289

Focus on Pathophysiology, Diagnosis and Management of Chronic Thromboembolic Disease

I. LANG, M. KNEUSSL

Definition

CTEPH is the result of single or recurrent pulmonary thromboemboli arising from sites of venous thrombosis. The natural history of pulmonary thromboemboli is to undergo total resolution, or resolution leaving minimal residua, with restoration of normal pulmonary haemodynamics. For reasons still unclear, thromboemboli in CTEPH patients fail to resolve and form endothelialised obstructions of the pulmonary vascular bed including the major branches.

Pathophysiology

Natural history

The majority of patients have a history of deep venous thrombosis (DVT) when carefully questioned. However, more than 60% of patients lack signs of past DVT at the time of diagnosis [1]. After an initial thromboembolic event that may be or may not be symptomatic the patients experience months to years of a 'honeymoon period' without any clinical symptoms. Gradually, however, dyspnea on exertion develops. Clinical deterioration parallels the loss of right ventricular functional capacity. While right ventricular hypertrophy develops, additional changes in the pulmonary vascular bed develop. These changes are histologically indistinguishable from pulmonary vascular lesions found in any other kind of pulmonary vascular hypertension [2]. These changes further increase pulmonary vascular resistance. It is suspected that the degree of these 'secondary' changes determines the capability to normalise pressures after successful pulmonary thromboendarterectomy. While the initial major vessel red thrombi transform into whitish adherent masses of granulation tissue, high pulmonary vascular resistance and slow flow through multiple irregular vascular channels lined with dysfunctional endothelium cause further apposition of fresh red thrombus. Due to segmental underperfusion, alveolar dead space increases. Finally, right ventricular failure ensues. Hypoxaemia becomes exaggerated by a combination of factors including a decline in cardiac output with a fall in mixed venous oxygen saturation, worsening ventilation-perfusion ratios, reopening of the foramen ovale, and development of small pulmonary arteriovenous fistulas in the lungs.

Pulmonary haemodynamics

The clinical 'honeymoon period' reflects the capacity of the right ventricle to overcome increased pulmonary vascular resistance. While right ventricular hypertrophy develops, additional changes in the pulmonary vascular bed develop. These changes are histologically indistinguishable from pulmonary vascular lesions found in any other kind of pulmonary vascular hypertension [2]. These changes further increase pulmonary vascular resistance. It is suspected that the degree of these 'secondary' changes determines the capability to normalise pressures after successful pulmonary thromboendarterectomy. As pulmonary vascular resistance (PVR) rises, left ventricular diastolic function deteriorates due to interventricular interdependence and diastolic forward movement of the interventricular septum. In contrast to acute right ventricular pressure rise, pericardial constriction does not appear to play a role in this process [3]. Right ventricular impairment is reversible with decrease of PVR [4].

Coagulation and fibrinolysis

No abnormalities of coagulation [1] or fibrinolysis [5] have been identified in patients with CTEPH. Recent data suggest that lupus anticoagulant (LAC), high levels of anticardiolipin, and anti-beta2-glycoprotein I antibodies are associated with chronic thromboembolic pulmonary hypertension [6]. Approximately 10% of CTEPH patients demonstrate LAC, and there exists an increased association with heparin-induced thrombocytopenia [7]. A recent study in a series of 20 CTEPH patients demonstrated no increased prevalence of the factor V Leiden mutation in CTEPH [8].

Cell biology of pulmonary artery and pulmonary arterial thromboemboli

Recent research has focused on local gene expression within pulmonary arterial thromboemboli and pulmonary arteries from CTEPH patients. By a candidate gene approach utilising in situ techniques, increased expression of plasminogen activator inhibitor type 1 was found in small thrombus neovessels, thus potentially promoting small vessel thrombosis and thrombus growth from within [9]. Furthermore, the expression of a potent inhibitor of Factor IXa and Factor XIa (i.e., protease nexin-2/amyloid beta-protein precursor, A beta PP) in the organised vascular occlusions harvested from patients with this disease was demonstrated [10]. Clot vessel haemorrhage is a feature of CTEPH thrombus histology and is speculated to be a powerful stimulator for angiogenesis.

Diagnosis

Clinical presentation

Exertional dyspnoea is the leading complaint. The key to diagnosis is to consider CTEPH in such cases in the absence of obvious reasons for dyspnoea.

Physical findings

In the absence of right ventricular failure, clinical findings are poor. Tricuspid regurgitation and pulmonary flow murmurs are the only findings.

Differential diagnosis

Primary pulmonary hypertension (PPH) must be ruled out. Female prevalence (male: female = 1:4), familial occurrence, past intake of appetite suppressant drugs, a normal or patchy non-segmentally abnormal ventilation-perfusion (V/Q) scan and vascular pruning on the angiogram are strong evidence for PPH. However, distal forms of CTEPH, and PPH with thrombi in the major pulmonary arteries complicate the diagnosis [11].

Further differential diagnoses to be ruled out are fibrosing mediastinitis, pulmonary arterial tumour or tumour invasion of the pulmonary arteries, or pulmonary arteritis [12]. In the moderately symptomatic patient left ventricular diastolic dysfunction with oxygen desaturation under exercise is a frequent differential diagnosis.

ECG

ECG is not diagnostic. When right heart failure develops, typical signs such as right bundle branch block and right axis deviation develop. Persistent negative precordial T-waves indicate right ventricular strain.

A classic cardiac stress test in the absence of right ventricular failure is normal.

Pulmonary function test and blood gas analysis

Pulmonary function tests are usually within normal limits. About 20% of patients have 'a restricitive defect' due to parenchymal scarring [13]. The transfer of CO (DL_{CO}) can be impaired for the same reason, but does not reflect the degree of vascular obstruction. While it may be reduced, a normal DL_{CO} does not exclude the diagnosis of CTEPH. Normalisation of DL_{CO} in the course of the disease probably reflects the extensive bronchial arterial collateral flow which may exceed 10% of the cardiac output in these patients. Arterial blood gas studies at rest and with exercise are important for patient evaluation. A decline in arterial PO_2 and widening of the $AADO_2$ are standard features under exercise, even with normal resting blood gases.

In the later stages of disease hypoxaemia becomes exaggerated by a combination of factors including a decline in cardiac output with a fall in mixed venous oxygen saturation, worsening ventilation-perfusion relations, opening of the foramen ovale, and development of small pulmonary arteriovenous fistulas in the lungs.

Chest X-ray

Lung fields are clear. On a closer look, areas of hypoperfusion may be seen. The hilar structures may be prominent and even interpreted as lymphomas. In extreme cases a reduction in vascular size may suggest agenesis of the pulmonary artery(ies). In some patients cavitary lesions persist or form newly at any time in the course of the disease in areas of old infarctions.

V/Q scan

In CTEPH a segmentally positive V/Q scan is diagnostic. In the absence of at least one segmental defect the diagnosis of CTEPH cannot be made. However, the severity of V/Q mismatches underestimates the severity of vascular occlusions. Although CTEPH is a vascular disorder, a ventilation scan must be performed. CTPEH patients with concomitant chronic obstructive pulmonary disease represent particular diagnostic challenges. In these patients spiral computed tomography and pulmonary angiography yield important diagnostic clues.

Post-operatively 'reverse' V/Q scan patterns are observed due to a vascular steal phenomenon diverting flow to the endarterectomised vascular compartments [14].

Exercise stress test

Exercise stress testing with arterial blood gas analysis is important for patients with normal resting pulmonary pressures and suspicion of unilateral disease. Frequently, desaturation with exercise is the first objective finding in patients who present early in evolution of their disease. Classic cardiac stress testing without measurement of arterial blood gases (or measurements of O_2 saturations by oximetry) usually yields negative results.

Echocardiography

Transthoracic echocardiography (TTE) is a readily accessible and very helpful tool for the diagnosis of CTEPH. Although the exact measurements of right ventricular dimensions is a difficult task, interventricular septal motion, right ventricular cavity dimensions, thickness of the right ventricular free wall and the velocity of tricuspid regurgitation allow the diagnosis of pulmonary hypertension to be made. Because cardiac output cannot be reliably estimated from echocardiography at the present time, the indication for surgery cannot be solely based on non-invasive pulmonary artery pressure measurements. In our experience, about 20% of CTEPH patients (usually young patients) present with normal or near normal right ventricular cavity dimensions.

Transoesophageal echocardiography (TEE) is helpful for the exclusion of an open or functionally open foramen ovale and thus helps to explain severe hypoxaemia in some patients. Furthermore, in 40% of patients proximal pulmonary arterial thrombus can be seen. Unfortunately, wall irregularities, scars and bands in the pulmonary artery cannot yet be visualised with this technique. In the majority of patients these signs are the only proximal signs of disease and can presently only be demonstrated by angioscopy.

Computed tomography

Spiral computed tomography with contrast medium is a valuable and indispensable diagnostic procedure for the diagnosis of CTEPH. However, because of limits in resolution beyond segmental arteries, distal vascular occlusions are not seen. In these instances and in all other cases, a mosaic perfusion pattern reflecting perfusion inequalities offers important diagnostic clues.

Lung biopsy

Because of a lack in specific pathological changes in CTEPH lung biopsy cannot provide differential diagnostic clues.

Right heart catheterisation

Right heart catheterisation must be performed in any case of suspected pulmonary hypertension. The assessment of pulmonary systolic, diastolic and mean pressures, pulmonary capillary wedge pressure, cardiac output and oxygen saturations are important for the calculation of shunts and pulmonary vascular resistance (PVR). Central venous saturation, PVR and cardiac output are the most important prognostic parameters in pulmonary hypertension regardless of aetiology. A PVR of > 300 dynes • s • cm^{-5} is required for pulmonary thromboendarterectomy.

Pulmonary angiography

Pulmonary angiography usually completes the diagnostic sequence. In general it is an indispensable examination. Experience over the past decade has indicated that pulmonary angiography can be carried out in any patient with pulmonary hypertension when a rigorous protocol is followed. Venous access may be from an arm, neck or femoral vein if cavography is performed first to rule out vena caval thrombosis. Usually, diagnostic right heart catheterisation is carried out prior to angiography. Selective injection of non-ionic contrast medium and re-strictive use of contrast medium in general guarantee that hemodynamic com-promise does not occur. In the case of the finding of bands and webs and vessel breakoffs the conventional pulmonary angiogram, and segmental defects in the digital angiogram, the procedure is concluded with the insertion of a vena caval filter.

The choice of the angiographic technique, i.e., conventional versus subtrac-tion pulmonary angiography is at the operator's discretion.

Treatment

Pulmonary thromboendarterectomy

Pulmonary thromboendarterectomy (PTE) is a classical bilateral endarterectomy in which the thrombus and the adjacent medial layer are carefully dissected and removed under general anaesthesia and on cardiopulmonary bypass with the pa-tient cooled to 20°C. To prevent bronchial arterial backflow into the operating field, dissections are performed under repeated periods of circulatory arrest. Complete endarterectomy of the pulmonary vascular bed is the goal. Meticulous post-operative care is demanded. A 24-hour mechanical ventilation period and fluid restriction are designed to prevent pulmonary reperfusion oedema. This life-threatening complication of PTE surgery is an acute lung injury pattern re-sulting from perfusion of a dysfunctional capillary bed in a chronically under-perfused lung segment.

Criteria for pulmonary thromboendarterectomy

A surgically accessible pulmonary thrombus (thrombi visible in the segmental arteries), a resting PVR of > 300 dynes • s • cm^{-5} or inadequate pressure rise un-der exertion and patient's consent are important criteria for a PTE listing.

Outcome

The patient's age, haemodynamics and clinical status, location of thrombus, and comorbidity determine post-operative outcome. Distal location of pulmonary thromboemboli doubles operative risk. Peri-operative mortality also depends on the surgeon's experience and post-operative care and is between 4 and 25% [15-17]. At the present time the most experienced PTE centre at the University of California at San Diego has performed over 1000 PTEs with a mortality rate as low as 4% in uncomplicated cases. Other than coumarin, patients do not usually require additional post-operative medication. Recurrent thromboembolism is a rare event. It is unexplained why some patients (approximately 10%) do not experience haemodynamic improvement despite removal of the thrombus.

Other treatments

Despite great progress in surgical techniques there are patients who cannot be operated on. Conventional therapy consists of diuretics, digitalis, anticoagulation and caval filters, chronic oxygen therapy and low-dose calcium antagonists. Inhaled prostaglandins are not known to improve haemodynamic status or survival and can be considered experimental at this time. Lung transplantation is a last treatment option.

References

1. Moser KM, Auger WR, Fedullo PF (1990) Chronic major-vessel thromboembolic pulmonary hypertension. Circulation 81:1735-1743
2. Moser KM, Bloor CM (1993) Pulmonary vascular lesions occurring in patients with chronic major vessel thromboembolic pulmonary hypertension. Chest 103:685-692
3. Blanchard DG, Dittrich HC (1992) Pericardial adaptation in severe chronic pulmonary hypertension. An intraoperative transesophageal echocardiographic study. Circulation 85:1414-1422
4. Dittrich HC, Chow LC, Nicod PH (1989) Early improvement in left ventricular diastolic function after relief of chronic right ventricular pressure overload. Circulation 80:823-830
5. Olman MA, Marsh JJ, Lang IM et al (1992) Endogenous fibrinolytic system in chronic large-vessel thromboembolic pulmonary hypertension. Circulation 86:1241-1248
6. Martinuzzo ME, Pombo G, Forastiero RR et al (1998) Lupus anticoagulant, high levels of anticardiolipin, and anti-beta2-glycoprotein I antibodies are associated with chronic thromboembolic pulmonary hypertension [In Process Citation]. J Rheumatol 25:1313-1319
7. Auger WR, Permpikul P, Moser KM (1995) Lupus anticoagulant, heparin use, and thrombocytopenia in patients with chronic thromboembolic pulmonary hypertension: a preliminary report. Am J Med 99:392-396
8. Lang IM, Klepetko W, Pabinger I (1996) No increased prevalence of the factor V Leiden mutation in chronic major vessel thromboembolic pulmonary hypertension (CTEPH) [letter]. Thromb Haemost 76:476-477
9. Lang IM, Marsh JJ, Olman MA et al (1994) Expression of type 1 plasminogen activator inhibitor in chronic pulmonary thromboemboli. Circulation 89:2715-2721
10. Lang IM, Moser KM, Schleef RR (1996) Expression of Kunitz protease inhibitor-containing forms of amyloid beta-protein precursor within vascular thrombi. Circulation 94:2728-2734
11. Moser KM, Fedullo PF, Finkbeiner WE, Golden J (1995) Do patients with primary pulmonary hypertension develop extensive central thrombi? Circulation 91:741-745
12. Kerr KM, Auger WR, Fedullo PF et al (1995) Large vessel pulmonary arteritis mimicking chronic thromboembolic disease. Am J Respir Crit Care Med 152:367-373
13. Morris TA, Auger WR, Ysrael MZ et al (1996) Parenchymal scarring is associated with restrictive spirometric defects in patients with chronic thromboembolic pulmonary hypertension. Chest 110:399-403

14. Olman MA, Auger WR, Fedullo PF, Moser KM (1990) Pulmonary vascular steal in chronic thromboembolic pulmonary hypertension. Chest 98:1430-1434
15. Jamieson SW (1998) Pulmonary thromboendarterectomy [editorial]. Heart 79:118-120
16. Iversen S (1994) Surgical treatment of thromboembolism-induced pulmonary hypertension. Z Kardiol 6:193-199
17. Klepetko W, Moritz A, Burghuber OC et al (1995) Chronic thromboembolic pulmonary hypertension and its treatment with pulmonary thrombendarterectomy. Wien Klin Wochenschr 107:396-402

EVIDENCE-BASED MEDICINE
PULMONARY SURFACTANT

Rationale for Exogenous Surfactant in Acute Respiratory Distress Syndrome

J.J. HAITSMA, B. LACHMANN

Acute Respiratory Distress Syndrome (ARDS) is characterized by respiratory dysfunction including hypoxemia and decreased lung compliance. The definition for ARDS according to the American-European Consensus Conference on ARDS [1] stipulates: 1. acute onset; 2. $PaO_2 < 200$ mmHg; 3. bilateral infiltrates as seen on a frontal chest radiograph; and 4. pulmonary artery wedge pressure < 18 mmHg or no clinical evidence of left atrial hypertension.

This definition, however, does not explain the basic physiology behind ARDS.

In ARDS increased alveolo-capillary permeability, often associated with damage to the alveolar epithelium, leads to high permeability edema. The mechanisms responsible for the injury to the alveolar-capillary membrane are complex and are still under discussion.

However, the capillary leakage combined with damage to the alveolar epithelium leads to an immediate, or moderately slow loss of active surfactant by inactivation or depletion from the alveoli and the small airways. Normally, the loss of active surfactant will be compensated by release of stored surfactant from type II cells. When the balance between production/release and loss/inactivation of surfactant favors the latter, the surface tension will rise to the air liquid interface. The alveoli will become susceptible to end-expiratory collapse and subsequent reopening at inspiration, if the applied inspirational pressure is high enough, giving way to dangerous shear forces. Shear forces are now widely accepted as the major reason for epithelial disrupture and loss of the barrier function of the alveolar membrane, and thereby attenuating the lung damage.

In summary, the progressive inactivation and loss of surfactant leads to collapse of the alveoli and subsequent atelectasis, increase in right-to-left shunt and finally, in a decrease in PaO_2.

In spite of increased sophistication in methods for respiratory support and knowledge of ARDS learned during the last twenty years, the incidence of ARDS is still 13 patients per 100,000 patients/year [2] and the mortality is still above 40% which is as high as it has always been.

As mentioned above, in ARDS the deficiency of (active) surfactant leads to the progressive deterioration of the lung function. If one can reverse the (active) surfactant deficiency one can expect also to improve lung function and ultimately this may reduce the mortality rate of ARDS. Therefore, it would be logical to supplement the ARDS lung with exogenous surfactant; this has been done with great success and with minimal side effects in more than 250,000 premature infants, since 1980, suffering from respiratory distress syndrome (RDS). But in neonatal RDS surfactant deficiency is the primary cause whereas in ARDS, it is secondary to lung injury. The injured lung already has high permeability edema leaking fibrinogen and other strong inhibitors of surfactant into the alveoli [3].

Thus can exogenous surfactant therapy overcome the potent inhibitors present in the lungs of ARDS patients?

Exogenous Surfactant Therapy, lessons from animal models

Surfactant replacement therapy has been described in various animal models. One of the most consistent and convenient models for ARDS and surfactant deficiency has been described by Lachmann et al. [4]. In this model surfactant deficiency is induced by repeated bronchoalveolar lavage (BAL) with warm saline. It has been postulated that, in the acute phase, this model reflects more a primary surfactant deficiency, as seen in neonatal RDS. But when animals are ventilated after lavage for 2 to 3 hours, a more severe lung injury has been shown to occur. This has been demonstrated by the increase in the protein concentration in the lungs, resulting in a more ARDS-like injury. The ensuing lung injury is characterized by acute quantitative surfactant deficiency and together with conventional mechanical ventilation, leads to impaired gas exchange, decreased lung compliance and decreased functional residual capacity, and increased permeability of the alveolo-capillary membrane resulting in edema leakage into the alveolus. The lavage model was the first to describe that surfactant can be used as a therapy for ARDS [5].

Besides the lavage model, there are several animal models, which mimic an ARDS-like lung injury pattern [6]. The hydrochloric acid instillation model [7] matches the clinical state of aspiration of gastric contents, leading to severe ARDS. Prolonged exposure to pure oxygen also results in a lung injury pattern resembling ARDS. Other animal models of ARDS which have their specific uses are: neurogenic ARDS, paraquat intoxication, oleic acid infusion, pulmonary infections, and immunological induced lung injuries.

All these models have instigated an enormous amount of research on how to use exogenous surfactant therapy to improve gas exchange and lung mechanics. The different animal models have led to a better understanding of delivery techniques, timing of administration and type of surfactant to be used.

Bolus administration is the most commonly used method of instillation for its ability to rapidly deliver large quantities of surfactant necessary to overcome the inhibitory effects of serum proteins present in the alveoli. Segerer et al. [8]

demonstrated in lung lavaged rabbits, a homogenous pulmonary surfactant distribution after bolus instillation, whereas distribution after slow tracheal infusion of exogenous surfactant was extremely uneven. This study also showed a distinct correlation between distribution of surfactant and pulmonary gas exchange. However, the disadvantage of bolus instillation technique is that a relatively large amount of fluid has to be instilled. However, Gilliard et al. [9] demonstrated that the volume of fluid in which surfactant is administered is rapidly absorbed. Thirty minutes after surfactant instillation, there was no significant difference between the lung weights of animals with lung injury receiving 5 ml and those receiving 50 ml of surfactant suspension. Aerosol delivery for exogenous surfactant has also been investigated, Lewis et al. [10] showed a more homogenous distribution pattern. However, they found that tracheally instilled surfactant was superior to aerosol surfactant in improving blood gases, whereas no difference in the improvement of lung mechanics was seen. Aerosol delivery is further complicated by the low quantities (6.1%) of surfactant deposited in the lung and the relatively long period of administration of the surfactant. Our study also showed that lavaging the lung with a diluted surfactant suspension (3.3 mg/ml, 30 ml/kg) prior to surfactant administration (100 mg/kg) was as effective as high bolus administration (250 mg/kg) in improving gas exchange in established lung injury due to acid aspiration [11].

Another important aspect regarding optimal surfactant therapy is the time elapsed between initial damage and start of the therapy. Our group showed that respiratory failure could be prevented when exogenous surfactant was given before deterioration of lung function (i.e. within 10 min after acid aspiration). Whereas after the development of respiratory failure exogenous surfactant served only to prevent further decline of lung function but did not restore gas exchange [7]. When treatment starts at a later stage of lung injury, the amount of inhibitory proteins that have accumulated in the lung require larger amounts of surfactant, or several consecutive administrations, to improve lung function.

Various surfactant preparations are already available on the market and are being used in the treatment of RDS in neonates. Studies performed in animal models under standardized conditions showed marked differences in efficacy in improving lung function among the various preparations [12]. Natural surfactants containing the hydrophobic proteins SP-B and SP-C, which are able to partly withstand the inactivation by plasma proteins, are more effective in improving lung function than artificial surfactants or natural surfactants with low amounts of SP-B and SP-C.

First clinical results

Although clinical data supports the use of surfactant in RDS, the amount of data concerning ARDS is limited and at most consists of a few case reports [13]. Recently, the results of the first multi-patient studies have been published. Walmarth et al. [14] studying 10 patients with established severe ARDS and sepsis, showed that bronchoscopic application of a natural surfactant (300 mg/kg) resulted in an "immediate, impressive, and highly significant improvement in arterial oxygenation in all patients, due to a marked reduction of the shunt flow". In half of the patients, a second dose (200 mg/kg) was required. A total of 8 patients survived the 14-day observation period, and 5 patients were weaned from the ventilator. All fatalities were not respiratory related.

Gregory and colleagues [15] studied four different dosages in 48 adults with ARDS. The results showed that maximum improvement in oxygenation, minimum ventilatory requirements, and the lowest mortality rate were obtained using four doses of 100 mg/kg of natural surfactant (total amount of 400 mg/kg). The administration of large volumes of surfactant suspension was generally well tolerated (up to 2,200 ml in a 48 h period).

Anzueto et al. [16] demonstrated that administration of aerosol artificial surfactant had no effect on mortality and lung function in a multicenter, randomized placebo-controlled trial in 725 patients with sepsis-induced ARDS. In this study it was speculated that one of the reasons for the lack of response could be that less than 25 mg of surfactant per kg bodyweight was actually delivered into the lungs due to the method of administration, which was only one-sixteenth of the dosage used by Gregory et al. [15].

Conclusion and future considerations

In adults with ARDS, increased alveolo-capillary permeability combined with inflammation is known to inactivate the functional alveolar surfactant. This causes the lung to fail as a gas exchange organ. The value of surfactant therapy is that functional impairment of active surfactant can be reversed by instillation of an excess of exogenous surfactant. Research data from both animal and preliminary clinical studies offer insight on how to optimize exogenous surfactant.

- Bolus instillation delivers large quantities of active surfactant into the lungs, whereas aerosol delivery delivers only low quantities of surfactant [10, 16]. To optimize exogenous surfactant therapy, bolus instillation is the preferred method; the large amount of fluid to the patient is, generally, well tolerated [9, 15].
- A bolus of exogenous surfactant should have a sufficiently high dosage to overcome the inhibitory effects of the plasma proteins [3, 14, 15]. Clinical data suggest 200 or 400 mg/kg of surfactant.
- The lack of response seen with the synthetic surfactant preparation used by Anzueto et al. [16] versus the clear improvement seen with the natural surfactants used by Gregory et al. [15] and Walmarth and colleagues [14], proves the complex nature of natural surfactant and the essential role of the surfactant proteins in the phospholipid monolayer. This observation is in

agreement with animal data from our group [12]. The preferred surfactant is a natural surfactant containing a sufficient amount of the surfactant proteins SP-B and SP-C.

- Animal data [7] and clinical experience in neonates with RDS suggest that surfactant therapy, when started as soon as possible, improves the effectiveness of exogenous surfactant therapy. The efficacy can be further enhanced by lavaging the lungs, prior to instillation of exogenous surfactant with a diluted surfactant suspension [11], thus removing some of the inhibitory proteins.

Although the rationale for surfactant therapy is clear, a question remains as to why it hasn't become standard practice as a therapeutic agent in ARDS.

First and foremost the high price of surfactant, a dosage of 100 mg/kg (standard in infants) would require at least 7-10 g of surfactant in adults, which is about US$ 40,000 per treatment.

Furthermore, more clinical trials are needed, which need to take into account the lessons learned from the animal models, and aimed to optimize surfactant therapy and establish the optimal therapeutic scheme (one dosage, several dosage, prior lavage, etc.).

References

1. Bernard GR, Artigas A, Brigham KL et al (1994) Report of the American-European Consensus conference on acute respiratory distress syndrome: definitions, mechanisms, relevant outcomes, and clinical trial coordination. Consensus Committee. J Crit Care 9:72-81
2. Luhr OR, Antonsen K, Karlsson M et al (1999) Incidence and mortality after acute respiratory failure and acute respiratory distress syndrome in Sweden, Denmark, and Iceland. The ARF Study Group. Am J Respir Crit Care Med 159:1849-1861
3. Seeger W, Stohr G, Wolf HR et al (1985) Alteration of surfactant function due to protein leakage: special interaction with fibrin monomer. J Appl Physiol 58:326-338
4. Lachmann B, Robertson B, Vogel J (1980) In vivo lung lavage as an experimental model of the respiratory distress syndrome. Acta Anaesthesiol Scand 24:231-236
5. Lachmann B, Jonson B, Lindroth M (1982) Modes of artificial ventilation in severe respiratory distress syndrome. Lung function and morphology in rabbits after wash-out of alveolar surfactant. Crit Care Med 10:724-732
6. Lachmann B, Van Daal G-J (1992) Adult Respiratory Distress Syndrome: Animal Models. In: Robertson B, Van Golde LMG, Batenburg JJ (eds) Pulmonary Surfactant: from molecular biology to clinical practice. Elsevier Science Publishers BV, pp 635-663
7. Eijking EP, Gommers D, So KL et al (1993) Prevention of respiratory failure after hydrochloric acid aspiration by intratracheal surfactant instillation in rats [see comments]. Anesth Analg 76:472-477
8. Segerer H, van Gelder W, Angenent FW (1993) Pulmonary distribution and efficacy of exogenous surfactant in lung-lavaged rabbits are influenced by the instillation technique. Pediatr Res 34:490-494
9. Gilliard N, Richman PM, Merritt TA (1990) Effect of volume and dose on the pulmonary distribution of exogenous surfactant administered to normal rabbits or to rabbits with oleic acid lung injury. Am Rev Respir Dis 141:743-747

10. Lewis JF, Tabor B, Ikegami M et al (l993) Lung function and surfactant distribution in saline-lavaged sheep given instilled vs. nebulized surfactant. J Appl Physiol 74:1256-1264
11. Gommers D, Eijking EP, So KL et al (1998) Bronchoalveolar lavage with a diluted surfactant suspension prior to surfactant instillation improves the effectiveness of surfactant therapy in experimental acute respiratory distress syndrome (ARDS). Intensive Care Med 24:494-500
12. Gommers D, van't Veen A, Verbrugge SJC et al (1998) Comparison of eight different surfactant preparations on improvement of blood gases in lung-lavaged rats. Appl Cardiopulm Pathophysiol 7:95-102
13. Gommers D, Lachmann B (1993) Surfactant therapy: does it have a role in adults? Clin Intensive Care 4:284-295
14. Walmrath D, Gunther A, Ghofrani HA et al (1996) Bronchoscopic surfactant administration in patients with severe adult respiratory distress syndrome and sepsis. Am J Respir Crit Care Med 154:57-62
15. Gregory TJ, Steinberg KP, Spragg R et al (1997) Bovine surfactant therapy for patients with acute respiratory distress syndrome. Am J Respir Crit Care Med 155:1309-1315
16. Anzueto A, Baughman RP, Guntupalli KK et al (1996) Aerosolized surfactant in adults with sepsis-induced acute respiratory distress syndrome. N Engl J Med 334: 1417-1421

Surfactant in the Airways: Function and Relevance in Asthma

J.M. HOHLFELD

Pulmonary surfactant reduces the surface tension at the air-liquid interface in the entire lung by forming a layer between the aqueous airway liquid and inspired air. The major component of surfactant, dipalmitoylphosphatidylcholine (DPPC), is an amphiphatic phospholipid. Its polar head region is associated with the aqueous hypophase whereas the hydrophobic fatty acid chains face the luminal air. Surfactant-specific proteins facilitate the arrangement of phospholipids in this layer, thereby optimizing surface tension reducing capacity. This important function prevents alveolar and airway collapse at end-expiration and thus allows cyclic ventilation of the lungs.

The pathogenetic relevance of surfactant was initially recognized in infant respiratory distress syndrome as a quantitative surfactant deficiency [1], but today biochemical and biophysical surfactant abnormalities have been reported in various lung diseases, such as acute respiratory distress syndrome, pneumonia, and cardiogenic lung oedema [2]. These disorders show an alveolar surfactant dysfunction. In contrast, the possible involvement of pulmonary surfactant in the pathophysiology of respiratory diseases with a predominant disturbance in the conducting airways, such as asthma has only recently been addressed [3]. Increased airway resistance in asthma which is commonly thought to be caused by smooth muscle constriction, mucosal oedema and secretion of fluid into the airway lumen, may partly be due to a poor function of pulmonary surfactant.

In the last decade, direct and indirect evidence has emerged for surfactant as a factor in the regulation of airway calibres. The physiologic aspects of airway mechanics that are related to the function of surfactant and its potential relevance in asthma will be discussed.

Physiologic aspects and functions of airway surfactant

The majority of airway surfactant originates from the alveoli. During expiration alveolar surfactant becomes extruded into adjacent conducting airways. In addition, local synthesis and release of phospholipids in tracheal epithelial cells has been demonstrated [4]. Surfactant-protein synthesis has also been shown in

Clara cells [5, 6]. Synthesis of surfactant components in the airways might indicate the possibility of local adaptation of the airway surfactant system.

Airway surfactant lowers surface tension at the air-liquid interface of conducting airways. This reduces the tendency of airway liquid to form bridges in the airway lumen (film collapse). In addition, a low surface tension minimizes the magnitude of negative pressure on the airway wall and its liquid layer which in turn reduces the tendency for airway wall ("compliant") collapse. Surface tension in the conducting airways has been shown to range between 25-30 mN/m. This causes transmural pressures of less than 1 cm H_2O whereby the patency of airways is maintained. By prevention of both, film collapse and compliant collapse, airway surfactant maintains airway structure and openness.

Surfactant also contributes to the regulation of airway fluid balance, improves bronchial clearance, act as a barrier of inhaled agents, and plays an important role in local immunomodulation. Firstly, the high surface pressure (low surface tension) of surfactant counteracts fluid influx into the airway lumen. Loss of surface activity would result in additional inward forces that cause fluid accumulation in the airway lumen. The influence of surfactant on airway liquid balance also prevents desiccation. Secondly, surfactant improves bronchial clearance by optimizing transport of particles and bacteria from the peripheral to the more central airways. Moreover, surfactant has been shown to enhance mucociliary clearance [7] partly by increasing ciliary beat frequency [8]. Thirdly, several studies have suggested that surfactant acts as a barrier to the diffusion of inhaled agents including bacteria, allergens and drugs [9, 10]. For example, depletion of the surfactant layer by lung lavage leads to augmented responses to drugs and allergens [11, 12]. In contrast, exogenous surfactant treatment lessens the response to bronchoconstrictor stimuli [13]. Besides various aspects of immunomodulation by surfactant components, there are some important findings relevant to asthma. Surfactant protein-A has been shown to bind to pollen grains [14]. Lymphocyte activity and proliferation can be downregulated by phospholipids and SP-A. Surfactant proteins SP-A and SP-D have also been demonstrated to bind to allergens and to reduce allergen-induced lymphocyte activation in a dose-dependent manner [15, 16]. To summarize, a good functioning surfactant stabilizes the airways, prevents luminal liquid accumulation, improves bronchial clearance, reduces the diffusion of bronchoconstrictors to the underlying mucosa, and reveals antiinflammatory properties. All these functions might be of potential benefit in asthma.

Surfactant dysfunction in the airways and asthma

Data on airway surfactant function have been derived using in-vitro models, animal experiments, and hitherto a few human studies. A simple method to estimate surfactant function of a cylindrical surface such as a narrow conducting airway, is the Capillary Surfactometer. This instrument simulates the morphology and function of a terminal conducting airway with a glass capillary that in a short section is particularly narrow with an ID of 0.3 mm [17-19]. It is there that liquid is likely to accumulate, but this can be prevented by a well-functioning pulmonary surfactant. A small volume (0.5 μL) of the liquid to be evaluated is deposited in this section. The lumen of the capillary will be totally blocked but, when pressure is raised at one end of the capillary, the liquid is extruded from the narrow section. It will not return if it contains well-functioning surfactant, but if the surfactant concentration is very low or functioning poorly, the liquid will return and again block the capillary lumen. Since there is a continuous flow of air through the capillary and pressure is recorded at the capillary inlet, the function of the surfactant can be evaluated. Pressure is zero if the capillary is open for free airflow, but there will be an increase in pressure when the liquid returns to block the narrow section. Pressure is recorded for 120 seconds and a computer calculates the percentage in time the capillary remains open. Well-functioning pulmonary surfactant will keep the capillary open 100%, showing an excellent ability to maintain airway patency, with a surfactant functioning very poorly, the value of 'Open in %' will be zero.

Liu et al. [17] found that surfactant-containing fluid allowed a free airflow through the tube whereas saline lead to spontaneous refilling of the capillary. The ability of surfactant to maintain free airflow was lost with the addition of albumin or fibrinogen (two potent surfactant inhibitors). Surfactant function was seriously affected by hydrolysis with phospholipase C, but not with phospholipase A_2 [18].

In a murine model of asthma it has been reported that guinea pigs, sensitized with ovalbumin, and then challenged with aerosolized antigen, reacted with a leakage of plasma proteins into the airways, a markedly increased airway resistance, and an altered surfactant performance indicating a dysfunction [20]. It has also been shown that prophylactic treatment of sensitized animals with intratracheal instillation of surfactant reduces the deteriorating lung function that otherwise would have developed [21]. In studies from another laboratory it was demonstrated that treatment of immunized guinea pigs with aerosolized surfactant alleviates an increase in airway resistance [22]. Moreover, in heterozygous SP-B deficient mice air trapping was observed, suggesting that airway obstruction might have been due to a surfactant dysfunction caused by the SP-B deficiency [23]. Recently, van de Graaf et al. [24] described that the bronchoalveolar lavage (BAL) levels of SP-A were lowered in patients with asthma. Kurashima et al. [25] reported that sputum samples from patients with asthma have a low surface activity.

We have recently investigated the inflammatory changes of bronchoalveolar lavage fluid and the performance of BALF surfactant in healthy controls ($n = 9$) and patients with mild allergic asthma ($n = 15$), before and after segmental allergen challenge [26]. BALF was obtained for baseline values, and 24 hours after challenge with saline solution in one lung segment and with allergen in another. Cell counts, phospholipid and protein concentrations, and ratios of small to large surfactant aggregates (SA/LA) were analyzed. Surface tension was determined with a Pulsating Bubble Surfactometer, and the ability of the BALF surfactant to maintain airway patency was assessed with a Capillary Surfactometer. Baseline values of controls and asthmatics were not different. Challenge with saline and antigen raised total inflammatory cells in both controls and asthmatics. Allergen challenge of asthmatics, but not of healthy volunteers, significantly increased eosinophils, proteins, SA/LA, surface tension at minimum bubble size, and diminished the time the capillary tube was open. Most likely, the reason for disturbed surfactant function was that proteins had invaded the airways as they reached a tenfold increase in concentration. Proteins have extensively been proven to inhibit surfactant function [27, 28]. Interestingly, a washing procedure with saline that removed water soluble inhibitors, such as the proteins, restored surfactant function. These data show that allergen challenge in asthmatics induces surfactant dysfunction, probably mainly due to inhibiting proteins. During an asthma attack narrow conducting airways may become blocked, which might contribute to increased airway resistance.

Therapeutic implications

Although there is no direct poof that surfactant dysfunction in human asthma causes airway obstruction the above mentioned and published data from the literature support the concept that a poorly functioning surfactant contributes to the pathophysiology or asthma. Thus, it is justified to investigate the potential role of surfactant therapy in asthma. There are two different ways to improve the surfactant balance in the airways. Firstly, various drugs that are commonly used in asthma therapy, like corticosteroids, β-adrenergic agents, and theophylline have been shown to stimulate surfactant synthesis or secretion [29-31]. However, it remains to be determined whether pharmacological stimuli can augment surfactant secretion the extent that could be clinically relevant. The overall effect of pharmacotherapy on surfactant function and its impact on asthma requires further investigation. Secondly, treatment with exogenous surfactant has been shown to improve allergic airway obstruction in animal models of asthma [21, 22]. Human data are rare. A small randomized controlled trial demonstrated a significant improvement of pulmonary function data after inhalation of surfactant in patients with acute asthma attacks [32]. In contrast, nebulized surfactant did nor alter airway obstruction and bronchial responsiveness to histamine in asthmatic children with mild airflow limitation [33]. A prospective randomized controlled trial of aerosolized synthetic surfactant (Exosurf) in 87 adult patients with stable chronic bronchitis revealed a significant improvement of forced expiratory volume in 1 second of 11%, a decrease of thoracic gas trapping by 6%, and an improvement of sputum transportability [34]. Taken together, these results demonstrate that exogenous surfactant therapy might have at least some beneficial effect in patients with asthma and obstructive airways disease. However, exogenous surfactant therapy is expensive and therefore still limited to research and case studies. Future investigations will help reveal relevant surfactant components with the best anti-obstructive effects and antiinflammatory capacity.

Conclusions - The potential relevance of surfactant in asthma

Pulmonary surfactant with an optimal function in the airways is important because it stabilizes the conducting airways, prevents fluid accumulation within the airway lumen, improves bronchial clearance, acts as a barrier to the uptake of inhaled agents, and has important immunomodulatory properties. In asthma, it has been demonstrated that there is surfactant dysfunction mainly due to inhibition by proteins present during the inflammatory process in the airways. Surfactant dysfunction in asthma adds to our understanding of the pathophysiology of airway obstruction in this respiratory disease. Therapeutic interventions that improve airway surfactant balance by stimulation of the endogenous surfactant system or by additional exogenous surfactant might be of benefit in reversing airway obstruction in asthma. Safe and effective ways of managing airway inflammation and airway obstruction with surfactant components may be helpful in asthma.

References

1. Avery ME, Mead J (1959) Surface properties in relation to atelectasis and hyaline membrane disease. Am J Dis Child 97:517-523
2. Günther A, Siebert C, Schmidt R (1996) Surfactant alterations in severe pneumonia, acute respiratory distress syndrome, and cardiogenic lung edema. Am J Respir Crit Care Med 153:176-184
3. Hohlfeld J, Fabel H, Hamm H (1997) The role of pulmonary surfactant in obstructive airways disease. Eur Respir J 10:482-491
4. Barrow RE (1990) Chemical structure of phospholipids in the lungs and airways of sheep. Respir Physiol 79:1-8
5. Auten RL, Watkins RH, Shapiro DL (1990) Surfactant apoprotein A (SP-A) is synthetized in airway cells. Am J Respir Cell Mol Biol 3:491-496
6. Voorhout WF, Veenendaal T, Kuroki Y (1992) Immunocytochemical localization of surfactant protein D (SP-D) in type II cells, Clara cells, and alveolar macrophages of rat lung. J Histochem Cytochem 40:1589-1597
7. De Sanctis GT, Tomkiewicz RP, Rubin BK (1994) Exogenous surfactant enhances mucociliary clearance in the anaesthetized dog. Eur Respir J 7:1616-1621
8. Kakuta Y, Sasaki H, Takishima T (1991) Effect of artificial surfactant on ciliary beat frequency in guinea pig trachea. Respir Physiol 83:313-322
9. Widdicombe JG (1997) Airway liquid: a barrier to drug diffusion? Eur Respir J 10:2194-2197
10. Hills BA (1996) Asthma: is there an airway receptor barrier? Thorax 51:773-776
11. So KL, Gommers D, Lachmann B (1993) Bronchoalveolar surfactant and intratracheal adrenaline. Lancet 341:120-121

12. Kiekhaefer CM, Kelly EAB, Jarjour NN (1999) Enhanced antigen-induced eosinophilia with prior bronchoalveolar lavage. Am J Respir Crit Care Med 159:A99
13. Hohlfeld J, Hoymann HG, Molthan J (1997) Aerosolized surfactant inhibits acetylcholine-induced airway obstruction in rats. Eur Respir J 10:2198-2203
14. Malhotra R, Haurum J, Thiel S (1993) Pollen grains bind to lung alveolar type II cells (A549) via lung surfactant protein A (SP-A). Biosci Rep 13:79-90
15. Wang JY, Kishore U, Lim BL (1996) Interaction of human lung surfactant proteins A and D with mite (Dermatophagoides pteronyssinus) allergens. Clin Exp Immunol 106:367-373
16. Wang JY, Shieh CC, You PF (1998) Inhibitory effect of pulmonary surfactant proteins A and D on allergen-induced lymphocyte proliferation and histamine release in children with asthma. Am J Respir Crit Care Med 158:510-518
17. Liu M, Wang L, Li E (1991) Pulmonary surfactant will secure free airflow through a narrow tube. J Appl Physiol 71:742-748
18. Enhorning G, Holm BA (1993) Disruption of pulmonary surfactant's ability to maintain openness of a narrow tube. J Appl Physiol 74:2922-2927
19. Enhorning G (1996) Pulmonary surfactant function in alveoli and conducting airways. Can Respir J 3:21-27
20. Liu M, Wang L, Enhorning G (1995) Surfactant dysfunction develops when the immunized guinea-pig is challenged with ovalbumin aerosol. Clin Exp Allergy 25:1053-1060
21. Liu M, Wang L, Li E (1996) Pulmonary surfactant given prophylactically alleviates an asthma attack in guinea-pigs. Clin Exp Allergy 26:270-275
22. Kurashima K, Fujimura M, Tsujiura M (1997) Effect of surfactant inhalation on allergic bronchoconstriction in guinea pigs. Clin Exp Allergy 27:337-342
23. Clark JC, Weaver TE, Iwamoto HS (1997) Decreased lung compliance and air trapping in heterozygous SP-B-deficient mice. Am J Respir Cell Mol Biol 16:46-52
24. van de Graaf EA, Jansen HM, Lutter R (1992) Surfactant protein A in bronchoalveolar lavage fluid. J Lab Clin Med 120:252-263
25. Kurashima K, Fujimura M, Matsuda T (1997) Surface activity of sputum from acute asthmatic patients. Am J Respir Crit Care Med 155:1254-1259
26. Hohlfeld J, Ahlf K, Enhorning G (1999) Dysfunction of pulmonary surfactant in asthmatics after segmental allergen challenge. Am J Respir Crit Care Med 159:1803-1809
27. Fuchimukai T, Fujiwara T, Takahashi A (1987) Artificial pulmonary surfactant inhibited by proteins. J Appl Physiol 62:429-437
28. Seeger W, Grube C, Günther A (1993) Surfactant inhibition by plasma proteins: differential sensitivity of various surfactant preparations. Eur Respir J 6:971-977
29. Dobbs LG, Mason RJ (1979) Pulmonary alveolar type II cells isolated from rats. Release of phosphatidylcholine in response to β-adrenergic stimulation. J Clin Invest 63:378-387
30. Ekelund L, Burgoyne R, Brymer D (1981) Pulmonary surfactant release in fetal rabbits as affected by terbutaline and aminophyllin. Scand J Clin Lab Invest 41:237-245
31. van Golde LMG (1985) Synthesis of surfactant lipids in the adult lung. Annu Rev Physiol 47:765-774
32. Kurashima K, Ogawa H, Ohka T (1991) A pilot study of surfactant inhalation in the treatment of asthmatic attack. Aerugi (Jpn J Allergol) 40:160-163
33. Oetomo SB, Dorrepaal C, Bos H (1996) Surfactant nebulization does not alter airflow obstruction and bronchial responsiveness to histamine in asthmatic children. Am J Respir Crit Care Med 153:1148-1152
34. Anzueto A, Jubran A, Ohar JA (1997) Effects of aerosolized surfactant in patients with stable chronic bronchitis. A prospective randomized controlled trial. JAMA 278:1426-1431

Alveolar Surfactant and Inflammatory Mediators

M. HALLMAN

Alveolar surfactant is a lipid protein complex that prevents atelectasis, decreases work of breathing, and promotes uniform expansion of alveoli allowing efficient gas exchange. In addition, the surfactant protects the alveoli and the small airways against edema and mechanical trauma. Surfactant also contains components that are involved in defense against microbes and xenobiotics. According to present hypothesis non-clonal innate immunity – an ancient non-vertebrate defense system – is important in host defense particularly in transcellular spaces. This system has evolved to function in a natural state of infectious and inflammatory diseases. The present methods of intensive care have been developed in the absence of the knowledge of the function of the host defense system. It is conceivable that the new and effective invasive treatment practices "fool" the innate immunity to trigger an inappropriate response that becomes destructive rather than protective to the host.

The surfactant system is of central importance in pulmonary gas exchange and important in pulmonary innate immunity. Investigation on the roles of inflammatory mediators may reveal new concepts of lung protection during intensive treatment.

Brief description of the surfactant system

Alveolar surfactant complex is synthesized, secreted and for the most part catabolized in type II alveolar cells. After intracellular transport, storage in lamellar inclusion bodies and exocytosis the surfactant undergoes aggregate transformation in the epithelial lining. Extracellular surfactant participates in dynamic reduction of surface tension in air-liquid interface. Eventually surfactant components are cleared and catabolized by type II cells and pulmonary alveolar macrophages (PAM), and reutilized by type II cells. Alveolar surfactant consists of dipalmitoyl phosphatidylcholine (DPPC), unsaturated phosphatidylcholine, phosphatidylglycerol, phosphatidylinositol and other minor lipids. Four so-called surfactant proteins that comprise up to 10% of the complex have unique features. Of the hydrophobic surfactant proteins, mature surfactant protein-B induces fast surface adsorption, spreading and surface stability of the phospholipids. Congenital absence of SP-B gene in man or SP-B gene deletion in mice results in fatal respiratory failure, characterized by abnormal structure of type II cells, abnormal composition and deficient surface activity of surfactant. SP-C is a small, type II cell-specific proteolipid that covalently binds two palmitate molecules, enhancing the surface adsorption of phospholipids. SP-C is expressed in the alveolar cells during early fetal life prior to the other surfactant components. The phenotype of absent SP-C gene expression has thus far not been described. SP-A is a C-type (i.e. collagenous) lectin. It binds to surfactant aggregates and together with SP-B, DPPC, phosphatidylglycerol and Ca^{++} form tubular myelin that is extremely surface active. However, mice lacking SP-A gene expression have no respiratory failure. Instead, they are prone to specific infections introduced to the respiratory tract (group B *Streptococcus* and respiratory syncytial virus). With the carbohydrate-binding domain, SP-A binds to specific microbes and increases their phagocytosis by alveolar macrophages *in vitro*. Hence SP-A is a component of the innate immunity. SP-D is another C-type lectin that binds to specific microbes and LPS. Thus far SP-D has not been shown to stimulate phagocytosis of pathogens. Although SP-D has apparently only small effects on surfactant metabolism and does not bind to surfactant complex (it binds phosphatidylinositol, however), deletion of SP-D gene expression resulted in an order of magnitude increase in the surfactant pool size, and to an emphysematous lung condition in adult mice. The roles of SP-D in homeostasis of the lung remain little understood.

Cytokines

Several cytokines are involved in alveolar growth, morphogenesis or differentiation of surfactant system. Cytokines are small proteins, produced by a variety of cells. They have biologic activity at a very low concentration (pikomolar – nanomolar) – apocrine, paracrine or endocrine activity being critically dependent on the concentration, on surface receptors, and on activities of other agonists and antagonists. Inflammatory cells particularly monocyte-macrophages produce very large quantities of proinflammatory cytokines as a result of contact with bacterial products or specific cytokines. Many cytokines have naturally occurring inhibitors (receptor antagonists, soluble receptors or decoy receptors) that moderate and suppress their activity.

In this brief review, several cytokines known to regulate production of surfactant components, are divided into two groups: those that are mainly expressed in the normal lung and those mainly associated with pathological conditions, i.e. during infection or inflammation (i.e. proinflammatory cytokines). The cytokines have a myriad of overlapping, often redundant functions that range from regulation of growth, differentiation, and defense against infection, regulation of immune cells, and many other roles. The effects of cytokines on the surfactant system range from promotion of alveolar cell growth, induction of surfactant synthesis to profound suppression of surfactant synthesis, metabolism and alveolar cell damage. Cytokines activate intracellular kinases and specific transcription factors and also induce secondary mediators including nitric oxide (NO), prostaglandins, leukotrienes and others. Nitric oxide and its metabolites have extensive interactions with the surfactant system, and PGE_2 influences the expression of a surfactant protein.

Cytokines having roles mainly in normal differentiation

Epidermal growth factor (EGF) and *transforming growth factor-α (TGF-α)* are related peptides that both bind to the EGF receptor with different affinities. EGF has been localized in respiratory epithelium [1], and increases also in lung effluent during prenatal development. TGF-α is a proinflammatory cytokine that is expressed in normal fetal airway epithelial cells at all levels. Administration of EGF to fetal rabbits and rhesus monkeys has been shown to increase surfactant phospholipids and SP-A in type II cells, in the amniotic fluid, and to increase the alveolarization and the stability of the premature lung [2-4]. As a result of the androgen-induced delay in the expression of EGF receptor level, female lung may respond more readily than the male lung [5]. Likewise antibody to EGF delays differentiation of surfactant. Mice lacking EGF receptor expression suffer from impaired epithelial development of several organs, including the lung. Some strains of EGF deficient mice die early due to respiratory failure associated with deficient airway branching and lack of alveolar epithelial differentiation [6]. After birth the bronchiolar epithelium in bronchopulmonary dysplasia (BPD; also called chronic lung disease, CLD) shows immunostaining suggesting a role of EGF abnormal regeneration of airways [1].

Transforming growth factor-β (TGF-β) belongs to the superfamily of more than 20 dimeric proteins of similar structure [7]. Three TGF-β isoforms and several other members of the superfamily are expressed in mammalian tissues. A major role of these highly conserved cytokines is to regulate the formation of extracellular matrix, increasing synthesis and secretion and decreasing the breakdown of a variety of extracellular matrix proteins. Thus an excess of TGF-β in tissues can lead to an unbalanced deposition of extracellular matrix and contribute to a variety of fibrotic lung disorders. TGF-β1, TGF-β2, and TGF-β3 are expressed in the lung during fetal and postnatal life. The *in situ* hybridization patterns of these three isoforms are distinct. High levels of TGF-β have been reported in epithelial lining fluid from normal humans. TGF-β inhibits the expression of SP-A in explants from human lung, and blocks the stimulatory effect of EGF on SP-A expression [3]. A TGF-β-like activity from lung fibroblasts inhibits surfactant phospholipid production by murine fetal type II cells in vitro. On the contrary, TGF-β1 null mice have a tendency to die *in utero*. Those developing to term have a multifocal fatal inflammatory disease affecting lung and heart [8].

Granulocyte-macrophage colony-stimulating factor (GM-CSF) is traditionally involved in regulation of hematopoiesis. GM-CSF that is expressed in alveolar and airway cells, increases in lung effluent more than 10-fold during the last trimester of fetal development [9]. GM-CSF tends to increase in lung effluent among infants developing BPD. Overexpression of GM-CSF by type II alveolar cells increases the alveolar cells (type II and PAM), but does not affect the pool size of surfactant [10]. On the other hand, administration of GM-CSF to the airways of the premature rabbits acutely increased the intracellular transport, exocytosis and extracellular pools of the surfactant phospholipids. In contrast at term, GM-CSF increased the turnover of surfactant phospholipids without affecting the pool size [11]. Mice lacking GM-CSF expression do not have deficiency in peripheral hematopoietic cells. Instead, adult animals develop pulmonary alveolar proteinosis that is characterized by accumulation of excessive quantities of surfactant components in alveolar spaces and in PAM [12], and abnormally slow turnover of surfactant components [13]. GM-CSF appears to have a role in proliferation and differentiation of the alveolar cells, although it does not influence the transcription of SPs.

Keratinocyte growth factor (KGF) is an epithelial cell-specific heparin-binding growth factor. KGF is necessary in embryonic differentiation of type II epithelial phenotype and in the induction SP-C expression [14]. In addition, KGF reduces bleomycin-induced [15] and acid instillation-induced [16] lung injury, increasing type II cell proliferation and SP mRNA expression.

Proinflammatory cytokines

Tumor necrosis factor-α (TNF-α) includes two structurally and functionally related proteins. TNF-α and TNF-β that bind to same receptors (types I and II), have similar activities. TNF-α is mainly produced in monocytes/macrophages and TNF-β in lymphoid cells. TNF-α is actively expressed in response to bacterial, viral, parasite, and endogenous (such as free oxygen radicals) toxins. Overproduction of TNF-α in infections, for instance during endotoxin shock, leads to severe toxicity. TNF-α enhances the production of many other cytokines and inflammatory mediators (NO, prostaglandins, acute phase proteins and others). Long term overproduction of TNF may lead to weight loss, anorexia, and excessive catabolism of proteins. TNF-α has also been implicated as a factor in pathogenesis of autoimmune disorders and of graft-versus-host disease. It serves as an immunostimulant and increases the host resistance.

Activated PAMs produce TNF-α and soluble TNF-α receptors [17]. TNF-α levels in lung effluent are elevated in newborn infants with nosocomial pneumonia, not in infants with respiratory distress syndrome in the newborne (RDS). During development of ARDS in trauma, shock or in sepsis the concentrations of TNF-α (but also soluble TNF receptors I and II serving as inhibitors) increase in BAL [18, 19]. Thus, because of increase in these inhibitors, little biologic

TNF activity was detected in BAL despite remarkable increase in TNF-α protein. Plasma concentrations of TNF-α are low in IRDS and in ARDS, except in septic shock.

TNF-α decreases the expression of human SP-A and SP-B mRNA and protein in adenocarcinoma cells [20]. TNF-α, administered intratracheally to adult mice reduces SP-C and SP-B mRNA and causes inflammatory lung disease [21]. Transgenic mice overexpressing TNF-α by type II alveolar cells under the control of human SP-C gene promoter develop leukocytotic alveolitis and progressive pulmonary fibrosis [22].

Interferon-γ (IFN-γ) is produced by activated macrophages or CD4 and CD8 T lymphocytes. It is a potent phagocytotic activator of macrophages, NK cells and neutrophils. IFN-γ also enhances lymphocyte functions. As shown in explants from human fetal lung, IFN-γ stimulates synthesis of SP-A mRNA and protein without affecting SP-B or SP-C mRNA [23].

Interleukin-1 (IL-1) family denotes three polypeptides that have rather little structural homology (30-50%), despite binding to the same cell surface receptors with similar affinity. Of the two IL-1 receptors, only the type I is involved in signaling, whereas type II receptor serves as a decoy receptor that either as a membrane bound or a soluble protein shunts the ligand away from type I receptor. IL-1α and IL-1β induce signal transduction, whereas IL-1ra serves as an inhibitor or moderator of IL-1 activity by binding to the receptor without causing signal transduction. In healthy organism the expression of IL-1α and IL-1β are generally low whereas the expression level of IL-1ra is more than one order of magnitude higher [24]. In PAM, IL-1α and IL-1β are induced, and IL-1ra expression increased in response to microbial products.

IL-1 activity and the individual peptides are increased in BAL from ARDS patients [25, 18] and in airway specimens of infants who develop BPD [26]. In intrauterine infection (IUI) the amniotic fluid contains increased concentrations of endotoxin (LPS) and proinflammatory cytokines [27]. At birth, very premature infants that are born due to IUI have increased IL-1 and several other proinflammatory cytokines in airway specimens. These infants have significantly decreased incidence of RDS, yet they have an increased risk to develop BPD [28]. Premature birth, the main cause of infant mortality and BPD, is the result of IUI in 30-60% of cases.

Recombinant human IL-1α given intra-amniotically (1500 or 150 ng per fetus) to immature rabbit fetuses caused a dose-dependent increase in the expression of SP-A and SP-B mRNA and protein, and an increase in the amount of DPPC in BAL, compared to vehicle treated animals in the opposite uterine horn. The rabbits delivered on d. 27.0 of pregnancy revealed strikingly increased dynamic compliance during a brief period of mechanical ventilation and homogenous aeration of the lung. In the controls, the low lung compliance and generalized atelectasis were consistent with severe RDS. IL-1ra (20 μg intra-amniotically) had no effect on expression of the SPs, suggesting no endogenous IL-1 activity [29]. Intra-amniotic IL-1α had no apparent toxicity, whereas intrafetal IL-1α (150 ng) caused fetal death [30]. Intra-amniotic IL-1α (125 µg) to immature ovine fetuses increased surfactant phospholipid in BAL, and increased lung compliance and gas exchange during brief period of mechanical ventilation. There was little evidence of lung inflammation [31].

The following findings indicate that IL-1 directly accelerates the differentiation of the surfactant system. Intra-amniotic IL-1α neither increased systemic levels of glucocorticoid nor caused a stress response [31]. IL-1 acutely increased the expression of SP-A and SP-B mRNA and protein as studied using explants from immature lung [32]. These effects on SPs are very similar to those observed after the intra-amniotic IL-1. Taken together, these findings suggest that in premature births due to IUI, IL-1 is responsible for the decreased incidence of RDS.

High activities of proinflammatory cytokines, including IL-1, are associated with ARDS and with the development of BPD in the premature. Consistent with the observed surfactant dysfunction in ARDS and in BPD, IL-1 suppressed rather than induced the expression of SP-C and SP-B in "mature" (i.e. term fetal and postnatal) lung explants. The suppression increased with the increase in IL-1α concentration [32]. The suppression of surfactant proteins by IL-1 is consistent with previous data indicating that intratracheal IL-1α given to adult rats results in high permeability lung edema and lung inflammation that was dependent on the dose of IL-1 [33]. These detrimental effects of IL-1 were expectedly reduced by administration of IL-1ra, and also by administration of N-acetylcysteine (an agent that increases cellular GSH levels) and dimethyl sulfoxide, a scavenger of hydroxyl radicals. Similar to TNF-α and LPC, administration of IL-1 protects against oxidant lung injury, when IL-1 is administered prior to the induction of oxidant injury [34].

Towards understanding the function of proinflammatory cytokines

The primary proinflammatory cytokines IL-1 and TNF have many additive or synergistic interactions. Other cytokines, such as IFN-γ and TGF-α may have a further additive effect. Likewise, cytokines with anti-inflammatory properties moderate the effects of proinflammatory cytokines specifically (IL-1ra antagonizing IL-1 or soluble TNF receptors antagonizing TNF-α) or by antagonizing the action of proinflammatory cytokines (TGF-β, IL-10, IL-6, IL-4, other cytokines). Other mediators, particularly glucocorticoid, also serve as anti-inflammatory agents.

The response elicited by the cytokines is strictly dependent on the host. In explants from near term fetal or postnatal lung, IL-1 and TNF-α additively inhibited the expression of SP-A, -B and -C. LPS that induces IL-1 and TNF-α in monocyte/macrophages, strongly inhibited the expression of SPs [35]. Dexamethasone (Dex 10^{-7}-10^{-9} M) acutely decreased the inhibitory effect of IL-1 and TNF-α [36]. These findings further imply the important role of proinflammatory cytokines in pathogenesis of surfactant defects in ARDS and in BPD.

In very immature lung *in vitro*, the effects of proinflammatory cytokines and anti-inflammatory agents on the expression of alveolar surfactant proteins are different. Neither TNF-α nor LPS had a detectable effect on SP-A, -B, or C, whereas IL-1 induced SP-A and -B, and moderately increased SP-C [35]. The switch from the IL-1-triggered induction of SP-A and SP-B to the IL-1-induced suppression of SP-B and SP-C took place at the same stage of fetal development than the onset of TNF-α- and LPS-induced suppression of SPs.

We propose that the alveolar epithelial cells of very immature lung respond to IL-1 from the amniotic fluid rather than to LPS. The inflammatory response of the immature alveolar structure is paradoxical: by accelerating surfactant maturity, IL-1 prevents RDS and prepares the fetus for postnatal survival [36, 28]. In contrast, exposure of the immature lung directly to microbial products neither induces lung maturity not elicits a proper inflammatory response. The fetuses either die *in utero* or develop fulminant hyperacute pneumonia if delivered prematurely. Lack of IL-1β and SP-A in airway specimens, very low inducible NO synthase and of nitrotyrosine immunoreactivities in PAM are characteristics of these premature infants that present with symptoms of severe RDS and persistence of fetal circulation shortly after birth. The appearance of IL-1β, SP-A, inducible NO synthase and nitrotyrosine in PAM during the recovery from hyperacute sepsis further suggests that IL-1 is a critical factor in the host defense of immature lung [37].

The proinflammatory cytokines induce free radicals, proteolytic enzymes, inhibit growth and induce lung fibrosis. They are likely to be involved in progression of respiratory disease to ARDS and in generation of clinical and pathologic characteristics of BPD. The decrease in formation of surfactant, induced by the proinflammatory cytokines (IL-1 and TNF-α in particular) is an ancient host defense mechanism. Surfactant defect causes an atelectatic sequestration of the infectious focus (i.e. localized pneumonia) as part of the alveolar host defense against generalized infection.

New therapies that limit the generalized proinflammatory cytokine response during invasive pulmonary treatment (without causing a generalized suppression of the cytokine response) remain to be discovered. New treatment that turns on the expression of surfactant components may prove to be important in prevention of progressive alveolar disease.

References

1. Stahlman MT, Orth DN, Gray ME (1989) Immunocytochemical localization of epidermal growth factor in the developing human respiratory system and in acute and chronic lung disease in the neonate. Lab Invest 60:539-547
2. Sundell HW, Gray ME, Serenius FS et al (1980) Effects of epidermal growth factor on lung maturation in fetal lambs. Am J Pathol 100:707-726
3. Whitsett JA, Weaver TE, Lieberman MA et al (1987) Differential effects of epidermal growth factor and transforming growth factor-β on synthesis of Mr = 35,000 surfactant-associated protein in fetal lung. J Biol Chem 262:7908-7913
4. Goetzman BW, Read LC, Plopper CG et al (1994) Prenatal exposure to epidermal growth factor attenuates respiratory distress syndrome in rhesus infants. Pediatr Res 35:30-36
5. Klein JM, Nielsen HC (1995) Androgen regulation of epidermal growth factor receptor binding activity during fetal rabbit lung development. J Clin Invest 91:425-431
6. Sibilia M, Wagner EF (1995) Strain-dependent epithelial defects in mice lacking the EGF receptor. Science 269:234-238
7. Roberts AB, Sporn MB (1992) Differential expression of the TGF-β isoforms in embryogenesis suggests specific roles in developing and adult tissues. Molec Reprod Devel 32:91-98
8. Kulkarni AB, Ward JM, Yaswen L et al (1995) Transforming growth factor-β 1 null mice. An animal model for inflammatory disorders. Am J Pathol 146:264-275
9. Bry K, Hallman M, Teramo K et al (1997) Granulocyte-macrophage colony-stimulating factor in amniotic fluid and in airway specimens of newborn infants. Pediatr Res 41:105-109
10. Huffman Reed JA, Rice WR, Zsengeller ZK et al (1997) GM-CSF enhances lung growth and causes alveolar type II epithelial cell hyperplasia in transgenic mice. Am J Physiol 273: L715-L725
11. Uy CC, Bry K, Lappalainen U, Hallman M (1999) Granulocyte-macrophage colony-stimulating factor increases surfactant phospholipid in premature rabbits (in press)
12. Dranoff G, Crawford AD, Sadelain M et al (1994) Involvement of granulocyte-macrophage colony-stimulating factor in pulmonary homeostasis. Science 264:713-716
13. Ikegami M, Ueda T, Hull W et al (1996) Surfactant metabolism in transgenic mice after granulocyte-macrophage colony-stimulating factor ablation. Am J Physiol 270:L650-L658
14. Shannon JM, Gebb SA, Nielsen LD (1999) Induction of alveolar type II cell differentiation in embryonic tracheal epithelium in mesenchyme-free culture. Development 126:1675-1688
15. Deterding RR, Havill AM, Yano T et al (1997) Prevention of bleomycin-induced lung injury in rats by keratinocyte growth factor. Proc Ass Amer Physicians 109:254-268
16. Yano T, Deterding RR, Simonet WS et al (1996) Keratinocyte growth factor reduces lung damage due to acid instillation in rats. Am J Respir Cell Mol Biol 15:433-442
17. Buch C, Gallati H, Pohlandt F, Bartmann P (1994) Increased levels of tumor necrosis factor alpha (TNF-alpha) and interleukin-1 β in tracheal aspirates of newborns with pneumonia. Infection 22:238-241
18. Suter PM, Suter S, Girardin E et al (1992) High bronchoalveolar levels of tumor necrosis factor and its inhibitors, interleukin-1, interferon, and elastase, in patients with adult respiratory distress syndrome after trauma, shock, or sepsis. Am Rev Respir Disease 145:1016-1022
19. Parsons PE, Moore FA, Moore EE et al (1992) Studies on the role of tumor necrosis factor in adult respiratory distress syndrome. Am Rev Respir Dis 146:694-700
20. Wispe JR, Clark JC, Warner BB et al (1990) Tumor necrosis factor-alpha inhibits expression of pulmonary surfactant protein. J Clin Invest 86:1954-1960
21. Bachurski CJ, Pryhuber GS, Glasser SW et al (1995) Tumor necrosis factor-alpha inhibits surfactant protein C gene transcription. J Biol Chem 270:19402-19407
22. Miyazaki Y, Araki K, Vesin C et al (1995) Expression of a tumor necrosis factor-α transgene in murine lung causes lymphocytic and fibrosing alveolitis. A mouse model of progressive pulmonary fibrosis. J Clin Invest 96:250-259
23. Ballard PL, Liley HG, Gonzales LW et al (1990) Interferon-γ and synthesis of surfactant components by cultured human lung. Am J Respir Cell Mol Biol 2:137-143

24. Dinarello CA (1991) Interleukin-1 and interleukin-1 antagonism. Blood 77:1627-52
25. Siler TM, Swierkosz JE, Hyers TM et al (1989) Immunoreactive IL-1 in bronchoalveolar lavage fluid of high-risk patients and patients with the adult respiratory distress syndrome. Exp Lung Res 15:881-894
26. Kotecha S, Wilson L, Wangoo A et al (1996) Increase in interleukin (IL)-1a and IL-6 in bronchoalveolar lavage fluid obtained from infants with chronic lung disease of prematurity. Pediatr Res 40:250-256
27. Gomez R, Ghezzi F, Romero R et al (1995) Premature labor and intra-amniotic infection: Clinical aspects and role of the cytokines in diagnosis and pathophysiology. Clin Perinatol 22:281-342
28. Watterberg KL, Demers LM, Scott SM, Murphy S (1996) Chorioamnionitis and early lung inflammation in infants in whom bronchopulmonary dysplasia developes. Pediatrics 97:210-215
29. Bry K, Lappalainen U, Hallman M (1997) Intra-amniotic interleukin-1 accelerates surfactant protein synthesis in fetal rabbits and improves lung stability after premature birth. J Clin Invest 99:2992-2999
30. Bry K, Lappalainen U, Hallman M (1997) Maturational effects of IL-1 on fetal lungs are dependent on route of cytokine administration. Pediatr Res 41:42
31. Emerson GA, Bry K, Hallman M et al (1997) Intra-amniotic interleukin-1 alpha treatment alters postnatal adaptation in premature lambs. Biol Neonate 72:370-379
32. Glumoff V, Väyrynen O, Kangas T, Hallman M (1999) Degree of lung maturity determines the direction of interleukin-1 induced effect on the expression of surfactant proteins. Am J Respir Cell Mol Biol (in press)
33. Leff JA, Baer JW, Bodman ME et al (1993) Interleukin-1-induced lung neutrophil accumulation and oxygen metabolite mediated lung leak in rats. J Appl Physiol 266:2-8
34. Repine JE (1994) Interleukin-1-mediated acute lung injury and tolerance to oxidative injury. Environ Health Prospect 102[Suppl 10]:75-78
35. Väyrynen O, Glumoff V, Kangas T, Hallman M (1999) Endotoxin-induced changes in expression of surfactant proteins are dependent on the degree of lung maturity. Pediatr Res 45:896
36. Glumoff V, Väyrynen O, Kangas T, Hallman M (1999) Expression of surfactant proteins. Interaction between interleukin-1 (IL-1) and dexamethasone (Dx). Pediatr Res 45:892
37. Aikio O, Vuopala K, Pokela M-L, Hallman M (1999) Diminished inducible nitric oxide synthase expression in fulminant early-onset neonatal pneumonia. Pediatrics (in press)

Role of Surfactant in Ventilation-Induced Lung Injury

S.J.C. Verbrugge, J.J. Haitsma, B. Lachmann

Physiology at the alveolo-capillary barrier

The alveolo-capillary barrier compromises three extracellular liquid compartments: 1) the vascular space, 2) the interstitial space and 3) the liquid in the lumen of the alveoli, which are separated by the capillary endothelium and the alveolar epithelium, respectively.

The exchange of hydrophillic solutions over the pulmonary capillary is determined by several factors: 1) the outward directing capillary hydrostatic pressure, 2) the inward directing oncotic pressure, 3) lymphatic drainage of the interstitium and 4) the alveolar surface tension [1, 2]. This last factor is determined by the attractive forces of the molecules at the air-liquid interface of the alveolus. These forces result in suctioning where the curvature of the alveolar wall at the border of a capillary is sharp; they decrease filtration where the pulmonary capillary bulges into the alveolus, supporting the capillaries like the hoops of a barrel [3]. The presence of surface tension at the air-liquid interface of the lung is believed to generate most of the observed negative pressure in the interstitial space in places where the capillary does not protrude into the alveolus.

Exchange of fluid also takes place over the alveolar epithelium between the interstitial and alveolar fluid compartment [2]. It compromises a balance between: 1) the interstitial pressure which is negative and favors fluid absorption from the alveolus, 2) a large oncotic pressure gradient generated by impermeability of the alveolar epithelium, 3) an active transport of sodium by the epithelium out of the lung lumen, and 4) the hydrostatic pressure of the fluid compartment in the alveolus lining the epithelial layer. This hydrostatic pressure is equal to the pressure of gas in the airspace, minus the amount of pressure which compensates for the collapse tendency of the alveolus ($p_{Collapse}$) caused by the retractive forces at the air-liquid interface of the alveolus. This collapse pressure is given by the law of LaPlace, $p_{Collapse} = 2\,\gamma/r$ (γ = surface tension at the air-liquid interface; r = radius of the alveolus) and is very low in the normal alveolus due to the low surface tension.

Disturbance of the fluid balance due to mechanical ventilation

Despite initial controversy about the role of mechanical ventilation in inducing lung injury [4]. It has now been clearly demonstrated in different animal models that mechanical ventilation at high peak inspiratory lung volumes can cause lung injury and edema, which does not fundamentally differ from that seen in human acute respiratory distress syndrome (ARDS) [5]. Pulmonary oedema is considered hydrostatic when there is an increased hydrostatic pressures and/or filtration and when the permeability of the endothelial barrier to protein is intact. It is considered high permeability oedema when it is caused by permeability of the endothelial barrier to protein. The distinction between the two is a grey area because increased permeability makes the lung more susceptible to increased hydrostatic pressures/filtration and, on the other hand, high capillary circumferential tensions eventually lead to permeability changes.

The changes to the epithelial and endothelial barrier due to mechanical ventilation have been extensively described [6]. Due to damage of both the epithelial and endothelial barrier, surfactant components may be lost into the bloodstream [7, 8]. More importantly, intra-alveolar protein will accumulate which results in dose-dependent inhibition of surfactant [9]. As surfactant is the rate-limiting factor in the transfer of proteins over the alveolo-capillary barrier, loss of surfactant function will lead to further protein infiltration. This may result in a self-triggering mechanism of surfactant inactivation. However, surfactant may also be primarily affected by mechanical ventilation.

Surfactant changes due to mechanical ventilation

In 1959 Mead demonstrated that mechanically ventilated dogs showed a progressive fall in pulmonary compliance [10]; such mechanical changes were related to the pulmonary surfactant system as shown by Greenfield and coworkers who demonstrated increased surface tensions of lung extracts in dogs ventilated at peak inspiratory pressures of 28-32 cm H_2O for 1 to 2 hours [11].

Two primary mechanisms of surfactant inactivation by mechanical ventilation have been described. First, mechanical ventilation was shown to enhance surfactant release from the pneumocyte type II into the alveolus [12]. Subsequently this material is lost into the small airways as a result of compression of the surfactant film when the surface of the alveolus becomes smaller than the surface occupied by the surfactant molecules [13, 14].

A second mechanism to describe surfactant changes associated with mechanical ventilation is based on the observation that changes associated with mechanical ventilation of the alveolar surface area result in the conversion of large surface active surfactant aggregates into small non-surface active surfactant aggregates [15, 16].

Surfactant changes due to mechanical ventilation are reversible as a result of a metabolically active process involving de novo production of surfactant. It probably involves a balance between secretion and production of large aggregates, and uptake clearance and reconversion of small aggregates in the pneumocyte type II [17].

Consequences of surfactant changes

Surfactant inactivation with an increase in alveolar surface tension results in a decrease in pericapillary pressure [18] and results in loss of supportive "hoop" function by surfactant on the capillary wall [3].

Surfactant dysfunction has also been shown to increase the permeability of the alveolo-capillary barrier to both small solutes (without other substantial changes to the alveolo-capillary barrier) and large solutes; in addition, increased surfactant content was shown to reduce permeability [19, 20]. These studies have indicated that surfactant has a primary role in the regulation of the permeability of the alveolo-capillary barrier to small solutes and protein.

It has become clear that microvascular injury secondary to ventilation occurs at much lower airway pressures and volumes in isolated perfused lungs with inactivated surfactant due to dioctyl succinate, as compared to ventilation of healthy lungs [21]. These studies suggest that lungs with an impaired surfactant system are more susceptible to overinflation than healthy lungs and that minor surfactant alterations, such as those produced by spontaneous ventilation during prolonged anesthesia are sufficient to synergistically increase the harmful effects of overinflation on permeability of the endothelial barrier.

Repeated collapse and reexpansion of alveoli due to surfactant changes

One idea of ventilation-induced lung injury and epithelial stretching goes back to the pioneering work of Mead who demonstrated that, due to pulmonary interdependence of the alveoli, the forces acting on the fragile lung tissue in non-uniformly expanded lungs are not only the applied transpulmonary pressures, but rather the shear forces that are present in the interstitium between open and closed alveoli [22]. An alveolus with surfactant impairment, which may be primarily caused by mechanical ventilation as described above, would be predisposed to end-expiratory alveolar collapse and would be prone to be affected by such 'shear forces'. Shear forces, rather than end-inspiratory overstretching, may well be the major reason for epithelial disrupture, loss of barrier function of the alveolar epithelium, and considerable increases in regional microvascular transmural pressure. Important evidence for these mechanisms comes from the findings that ventilation at low lung volumes can also augment lung injury in lungs with an impaired surfactant system [23] and the fact that surfactant changes make the lung vulnerable to lung parenchymal injury by mechanical ventilation [24].

Effects of positive end-expiratory pressure (PEEP)

It has now been unequivocally demonstrated in different animal models that ventilation with PEEP at lower tidal volumes results in less oedema than ventilation without PEEP and a higher tidal volume for the same peak or mean airway pressure [6]. PEEP has also been shown to prevent alveolar flooding and reduce endothelial and epithelial injury [6].

How to explain the beneficial effects of PEEP?

Several experiments in closed-chest animals have suggested that PEEP reduces microvascular filtration pressure due to a decrease in cardiac output. The effect of PEEP in reducing protein infiltration and permeability of the alveolo-capillary barrier has therefore been attributed to a decrease in lung capillary hydrostatic pressure with a reduction in filtration pressure [25].

Other experiments have shown a reduction in conversion rate of active into non-active surfactant aggregates due to PEEP suggesting that the beneficial effect of PEEP in reducing protein infiltration after overinflation is partially attributable to a reduced filtration by surfactant preservation [16].

Two basic mechanisms have been described in literature which explain the surfactant preserving effect of PEEP during mechanical ventilation. Studies by Wyszogrodski et al. have shown that PEEP prevents a decrease in lung compliance and surface activity of lung extracts, indicating a preventive of loss of alveolar surfactant function during lung overinflation [13]. It has been suggested that PEEP prevents alveolar collapse thus keeping the end-expiratory volume of alveoli at a higher level, and preventing excessive loss of surfactant in the small airways by a squeeze-out mechanism during expiration [26]. Successive studies by Veldhuizen and colleagues have shown that the rate of conversion of large surfactant into small aggregates is dependent on tidal volume and time [15]; changing the respiratory rate [15] or the level of PEEP [27] did not affect surfactant conversion. These studies suggest that the preservation of the surfactant system by PEEP comes from the reduction in cyclic changes in surface area by PEEP.

To further test the hypothesis that reduced filtration due to surfactant preservation is responsible for the reduction of edema by PEEP, we conducted a study in which high peak inspiratory pressure ventilation without PEEP was preceded by administration of high amounts of exogenous surfactant [28]. It was shown that an amount of 200 mg/kg bodyweight surfactant preserved oxygenation and lung mechanics after 20 minutes of overinflation at high peak inspiratory pressures without PEEP. Although 400 mg/kg bodyweight surfactant did not reduce the lung tissue content of Evans blue dye, it was shown to reduce its intra-alveolar accumulation [28]. These data provide strong evidence that, besides peak inspiratory overstretching after lung overinflation, surfactant inactivation plays a key role in ventilation-induced intra-alveolar edema formation and that the effect of PEEP in reducing lung permeability to protein is at least partially attributable to its effect on preservation of the surfactant system.

The utilization of PEEP to splint open the airways and alveoli at end-expiration in surfactant- deficient lungs may markedly reduce lung injury. It has been demonstrated that surfactant impairment ventilation strategies keep the alveoli open throughout the respiratory cycle with high levels of PEEP, induces significantly less morphological injury with better preservation of pulmonary compliance than strategies in which alveolar collapse is allowed at end-expiration [29].

Conclusion

Surfactant changes play a key role in maintaining the normal fluid balance of the alveolo-capillary barrier and may play an important role in the mechanism of ventilation-induced lung injury. It has become clear that early surfactant changes, which may be induced by mechanical ventilation itself, predispose lungs to ventilation-induced lung injury due to repeated opening and closure of alveolar units. The studies reviewed in this article support the use of mechanical ventilation strategies which avoid both continuous alveolar overdistension, repeated collapse, and reexpansion of alveoli. Keeping all alveoli open at end-expiration should cause the smallest possible pressure amplitudes. Such ventilation strategies will prevent ventilation-induced surfactant changes and may (partially) prevent the pathophysiological changes, morbidity and mortality associated with mechanical ventilation.

References

1. Gommers D, Lachmann B (1993) Surfactant therapy: does it have a role in adults? Clinical Intensive Care 4:284-295
2. Walters DV (1992) The role of pulmonary surfactant in transepithelial movement of fluid. In: Robertson B, van Golde LMG, Batenburg JJ (eds) Pulmonary surfactant: from molecular biology to clinical practice. Elsevier, Amsterdam, 193-213
3. West JB, Mathieu-Costello O (1992) Stress failure of pulmonary capillaries: role in lung and heart disease. Lancet 340:762-767
4. Nash G, Bowen JA, Langlinais PC (1971) "Respirator lung": a misnomer. Arch Pathol 21:234-240
5. Bachofen M, Weibel ER (1982) Structural alternations of lung parenchyma in the adult respiratory distress syndrome. In: RC Bone (ed) Clinics in chest medicine. Saunders WB, Philadelphia, 35-56

6. Dreyfuss D, Saumon G (1998) Ventilator-induced lung injury. Lessons from experimental studies. Am J Resp Crit Care Med 157:294-323

7. Doyle IR, Nicholas TE, Bersten AD (1995) Serum surfactant protein-A levels in patients with acute cardiogenic pulmonary edema and adult respiratory distress syndrome. Am J Resp Crit Care Med 152:307-317

8. Robertson B, Curstedt T, Herting E et al (1995) Alveolo-to-vascular leakage of surfactant protein A in ventilated immature newborn rabbits. Biol Neonate 68:185-190

9. Lachmann B, Eijking EP, So KL, Gommers D (1994) In vivo evaluation of the inhibitory capacity of human plasma on exogenous surfactant function. Intens Care Med 20:6-11

10. Mead J, Collier C (1959) Relationship of volume history of lungs to respiratory mechanics in anesthetised dogs. J Appl Physiol 14:669-678

11. Greenfield LJ, Ebert PA, Benson DW (1964) Effect of positive pressure ventilation on surface tension properties of lung extracts. Anesthesiology 25:312-316

12. Faridy EE, Permutt S, Riley RL (1966) Effect of ventilation on surface forces in excised dogs' lungs. J Appl Physiol 21:1453-1462

13. Wyszogrodski I, Kyei-Aboagye K, Taeusch Jr W, Avery ME (1975) Surfactant inactivation by hyperinflation: conservation by end-expiratory pressure. J Appl Physiol 38:461-466

14. Faridy EE (1976). Effect of ventilation on movement of surfactant in airways. Resp Physiol 27:323-334

15. Veldhuizen RAW, Marcou J, Yao LJ et al (1996) Alveolar surfactant aggregate conversion in ventilated normal and injured rabbits. Am J Physiol 270:152-158

16. Verbrugge SJC, Böhm SH, Gommers D et al (1998) Surfactant impairment after mechanical ventilation with large alveolar surface area changes and effects of positive end-expiratory pressure. Br J Anaesth 80:1-5

17. Magoon MW, Wright JR, Baritussio A et al (1983) Subfractions of lung surfactant. Implications for metabolism and surface activity. Biochim Biophys Acta 750:18-31

18. Albert RK, Lakshminarayan S, Hildebrandt J et al (1979) Increased surface tension favors pulmonary edema formation in anaesthetized dogs' lungs. J Clin Invest 63:1015-1018

19. Bos JAH, Wollmer P, Bakker W et al (1992) Clearance of ^{99m}Tc-DTPA and experimentally increased alveolar surfactant content. J Appl Physiol 72:1413-1417

20. Verbrugge SJC, Gommers D, Bos JAH et al (1996) Pulmonary ^{99m}Tc-human serum albumin clearance and effects of surfactant replacement after lung lavage in rabbits. Crit Care Med 24:1518-1523

21. Coker PJ, Hernandez LA, Peevy KJ et al (1992) Increased sensitivity to mechanical ventilation after surfactant inactivation in young rabbit lungs. Crit Care Med 20:635-640

22. Mead J, Takishima T, Leith D (1970) Stress distribution in lungs: a model of pulmonary elasticity. J Appl Physiol 28:596-608

23. Muscerede JG, Mullen JBM, Gan K, Slutsky AS (1994) Tidal ventilation at low airway pressures can augment lung injury. Am J Resp Crit Care Med 149:1327-1334

24. Taskar V, John E, Evander P et al (1997) Surfactant dysfunction makes lungs vulnerable to repetitive collapse and reexpansion. Am J Resp Crit Care Med 155:313-320

25. Dreyfuss D, Saumon G (1993) Role of tidal volume, FRC and end-inspiratory volume in the development of pulmonary edema following mechanical ventilation. Am Rev Resp Dis 148: 1194-1203

26. Tyler DC (1983) Positive end-expiratory pressure: a review. Crit Care Med 11:300-308

27. Ito Y, Veldhuizen RAW, Yao LJ et al (1997) Ventilation strategies affect surfactant aggregate conversion in acute lung injury. Am J Resp Crit Care Med 155:493-499

28 Verbrugge SJC, Šorm V, Gommers D, Lachmann B (1998) Exogenous surfactant preserves lung function and reduces alveolar Evans Blue dye influx in a rat model of ventilation-induced lung injury. Anesthesiology 89:467-474

29. Lachmann B, Danzmann E, Haendly B, Jonson B (1982) Ventilator settings and gas exchange in respiratory distress syndrome. In: Prakash O (ed) Applied physiology in clinical respiratory care. Martinus Nijhoff publishers, The Hague, 141-176

UPDATE ON ARDS

Has ARDS Epidemiology Changed in the Last 30 Years?

A. Artigas

Acute lung injury (ALI) and acute respiratory distress syndrome (ARDS) are a major cause of morbidity and mortality in critically ill patients. Despite recent advances, major questions remain about ways to identify patients at high risk for ALI/ARDS, the true incidence and prevalence of ALI/ARDS, the critical factors involved in the pathogenesis of ALI/ARDS, and individual host factors that influence whether a patient develops ALI/ARDS.

In spite of the advances in understanding, ARDS remains a syndrome with signs and symptoms that are periodically reviewed and rearranged. However, without any real insight regarding aetiology and with no reliable biologic markers to serve as the gold standard, it is impossible to do consistent epidemiologic studies. We believe that much of the controversy concerning ARDS is explained by the lack of a satisfactory definition of this elusive syndrome. How can we collect, much less compare epidemiologic data and mortality figures when there is no uniformly accepted (and used) definition? How can we study basic pathophysiologic mechanisms, understand its course and above all, evaluate new therapeutic approaches in what appeared now to be an amalgam of many different disorders?

Definition

The American-European Consensus Conference [1] recommended that ALI be defined as a syndrome of inflammation and increasing permeability that is associated with clinical, radiologic and physiologic abnormalities that cannot be explained by, but may coexist with left atrial or pulmonary capillary hypertension and that ARDS be defined as a more severe form of ALI. It was also recommended that the distinction in severity should be based solely on differences in oxygenation. Disturbances in gas exchange usually represent sum total effect of numerous processes and they are not just the manifestation of alveolar damage. Although such an operational definition may be useful in designing clinical studies, some authors believed that it is important to recall the functional and pathologic derangement that results in ARDS [2]. The chest radiograph and the use of pulmonary artery catheters to define the extent (bilateral) and characteristics of pulmonary oedema from increased-permeability pulmonary oedema are also controversial and need to be standardized [3].

Importance of ALI and ARDS as clinical problems

ALI and ARDS affect many patients each year but the exact incidence remains uncertain. The National Institute of Health estimated in 1972 the incidence of ARDS in the USA at 150,000 new cases per year (64 cases/10^5 population) [4]. Recent studies suggest a much lower incidence from 1.5 to 14 cases/10^5 population or 4,800 to 36,920 new cases per year in the US [5-10]. However, critical review of these studies raises methodologic concerns regarding patient identification, definitions, and on the population studied. More recently using prospectively the ALI/ARDS Consensus Conference definition, an incidence of 77.6/10^5 population/year of intubated patients with mechanical ventilation longer than 24 hours and 13.5/10^5 population/year for ARDS patients has been reported [11].

A wide variety of conditions have been reported associated with ARDS. Two relatively large single center studies have prospectively examined carefully risk conditions for ARDS and identified the incidence of the syndrome for each of these conditions [12, 13]. These studies suggest that the conditions with the highest incidence of ARDS include severe sepsis or sepsis syndrome (43%), severe trauma (25%) and aspiration of gastric contents (22%) with a global incidence of 26% among at risk patients. Although these prospective investigations provide an incidence of ARDS occurring with specific risk factors found at the two institutions involved in the studies, others may differ considerably in their patient population and risk conditions for ARDS.

The onset of ARDS substantially increases overall mortality (3-fold higher) for critically ill patients [13]. The mortality associated with ARDS ranges from about 30% to more than 60% among the different centers. Recently, an analysis of temporal trends in ARDS fatality at one institution indicated a decline from 1989 to a low of 30% in 1996 [14]. Nevertheless the mortality rate reported in recent large multi-trial study remains between 40-50%. The early mortality (within the first 3 days) has not changed, but there has been a major decline in late mortality suggesting a decrease in deaths due to complications following ARDS onset [15].

The European ARDS study demonstrated that the most important prognostic factors were age, cause of ARDS, pre-existing disease, the early time-course of lung function, a high systolic PAP and a low diastolic SAP. Trauma and younger patients were associated with a lower mortality rate. The initial response to mechanical ventilation identified the capability of ALI patients to improves gas exchange associated with a better outcome [16-18]. The introduction of standard and accurate methods of scoring the severity of respiratory failure and the disturbances of overall physiology with or without specific biological markers of lung injury may help to predict mortality, to stratify patients with ALI for comparison of patient population and to examine the efficiency of therapeutic interventions. Recently different authors demonstrated that successful estimation of risk of hospital mortality in patients with ALI can be obtained using a general severity score (SAPS II, MPM II or APACHE III) that accounts for both important pulmonary and extrapulmonary organ system dysfunction [19, 20]. Recently the American-European Consensus Conference on ARDS proposed the GOGA stratification system, which deals with all the aspects of ALI, and incorporates additional important prognostic factors [17].

Sequelae

An early impression held by many investigators and clinicians was that the sequelae after an ARDS are minimal and pulmonary function in most survivors returned to normal or near normal levels by 6 months following endotracheal extubation [22, 23]. Although most patients markedly improved their pulmonary function during recovery, approximately half continued to have abnormal pulmonary function. This is either a mild restrictive impairment, a bronchial hyperreactivity and sometimes a mild impairment in lung diffusing capacity. It is not clear which factors during the acute disease can be related with the long-term functional sequelae. Finally, survivors of ARDS continue to have impairments in overall physical and psychosocial function but these are mild, and are not related to their pulmonary condition, but are often related to other aspects of their acute injury or illness.

In conclusion ALI/ARDS is a relevant national health problem associated to a high number of death per year similar to breast cancer and AIDS. The magnitude of this public health problem posed by ALI/ARDS needs to increase our efforts and the support from national governments to improve outcome in patients who will have a chance to return to work and lead a normal life.

References

1. Bernard GR, Artigas A, Brigham K et al (1994). The American-European consensus conference on ARDS. Am J Respir Crit Care Med 149:818-824
2. Kollef MH, Schuster DP (1995) The acute respiratory distress syndrome. N Engl J Med 332:27-37
3. Artigas A (1999) Definition and diagnosis of acute respiratory distress syndrome. In: Mancebo J, Blanch L (eds) Syndrome de détresse respiratoire aigüe en réanimation. Elsevier, Paris, pp 15-29
4. National Health Institute (1972) Task force report on problems, research, approaches, needs. The Lung Program. Washington DC. US Government Printing Office, DHEW Publication No (NIH) 73-432:165-180

5. Webster NR, Cohen AT, Nunn JF (1988) Adult respiratory distress syndrome - How many cases in the UK? Anaesthesia 43:923-926
6. Villar J, Slutsky AS (1989) The incidence of the adult respiratory distress syndrome. Am Rev Respir Dis 140:814-816
7. Thomsen GE, Morris AH (1995) Incidence of the adult respiratory distress syndrome in the state of Utah. Am J Respir Crit Care Med 152:965-971
8. Evans BH, Wachter JP, Wiener-Kronish, Luce JM (1988) Incidence of the adult respiratory distress syndrome in an urban population. Am Rev Respir Dis 137:A469
9. Lewandowski K, Metz J, Deutschmann C et al (1995) Incidence, severity and mortality of acute respiratory failure in Berlin, Germany. Am J Respir Crit Care Med 151:1121-1125
10. Reynolds HN, McCunn M, Borg U et al (1998) Acute respiratory distress syndrome: estimated incidence and mortality rate in a 5 million-person population base. Crit Care 2:29-34
11. Luhr OR, Antonsen K, Karlsson M et al (1999) Incidence and mortality after acute respiratory failure and acute respiratory distress syndrome in Sweden, Denmark, and Iceland. Am J Respir Crit Care Med 159:1849-1861
12. Fowler AA, Hamman RF, Good JT et al (1983) Adult respiratory distress syndrome: Risk with common predispositions. Ann Inter Med 98:593-597
13. Hudson LD, Milberg JA, Anardi D, Maunder RJ (1995) Clinical risks for development of acute respiratory distress syndrome. Am J Respir Crit Care Med 151:293-301
14. Milberg JA, Davis DR, Steinberg KD, Hudson LD (1995) Improved survival of patients with acute respiratory distress syndrome (ARDS). JAMA 273:306-309
15. Hudson LD, Steinberg KP (1998) Epidemiology of ARDS. Incidence and outcome: a changing picture. In: Marini JJ, Evans TW (eds) Acute lung injury. Springer, Berlin, pp 3-15
16. Artigas A, Carlet J, Le Gall JR et al (1991) Clinical presentation, prognostic factors and outcome of ARDS in the European Collaborative Study (1985-1987). In: Zapol W, Lemaire F (eds) Adult respiratory distress syndrome. Marcel Dekker, New York, pp 37-63
17. Artigas A (1998) Prognostic factors and outcome of acute lung injury. In: Marini JJ, Evans TW (eds) Acute lung injury. Springer, Berlin, pp 16-38
18. Squara P, Dhainaut JF, Artigas A et al (1998) Haemodynamic profile in severe ARDS: results of the European Collaborative ARDS Study. Intensive Care Med 24:1018-1028
19. Knaus WA, Sun X, Hakim RB, Wagner DP (1994) Evaluation of definitions for adult respiratory distress syndrome. Am J Respir Crit Care Med 150:311-317
20. Mancebo J, Artigas A (1987) A clinical study of the adult respiratory distress syndrome. Crit Care Med 15:243-246
21. Artigas A, Lemeshow S, Rue M et al (1994) Risk stratification and outcome assessment of patients with acute lung injury. Am J Respir Crit Care Med 149:A1029
22. McHugh LG, Milberg JA, Whitcomb ME et al (1994) Recovery of function in survivors of the acute respiratory distress syndrome. Am J Respir Crit Care Med 150:90-94
23. Artigas A (1984) Evaluation de la fonction pulmonaire des malades survivant à un syndrome de détresse respiratoire aigüe de l'adulte. In: Lemaire F (ed) Le syndrome de détresse respiratoire aigüe de l'adulte. Masson, Paris, pp 125-136
24. Schelling G, Stoll C, Haller M et al (1998) Health-related quality of life and posttraumatic stress disorder in survivors of the acute respiratory distress syndrome. Crit Care Med 651-659
25. Weinert CR, Gross CR, Kangas JR et al (1997) Health-related quality of life after acute lung injury. Am J Respir Crit Care 156:1120-1128

Mechanism of ARDS

L. Brazzi, P. Pelosi, L. Gattinoni

Initially described more than 25 years ago [1] in 12 patients, adult respiratory distress syndrome (ARDS) is classically defined as an acute, severe alteration in lung structure and function characterized by hypoxemia, low-compliance lungs with low functional residual capacity, and diffuse radiographic infiltrates due to increased lung microvascular permeability.

It is now clear that within ARDS, different clinical entities characterized by different underlying pathologies and responses to treatment exist. We will focus not only on the more recent discoveries regarding the pathophysiology of the syndrome, but also on the methods available to maximize the efficacy of the commonly used therapeutical maneuvres.

Pathogenesis

It is well known that whenever an insult is applied to the lung, a host response is triggered resulting in lung inflammation. It is useful to consider this kind of pathogenesis as consisting of two pathways: the first due to the effect of an insult directly applied to lung cells (direct insult); the second occurring when pulmonary lesions result from an acute systemic inflammatory response (indirect insult). It is important to emphasize that the prevalent damage following the direct insult is intra-alveolar, with "occupation" of pulmonary units by biological material as intra-alveolar edema, fibrin, collagen, neutrophils, aggregates and hemorrhage. The clinical term often used to define this pattern is "pulmonary consolidation". Alternatively, pulmonary lesions may indirectly originate, via blood stream, by mediators released from extrapulmonary foci, as during peritonitis, pancreatitis and various abdominal diseases. The primary target, in this case, is pulmonary endothelial cells. The activation of the inflammatory network results in increased permeability of the endothelial barrier and cell recruitment (monocytes, PMN, platelets and others); consequently, the prevalent damage is represented by microvessel congestion and interstitial edema while intra-alveolar spaces are relatively spared.

It is likely that direct and indirect insults of various degrees coexist and, when acute lung inflammation occurs, either intra-alveolar or interstitial edema characterize the "early" phases of ARDS. After approximately one week, during "intermediate" ARDS, death of type I cells together with dysfunction of the remaining type II cells contribute to maintain lung edema, thus further distorting lung mechanical properties. Endothelial dysfunction and death contribute to plasma and cell transfer from the vascular compartment to the lung, while basement membrane collagen exposed to platelets leads to intravascular coagulation, further compromising lung function. Meanwhile, under the influence of a set of newly synthesized growth factors, interstitial fibroblasts differentiate into myofibroblasts and migrate into alveolar clots, thus initiating a fibroproliferative response that progressively leads to fibrous, not-compliant lung ("late" ARDS lung).

Lung structure and function

Most of our recent understanding of the pathophysiology of ARDS derives from computed tomography (CT). Before the introduction of CT technology, the imaging of ARDS was limited to chest X-ray, which showed a widespread and bilateral appearance of "pulmonary infiltrates". ARDS was then considered as a homogeneous alteration of the lung parenchyma, with reduced gas content and characterized by "abnormal stiffness". CT completely changed this model. It has been observed that the densities, which reflect the ratio of gas volume to total lung volume (i.e. gas volume/[tissue volume + gas volume]) are primarily distributed in the dependent lung regions [2, 3]. The non-dependent lung regions were relatively normally inflated, while the intermediate regions were poorly inflated (Fig. 1). Quantitative analysis with CT revealed that the ARDS lung is characterized by "normally inflated tissue", which can be quantified in grams (typically, in severe ARDS, 200-400 grams), "poorly aerated tissue" and "non-aerated tissue" (collapsed or consolidated) for a total lung weight of 2000-4000 grams, compared to 1000-1200 grams normal lung weight [4]. These observations led to the baby lung model as the amount of residual, normally inflated lung had the dimensions of a lung of a 5-6-year-old baby. The baby lung has the following characteristics: it is small and not stiff, as its specific compliance is near normal; it is located in the non-dependent lung regions, and it is associated with a various amount of abnormal lung, in part poorly inflated and in part collapsed or consolidated. Accordingly, ARDS lung could be modeled as a mixture of three zones: normally inflated (the baby lung, non-dependent), recruitable (i.e. openable with adequate pressure), and consolidated (i.e. alveolar occupation, not openable with pressure). This model, however, implies that part of the lung is normal (the baby lung) and that it is anatomically located in the non-dependent regions, spared by the disease process. However, when patients were studied in the prone position, we observed a redistribution of densities from dorsal to ventral (Fig. 2) [5]. The original baby lung model did not hold true, as

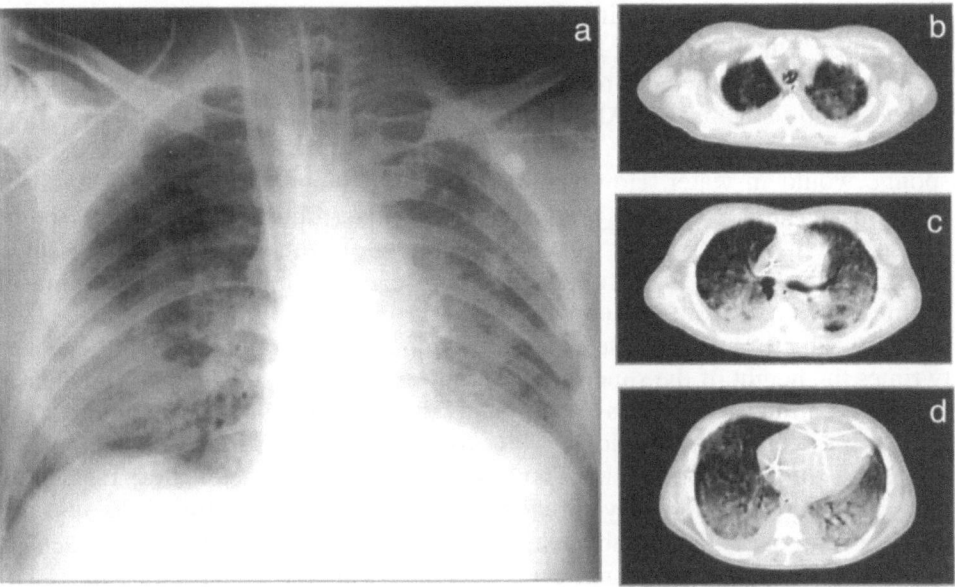

Fig. 1a-d. Conventional radiography (a) and CT of the lungs (b-d) of an ARDS patient in the early phase. b Apex. c Hilum. d Base. While the chest radiograph shows mainly a diffuse involvement, the CT scans clearly demonstrate a predominantly dependent distribution of the densities

End Expiration

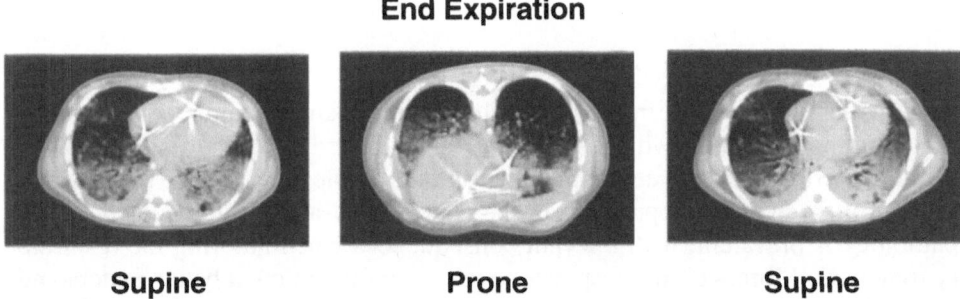

Supine   **Prone**   **Supine**

Fig. 2. Representative CT images in supine, prone and after return to supine position of an ARDS patient. Note the typical redistribution of lung densities in the prone position

now the inflated tissue (the baby lung) was still non-dependent, but the anatomical regions were not the same (the baby lung was in the dorsal regions in prone position and in the ventral regions in supine position). To understand the mechanism of density redistribution, we studied the regional characteristics of ARDS lung with CT.

The most important finding from the regional analysis was that the "excess tissue mass", likely deriving from edema, was not distributed according to gravity, but evenly distributed throughout the parenchyma, from ventral to dorsal in supine position. Thus, the ARDS lung, characterized by diffuse increased permeability (the whole lung is diseased), increases its edema in each level, as a sponge would in water. However, the increased lung mass, in a gravitational field, means increased lung weight, and the most dependent levels are compressed by increased weight of the levels above. In other words, if we assume that the lung behaves as a fluid, each lung level, from sternum to vertebra in supine position, is compressed by the pressure exerted by the level above. This pressure, called "superimposed pressure", equals, as in a fluid model, the density times the height of the superimposed lung. This model accounts for the density redistribution seen in prone position, as the gravitational forces compress the previously open ventral regions, while the dorsal regions become decollapsed. Therefore the sponge model presents the following characteristics: the whole lung is altered; the normally inflated tissue (baby lung) is still in the non-dependent regions; and the baby lung is not an anatomical reality, but instead a functional concept. This sponge model seems particularly appropriate in ARDS from indirect insult, where the diffuse permeability leads to diffuse interstitial edema and collapse. This model, however, is less applicable in ARDS due to direct insult, where the prevalent phenomenon is likely consolidation with occupation of pulmonary units, and the amount of recruitable lung (i.e. previously collapsed) is scarce.

Response to therapeutical maneuvers

As previously discussed, in the ARDS lung three main anatomic conditions coexist: pulmonary units which are open, consolidated or collapsed. CT per se cannot discriminate between consolidation and collapse, however, the response to controlled changes of pressure in the airway may allow inferences on which pathology is prevalent, with relevant consequences when tailoring the respiratory treatment. Moreover, the response to pressure may allow a better understanding of the mechanism through which PEEP acts and tidal volume is distributed.

Mechanisms of PEEP

Keeping the lung open

The primary role of PEEP in ARDS is to keep open, at end expiration, pulmonary units which otherwise collapse. For years, there has been a search for the "best PEEP", implying that in each ARDS there is an ideal level of pressure. CT clearly showed that such a level does not exist, and that PEEP is always a compromise between lung stretching and lung recruitment. In fact, by studying a series of patients with PEEP levels from 0 to 20 cm H_2O and performing the regional quantitative analysis of the gas/tissue ratio, it has been found, as expected from the sponge model, that the various levels of the same lung, from sternum to vertebra, require different levels of PEEP to stay open [6]. According to the sponge model, in fact, the superimposed pressure over a given lung level is a function of density of the level above times height. It follows that the PEEP required to keep open the ventral regions (in supine position) is 0 cm H_2O (no compression, no atelectasis). In the middle lung, the PEEP necessary to counteract the superimposed pressure will be higher and will be highest in the most dependent lung regions. It follows that, to keep open the most dorsal regions, the most ventral regions will be overexpanded, consequently the PEEP is never "best", but it is always a compromise.

Redistribution of ventilation/perfusion

While the mechanism of PEEP is quite straightforward in the sponge model, which closely fits ARDS due to extrapulmonary diseases (interstitial edema and collapse), the mechanism of its beneficial effects on oxygenation are far less clear in ARDS due to pulmonary disease, such as diffuse pneumonia (prevalent consolidation), as well as in late phases of ARDS. In both these conditions the compression atelectasis and the possibilities of recruitment are scarce [7, 8] even if PEEP is still necessary to optimize oxygenation. Although not proven, we believe that the mechanism is different from "keeping open" and possibly it consists, prevalently, in a redistribution of ventilation from ventral to dorsal regions (and not in a true recruitment). In fact, PEEP, overstretching the non-dependent regions, decreases their compliance, and ventilation may be diverted towards the middle and dependent regions, increasing the VA/Q ratio of the poorly inflated regions.

Mechanism of lung opening

When delivering a tidal volume in ARDS lung, two phenomena may occur: inflation and recruitment. Recruitment is defined as the inflation of previously not-inflated regions. It has been known for years that the pressures required to open are greater than those required to keep open the pulmonary units. As previously discussed, ARDS is characterized by consolidation and/or collapse, with different prevalence according to direct or indirect pathogenic pathway. It is worth emphasizing, however, that two kinds of collapse may coexist, one due to collapse of the small airways and one, the true alveolar collapse, due to a complete reabsorption of gases.

The distinction between small airways and alveolar collapse is important, as the pressure required for opening may be greatly different, 10-20 cm H_2O in small airways collapse and 30-35 cm H_2O pressure in alveolar collapse due to gas reabsorption [9]. Consequently, there is a complete range of opening pressures in ARDS from 0-1 cm H_2O to initially inflate open units, to 10-20 cm H_2O transmural pressure to counteract the small airway collapse, and up to 30-35 cm H_2O transmural pressure to revert the alveolar collapse. At the end of the spectrum there is the consolidation, in which opening is just impossible because of the occupation of the pulmonary units.

Mechanisms of distribution of tidal volume

Distribution of the insufflated volume is function of two factors, the regional airway resistances and the regional compliance. CT in static conditions allows making inferences about the regional compliance variations. We found that in ARDS the distribution of insufflated tidal volume is a function of PEEP. In fact, we found that by increasing PEEP from 0 to 20 cm H_2O, the amount of tidal volume distributed in non-dependent lung versus the amount distributed to the dependent lung decreased from 2.5:1 to approximately 1:1, i.e. the ventilation becomes more homogeneous and this phenomenon is always associated with better oxygenation [10]. The mechanism of the redistribution of the insufflated tidal volume with PEEP is as follows: in the most ventral regions, which are already open, increasing PEEP causes a progressive stretching of the pulmonary units, with decrease of their compliance; in the most dorsal regions, PEEP keeps open (i.e. maintains the recruitment of) pulmonary units otherwise collapsing and increases the compliance as more pulmonary units are available for inflation. The final effect depends on the balance between stretching and recruitment phenomena. Decreasing the non-dependent compliance and increasing the dependent compliance makes the compliance distribution more homogeneous, with consequent more homogeneous ventilation distribution.

Positioning

An important maneuver, increasingly used in ARDS, is to position the patients prone [11]. In Fig. 2 we already showed the effects on density redistribution from dorsal to ventral occurring in the majority of the patients when prone. It is worth reminding that this effect is not due to a different distribution of edema. In fact, in ARDS the interstitial edema, rich in proteins, is not "free" to move throughout the lung parenchyma. Instead, the density distribution, according to the sponge model, is due to "squeezing" out the gas from the dependent lung regions due to the superimposed pressure.

The density redistribution is more pronounced in ARDS due to extrapulmonary disease, since the consolidated part and pneumonia foci maintain their position both in supine and prone positions. The prone position, in about 60-70% of ARDS patients, is associated with increased oxygenation. Several mechanisms are likely involved, and are not necessarily the same in ARDS from pulmonary or extrapulmonary disease. In extrapulmonary disease, the amount of decollapsed tissue in prone is greater than in supine while the amount of collapsed tissue is low due to differences in anatomical lung and heart shape between supine and prone position [12]. On the other hand, in ARDS from pulmonary disease, we found that changes in thoracic compliance play a substantial role. In fact, in prone position, for anatomical reasons, the dorsal component of chest wall is stiffer than the anterior wall and the tidal volume is more distributed towards the ventral and abdominal regions, where the lesions are predominant [13]. Indeed, human and animal studies conclude that a more homogeneous inflation/ventilation is the main mechanism of oxygenation improvement in prone position.

Conclusions

The existing data strongly suggest that different therapeutic effects could be expected according to the individual type and the stage of the different cases of ARDS. Care should hence be taken, when approaching ARDS patients, not only to imaging and mechanical properties of the lungs but even to the pathogenesis of syndrome that, in some cases, could play a major role in suggesting the best therapeutical approach to be used to reduce the iatrogenic cost of the therapy itself.

References

1. Ashbaugh DG, Bigelow DB, Petty TL, Levine BE (1967) Acute respiratory distress in adult. Lancet 2:319-323
2. Gattinoni L, Mascheroni D, Torresin A et al (1986) Morphological response to positive end-expiratory pressure in acute respiratory failure. Intensive Care Med 12:137-142
3. Maunder RJ, Shuman WP, McHugh JW et al (1986) Preservation of normal lung regions in adult respiratory distress syndrome: analysis by computed tomography. JAMA 255:2463-2465
4. Gattinoni L, Pesenti A, Avalli L et al (1987) Pressure-volume curve of total respiratory system in acute respiratory failure. Am Rev Respir Dis 136:730-736
5. Gattinoni L, Pelosi P, Vitale G et al (1991) Body position changes redistribute lung computed tomographic density in patients with acute respiratory failure. Anesthesiology 74:15-23
6. Gattinoni L, D'Andrea L, Pelosi P et al (1993) Regional effects and mechanism of positive end-expiratory pressure in early adult respiratory distress syndrome. JAMA 269:2122-2127
7. D'Angelo E, Calderini E, Robatto FM et al (1997) Lung and chest wall mechanics in patients with acquired immunodeficiency syndrome and severe Pneumocystis carinii pneumonia. Eur Respir J 10:2343-2350
8. Winer-Muram HT, Steiner RM, Gurney JW et al (1998) Ventilator-associated pneumonia in patients with acute respiratory distress syndrome: CT evaluation. Radiology 208:193-199
9. Glaister DH, Schroter RC, Sudlow MF et al (1973) Transpulmonary pressure gradient and ventilation distribution in excised lungs. Respir Physiol 17:347-364
10. Gattinoni L, Pelosi P, Crotti S et al (1995) Effects of positive end-expiratory pressure on regional distribution of tidal volume and recruitment in adult respiratory distress syndrome. Am J Respir Crit Care Med 151:1807-1814

11. Albert RK (1996) Positioning and the patient with acute respiratory distress syndrome. Curr Opin Crit Care 2:67-72
12. Gattinoni L, Pelosi P, Valenza F et al (1994) Patient positioning in acute respiratory failure. In: Tobin MJ (ed) Principles and practice of mechanical ventilation. McGraw Hill, New York, pp 1067-1076
13. Pelosi P, Tubiolo D, Mascheroni D et al (1998) Effect of the prone position on respiratory mechanics and gas exchange during acute lung injury. Am J Respir Crit Care 157:387-393

Dynamics of Recruitment and Collapse of the Lung in Models of ARDS

P. NEUMANN, G. HEDENSTIERNA

In acute respiratory failure, mechanical ventilation is usually required in order to restore an acceptable gas exchange and to relieve the patient from the increased work of breathing. However, there is evidence from experimental studies that mechanical ventilation itself can induce lung damage by overdistension and repeated opening and closing of alveolar units [1, 2]. Mechanical ventilation may thus be a contributing factor to lung function deterioration during the course of ARDS and this concern prompted the recommendation of a consensus conference on mechanical ventilation to limit the end-inspiratory plateau pressure to 35-45 cm H_2O [3]. Consequently, pressure-controlled ventilation (PCV) has gained widespread popularity in order to limit the end-inspiratory airway pressure. If oxygenation is not acceptable, one may improve gas exchange by either increasing PEEP or extending the inspiratory time interval. Both manoeuvres increase the mean airway pressure, which is a major determinant of oxygenation in acute lung injury [4]. In order to optimise PCV, it is desirable to know the time course of lung collapse during expiration, so that an expiratory time can be chosen that minimises lung collapse, and still allows the lung to expire. During inspiration, complete reopening of collapsed lung tissue should ideally be accomplished with an inspiratory time interval as short as possible in order to reduce the risk of barotrauma.

ARDS is heterogeneous since it may develop due to different underlying causes such as sepsis, multiple trauma, lung contusion, near drowning, aspiration, etc. [5]. Consequently, different ARDS models have been developed such as endotoxin infusion [6], which resemble ARDS associated with sepsis, repeated lung lavage [7], which causes surfactant depletion as seen in the respiratory distress syndrome of the newborn and oleic acid injection [8], which was originally developed as a model of fat embolism syndrome. These three models have different characteristics. Endotoxin infusion induces an inflammatory response with accumulation of granulocytes and lymphocytes in the pulmonary microcirculation and damage of pulmonary endothelial cells, which finally leads to a proteinaceous edema [6, 9].

Repeated lung lavage causes surfactant depletion with dilated pulmonary lymphatics and thickened alveolo-capillary membranes, but no morphological damage to alveolar or perivascular cells and hyaline membranes [10].

Oleic acid injection produces a syndrome of acute endothelial and alveolar epithelial cell necrosis causing alveolar proteinaceous edema, without an initial inflammatory response [8].

In a first study from our group [11], the dynamics of lung collapse and recruitment were analysed with computerised tomography in the three above mentioned lung injury models using different breath holding procedures. In a second study [12], lung collapse and recruitment were further investigated only in the oleic acid model, since it caused the most severe lung injury [11], and thus seems to be an appropriate model to study "the worst case".

Lung collapse as exponential wash-in and wash-out functions

Lung collapse and recruitment follow an exponential wash-out (recruitment) and wash-in (lung collapse) function [11, 13]. Thus, during inspiration the rate of recruitment decreases progressively with diminishing atelectasis and during expiration atelectasis rises towards a limiting value at a rate which decreases progressively with the reduction of aerated lung tissue.

A wash-out function has the general form $y = y_0 \cdot e^{-t/\tau}$ where the quantity of the variable y at time 0 (y_0), the time constant (τ) and the elapsed time period (t) [14]. After 1 time constant, y will have fallen to 1/e of its initial value or approximately 37% of y_0. After $2 \cdot \tau$ a change is 86.5% complete, after $3 \cdot \tau$ it is 95% and after $4 \cdot \tau$ it is 98.2% complete. The half life, which is the time required for y to change to half of its previous value, is $0.69 \cdot \tau$.

A wash-in function has the general form: $y = y_{infinit} \cdot (1 - e^{-t/\tau})$ [14], where $y_{infinite}$ is the limiting value which would be attained only at infinite time. For an explanation of τ and t refer to the wash-out function above.

τ is ideally suited to compare the rate at which changes of atelectasis occur during prolonged breathing since τ is independent from the size of atelectasis. Thus, it allows to compare the dynamics of lung collapse and recruitment in subjects with different amounts of atelectasis.

Comparison of endotoxin-, lavage- and oleic acid-induced lung injury

Lung collapse occurred significantly faster in endotoxin- and oleic acid- compared to lavage-induced lung injury. During a prolonged expiration (40 s) without PEEP, τ was in the range of 10 to 20 seconds for the lavage model, but averaged only 2.5-4.5 seconds for endotoxin and oleic acid-induced lung injury [11]. Although, the use of PEEP reduces the amount of atelectasis, PEEP may decrease τ [11], presumably because it preferentially stabilises lung areas which are only moderately injured and would collapse rather slowly without PEEP. Thus, τ averaged only 0.86 seconds during mechanical ventilation with PEEP ≥ 10 cm H_2O in the oleic acid model [12].

During inspiration, in contrast, τ was between 0.7 and 1.8 seconds for all three lung injury models but time constants tended to be longer after oleic acid injection compared to the other two models. There was no correlation between time constants and the severity of lung injury as assessed by the PaO_2/FiO_2 ratio. Repeated lung lavage, characterised by long expiratory ($\tau \sim 10\text{-}20$ s) and short inspiratory time constants ($\tau \sim 0.75$ s), which means that the lungs collapse slowly but reopen fast, caused severe impairment of gas exchange with a PaO_2/FiO_2 ratio of approximately 100 mmHg during ventilation without PEEP. In the endotoxin model, in contrast, lung injury was only moderate (PaO_2/FiO_2 ratio ~ 300 mmHg), but damaged lung parenchyma had the tendency to collapse or become flooded very rapidly ($\tau \sim 3\text{-}4.5$ s) while recruitment ($\tau \sim 0.75$ s) occurred at a comparable rate to lavage-induced lung injury. Oleic acid injection caused the most severe abnormalities of gas exchange with expiratory time constants ($\tau \sim 2.5\text{-}3.6$ s) similar to the endotoxin model and its inspiratory time constants were the longest of all three lung injury models ($\tau \sim 1\text{-}1.8$ s).

Discussion and conclusion

These differences during lung collapse and recruitment may be important in the field of mechanical ventilatory support for acute respiratory failure. Recently, the "open lung approach" has gained widespread popularity in experimental [15-17] and clinical studies [18]. However, the feasibility of such an approach may also depend on the type of lung injury studied. In the lavage model, an inspiratory airway pressure of 40-50 cm H_2O, commonly used for recruitment manoeuvres in the open lung approach, will almost completely re-expand collapsed lung tissue after a few seconds. Thereafter, surfactant depleted lungs can easily be stabilised by short expiratory time intervals as used in inverse ratio ventilation because they collapse rather slowly. In addition, a PEEP of only 5 cm H_2O reduces end-expiratory atelectasis by 50% [11]. Thus, a moderate end-expiratory pressure may also be sufficient to maintain open lung conditions. In the oleic acid model, in contrast, higher airway pressures are needed for complete recruitment compared to lavage-induced lung injury [11], and this may increase the risk of barotrauma during effective recruitment manoeuvres. Thereafter, the lungs will collapse rapidly when the airway pressure falls below 20 cm H_2O [12], and furthermore a PEEP level of 5 cm H_2O reduces end-expiratory atelectasis by approximately only 10% [11]. Consequently, a high extrinsic PEEP of about 20-25 cm H_2O seems necessary in order to keep oleic acid-injured lungs open, unless very short expiratory time intervals (~ 0.5 s) are used. This last approach, however, would inevitably lead to high frequency ventilation or extreme settings during inverse ratio ventilation. Long inspiratory time intervals, as occasionally used in inverse ratio ventilation, seem to be unnecessary to open up lung tissue, since recruitment occurs mainly during the beginning of an inspiration due to the exponential time course.

In conclusion, researchers should be aware of the different time course of recruitment and de-recruitment phenomena in different types of lung injury, because it may affect the results of studies comparing different ventilatory modes in the treatment of acute respiratory failure. Different dynamics of lung collapse and recruitment may also contribute to the well known clinical observation that gas exchange may improve rapidly in some patients if inspiration is prolonged and expiration is shortened.

References

1 Pelosi P, Gattinoni L (1996) Mechanical ventilation in adult respiratory distress syndrome: a good friend or a secret killer? Curr Opin Anaesthesiol 9:515-522
2. Sykes MK (1991) Does mechanical ventilation damage the lung? Acta Anaesthesiol Scand [Suppl]35:35-39
3. Slutsky AS (1994) Consensus conference on mechanical ventilation - January 28-30, 1993 at Northbrook, Illinois, USA. Part 2. Intensive Care Med 20:150-162
4. Marini JJ, Ravenscraft SA (1992) Mean airway pressure: Physiologic determinants and clinical importance. Part 2. Clinical implications. Crit Care Med 20:1604-1616
5. Bernard GR, Artigas A, Brigham KL et al (1994) Report of the American-European consensus conference on ARDS: definitions, mechanisms, relevant outcomes and clinical trial coordination. Intensive Care Med 20:225-232
6. Brigham KL, Meyrick B (1986) Endotoxin and lung injury. Am Rev Respir Dis 133:913-927
7. Lachmann B, Robertson B, Vogel J (1980) In vivo lung lavage as an experimental model of the respiratory distress syndrome. Acta Anaesthesiol Scand 24:231-236
8. Schuster DP (1994) ARDS: clinical lessons from the oleic acid model of acute lung injury. Am J Respir Crit Care Med 149:245-260
9. Borg T, Alvfors A, Gerdin B et al (1985) A porcine model of early adult respiratory distress syndrome induced by endotoxaemia. Acta Anaesthesiol Scand 29:814-830
10. Nielsen JB, Sjostrand UH, Edgren EL et al (1991) An experimental study of different ventilatory modes in piglets in severe respiratory distress induced by surfactant depletion. Intensive Care Med 17:225-233
11. Neumann P, Berglund JE, Mondejar EF et al (1998) Dynamics of lung collapse and recruitment during prolonged breathing in porcine lung injury. J Appl Physiol 85:1533-1543
12. Neumann P, Berglund JE, Mondejar EF et al (1998) Effect of different pressure levels on the dynamics of lung collapse and recruitment in oleic-acid-induced lung injury. Am J Respir Crit Care Med 158:1636-1643
13. Rothen HU, Neumann P, Berglund JE et al (1999) Dynamics of re-expansion of atelectasis during general anaesthesia. Br J Anaesth 82:551-556
14. Nunn JF (1993) Nunn's applied respiratory physiology. Butterworth-Heinemann, Oxford
15. Lichtwarck Aschoff M, Nielsen JB, Sjostrand UH (1992) An experimental randomized study of five different ventilatory modes in a piglet model of severe respiratory distress [see comments]. Intensive Care Med 18:339-347
16. Lichtwarck Aschoff M, Markström A, Hedlund AJ (1996) Oxygenation remains unaffected by increased inspiration-to-expiration ratio but impairs hemodynamics in surfactant-depleted piglets. Intensive Care Med 22:329-335
17. Markström A, Lichtwarck Aschoff M, Svennson B et al (1999) Ventilation with constant versus decelerating inspiratory flow in experimentally induced acute respiratory failure. Anesthesiology 84:882-889
18. Amato MB, Barbas CS, Medeiros DM et al (1998) Effect of a protective-ventilation strategy on mortality in the acute respiratory distress syndrome [see comments]. N Engl J Med 338: 347-354

Regional Lung Blood Flow and Inhalation of Nitric Oxide

G. Hedenstierna, K. Hambraeus Jonzon, F. Fredén

It did not take long after it was discovered that nitric oxide is produced in the vascular wall of endothelial cells and that it has a powerful vasodilatory effect until efforts were made to modify the pulmonary vascular tone by either inhaling NO or blocking its endogenous production by means of an NO synthase inhibitor. Thus, lambs were exposed either to hypoxic gas or to a thromboxane analogue in order to constrict the vessels and subsequent inhalation of 5-80 parts per million (ppm) of NO was shown to relax the pulmonary vessels in a dose-dependent manner [1, 2]. In similar experiments, healthy humans exposed to hypoxic gas (12% O_2) did also respond with pulmonary vasorelaxation back to baseline on inhalation of NO in doses of 5-40 ppm [3]. The inhalation of NO, however, did not affect systemic arterial pressure, neither in the lambs nor in the human volunteers. This can be explained by the avid binding of NO to haemoglobin (met-haemoglobin) which does not exert an NO vasoactive effect. In similar experiments in patients with acute respiratory failure, inhalation of NO could also lower pulmonary artery pressure in the presence of pulmonary hypertension [4]. Moreover, in these patients an improvement in arterial oxygenation was also seen which may be due to a redistribution of lung blood flow to ventilated regions from non-ventilated shunt areas. This is because inhaled NO will only exert its dilatory effect in those lung regions reached by NO. This is different from the effect of a systemically administered vasodilator, for example, sodium nitroprusside, nitroglycerine or prostacycline. These will dilate vessels both in ventilated and non-ventilated lung regions, usually with a more powerful relaxant effect in the non-ventilated shunt regions because their preceding hypoxic vasoconstriction. Moreover, a systemic hypotension may also develop. Thus, for the first time it seemed as if a drug exerted its effect only on pulmonary circulation and ventilated lung regions. Subsequent studies on nebulisation of the airways using prostacycline has also been shown to exert its effect solely where it has been deposited in the lung; similar to inhaled NO [5]. In neonates with the persistent pulmonary hypertension a dramatic fall in the pulmonary artery pressure and increasing PaO_2 was observed NO inhalation [6], raising high expectations on the usefulness of NO as a life saving drug in adult and in neonatal ARDS.

Although, initial experiments were carried out with inhaled NO concentrations of approximately 40 ppm, subsequent dose-response tests in patients in respiratory failure showed that a full response could be obtained with as low doses at 1 ppm [7].

A number of multicenter trials were subsequently set up to analyse the possible beneficial effects of inhaled NO, in particular in patients with neonatal or adult respiratory distress syndrome. The trial on neonatal intensive care patients, the NINOS study, showed that extra corporeal membrane oxygenation was significantly less in patients that received i-NO than in an otherwise similarly treated control group, but outcome did not differ between the two groups [8]. This was considered a partial success and the U.S. Food and Drug Administration approved i-NO for neonatal intensive care. However, there are differences in response to i-NO which depend on the underlying disease. Thus, persistent pulmonary hypertension seems to respond much more favourably to i-NO than for example congenital diaphragmatic hernia with pulmonary dysplasia [9].

The trials in adult respiratory distress turned out to be even less successful. Thus in a total 185 patients, no difference could be seen between the i-NO group and the control group in terms of survival period without ventilator and treatment period in intensive care unit. However, a subgroup analysis showed that the group that received i-NO at a concentration of 5 ppm lived longer off the ventilator than the control group [10]. These results certainly curtailed interest in i-NO therapy as seen from an editorial to the adult multicenter trial [11]. It may be that the trials were executed too early since there is far from a full understanding of the effects of i-NO and possible compensatory mechanisms in the regulation of pulmonary vascular tone that may occur when initiating i-NO. Moreover, as many as 40% of the patients were non-responders to i-NO, i.e. they did not improve their PaO_2 by 20% or more. The reasons for not responding to i-NO are not yet fully understood. It is obvious however, that i-NO can only relax pulmonary vessels if they are preconstricted, i.e. are exposed to an increased tone. Any other cause of a pulmonary hypertension such as vascular occlusion by various emboli, vascular remodelling with narrowing of the vascular lumen and increased left atrial pressure are not amenable to i-NO. It may also be that the inhaled NO cannot reach its target, the vascular smooth muscle, because of increased diffusion distances in the event of oedema, or is scavenged by compounds that inactivate NO. It has been shown that septic shock is seen in more non-responses to i-NO than other forms of ARDS [12]. In our experiments we have seen that rabbits with airways preconstricted by methacholine respond bronchial relaxation to i-NO, but not after nebulization of the airway of hypertonic saline [13]. Such nebulizations cause an epithelial hypertonic oedema. However, it is unlikely that the lack of an effect of i-NO was caused by diffusion impairment since concentrations of NO as high as 300 ppm did not exert any effect. That concentration should overcome a diffusion impairment. In subsequent experiments on isolated guinea pig tracheas mounted into a perfusion bath, the addition of hypertonic saline to the luminal side attenuated or eliminated the dilatory effect of an NO donor, sodium nitroprusside (SNP) [14]. However, if the hypertonic saline was given to the extraluminal side, SNP exerted full effect. This speaks strongly against any diffusion impairment but points to a scavenging effect by the oedema or one of its components. To what extent this may apply to vascular oedema in ARDS remains to be shown.

Blocking the endogenous NO production by an NO synthase inhibitor given intravenously will cause systemic and pulmonary hypertension. In a rabbit experiment where each lung was ventilated separately, one-lung hypoxia caused a redistribution away from the hypoxic lung and this redistribution was enhanced by intravenous administration of an NO synthase blocker [15]. This indicates that endogenous NO plays a role in the hypoxic pulmonary vasoconstrictor response (HPV). Similar results were obtained in pig experiments where the left lower lobe was ventilated separately with hypoxic (5%) gas [16]. The hypoxia per se reduced left lower lobar perfusion to 25% of baseline and an intravenous NO synthase blocker reduced it further, to 12%. Since i.v. administration of the blocker will eliminate any NO production also in the well oxygenated lung regions, promoting vasoconstriction, replacement of NO was done by inhalation via the airways. This resulted in lowering of the PA-pressure, as expected, and a further redistribution of blood flow away from the hypoxic left lower lobe that was now perfused by no more than 3% of the baseline share of blood flow. Thus, manipulation of the NO system has marked effects on regional lung blood flow, at least in animal experiments!

Unilateral inhalation of NO has also been tested in man during one-lung anesthesia. However, the results have been varying and often modest. The aim of the experiment was to cause a redistribution of blood flow from the non-ventilated, hypoxic lung to the other, ventilated, hyperoxic lung. Thus, some studies have shown a certain increase in PaO_2, suggestive of such redistribution, whereas others have not [17-20]. However, it should be understood that PaO_2 may not be a good measure of any redistribution between the lungs since there may also be a redistribution of blood flow within the lung that receives NO. The only study so far that has made direct measurement of the blood flow to each lung during varied individual ventilation in anesthetised man is the one by Hambraeus-Jonzon et al. [21]. The fractional blood flow to each lung was measured by infusing a poorly soluble gas, sulphurhexa-fluoride (SF6), into a systemic vein and collecting expired gas from each lung separately and analysing it for SF6. Some interesting results where obtained. Thus, when both lungs were ventilated with hyperoxic or normoxic gas and i-NO was given to one lung, no effect on the distribution of blood flow between the lungs was seen. If, on the other hand, one lung was ventilated with hypoxic gas (5% O_2) and the other one with hyperoxic gas, then i-NO given to the hyperoxic lung caused a redistribution of blood flow with a decrease in hypoxic lung blood flow from 30 to 25% of cardiac output. It thus seems as if the effect of regional i-NO depends on the oxygen concentration in the regions that do not receive i-NO.

To study whether regional NO can exert a distant effect, pig experiments were executed by Hambraeus Jonzon et al. (on-going study). In pigs with left lower lobar hypoxia, endogenous NO production increased as evidenced by an increased NO synthase activity in lung tissue and an increased concentration of expired NO from that lobe. The inhalation of NO to the hyperoxic right lung and left upper lobe, however, down-regulated the NO synthase activity and decreased the expired NO in the left lower lobe. To see whether this was an effect that was mediated via the blood or a neurogenic reflex, and to analyse the effects on the pulmonary vascular tone, blood was cross circulated between two pigs. One pig was ventilated with hyperoxic gas and received i-NO during part of the study. The other pig was ventilated with hyperoxic gas to the right lung and left upper and middle lobes whereas the left lower lobe received a hypoxic gas, similar to previous experiments. Blood was cross circulated between the pigs at a rate of 500 ml/min. When the first pig received i-NO the pulmonary artery pressure went up in the second pig and the pulmonary vascular resistance was increased. The vasoconstriction seemed to be stronger in the hypoxic left lower lobe than in the hyperoxic regions. Thus, a distant, blood borne effect was demonstrated. Such a dual effect of i-NO, both relaxing vessels in ventilated lung and constricting vessels in non-ventilated tissue demonstrates that the effect of inhaled NO is not as simple as believed. The dual effect may also explain why there may be a dissociation between improvement in PaO_2 and decrease in pulmonary artery pressure. The larger the share of lung that does not receive NO because of collapse and consolidation, the larger will the redistribution of blood flow be with subsequent possible improvement in PaO_2. At the same time, the effect on pulmonary artery pressure will be successively decreasing, since the non-ventilated parts may constrict rather than relax, opposing the relaxant effect in he ventilated parenchyma. However, these results have been obtained in pigs and to what extent they can be extrapolated to other species including man is not clear.

In summary, manipulation of the nitric oxide system, by blocking endogenous NO production or administering NO by inhalation, may have marked effects on regional lung blood flow. However, nitric oxide is just one of several vasoactive substances and its manipulation will most likely cause a number of compensatory effects that will render it difficult to detect the effect of NO on pulmonary vascular pressure and arterial oxygenation. Before we have a fuller insight into these mechanisms, the administration of endogenous NO, or the blockage of endogenous NO, as a therapeutical means must also be considered. The multicenter studies on i-NO that have been conducted with rather meagre results may therefore have been more of an obstacle to our interest and understanding of vasoregulation than a help in intensive care.

References

1. Frostell C, Fratacci MD, Wain JC et al (1991) Inhaled nitric oxide. A selective pulmonary vasodilator reversing hypoxic pulmonary vasoconstriction [published erratum appears in Circulation 1991 Nov;84(5):2212]. Circulation 83(6):2038-2047
2. Fratacci MD, Frostell CG, Chen TY et al (1991) Inhaled nitric oxide. A selective pulmonary vasodilator of heparin-protamine vasoconstriction in sheep. Anesthesiology 75(6):990-999
3. Frostell CG, Blomqvist H, Hedenstierna G et al (1993) Inhaled nitric oxide selectively reverses human hypoxic pulmonary vasoconstriction without causing systemic vasodilation [see comments]. Anesthesiology 78(3):427-435
4. Rossaint R, Falke KJ, Lopez F et al (1993) Inhaled nitric oxide for the adult respiratory distress syndrome [see comments]. N Engl J Med 328(6):399-405
5. Walmrath D, Schneider T, Schermuly R et al (1996) Direct comparison of inhaled nitric oxide and aerosolized prostacyclin in acute respiratory distress syndrome. Am J Respir Crit Care Med Mar 153(3):991-996
6. Kinsella JP, Neish SR, Shaffer E, Abman SH (1992) Low-dose inhalation nitric oxide in persistent pulmonary hypertension of the newborn [see comments]. Lancet 340(8823):819-820
7. Gerlach H, Pappert D, Lewandowski K et al (1993) Long-term inhalation with evaluated low doses of nitric oxide for selective improvement of oxygenation in patients with adult respiratory distress syndrome [see comments]. Intensive Care Med 19(8):443-449
8. The Neonatal Inhaled Nitric Oxide Study Group (1997) Inhaled nitric oxide in full-term and nearly full-term infants with hypoxic respiratory failure. N Engl J Med 336:597-604
9. Mercier JC, Lacaze T, Storme L et al (1998) Disease-related response to inhaled nitric oxide in newborns with severe hypoxaemic respiratory failure. French Paediatric Study Group of Inhaled NO. Eur J Pediatr 157(9):747-752
10. Dellinger R, Zimmermann J, Taylor R, Straube CEA (1998) Effects of inhaled nitric oxide in patients with acute respiratory distress syndrome: Results of a randomized phase II trial. Crit Care Med 26(1):15-23
11. Zapol W (1998) Nitric oxide inhalation in acute respiratory distress syndrome: it works, but can we prove it? Crit Care Med 26(1):2-3
12. Manktelow C, Bigatello LM, Hess D, Hurford WE (1997) Physiologic determinants of the response to inhaled nitric oxide in patients with acute respiratory distress syndrome. Anesthesiology 87:297-307
13. Högman M, Hjoberg J, Hedenstierna G (1998) Increased airway osmolarity inhibits the action of nitric oxide in the rabbit. Eur Respir J 12(6):1313-1317
14. Hjoberg J, Högman M, Hedenstierna G (1999) Hyperosmolarity reduces the relaxing potency of nitric oxide donors in guinea-pig trachea. Br J Pharmacol 127(2):391-396
15. Sprague RS, Thiemermann C, Vane JR (1992) Endogenous endothelium-derived relaxing factor opposes hypoxic pulmonary vasoconstriction and supports blood flow to hypoxic alveoli in anesthetized rabbits. Proc Natl Acad Sci USA 89(18):8711-8715
16. Fredén F, Wei SZ, Berglund JE et al (1995) Nitric oxide modulation of pulmonary blood flow distribution in lobar hypoxia. Anesthesiology 82(5):1216-1225
17. Rich GF, Lowson SM, Johns RA et al (1994) Inhaled nitric oxide selectively decreases pulmonary vascular resistance without impairing oxygenation during one-lung ventilation in patients undergoing cardiac surgery. Anesthesiology 80(1):57-62
18. Wilson WC, Kapelanski DP, Benumof JL et al (1997) Inhaled nitric oxide (40 ppm) during one-lung ventilation, in the lateral decubitus position, does not decrease pulmonary vascular resistance or improve oxygenation in normal patients. J Cardiothorac Vasc Anesth 11(2): 172-176
19. Hartigan P, Formanek V, Sheman S et al (1996) Inhaled NO fails to improve gas exchange during one-lung ventilation (abstr). Anesthesiology 85:A1165
20. Booth J, Powrosnyk A, Oduru A et al (1995) Effect of nitric oxide on arterial oxygenation and pulmonary shunt during one-lung ventilation (abstr). Anesthesiology 83:A1201
21. Hambraeus Jonzon K, Bindslev L, Frostell C, Hedenstierna G (1998) Individual lung blood flow during unilateral hypoxia: effects of inhaled nitric oxide. Eur Respir J 11:565-570

AIRFLOW LIMITATION

Mechanisms and Detection of Tidal Expiratory Flow Limitation

J. MILIC-EMILI

The highest pulmonary ventilation that a subject can achieve is ultimately limited by the highest flow rates that can be generated. Most normal subjects and endurnance-trained athletes do not exhibit expiratory flow limitation even during maximal exercise [1, 2]. In contrast, patients with chronic obstructive pulmonary disease (COPD) may exhibit flow limitation even at rest, as first suggested by Hyatt [1]. This was based on his observation that patients with severe COPD often breathe tidally along their MEFV curve. The presence of expiratory flow limitation during tidal breathing promotes dynamic pulmonary hyperinflation, with concomitant increase of inspiratory work, impairment of inspiratory muscle function and adverse effects on hemodynamics [3], and may contribute to dyspnea [4].

Conventionally, flow limitation (FL) is assessed by comparison of the tidal expiratory flow-volume ($\dot{V}$-V) curves with the corresponding MEFV curves: patients in whom, at comparable lung volumes, tidal flows are similar to those obtained during the forced expiratory vital capacity (FVC) maneuver are considered FL [1]. As discussed below, this approach has both theoretical and practical limitations. Nevertheless, this analysis has been the kernel for understanding respiratory dynamics. Accordingly it is useful to review it in some detail.

Figure 1 depicts the flow-volume ($\dot{V}$-V) loops at rest and during maximal exercise, together with the corresponding maximal $\dot{V}$-V curves, of a normal subject and a patient with severe airway obstruction. In the normal subject, even during maximal exercise, the flows are less than maximal (i.e. there is no flow limitation). In this case, the increase of tidal volume during exercise is obtained as a result of both an increase in end-inspiratory and a decrease in end-expiratory lung volume compared to rest, and the work of breathing during exercise is sustained by activity of both inspiratory and expiratory muscles. In contrast, in patients with severe airway obstruction maximal expiratory flows may be reached even at rest. In this case, the increase of tidal volume during exercise must be accompanied by increases in end-expiratory volume and inspiratory flow [6, 7]. This pattern of breathing, in which the ratio of inspiratory time to total cycle duration falls to 0.3 or less as compared to normal values of 0.4 to 0.5, may be considered an adaptation to expiratory flow limitation. However, the increase in volume is associated with an expansion of the thoracic

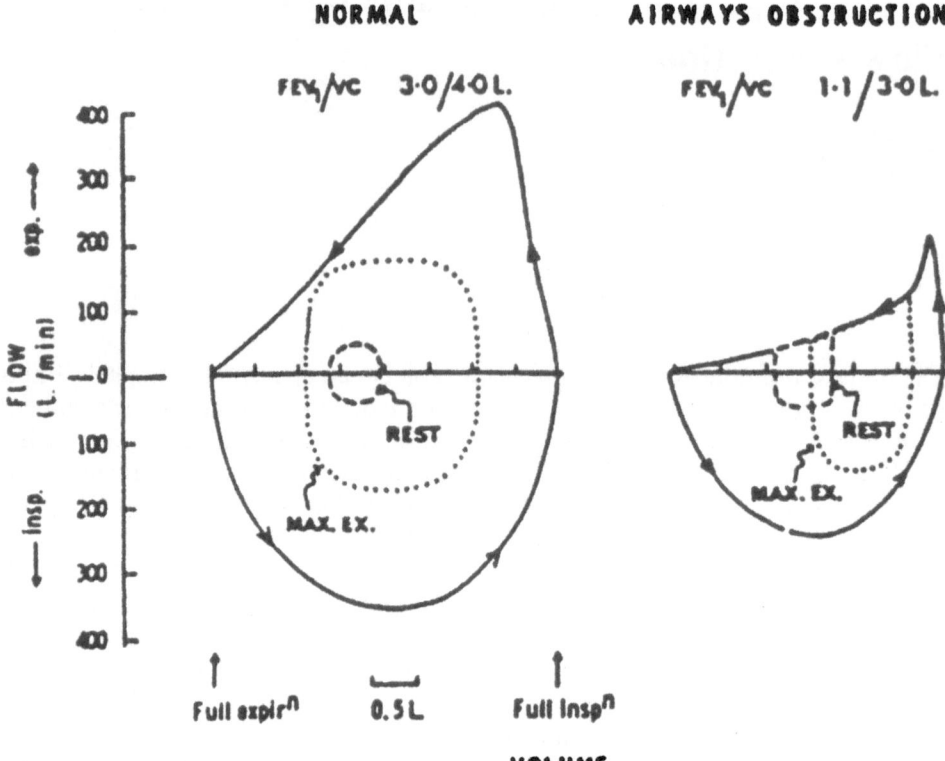

Fig. 1. Flow-volume curves obtained from a normal subject and a patient with chronic obstructive pulmonary disease. Spontaneous flow-volume loops at rest (*dashed lines*) and maximum exercise (Max Ex, *dotted lines*) are compared with maximum flow-volume loops (*outer solid lines*). FEV_1, forced expiratory volume in one second; VC, vital capacity (from Leaver DG, Pride NB (1971) Flow-volume curves and expiratory pressures during exercise in patients with chronic airways obstruction. Scand J Respir Dis [Suppl]77:23-27 *with permission*)

cage to a point where the inspiratory muscles operate inefficiently. Furthermore, the dynamic hyperinflation causes a) an increase in inspiratory work through a decrease in static compliance of the respiratory system, as patients now breathe along a flatter portion of the static volume-pressure curve; and b) a high inspiratory threshold load due to the need to generate additional pressure before inspiratory flow can begin (this threshold pressure has been labelled intrinsic PEEP) [3]. With severe dynamic hyperinflation, this phenomenon becomes self-limiting because the changes in volume and inspiratory flow require too high force development by the inspiratory muscles. Thus, in patients with severe airway obstruction inspiratory muscle fatigue may limit exercise performance. This explains why detection of tidal expiratory flow limitation is of great clinical importance.

The conventional approach for detecting expiratory flow limitation illustrated in Fig. 1, however, has an important practical limitation because, as a result of thoracic gas compression during the FVC maneuver, the tidal and maximal V̇-V curves have to be measured with a body plethysmograph [8]. This implies that such measurements are usually confined to resting breathing in sitting position. Apart from this, there are several other factors which make assessment of flow limitation based on comparison of tidal and maximal V̇-V curves problematic: a) volume-dependent changes in airway resistance and lung recoil during the maximal inspiration prior to the FVC maneuver, and b) time-dependent viscoelastic behavior of pulmonary tissues and time-dependent lung emptying due to time constant inequality [9, 10]. These mechanisms imply that the maximal flows which can be reached during expiration depend on the volume and time history of the preceding inspiration. Furthermore, since axiomatically the previous volume and time history varies between tidal and maximal inspiration, assessment of flow limitation based on comparison of tidal and maximal V̇-V curves commonly leads to erroneous conclusions, even if the measurements are made with body plethysmography [11, 12]. Recently, however, an alternate technique (NEP, negative expiratory pressure method) has been introduced to detect expiratory flow limitation during tidal breathing, which does not require either performance of FVC maneuvers on the part of the patient or a body plethysmograph [13, 14]. Accordingly, this method can also be applied to mechanically ventilated patients [13]. The NEP method has been validated by concomitant determination of iso-volume flow-pressure relationships [13].

NEP method for detection of expiratory flow limitation

Figure 2 illustrates the experimental setup used to detect expiratory flow limitation with NEP. It consists of a pneumotachograph and a Venturi device capable of generating a negative pressure when connected to a source of compressed air. The Venturi device is activated by opening a rapid solenoid valve [4]. The NEP method consists in applying negative pressure at the mouth during tidal expiration (usually about -3 to -5 cm H_2O) and comparing the ensuing V̇-V curve with that of the previous control expiration. Therefore, with this technique the volume and time history, as well as the intrathoracic pressures, during the expiration with NEP are the same as in the preceding control breath [15]. If application of NEP elicits increased flow over the entire range of the control tidal volume, the patient is not flow limited (Fig. 3, left panel). In contrast, if with NEP the subject exhales along part or the entire control V̇-V curve, flow limitation (FL) is present (Fig. 3, middle and right panels). The FL portion of the tidal expiration can be expressed as percentage fraction of the control tidal volume ($\%V_T$). In the two FL subjects in Fig. 3, flow limitation amounted to 45 and 68% V_T, respectively. If expiratory flow limitation is present when NEP is applied, there is a transient increase of flow (spike in Fig. 3, right panel), which

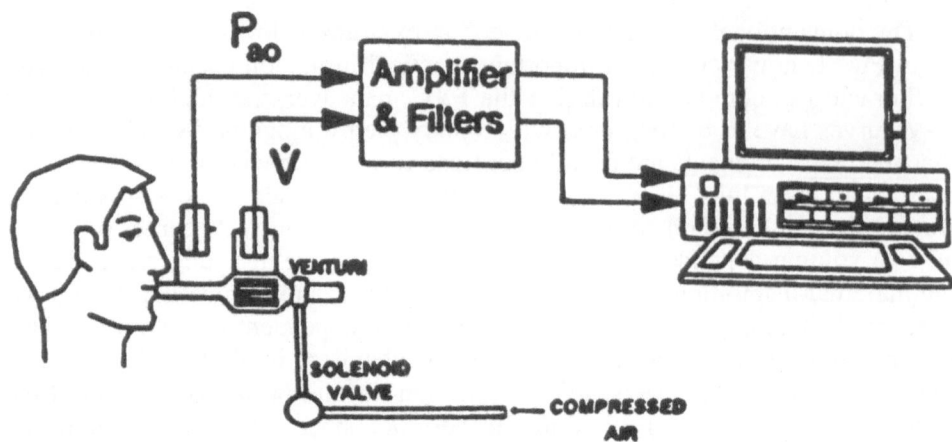

Fig. 2. Schematic diagram of equipment setup for NEP test. Pao, pressure at airway opening; $\dot{V}$, flow. Volume is obtained by numerical integration of $\dot{V}$ signal. During the study, the time course of flow, volume and pressure are continuously monitored on the screen of the computer, together with the corresponding flow-volume curves (from Eltayara L, Becklake MR, Volta CA et al (1996) Relationship of chronic dyspnea and flow limitation in COPD patients. Am J Respir Crit Care Med 154:1726-1734 *with permission*)

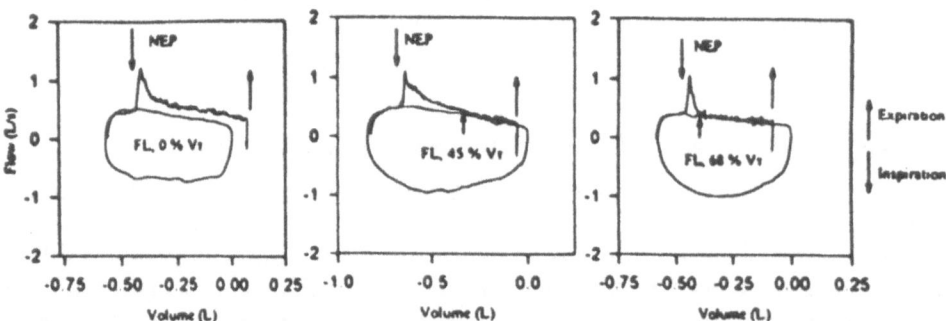

Fig. 3. Flow-volume loops of NEP test breaths and preceding control breaths in three representative COPD patients seating at rest. No flow limitation (FL) (*left panel*), FL over last 45% of control expired tidal volume (V_T) (*middle panel*), FL over 68% V_T (*right panel*). *Long arrows* indicate onset of NEP. *Short arrows* indicate onset of FL. Zero volume is end-expiratory lung volume of control breaths (from Eltayara L, Becklake MR, Volta CA et al (1996) Relationship of chronic dyspnea and flow limitation in COPD patients. Am J Respir Crit Care Med 154:1726-1734 *with permission*)

mainly reflects enhanced dynamic airway compression and sudden reduction in volume of the compliant oral and neck structures [14, 15]. Such spikes are useful markers of FL.

Flow limitation and chronic dyspnea

Intuitively one would expect patients with the most severe airway obstruction, as assessed with routine lung function measurements, to be the most dyspneic. However, some patients with severe airway obstruction are minimally symptomatic, whereas others with little objective dysfunction appear to be very dyspneic [16]. In fact, many studies have shown that the correlation between chronic dyspnea and FEV_1 is weak [4]. In contrast, flow limitation as measured with the NEP technique is a much better predictor of chronic dyspnea then FEV_1 [4, 11, 12].

Using the NEP technique, it has been shown that assessment of FL based on comparison of tidal with maximal $\dot{V}$-V curves has been found inaccurate even when volume was measured with a body plethysmograph in order to avoid thoracic gas compression artifacts [11, 12].

Flow limitation and exercise capacity

Since in COPD the reduced exercise capacity shows only a weak relation to FEV_1 and FVC [4, 17], it has been concluded that other factors, such as peripheral muscle weakness, deconditioning and impaired gas exchange play a predominant role to reduced exercise tolerance [18]. A recent study, however, has shown that in COPD there is a relatively strong correlation ($r = 0.81$) between the resting inspiratory capacity (IC) and the exercise capacity [19]. Accordingly, lung function impairment is probably an important cause of decreased exercise tolerance in many COPD patients. Indeed, because of expiratory flow limitation, the maximal tidal volume (and hence ventilation) is necessarily closely related to resting IC [15].

Conclusion

The NEP technique provides a simple and reliable tool for detecting expiratory flow limitation both at rest and during exercise. The method does not require body plethysmography, does not depend on patient cooperation and coordination, and can be applied in any desired body posture.

Acknowledgement: We thank Ms. Angie Bentivegna for typing this manuscript.

References

1. Hyatt RE (1961) The interrelationship of pressure, flow and volume during various respiratory manoeuvers in normal and emphysematous patients. Am Rev Respir Dis 83:676-683
2. Mota S, Casan P, Drobnic F et al (1999) Expiratory flow limitation during exercise in competition cyclists. J Appl Physiol 86:611-616
3. Gottfried SB (1991) The role of PEEP in the mechanically ventilated COPD patient. In: Roussos C, Marini JJ (eds) Ventilatory Failure. Springer, Berlin, pp 392-418
4. Eltayara L, Becklake MR, Volta CA et al (1996) Relationship of chronic dyspnea and flow limitation in COPD patients. Am J Respir Crit Care Med 154:1726-1734
5. Leaver DG, Pride NB (1971) Flow-volume curves and expiratory pressures during exercise in patients with chronic airways obstruction. Scand J Respir Dis [Suppl]77:23-27
6. Stubbing DG, Pengelly LD, Morse JLC et al (1980) Pulmonary mechanics during exercise in subjects with chronic air-flow obstruction. J Appl Physiol 49:511-515
7. Grimby G, Stiksa J (1970) Flow-volume curves and breathing patterns during exercise in patients with obstructive lung disease. Scan J Clin Lab Invest 25:303-313
8. Ingram RH Jr, Schilder DP (1966) Effect of gas compression on pulmonary pressure, flow and volume relationship. J Appl Physiol 47:1043-1050
9. Koulouris NG, Rapakoulias P, Rassidakis A et al (1995) Dependence of FVC manoeuvre on time course of preceding inspiration in patients with restrictive lung disease. Eur Respir J 8: 306-313
10. D'Angelo E, Robatto E, Calderini M et al (1991) Pulmonary and chest wall mechanics in anaesthetized paralyzed humans. J Appl Physiol 70:2602-2610
11. Murciano D, Pichot M-H, Boczkowski J et al (1997) Expiratory flow limitation in COPD patients after single lung transplantation. Am J Respir Crit Care Med 155:1036-1041
12. Boczkowski J, Murciano D, Pichot M-H et al (1997) Expiratory flow limitation in stable asthmatic patients during resting breathing. Am J Respir Crit Care Med 156:752-757
13. Valta P, Corbeil C, Lavoie A et al (1994) Detection of expiratory flow limitation during mechanical ventilation. Am J Respir Crit Care Med 150:1311-1317
14. Koulouris NG, Valta P, Lavoie A et al (1995) A simple method to detect expiratory flow limitation during spontaneous breathing. Eur Respir J 8:306-313
15. Koulouris NG, Dimopoulou I, Valta P et al (1996) Detection of expiratory flow limitation during exercise in COPD patients. J Appl Physiol 82:723-731
16. Fletcher CM (1961) Bronchitis: an international symposium. Assen: The Netherlands Discussion. Thomas CC (ed), Springfield IL, pp 212-214
17. Jones NG, Jones G, Edwards RHT (1971) Exercise tolerance in chronic airway obstruction. Am Rev Repir Dis 103:477-494
18. Gosselink R, Troosters T, Decramer M (1997) Exercise training in COPD patients: the basic questions. Eur Respir J 10:2884-2891
19. Murariu C, Ghezzo H, Milic-Emili J et al (1998) Exercise limitation in obstructive lung disease. Chest 114:965-968

Clinical Consequences of the Airflow Limitation

C. Tantucci, A. Ferretti, V. Grassi

The term *airflow limitation* or better *expiratory flow limitation* refers to a functional condition in which the expiratory flow cannot augment at a given lung volume. Hence, it should not be used as a synonymn for airway obstruction which simply reflects an increase in the airway resistance leading to a reduced expiratory flow rate (Fig. 1).

It follows that expiratory flow limitation (EFL) is present only when the expiratory flow cannot be increased by increasing pleural and therefore alveolar pressure at a given lung volume.

EFL is normally observed in healthy subjects as well as in patients with respiratory disorders during maximal forced expiratory manoeuvre, where, after the peak expiratory flow (PEF), isovolumic expiratory flow rates do not increase by increasing expiratory effort and, thus, are maximal [1].

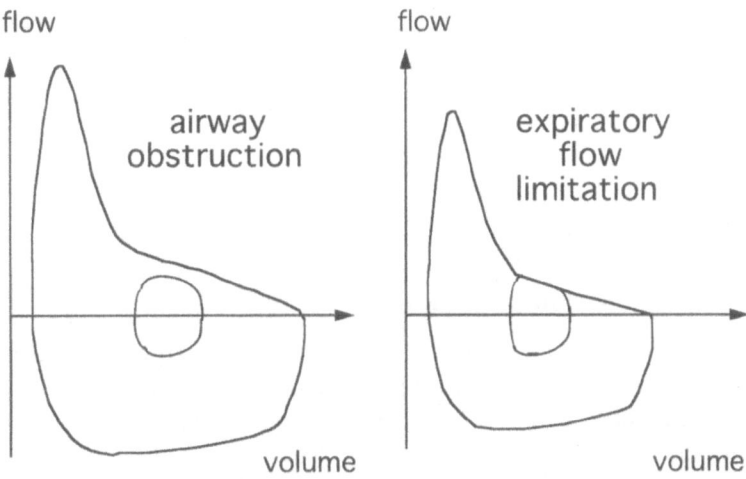

Fig. 1. The relationship between maximal and resting tidal flow/volume loops is schematically depicted in the presence of airway obstruction (*left panel*) and expiratory flow limitation (EFL) (*right panel*). Whereas airway obstruction implies a reduction in maximal expiratory flow rates, EFL at rest reflects the impossibility to increase the expiratory flow at a lung volume corresponding to the resting tidal volume

In contrast, EFL never occurs during tidal breathing at rest in normal subjects, regardless of age, both in supine and sitting-standing position [2, 3] and in most young athletes even at maximal exercise [4].

At times, however, EFL may abnormally be present during tidal breathing both during effort and also at rest.

The following review will focus on the pathophysiological and clinical aspects related to the presence of tidal EFL.

Pathophysiology

The development of tidal EFL is functionally relevant because under the prevailing conditions (e.g.: during exercise, at rest either in the supine or seated position) EFL is associated to or promotes pulmonary dynamic hyperinflation (DH) by prolonging the time required for the respiratory system to reach its relaxation volume (Vr) during expiration [5, 6]. Moreover, when EFL occurs, the expiratory flow may be increased only by increasing the absolute lung volume.

Indeed, in the presence of tidal EFL, even if resting DH can be avoided if the expiratory time (Te) is long enough for Vr to be reached, the end-expiratory lung volume (EELV) is more often dynamically raised at rest (Fig. 2) and invariably increases with increasing ventilatory demand which requires greater tidal volume and faster breathing frequency with shorter Te [7, 8].

DH implies a positive alveolar end-expiratory pressure (PEEPi) with a concomitant increase in inspiratory work due to PEEPi acting as a threshold load, impairment of the function of the inspiratory muscles which are functionally weaker and adverse effects on hemodynamics [9]. These factors together with flow-limiting dynamic airway compression during breathing may contribute to the dyspnea sensation [10].

Clinical aspects

Expiratory flow limitation at rest

The presence of resting tidal EFL represents an unfavourable functional condition which tends to be associated with a marked increase in airway resistance and therefore, is more commonly found in patients suffering from moderate-to-severe chronic obstructive pulmonary disease (COPD) [2, 5, 6] (Fig. 2) and bronchial asthma [5, 11]. Despite this general picture, changes in conventional indices of airway obstruction such as FEV_1, FEV./FVC and PEF, derived from full maximal flow/volume curve, are not useful to predict tidal EFL [2, 6, 11] and the adoption of special techniques is needed to accurately assess EFL in these patients [2, 12].

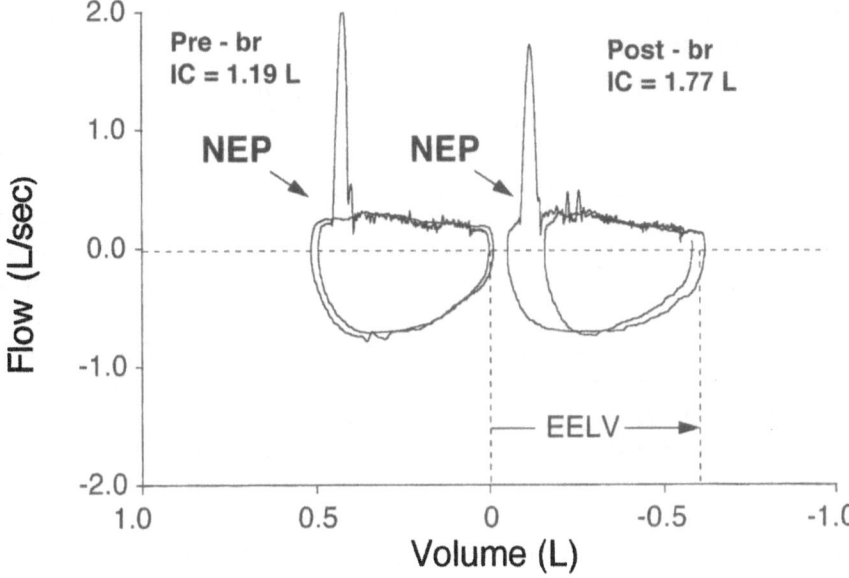

Fig. 2. In a representative COPD patient, tidal flow/volume loops and the corresponding test breath with application of negative expiratory pressure (NEP) are shown at rest, both in basal conditions (Pre-br) and after administration of bronchodilator (Post-br). According to the NEP method, complete EFL is present at baseline since the flow during NEP impinges on the control expiratory flow throughout the ensuing expiration (*loops at left*). After bronchodilator, although EFL persists, the reduction in end-expiratory lung volume (EELV), reflecting a decrease in dynamic pulmonary hyperinflation (DH), documents the presence of DH in basal conditions (*loops at right*). Modified from [24]

In COPD patients EFL at rest has been found to correlate with chronic dyspnea better than with routine spirometric indices [13]. This finding is not surprising because tidal EFL more than airway obstruction *per se* entails a greater risk of DH. DH, throughout its adverse effects on respiratory system mechanics and inspiratory muscle function, has been increasingly recognized as a main mechanism in the generation of dyspnea either at rest or during effort in COPD patients [7, 14].

During episodes of acute respiratory failure (ARF) COPD patients are prone to develop DH even in the absence of EFL because of both increased airway resistance with longer time constant of the respiratory system and rapid and shallow breathing with reduction in Te [9]. Moreover, higher ventilatory requirements due to fever, increased physiologic dead space and deterioration of gas exchange facilitate the occurrence of DH.

In the presence of EFL, however, all these factors may cause a catastrophic increase in DH which cannot be sustained for long during spontaneous breathing without acutely fatiguing the respiratory muscles, leading to the adoption of mechanical ventilation because of ventilatory failure.

In this respect, it should be stressed that almost all COPD patients mechanically ventilated for ARF invariably exhibit tidal EFL, since further increase in expiratory flow resistance is induced by endotracheal tube, expiratory circuit of the ventilator, and additional equipment, if any [15]. If these patients are sedated and paralyzed during controlled mechanical ventilation, the observation of the expiratory profile of the tidal flow/volume curve may suggest the presence of EFL by showing a distinct inflection point after which the expiratory limb of the flow/volume curve becames convex toward the volume axis over the entire EFL range of the tidal volume [15]. This is relevant when a form of assisted mechanical ventilation is started because under these circumstances the inspiratory work could be still very high for these patients, while an external PEEP, applied to counterbalance PEEPi, might reduce the threshold load without increasing the EELV.

Except for patients with chronic asthma (i.e.: with uninterrupted, long-lasting bronchial obstruction) [5], tidal EFL is seldom observed at rest in asthmatic subjects [11], unless under severe and prolonged attacks. In clinically stable patients with restrictive respiratory disorders EFL is very uncommon during resting breathing [16]. Data available in massive obesity [17, 18] and chronic congestive heart failure [19] indicate that tidal EFL is rarely present at rest in these conditions, at least in a seated position.

Expiratory flow limitation and posture

Tidal EFL occurring only in the supine position reflects a functionally less severe condition, although EFL during recumbency might be, at least in part, responsible for the onset of orthopnea in many patients.

On assuming the supine position the EELV decreases, tidal breathing occurs at a lower lung volume and the corresponding maximal expiratory flows are consequently reduced [20, 21]. Therefore, tidal EFL should be more easily observed in patients with obstructive lung disease when in the lying position. Indeed, both in COPD and asthmatic patients, tidal EFL has been more frequently detected in the supine than in the seated position [2, 6, 11]. Also in subjects who have a decreased expiratory reserve volume (ERV), the assumption of the supine posture could be potentially associated with the presence of EFL. This has been recently shown in massively obese subjects (Fig. 3) and patients with acute worsening of chronic heart failure (CHF) who exhibited tidal EFL essentially when recumbent [17, 19]. In all instances, the development of EFL in the supine position would prevent the EELV from reaching Vr, leading to dynamic hyperinflation and PEEPi. In line with this reasoning, a group of grossly obese subjects who developed EFL with recumbency, had a significant increase in PEEPi and diaphragmatic activity on shifting to the supine position [18]. Since this

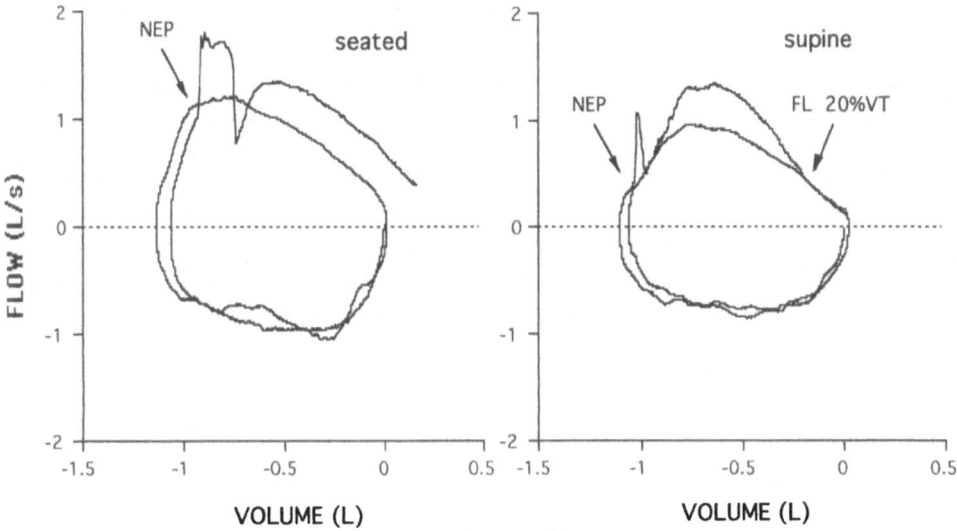

Fig. 3. Tidal flow-volume loops with the corresponding NEP test breath are shown during resting breathing both in seated (*left panel*) and supine position (*right panel*) in a representative healthy obese subject. Partial EFL encompassing 20% of the tidal volume is detected in the supine position (*right panel*), while is absent in the seated position (*left panel*) (VT = tidal volume). Modified from [17]

threshold load on the inspiratory muscles has been related to the dyspnea sensation [7, 14], the occurence of the supine EFL might play a role in eliciting orthopnea. Limited data suggest a fairly good correlation between the presence of EFL in the supine position and orthopnea both in morbidly obese subjects and in CHF patients [17, 19].

Expiratory flow limitation and exercise

While in normal subjects there is no evidence of tidal EFL during incremental exercise up to submaximal levels (90% of maximum predicted workload), and the EELV does not increase but rather decreases [8, 22], most of a group of mild-to moderate COPD patients (FEV_1 = 58 ± 20 %pred) exhibited tidal EFL and became dynamically hyperinflated according to a progressive decrease in the inspiratory capacity (IC) at light-to-moderate exercise [8]. Moreover, COPD patients who were flow limited at rest, showed a reduced maximal oxygen consumption ($\dot{V}O_2max$) amounting to 69 ± 7 %pred which was associated with a lower maximal tidal volume (Vtmax), probably indicating that a more severe DH occurred during exercise in this subset of patients. This was not the case in most of the other COPD patients who were non flow limited at rest. Since DH throughout its adverse effects on lung and chest wall mechanics, inspiratory muscle strength and neuro-ventilatory coupling, has been stressed as a key determinant of exertional dyspnea in COPD patients [7, 23], it is conceivable that COPD patients in whom tidal EFL is present at rest or quickly develops during exercise, should experience more dyspnea at equivalent, low work rates as compared to those without EFL. Consistent with this hypothesis, preliminary results indicate that breathlessness measured at the end of a 6-min steady state exercise performed by a cycloergometer at comparable effort (33% of the maximal workload) is greater in flow limited than in non flow limited COPD patients with similar degree of airway obstruction during resting breathing [24].

References

 1. Hyatt RE, Schilder P, Fry DL (1958) Relationship between maximum expiratory flow and degree of lung inflation. J Appl Physiol 13:331-336
 2. Koulouris NG, Valta P, Lavoie A et al (1995) A simple method to detect expiratory flow limitation during spontaneous breathing. Eur Respir J 8:306-613
 3. Grassi V, Cossi S, Leonardi R, Tantucci C (1998) The aging lung: Functional aspects. Aging Clin Exp Res 10(2):141
 4. Mota S, Casan P, Drobnic F et al (1997) Expiratory flow limitation in elite cyclists during exercise. Eur Respir J 10;S25:1594, pp 250s
 5. Pellegrino R, Brusasco V (1997) Lung hyperinflation and flow limitation in chronic airway obstruction. Eur Respir J 10:543-549
 6. Tantucci C, Duguet A, Similowski T et al (1998) Effect of salbutamol on dynamic hyperinflation in chronic obstructive pulmonary disease patients. Eur Respir J 12:799-804
 7. O'Donnell DE, Webb KA (1993) Exertional breathlessness in patients with chronic airflow limitation. The role of lung hyperinflation. Am J Respir Crit Care Med 148:1351-1357
 8. Koulouris NG, Dimopoulou I, Valta P et al (1997) Detection of expiratory flow limitation during exercise in COPD patients. J Appl Physiol 82(3):723-731
 9. Gottfried SB (1991) The role of PEEPi in the mechanically ventilated COPD patient. Roussos C, Marini JJ (eds) Ventilatory failure. Springer, Berlin, pp. 392-418
10. O'Donnell DE, Sanii R, Anthonisen NR, Younes M (1987) Effect of dynamic airway compression on breathing pattern and respiratory sensation in severe chronic obstructive pulmonary disease. Am Rev Respir Dis 135:912-918
11. Boczkowski G, Murciano D, Pichot M-H et al (1997) Expiratory flow limitation in stable asthmatic patients during resting breathing. Am J Respir Crit Care Med 1564:752-757
12. Valta P, Corbeil C, Lavoie A et al (1994) Detection of expiratory flow limitation during mechanical ventilation. Am J Respir Crit Care Med 150:1311-1317
13. Eltayara L, Becklake MR, Volta CA, Milic-Emili J (1996) Relationship between chronic dyspnea and expiratory flow limitation in patients with chronic obstructive pulmonary disease. Am J Respir Crit Care Med 154:1726-1734
14. O'Donnell DE, Webb KA (1992) Breathlessness in patients with severe chronic airflow limitation. Physiologic correlations. Chest 102:824-831
15. Gottfried SB, Rossi A, Higgs BD et al (1985) Noninvasive determination of respiratory system mechanics during mechanical ventilation for acute respiratory failure. Am Rev Respir Dis 131:414-420
16. Baydur A, Milic-Emili J (1997) Expiratory flow limitation during spontaneous breathing. Comparison of patients with restrictive and obstructive respiratory disorders. Chest 112:1017-1023

17. Ferretti A, Giampiccolo P, Brighi N et al (1998) Expiratory flow limitation and orthopnea sensation in obese subjects. Eur Respir J 12;S28, pp 151s
18. Pankow W, Podszus T, Gutheil T et al (1998) Expiratory flow limitation and intrinsic positive end-expiratory pressure in obesity. J Appl Physiol 85:1236-1243
19. Duguet A, Tantucci C, Thomas D et al (1997) Expiratory flow limitation and orthopnea in patients with acute left heart failure. Am J Respir Crit Care Med 155;No.4:A368.
20. Agostoni E, Mead J (1964) Statics of the respiratory system. Macklem PT, Mead J (eds) Handbook of Physiology. Section 3. Vol I, The Respiratory System: Mechanics of Breathing. Bethesda, American Physiological Society, pp. 387-409
21. Castile R, Mead J, Jackson A et al (1982) Effect of posture on flow-volume curve configuration in normal humans. J Appl Physiol 53:1175-1183
22. Beck KC, Staets BA, Hyatt RE, Babb TG (1991) Dynamics of breathing during exercise. Whipp BJ, Wassermann K (eds) Exercise. Marcel Dekker, New York, pp. 67-97
23. Belman MJ, Botnick WC, Shin JW (1996) Inhaled bronchodilators reduce dynamic hyperinflation during exercise in patients with chronic obstructive pulmonary disease. Am J Respir Crit Care Med 153:967-975
24. Boni E, Corda L, Damiani GP et al (1998) Volume effect and exertional dyspnea after bronchodilator in COPD patients with and without expiratory flow limitation. Eur Respir J 12; S28, pp 151s

Mechanisms of Intrinsic PEEP

W.A. ZIN

In treating a patient presenting respiratory functional impairment, the physician is left with the task of running tests to determine whether there is a mechanical component to the illness. One abnormality that must be sought is the intrinsic positive end-expiratory pressure (PEEPi).

Intrinsic PEEP [1, 2] is the difference between alveolar pressure and the pressure at the airway opening at the end of expiration. It has also been termed auto-PEEP [3], occult PEEP [3], inadverted PEEP [4], endogenous PEEP, and internal PEEP.

Although not difficult to accomplish, the precise determination of PEEPi and the subsequent interpretation of the results demand awareness of exact theoretical and methodological concepts [5, 6].

Etiology

Intrinsic PEEP can result from one the following phenomena [6, 7]:

– Dynamic hyperinflation;
– Expiratory muscle activity; and,
– Dynamic hyperinflation associated with expiratory muscle activity.

Dynamic hyperinflation

Dynamic hyperinflation represents the inability of lung volume to return to FRC (volume at which elastic recoil equals external PEEP) before the subsequent inspiration takes place [8].

Dynamic hyperinflation and the ensuing PEEPi can be characterized by: Alveolar pressure remaining greater than extrinsic PEEP throughout expiration; expiratory flow can be detected up to the beginning of the subsequent inspiration, unless airways collapse is present; it occurs in the presence of high expiratory resistance or expiratory flow limitation; and it is influenced by respiratory system compliance, lung volume at the beginning of expiration, and expiratory duration.

Dynamic hyperinflation can be most frequently caused by either slow pulmonary emptying or an inadequate ventilator setting. In the former case, the patient's mechanical characteristics, for instance, high expiratory resistance, can slow down expiration. Another cause of slow pulmonary emptying rests on the physical characteristics of the ventilation tubing: narrow tracheal tube, kinks along the expiratory circuit, liquid accumulation in the tubing, connectors, and valves. The ventilator setting can contribute to dynamic hyperinflation to the extent that a high respiratory frequency and the use of an elevated I:E ratio may yield a too short expiratory duration, thus impairing lung emptying. In the same context, if tidal volume is high, one should bear in mind the need to adjust expiratory duration accordingly [5-9].

Among the consequences of dynamic hyperinflation one could stress: the respiratory system will cycle at volumes closer to TLC, where compliance is decreased [10]; interference with the ventilator triggering in assisted and pressure support modes may occur [9, 10]; respiratory work during weaning attempts will increase [11, 12]; haemodynamics is jeopardized as if caused by external PEEP [13, 14]; and the pressure gradient required to generate tidal breathing may be overestimated, thus leading to underestimation of respiratory system compliance [1, 6].

Expiratory muscle activity

Expiratory muscle activy can produce interesting features: alveolar pressure results from the interaction between respiratory system elastic recoil pressure and the pressure generated by the active expiratory muscles; only the active patient can generate PEEPi under these circumstances; in this condition PEEPi can occur at FRC, or even at smaller lung volumes; concomitant dynamic hyperinflation is not mandatory; the magnitude of PEEPi generated by expiratory muscle activity does not represent the amount of dynamic hyperinflation; and, expiratory muscle activity frequently occurs in the face of increased respiratory neuromuscular drive and/or expiratory resistance.

As a consequence of expiratory muscle activity: the respiratory system will not cycle near TLC - in this case lung volume may be smaller than FRC; ventilator triggering will not be jeopardized; inspiratory muscular work will not increase - it may even decrease; compliance will not be underestimated - it may be overestimated instead; and the use of external PEEP is not recommended because it may thwart expiratory muscle function.

Dynamic hyperinflation associated with expiratory muscle activity

When the two aforementioned conditions are associated, the characteristics of both intermingle. For instance, expiratory muscle activity may worsen expiratory flow limitation and the use of external PEEP is not recommended because it may add an extra load to the system. Hence, the magnitude of the resulting PEEPi represents the addition of the effects of both dynamic hyperinflation and expiratory muscle activity. As a consequence of this complex interaction, to date consensus has not been reached on the optimal method of correcting for the effect of expiratory muscle activity in order to arrive at a more accurate estimate of the true elastic recoil pressure of the respiratory system [6].

Measurement

Intrinsic PEEP can me determined under both static and dynamic conditions: Static PEEPi is measured when no movement can be detected - it is believed that it would provide an average value of all pulmonary PEEPi's [3]. Dynamic PEEPi is determined during respiratory movement - it might represent the smallest PEEPi that could be found in the uneven lung [1, 15].

In the presence of dynamic hyperinflation or expiratory muscle activity PEEPi can be determined under passive breathing as well as during active ventilation.

Passive ventilation

Under passive ventilation PEEPi can be determined using one of four methods: end-expiratory airway occlusion, plateau pressures, apnea, and extrinsic PEEP.

- End-expiratory airway occlusion: The airways are occluded at end expiration, and the pressure difference obtained from the values taken before and during the occlusion equals PEEPi [3].
- Plateau pressures: Initially the airways are occluded at end inspiration during a regular breathing cycle, and the plateau pressure is determined. Then, ventilation is interrupted for 20 seconds. In the following inspiration plateau pressure is measured again. The difference between the two pressure values equals PEEPi.
- Apnea: Initially inspiration is impeded for 20 to 30 seconds, while exhaled gas volume (previously dynamically withheld in the lungs) is being measured. Thereafter this volume is divided by the respiratory system compliance. The resulting pressure value equals PEEPi [16-18].
- Extrinsic PEEP: Starting from ZEEP, extrinsic PEEP is progressively augmented up to a point when an increase in lung volume and/or peak airway pressure can be detected. This PEEP value represents PEEPi. It should be noted that this method is valid solely in the presence of dynamic compression of the airway. Therefore, it can not be used when a simple increase in expiratory resistance occurs [19].

Active ventilation

During active ventilation two methods can be employed to quantify PEEPi: end-expiratory airway occlusion and pressure variation between onsets of inspiratory effort and flow.

- End-expiratory airway occlusion: The airways are occluded at the end of a spontaneous expiration. This occlusion is maintained for one to three inspiratory efforts. The difference between the pressure values obtained before the occlusion and after inspiratory muscle relaxation equals PEEPi [3, 15].

- Pressure variation between the onsets of inspiratory effort and flow: Airflow and pressure (oesophageal or transpulmonary) are recorded. Pressure is read both at the onset of the inspiratory effort and when flow is nil at the beginning of inspiration. This pressure gradient represents PEEPi [1].

Dynamic hyperinflation and expiratory muscle activity

Recently it has been recognized that expiratory muscle activity may add its effects to dynamic hyperinflation [20, 21] in generating PEEPi. This association leads to a less accurate measurement of the elastic recoil pressure of the lung, and, consequently, of PEEPi.

The first approch to estimating elastic recoil pressure PEEPi recordings was introduced in 1994 [22]. The negative deflection in gastric pressure (Pga) is subtracted from the negative deflection in Poes during the interval between the onset of an increase in transdiaphragmatic pressure (Pdi) and the onset of inspiratory flow.

In 1995 two methods were proposed to correct for the contribution of expiratory muscle activity of measured PEEPi values, as determined by the pressure variation between the onsets of inspiratory effort and flow [21]. The first approach is to subtract the total fall in Pga from the initial decrease in Poes, based on the assumption that the fall in Pga is solely due to abdominal muscle relaxation. However, a fall in Pga could also result to some degree from diaphragmatic dysfunction associated with excessive accessory muscle recruitment. This method also ignores possible contributions from the expiratory rib cage muscles. The second approach subtracts the rise in Pga (from the end-inspiratory value to the peak end-expiratory value) from the initial decrease in Poes. This method is based on the assumption that the diaphragm has no phasic activity during expiration and functions as a passive membrane. It ignores the postinspiratory activity of the diaphragm, and may also underestimate activity of expiratory intercostal muscles.

In conclusion, although simple to be identified and measured under certain conditions, PEEPi may prove to be an elusive mechanical parameter, whose existence can impair respiratory and cardiovascular function.

References

1. Rossi A, Gottfried SB, Zocchi L et al (1985) Measurement of static compliance of the total respiratory system in patients with acute respiratory failure during mechanical ventilation. The effect of "intrinsic" PEEP. Am Rev Respir Dis 131:672-767
2. Rossi A, Polese G, Brandi G et al (1995) The intrinsic positive end expiratory pressure (PEEPi): physiology, implications, measurement, and treatment. Intens Care Med 21:522-536
3. Pepe PE, Marini JJ (1982) Occult positive end-expiratory pressure in mechanically ventilated patients with airflow obstruction: The auto-PEEP effect. Am Rev Respir Dis 126:166-170
4. Bancalari E (1986) Inadvertent positive end-expiratory pressure during mechanical ventilation. J Pediatr 108:567-569
5. Rossi A, Polese G, Milic-Emili J (1997) Monitoring respiratory mechanics in ventilator-dependent patients. In: Tobin MJ (ed) Principles and practice of intensive care monitoring. McGraw-Hill, New York, pp 553-596
6. Tobin MJ (1997) Monitoring respiratory mechanics in spontaneously breathing patients. In: Tobin MJ (ed) Principles and practice of intensive care monitoring. McGraw-Hill, New York, pp 617-654
7. Marini JJ (1988) Monitoring during mechanical ventilation. Clin Chest Med 9:73-100
8. Marcy TW, Marini JJ (1994) Respiratory distress in the ventilated patient. Clin Chest Med 15:55-73
9. Marcy TW, Marini JJ (1992) Modes of mechanical ventilation. Curr Pulmonol 13:43-90
10. Amato MBP, Barbas CSV, Bonassa J et al (1992) Volume-assured pressure support ventilation (VAPSV). Chest 102:1225-1234
11. Hubmayr RD, Abel MD, Rehder K (1990) Physiologic approach to mechanical ventilation. Crit Care Med 18:103-113
12. Eissa NT, Milic-Emili J (1991) Modern concepts in monitoring and management of respiratory failure. Respiratory mechanics. Anesthesiol Clin N Am 9:199-218
13. Harken AH, Brennan MF, Smith B et al (1974) The hemodynamic response to positive end-expiratory pressure ventilation in hypovolemic patients. Surgery 76:786-793
14. Whittenberg JL, McGregor M, Berglund E et al (1960) Influence of the state of inflation of the lung on pulmonary vascular resistance. J Appl Physiol 15:878-882
15. Petrof BJ, Legaré M, Goldberg P et al (1990) Continuous positive airway pressure reduces work of breathing and dyspnea during weaning from mechanical ventilation in severe chronic obstructive pulmonary disease. Am Rev Respir Dis 141:281-289
16. Kimball WR, Leith DE, Robins AG (1982) Dynamic hyperinflation and ventilator dependence in chronic obstructive pulmonary disease. Am Rev Respir Dis 126:991-995
17. Ranieri VM, Eissa NT, Corbeil C et al (1991) Effects of positive end-expiratory pressure on alveolar recruitment and gas exchange in patients with the adult respiratory distress syndrome. Am Rev Respir Dis 144:544-551
18. Tuxen DV, Lane S (1987) The effects of ventilatory pattern on hyperinflation airway pressures, and circulation in mechanical ventilation of patients with severe airflow obstruction. Am Rev Respir Dis 136:872-879
19. Tobin MJ, Lodato RF (1989) PEEP, auto-PEEP and waterfalls (editorial). Chest 96:449
20. Ninane V, Yernault J-C, De Troyer A (1993) Intrinsic PEEP in patients with chronic obstructive pulmonary disease: role of expiratory muscles. Am Rev Respir Dis 148:1037-1042
21. Lessard MR, Lofaso F, Brochard L (1995) Expiratory muscle activity increases intrinsic positive end-expiratory pressure independently of dynamic hyperinflation in mechanically ventilated patients. Am J Respir Crit Care Med 151:562-569
22. Appendini L, Patessio A, Zanaboni S et al (1994) Physiologic effects of positive end-expiratory pressure and mask pressure support during exacerbations of chronic obstructive pulmonary disease. Am J Respir Crit Care Med 149:1069-1076

Static and Dynamic Intrinsic PEEP and Respiratory Mechanics in Mechanically Ventilated COPD Patients

V. Antonaglia, A. Peratoner, L. De Simoni

In 1982, Pepe and Marini [1] pointed out the clinical importance of dynamic increase in end-expiratory lung volume and positive end-expiratory alveolar pressure in mechanically ventilated patients with airflow obstruction. This end-expiratory pressure was termed "occult, auto or intrinsic PEEP" (PEEPi) and is due to the positive end-expiratory elastic recoil pressure of the total respiratory system consequent to incomplete lung emptying. In patients with severe airflow obstruction, because the rate of the lung emptying is slow relative to the available expiratory duration, the expiration is interrupted by the subsequent breath before the relaxation volume of the respiratory system (Vr) is reached. The increase in end expiratory lung volume above Vr is termed dynamic pulmonary hyperinflation. Dynamic hyperinflation and PEEPi were detected not only in ventilated patients with airway obstruction but also in ventilated patients with other disorders [2-4] and in all ventilatory conditions in which a short expiratory time is used, as inverse ratio ventilation (5, 6].

Deleterious effects of high values of PEEPi were observed on cardiac output and oxygen transport [1], work of the respiratory muscles during inspiratory efforts expended by the patients in assisted modes of mechanical ventilation [2, 7-10] as well as during weaning and spontaneous ventilation [11, 12]. In effect PEEPi functions as an inspiratory threshold load [13]. Therefore, it has been suggested by several authors that PEEPi should be routinely monitored in all mechanically ventilated patients [2, 14-20]. Monitoring PEEPi is of particular importance in expiratory flow limited COPD patients during assisted or spontaneus ventilation, because it is possible to assess the response to the application of external PEEP or CPAP [7, 21, 22].

Static and dynamic PEEPi

The measurement of PEEPi can be performed under static and dynamic conditions by airway occlusion at end-expiration (PEEPi,stat) and by recording the value in airway pressure corresponding to zero flow at the begin of lung inflation (PEEPi,dyn).The plateau in airway pressure during end-expiratory occlusion, PEEPi,stat represents the average PEEPi of the pulmonary districts with different time constants after a sufficient equilibration time between regional alveolar and airway opening pressure. The value of airway pressure at zero inspiratory flow, PEEPi,dyn corresponds to the lowest PEEPi in the districts with the shortest time constants and will underestimate PEEPi,stat in the presence of significant time constant inequalities [12]. Originally, both measurements were performed on the airway pressure in mechanically ventilated patients, the greater part of whom were COPD patients, and only a modest and not significant difference between the values of PEEPi,dyn and PEEPi,stat was observed [23]. Therefore, in the clinical intensive care setting PEEPi was routinely measured under static conditions by the customary manoeuvre of end-expiratory occlusion. A discrepancy between the values of PEEPi,dyn and PEEPi,stat was observed in PEEPi in spontaneously breathing COPD patients using a modified method [12] compared to that previously used [23]. The value of the drop in oesophageal pressure at zero inspiratory flow was referred to as dynamic PEEPi and was compared to that of plateau of airway pressure between occluded efforts corresponding to the elastic recoil pressure of the respiratory system. PEEPi,dyn levels were lower than the corresponding PEEPi,stat values and a positive correlation was found between the values of PEEPi,dyn and PEEPi,stat. This discrepancy was imputed to mechanical dynamic factors and expiratory muscle recruitment and tonic inspiratory muscle activity [12, 24-26].

More recently, using the original method a significant difference between the measurements of PEEPi,dyn and PEEPi,stat was reported in animals after administration of metacholine [27] and in sedated, paralysed patients with severe airway obstruction but not in mechanically ventilated patients with other disorders [28]. Maltais et al. [28] used the ratio PEEPi,dyn/PEEPi,stat to assess the degree of discrepancy between the static and dynamic measurements of PEEPi in the two groups. In COPD patients, the average ratio was 0.36 ± 0.06. They related the ratio PEEPi,dyn/PEEPi,stat to parameters of respiratory mechanics obtained by end-inspiratory airway occlusion and found that the ratio PEEPi, dyn/PEEPi,stat was inversely correlated to the slow decay after end-inspiratory airway occlusion, i.e. the end-inspiratory stress adaptation, reflecting the viscoelastic pressure dissipation and regional time constant inequalities. Because no correlation was found between PEEPi,dyn/PEEPi,stat and other mechanics parameters, the authors suggested that the discrepancy between dynamic and static PEEPi is related to regional differences in mechanical properties within the lung and/or increased viscoelastic pressure losses and that the discrepancy was not found previously because there were important differences in the severity of the airway obstruction of the patients and in the technical equipment between the two studies [23, 28].

PEEP applied through the external ventilator circuit has been used to decrease the work of breathing during asssisted or spontaneous breathing modes in patients with severe COPD and flow limitation [7, 21, 22]. "Critical PEEP" is the term given to the value of external PEEP which impedes expiratory flow and promotes further hyperinflation. In agreement with basic physiological principles characterising flow limitation, the value of critical PEEP is somewhat lower than the existing value of PEEPi,stat. In the present context, the critical PEEP should be equivalent to PEEPi,dyn. The ratio PEEPi,dyn/PEEPi,stat obtained in the study by Maltais et al. [28] was considerably lower than that observed between critical PEEP and PEEPi,stat in previous studies, which amounted to as much as 75% [7, 12, 29, 30]. The reasons for this discrepancy are not entirely clear. Excessive resistive pressure losses across the more proximal airways as well as the endotracheal tube and ventilator circuit [33] and the re-expansion of conducting airways dynamically compressed during the preceding expiration [28] might play a role.

In order to determine the entity of the ratio PEEPi,dyn/PEEPi,stat in mechanically ventilated patients, an important point is the baseline ventilatory setting. In mechanically ventilated COPD patients, using the same minute ventilation, Ve, at different values of respiratory rate or inspiratory time, we observed a wide range of the ratio PEEPi,dyn/PEEPi,stat.

Can the PEEPi,dyn/PEEPi,stat ratio be used to assess the degree of disease in mechanically ventilated COPD patients?

In the past, excluding the P_1-P_2 difference, significant relationships were not found between the other mechanical parameters of the respiratory system obtained with end-inspiratory occlusion and the PEEPi,dyn/PEEPi,stat ratio. Presumably, as for the relationship between the P_1-P_2 difference and PEEPi,dyn/PEEPi,stat, Maltais et al. [28] compared total and interrupted resistances to the PEEPi,dyn/PEEPi,stat ratio in all patients, whether with obstructed airway or not. Because the values of the resistances in patients without airway obstruction were low, they did not found significant relationships.

To determine whether the discrepancy between dynamic and static PEEPi in mechanically ventilated COPD patients depends on the severity of airway obstruction, we studied the values of PEEPi,stat and PEEPi,dyn in a population of 10 COPD patients in acute respiratory failure, who were admitted to the intensive care unit of Cattinara Hospital requiring orotracheal intubation and mechanical ventilation for infection of the upper respiratory tract. In other words, the aim of our study was to assess whether the ratio PEEPi,dyn/PEEPi,stat can be used to demonstrate the degree of disease of mechanically ventilated COPD patients. We found the difference between PEEPi,stat and PEEPi,dyn was statistically significant ($p < 0.002$). The relationship between PEEPi,stat and PEEPi,dyn-values was described by the regression equation: PEEPi,dyn = 0.34 x PEEPi,stat + 0.3 $r = 0.889$ ($p < 0.0001$). Table 1 also depicts the mean values of standard mechanics' parameters obtained during baseline ventilation by end-inspiratory airway occlusion.

Table 1. Respiratory mechanics' variables of the 10 COPD patients during baseline ventilation

$PEEP_{i,stat}$ (cm H_2O)	$PEEP_{i,dyn}$ (cm H_2O)	$PEEP_{i,dyn/stat}$	$E_{st,rs}$ (cm $H_2O \cdot L^{-1}$)	$E_{dyn,rs}$ (cm $H_2O \cdot L^{-1}$)	R_{rs} (cm $H_2O \cdot L^{-1} \cdot s$)	$R_{int,rs}$ (cm $H_2O(L^{-1} \cdot s)$	ΔP (cm H_2O)
7.1	2.91	0.41	15.1	23.9	14.88	8.22	3.89
4.18	1.66	0.13	3.1	5.8	6.84	4.70	1.41

Values are means ± SD. Values correspond to the average of 3 tests; $_{rs}$, total respiratory system; $E_{st,rs}$ static elastance; $E_{dyn,rs}$ dynamic elastance; R_{rs} resistance; $R_{int,rs}$ interrupted resistance; ΔP difference P_1-P_2

A significant inverse relationship was found between the difference P_1-P_2, Rrs, and Rint,rs and the ratio PEEPi,dyn/PEEPi,stat: (y = −6.5 x +6.8, r = −0.58) (p = 0.048), (y = −38.5 x +33, r = −0.78) (p = 0.0025), (y = −23.7 x +19.6, r = −0.67) (p = 0.017), respectively. No correlation was found between the static and dynamic elastance respiratory system and PEEPi,dyn/PEEPi,stat.

The present investigation confirms that PEEPi,dyn understimates PEEPi,stat in COPD patients. As in the study by Maltais and coworkers [28], using a similar protocol, data analysis, and equipment we found a significant difference between the measurements of PEEPi,dyn and PEEPi,stat (p < 0.002). The mean values of total and interrupter resistances were significantly less than those of the patients with airway obstruction in the study by Maltais and coworkers [28], but similar to those of the patients in the earlier study [23]. In this regard, the total resistances, Rrs, and the interrupted resistances, Rint,rs, averaged 13.7 ± 2.4 and 7.4 ± 1.5 cm $H_2O \cdot L^{-1}$, respectively, for 7 of the 10 previously reported patients in whom these results were available [23]. Consequently, the lack of significant difference between the dynamic and static measurements of PEEPi found in this study [23] is not imputable to important differences in the severity of airway obstruction between the population studied and that of Maltais's investigation, but presumably to technical issues in the former noted in the investigation of Maltais and coworkers [28].

In the present investigation the relationship between PEEPi,stat and PEEPi,dyn-values was described by the regression equation: PEEPi,dyn = 0.34 x PEEPi,stat + 0.3. In the previous study of mechanically ventilated COPD patients [23, 28] the relationship between PEEPi,stat and PEEPi,dyn-values was not reported. If we compare the regression equation of the present invesigation to the equation previously published by Petrof and coworkers [12] and Van den Berg and coworkers [31] in spontaneously breathing COPD patients, it can be seen that the slope of the regression equation in ventilated patients is less steep.

In contrast to the investigation of Maltais and coworkers [28], we found a significant inverse relationship between Rrs and Rint,rs to PEEPi,dyn/PEEPi,stat. Presumably, as stated before, this was because they studied the resistances in all patients, with airway obstruction or not, and the low resistances in the non-obstructed patients obfuscated potentially significant relationships. The total or maximal resistance of the respiratory system, Rrs, can be partitionated into ohmic, interrupter resistance Rint,rs and additional resistance, ΔRrs, obtained as P_1-P_2 divided by the corresponding end-inspiratory flow. We found a better relationship between Rint,rs and the ratio PEEPi,dyn/PEEPi,stat ($r = -0.67$ $p = 0.017$) than between the difference P_1-P_2 or the additional resistances and this ratio ($r = -0.58$ $p = 0.049$).

In the study by Maltais and coworkers [28] the mean value of the ratio PEEPi,dyn/PEEPi,stat (0.36 ± 0.06) of the patients with airway obstruction was less than that of the present investigation (0.41 ± 0.13). This is probably the result of the higher values of the difference P_1-P_2 and resistances observed in airway obstructed patients in Maltais's study. The mean values of the difference P_1-P_2, Rrs, and Rint,rs were higher than those of the present investigation by 66, 63 and 45%, respectively.

Conclusion

We found significant relationships between the PEEPi,dyn/PEEPi,stat ratio and the resistances of the respiratory system. Thus, the PEEPi,dyn/PEEPi,stat ratio should be considered indicative of the degree of disease in COPD patients.

Since the ratio can have the same value when PEEPi,dyn and PEEPi,stat both have low values or both have high values, it is important to "weigh" this ratio by the value of PEEPi,stat and compare it to the standard mechanics' parameters.

The "weighted" ratio PEEPi,dyn/PEEPi,stat should be studied at different ventilatory settings to confirm the relationships between it and the corresponding respirory parameters. If at PEEPi,dyn/PEEPi,stat the ratio is confirmed in these conditions as an expression of the degree of disease in ventilated COPD patients, it should be used to monitor the time-course of acute ventilatory failure and responsiveness to therapy.

References

1. Pepe PE, Marini JJ (1982) Occult positive end-expiratory pressure in mechanically ventilated patients with airflow obstruction: the auto-PEEP effect. Am Rev Respir Dis 126:166-170
2. Gottfried SB, Rossi A, Milic-Emili J (1986) Dynamic hyperinflation, intrinsic PEEP, and the mechanically ventilated patient. Intensive and Critical Care Digest 5:30-33
3. Broseghini C, Brandolese R, Poggi R et al (1988) Respiratory mechanics during the first day of mechanical ventilation in patients with pulmonary edema and chronic airway obstruction. Am Rev Respir Dis 138:355-361
4. Broseghini C, Brandolese R, Poggi R et al (1988) Respiratory resistance and intrinsic positive end-expiratory pressure in patients with the adult respiratory distress syndrome Eur Respir J 1:726-731

5. Abraham E, Yoshihara G (1989) Cardiorespiratory effects of pressure controlled inverse ratio ventilation in severe respiratory failure. Chest 96:1356-1359
6. Mercat A, Titiriga M, Anguel N et al (1997) Inverse ratio ventilation in acute respiratory distress syndrome. Am J Respir Crit Care Med 155:1637-1642
7. Smith TC, Marini JJ (1988) Impact of PEEP on lung mechanics and work of breathing in severe airflow obstruction. J Appl Physiol 65:1488-1499
8. Fernandez R, Benito S, Blanch LL (1988) Intrinsic PEEP: a cause of inspiratory muscle ineffectivity. Intensive Care Med 15:51-52
9. Braschi A, Iotti G, Rodi G et al (1988) Dynamic pulmonary hyperinflation during intermittent mandatory ventilation. Intensive Care Med 14:284-287
10. Rossi A, Brandolese R, Milic-Emili J et al (1990) The role of PEEP in patients with chronic obstructive pulmonary disease during assisted ventilation. Eur Respir J 3:818-822
11. Calderini E, Petrof B, Gottfried SB (1989) Continuous positive airway pressure improves efficacy of pressure support ventilation in severe COPD. Am Rev Respir Dis 139:A155
12. Petrof BJ, Legare M, Goldberg P et al (1990) Continuous positive airway pressure reduces work of breathing and dyspnea during weaning from mechanical ventilation in severe chronic obstructive pulmonary diseases. Am Rev Respir Dis 141:281-289
13. Campbell FJM, Dikinson CJ, Dinnick OP, Howell JBL (1964) The immediate effects of threshold loads on the breathing of men and dogs. Clin Sci 172:321-331
14. Fleury B, Murciano C, Talamo C et al (1985) Work of breathing in patients with chronic obstructive pulmonary disease in acute respiratory failure. Am Rev Respir Dis 131:822-827
15. Gottfried SB, Rossi A, Higgs BD et al (1985) Non-invasive determination of respiratory system mechanics during mechanical ventilation for acute respiratory failure. Am Rev Respir Dis 131:414-420
16. Brown DG, Pierson DJ (1986) Auto-PEEP is a common in mechanically ventilated patients: a study of incidence, severity, and detection. Respir Care 31:1069-1074
17. Gottfried SB, Milic-Emili J (1986) Non-invasive monitoring of respiratory system mechanics. In: Cherniack NS, Nochomovitz M (eds) Non-invasive respiratory monitoring. Churchill Livingston, New York, pp 59-82
18. Benson MS, Pierson DJ (1988) Auto-PEEP during mechanical ventilation of adults. Respir Care 33:557-565
19. Marini JJ (1988) Monitoring during mechanical ventilation. Clin Chest Med 9:73-100
20. Patel H, Yang K (1995) Variability of intrinsic positive end-expiratory pressure in patients receiving mechanical ventilation. Crit Care Med 23:1074-1079
21. Gay CG, Rodarte JR, Hubmayr RD (1989) The effects of positive expiratory pressure on isovolume flow and dynamic hyperinflation in patients receiving mechanical ventilation. Am Rev Respir Dis 139:621-626
22. Ranieri MV, Giuliani R, Cinella G et al (1993) Physiologic effects of positive end-expiratory pressure in patients with chronic obstructive pulmonary disease during acute ventilatory failure and controlled mechanical ventilation. Am Rev Respir Dis 147:5-13
23. Rossi A, Gottfried SB, Zocchi L et al (1985) Measurement of static compliance of the total respiratory system in patients with acute respiratory failure during mechanical ventilation: the effect of intrinsic positive end-expiratory pressure. Am Rev Respir Dis 131:672-677
24. Ninane V, Yernault JC, De Troyer A (1993) Intrinsic PEEP in patients with chronic obstructive pulmonary disease: role of expiratory muscles. Am Rev Respir Dis 148:1037-1042
25. Lessard MR, Lofaso F, Brochard L (1995) Expiratory muscle activity increases intrinsic positive end-expiratory pressure independently of dynamic hyperinflation in mechanically ventilated patients. Am J Respir Crit Care Med 151:562-569
26. Yan S, Kayser B, Tobiasz M, Sliiwinski P (1996) Comparison of static and dynamic intrinsic positive end-expiratory pressure using the Campbell Diagram. Am J Respir Crit Care Med 154:938-944

27. Hernandez P, Navalesi P, Maltais F et al (1994) Comparison of static and dynamic measurements of intrinsic PEEP in anesthetized cats. J Appl Physiol 76:2437-2442
28. Maltais F, Reissmann H, Navalesi P et al (1994) Comparison of static and dynamic measurements of intrinsic PEEP in mechanically ventilated patients. Am J Respir Crit Care Med 150: 1318-1324
29. Gay PC, Rodarte JR, Hubmayr RD (1989) The effects of PEEP on isovolume flow and dynamic hyperinflation in patients receiving mechanical ventilation. Am Rev Resp Dis 139: 621-626
30. Ranieri VM, Giuliani R, Cinella G et al (1993) A physiologic effects of PEEP in patients with COPD during acute respiratory failure and controlled mechanical ventilation. Am Rev Resp Dis 147:5-13
31. Van Den Berg B, Aerts JGJV, Bogaard JM (1995) Effect of continuous positive airway pressure in patients with chronic obstructive pulmonary disease depending on intrinsic PEEP levels. Acta Anaesthesiol Scand 39:1097-1102

Respiratory Rehabilitation

R. Brandolese, U. Andreose

Medicine has passed through different periods during its evolutionary process: unthinking medicine, empirical medicine, sacerdotal, magic and finally rationale medicine. Description of breathing exercise dates back to 2500 years BC during the period of empirical medicine. The first therapeutic respiratory description goes back to Tissot's work in 1781 [1]. In 1950 institutions dedicated to rehabilitation of patients affected by lung disease (tubercolosis) or by neuromuscular respiratory paralysis (poliomyelitis) appeared.

Actually the prevalence of different intrinsic lung disease such as chronic obstructive pulmonary disease (COPD) and other diseases involving the spinal cord and neuromuscular junction create an increasing demand on respiratory rehabilitation units. Pulmonary rehabilitation has been defined as "multidimensional continuum of services directed to the patient with pulmonary disease and family, usually by a multidisciplinary specialists, with the goal to achieve and maintain the individual maximal level of independence and functioning in the community" [2]. Pulmonary rehabilitation can be applied to COPD patients, to patients with neuromuscular diseases and/or to patients with breathing disorders during sleep and finally to subjects affected by medical, trauma brain injuries, stroke complicating their original disease with pulmonary dysfunction or insufficiency.

Rehabilitation in COPD patients

In Europe COPD is the fourth leading cause of death. Its incidence, in the world, is increasing rapidly and it is becoming a social disease because 50% of patients are work-limited whereas 25% are bed disabled [3].

Pathophysiology

COPD can be defined as a disorder characterized by abnormal tests of expiratory flow that do not change markedly over a period of several months. Cigarette smoke is the predominant cause of the disease in COPD patients because of chronic bronchitis and emphysema. Moreover, asthma and cystic fibrosis lead to the development of COPD [4].

Expiratory flow obstruction may be due to four mechanisms:

1. intraluminal secretions
2. bronchial wall thickening
3. smooth muscle hypertrophy
4. bronchoconstriction and loss of airway supporting structure

These pathological characteristics may affect airway responsiveness, lung mechanics, the respiratory muscles, gas exchange, control of breathing and pulmonary circulation.

The two major mechanical alterations of the lung in COPD are an increase in airway resistance and loss of elastic recoil pressure of the lung. Expiratory flow-limitation causes air trapping and is also responsible for pulmonary dynamic hyperinflation and intrinsic PEEP (PEEPi) [4]. An increase in the total lung capacity determines a shortening in the diaphragm fibers causing the diaphragm to work in a disadvantageous position with respect to its length-tension relationship. Moreover the presence of PEEPi causes an added elastic inspiratory threshold load that has to be overcome by the inspiratory muscles to initiate the inspiration. Consequently, the work of breathing is enhanced. The increased inspiratory load causes an increase in the central respiratory drive with a rapid shallow breathing pattern and chest wall-abdomen compartment asynchrony [5].

Hypoxemia develops as a result of VA/Q mismatching whereas the onset of hypercapnia, associated with an ominous prognosis, may be due to a combination of high inspiratory loads and muscle weakness but, also, to a ventilatory strategy made by the patients in order to spare their inspiratory muscles. COPD patients have a decreased capability to perform normal physical tasks because of decreased ventilatory reserve [6], hypoxemia dysfunction of respiratory muscles and a comprised function in right ventricular secondary to pulmonary hypertension. FEV1, maximal voluntary ventilation (MVV), Maximal inspiratory pressure (Pimax), are well-established predictors of exercise in COPD patients.

Standard medical treatment is a cornerstone in management of COPD patient during acute exacerbation of the disease and it is important to alleviate symptoms that usually persist during subacute and chronic phase. Pharmacological management includes the use of methylxantines that act as bronchodilators and these appear to ameliorate the endurance of the diaphragm to fatigue [7]. Moreover beta agonists, systemic and inhaled glucocorticoid, mucolytics antibiotics are widely used in COPD patients.

Significant weight loss occurs in 20-70% of COPD patients presenting evidence of clinical undernourishment and impaired nutritional status. Undernourishment is associated to a greater morbidity and mortality and to an elevated incidence of infections. Undernourishment can lead to respiratory muscles atrophy and decrease exercise capacity [8].

Patient selection

Any patient with symptomatic chronic lung disease is a candidate for pulmonary rehabilitation. Age alone should not be used as a criterion for respiratory rehabilitation program. Lung function measurements are weak predictors of symptoms, function and improvement of clinical status. Pulmonary rehabilitation is has not to be considered a primary mode of respiratory therapy and patients must not suffer from an unstable clinical condition that would limit their capability to participate in rehabilitation. The ideal patient for respiratory rehabilitation may be one with moderate or moderately severe lung disease, stable on standard medical therapy, not limited by other clinical conditions, willing and motivated to participate in a rehabilitation program [9].

Components of a pulmonary rehabilitation program

Breathing retraining

Rapid shallow breathing is a common respiratory pattern in COPD patients. Small tidal volume causes an increase of VD/VT ratio; and consequently, a decrease in alveolar ventilation. The short expiratory time exhibited because of the increased respiratory rate does not permit a complete exhalation of the tidal volume in the presence of augmented expiratory flow resistance so that the dynamic hyperinflation appears and hence PEEPi.

Patients with chronic airway obstruction (CAO), have an altered pattern of recruitment of the respiratory muscles in which the activity of inspiratory muscle of rib cage is predominant, so that during inspiration a paradoxical inward of the upper abdominal wall is visible [10].

Instruction in breathing technique such as pursed lip and diaphragmatic breathing may help to improve to the ventilatory pattern and gas exchange and assist patients to control the symptoms of breathlessness [11]. These technique are performed in supine position or in moderate "antitrendelemburg" in order to decrease the flow limitation by increasing the functional residual capacity (FRC). In this posture, in fact, the diaphragm is pulled into a lower part of the abdomen so enhancing the height of the lungs.

Airway secretion elimination

COPD patients, usually, are unable to perform an effective cough and hence to ensure airway patency. Chest percussion and postural drainage can be useful to mobilize secretions especially in those patients with a lot of sputum production more than 30-40 ml/day [12]. Application of positive end expiratory pressure (PEEP) is used in order to increase the volume closure capacity by increasing functional residual capacity (FRC) by recruiting to the ventilation the small airways occupied by retrained secretions. The optimal level of PEEP externally applied is based, empirically, on the degree of comfort or discomfort exhibited by the patient with application of increasing level of PEEP [13]. Other techniques have been proposed to mobilize pulmonary secretions such as flutter breathing, mechanical vibration or oscillation applied to the thorax or directly to the airways. However, controlled studies have been done to demonstrate clinical benefit.

Inspiratory resistive exercise

Endurance training has been performed successfully with voluntary isocapnic hyperventilation, inspiratory resistive loading and inspiratory threshold load [14]. Some authors reported an improved respiratory muscles function and reduced dyspnea after 8 weeks of inspiratory resistance training [15]. But, in general, the efficacy of this rehabilitation technique, has not been consistently demonstrated and such training cannot be widely recommended for general application in pulmonary rehabilitation.

Exercise induced hypoxemia

The occurrence of hypoxemia during exercise is a major problem in planning a safe rehabilitative program. Normal healthy individuals do not develop hypoxemia during exercise and COPD patients present an unpredictable value of PaO_2 during exercise. Hence, it is important to assess arterial oxygenation in order to avoid a dangerous hypoxemia and make possible to continue the exercise training by administering oxygen. The most widely accepted guideline for delivering oxygen during training is SaO_2 at less than 90% [16].

Respiratory muscles rest

In the diagram model of Bellamare-Grassino predicting the occurrence of respiratory muscle fatigue with different inspiratory loadings combined with different duration of inspiratory time, COPD patients, in stable condition, usually breath near to the fatigue zone and relatively minor changes in the pattern of breathing compel them to ventilate through the line that separate the fatigue from the non-fatigue area (critical zone). In this condition, periods of exercise and muscular rest are mandatory as a basic principle of respiratory rehabilitation. The diaphragm is put at rest using assisted mechanical ventilation by facial and/or nasal mask (non invasive positive pressure ventilation, NIPPV). NIPPV not only spares the inspiratory muscles but, also acts as a pneumatic splint that prevents airway collapse [17].

Results of pulmonary rehabilitation

The results of pulmonary rehabilitation may be expressed as follows:

Reduced:
- use of medical resources
- hospitalization
- respiratory symptoms
- psychological symptoms

Improved:
- quality of life
- exercise tolerance
- endurance

However there is no change in lung function and survival. Many studies indicate that respiratory rehabilitation results in significant improvement in ambulation capacity, exercise endurance, and maximum inspiratory pressure. The benefits of pulmonary rehabilitation on exercise performance and quality of life persist up to 12-18 months [18].

Rehabilitation of restrictive pulmonary disease

Restrictive pulmonary disease is due to:
1. primary parenchymal disease
2. surgical removal of lung parenchyma
3. disease of the pleura
4. disease of the chest wall
5. respiratory muscle weakness

The features of restrictive pulmonary disease are:
- low vital capacity
- decreased TLC
- increased respiratory rate
- increased pulmonary elastance
- increased elastic work of breathing

Thoracic deformities, obesity, hypopharyngeal collapse during sleep alter chest wall and lung mechanics increasing the mechanical workload for the inspiratory muscles. Unable to sustain a prefixed minute ventilation they become fatigued [19]. Original pulmonary deterioration is exacerbated by acute respiratory tract infection which can promote lung scarring; and because of repeated pneumonia patients with restrictive pulmonary disease worsen with aging or disease progression. For instance in Duchenne muscular dystrophy VC is lost at a rate of 250 ml per year. Patients with amyotrophic lateral sclerosis may lose their VC at a rate of 1000 ml per year; and with the loss of VC the patient is unable to perform sighs so that microatelectasis develop [20]. To overcome the increased elastic recoil pressure of total respiratory system the elastic work remarkably enhances. In patients with restrictive pulmonary disease who are mechanically ventilated because bronchopneumonia, we have found values of respiratory system compliance as low as 25 ml/cm H_2O. This signifies that the elastic workload for the respiratory muscles has to be incréased four times in comparison to that performed in normal subjects. This work appears to be too high to become sustained for a long period of time. The first significant blood gas alteration with restrictive pulmonary disease is hypercapnia usually associated to hypoxemia. Unless treated, this results in cor pulmonale and cardiac arrhythmias. Hypercapnia occurs when VC decrease below 40-50% of predicted value [21].

Patient with restrictive pulmonary disease have greater weakness in the expiratory than inspiratory muscles. Consequently, they have great difficulty to clear secretions and to cough.

Treatment

Maintenance of respiratory muscle strength and endurance

Shortly daily sessions of inspiratory resistance exercises performed in patients with neuromuscular disease have no effect on spirometry or maximum inspiratory or expiratory pressure but improve respiratory muscle endurance [22]. Improvement in endurance occurs in those patients in which VC is more than 30% of predicted. No improvement has been shown in patients with a reduction in VC under 30% of predicted.

Moreover there is no evidence that the ameliorated maximum inspiratory and expiratory pressures preserve muscular function i.e. delaying the time when the patient will require ventilatory aid. The training itself may de dangerous for patients in advanced stage of the illness.

Glossopharyngeal breathing (GPB)

Glossopharyngeal method is a non-invasive method to support ventilation: The patient is instructed to perform a deep breath and then to augment it by GPB. The tongue and glossopharyngeal muscles propel a bolus of 50-100 ml of air past the vocal cord. The vocal cords, after each bolus close; one breath consists of 5-10 gulps. A GPB rate of 12-12 min is able to provide patients with little VC with normal tidal volume and hours of ventilator-free time [23].

Airway secretion clearance

Patients with respiratory muscle weakness are clearly unable to generate pressures as high as 140-150 cm H_2O necessary to perform an efficacious cough. Chest percussion and postural drainage are widely prescribed methods to facilitate elimination of airway secretions, but there is no controlled study that demonstrates the efficacy of these methods in reducing morbidity and mortality.

A lot of manually assisting coughing methods have been proposed They are effective in removing secretions because the manual manoeuvre is able to produce an expiratory peak flow of 300L/min [24]. But, these methods are quite inadequate in patients with scoliosis. Then the mechanical insufflator-exufflator devices are indicated and effective.

Noninvasive ventilatory support

Intermittent positive pressure ventilation can be provided by different systems:
– Mouthpiece intermittent positive pressure ventilation (IPPV)
– Nasal IPPV
– Oronasal IPPV
– Body ventilators
– Intermittent abdomen pressure ventilator
– Negative pressure body ventilators

These techniques must not be strictly considered as part of the respiratory rehabilitative program, better they are therapeutic tools widely used in patients with advanced state of muscular weakness or dysfunction [25].

Conclusion

Benefits of comprehensive pulmonary rehabilitation have been demonstrated, but many questions remain unanswered. Great efforts have been addressed to COPD rehabilitative area. COPD is a chronic, progressive and irreversible disease with an insidious onset. The goals of medical therapy are:
– to slow the disease progression
– to improve lung function

Standard medical treatment is useful to stabilize the patients but it is unlikely that the progression of the disease stop. Perhaps pulmonary rehabilitation program could have an important role in ameliorating the survival rate of COPD patients. Many of the important benefits of respiratory rehabilitation are in the area related to behavioural aspects of COPD condition. It is difficult to measure the quality of life after a rehabilitation respiratory program because life satisfaction depends rather on personal preferences and the patients affected by an important disease are able to reset themselves to a lesser degree of precedent quality of life so that they are equally satisfied.

Dyspnea is an important symptom in COPD patients and is a central target in pulmonary rehabilitation programs. Exercise testing and physical reconditioning are considered important components but additional information needs to be obtained on the optimal methods for performing exercise testing especially in those patients that during exercise develop hypoxemia.

Rehabilitative respiratory programs request a multidisciplinary approach and a significant effort needs to be done from both patients and staff in order to understand and individualize specific rehabilitation techniques for different patients.

Actually there is agreement on the validity of rehabilitation respiratory programs as a means to improve the functional status and reduce disability in an increasing number of patients with chronic lung disease in an aging population.

References

1. Hass F, Hass A (1991) A history of pulmonary rehabilitation. In: Pulmonary therapy and rehabilitation: principles and practice, 2nd ed. Philadelphia, Williams and Wilkins, pp 179-195
2. Fishman AP (1996) The chest physician and physiatrist. In: Bach JR (ed) Pulmonary rehabilitation: the obstructive and paralytic conditions. Hanley and Belfus, Philadelphia, pp 1-12
3. Higgins ITT (1988) Epidemiology of bronchitis and emphysema. In: Fishman AP (ed) Pulmonary diseases and disorders, 2nd ed. McGraw-Hill, New York, pp 1159-1171
4. Mahler AD (1993) Chronic obstructive pulmonary disease. In: Mahler AD (ed) Pulmonary disease in the elderly patient. Marcel Dekker, New York, pp 159-188
5. Begin P, Grassino A (1991) Inspiratory muscle dysfunction and chronic hypercapnia in chronic obstructive pulmonary disease. Am Rev Respir Dis 143:905-912
6. Dillard AT, Piantadosi S, Rajagopal JR (1989) Determinants of maximal exercise capacity in patients with chronic airflow obstruction. Chest 96:267-281
7. Vitres N, Aubier M, Murciano D et al (1984) Effects of aminophylline on diaphragmatic fatigue during acute respiratory failure. Am Rev Respir Dis 129:396-402
8. Lewis MI (1996) Nutrition and chronic obstructive pulmonary disease: a clinical overview. In: Bach JR. Pulmonary rehabilitation: the obstructive and paralytic conditions. Hanley and Belfus, Philadephia, pp 156-172
9. Ries AL (1993) Pulmonary rehabilitation. In: Mahler AD (ed) Pulmonary disease in the elderly patient. Marcel Dekker, New York, pp 219-237
10. Fartinez FJ, Couser JL, Celli BR (1990) Factors influencing ventilatory muscle recruitment in patients with chronic airflow obstruction. Am Rev Respir Dis 142:276-282
11. Mueller RE, Petty TL, Filley GF (1970) Ventilation and arterial blood gas changes induced by pursed lip breathing. J Appl Physiol 28:784-789
12. Kiriloff LH, Owens GL, Roger RM, Mazzocco MG (1985) Does physical therapy work. Chest 88:436-444
13. van der Schans CP, van der Mark THW, de Vries G et al (1991) Effect of positive expiratory pressure breathing in cystic fibrosis. Thorax 46:252-256
14. Pardy RL, Reid WD, Belman MJ (1989) Respiratory muscle training. Clin Chest Med 9: 287-295

15. Levine S, Weiser P, Gille J (1986) Evaluation of a ventilatory muscle endurance training program in the rehabilitation of patients with chronic obstructive pulmonary disease. Am Rev Respir Dis 133:400-406
16. Dean NC, Brown JK, Himelman RB et al (1992) Oxygen may improve dyspnea and endurance in patients with chronic obstructive pulmonary disease. Am Rev Respir Dis 146: 941-945
17. Mezzanotte WS, Tangel DJ, Fox AM et al (1994) Nocturnal nasal continuous positive pressure ventilation in patients with chronic obstructive pulmonary disease. Chest 106:1100-1108
18. Ries AL, Kaplan RM, Limberg TM, Prewitt LM (1995) Effect of pulmonary rehabilitation on physiologic and psychosocial outcomes in patients with chronic obstructive pulmonary disease. Ann Inter Med 122:823-832
19. Bach JR, Alba AS (1990) Management of chronic alveolar hypoventilation by nasal ventilation. Chest 97:52-57
20. Gibson GJ, Pride NB, Newsom-Davies J, Loh LC (1977) Pulmonary mechanics in patients with respiratory muscle weakness. Am Rev Respir Dis 115:389-395
21. Braun NMT, Arora NS, Rochester DF (1983) Respiratory muscle and pulmonary function in polymyositis and other proximal myopathies. Thorax 36:616-623
22. Di Marco AF, Kelling JF, Di Marco MS et al (1985) The effect of inspiratory resistive training on respiratory muscle function in patients with muscular dystrophy. Muscle Nerve 8:284-290
23. Bach JR (1998) Rehabilitation of the patients with respiratory dysfunction. In: Delisa J (ed) Rehabilitation medicine. Lippincott-Raven, Philadelphia, pp 1359-1378
24. Massery M (1996) Manual breathing and coughing aids. Phys Med Rehabil Clin North Am 7: 407-422
25. Bach JR, Alba AS (1990) Noninvasive options for ventilatory support of traumatic high level quadriplegic. Chest 98:613-619

PERIOPERATIVE MEDICINE

EVOLUTION OF THE USE
OF ANAESTHETIC DRUGS

Clinical Biochemistry of N_2O: Recent Advances

J. RUPREHT

Contrary to the beliefs on the use of nitrous oxide (N_2O) of ten years ago, the role of N_2O in medicine has been established. More than ever, N_2O is being used during total intravenous anaesthesia but to the anaesthesia researcher, N_2O is of greater importance. N_2O has proven to be a most excellent agent to study the phenomenon of acute tolerance to drugs which alter functioning of the brain [1]. There have been developments in the mechanism of the N_2O-anaesthetic action [2] pointing towards a GABA-receptor related mechanism and to the fact that the reversible general anaesthetic effect may be more of an intracellular phenomenon than an extracellular one. Earlier experiments indicate that N_2O-antinociceptive effect can be enhanced biochemically [3]. This, however, has not been followed by studies which would demonstrate if indeed, it is possible to improve N_2O performance in clinical practice.

Occasional case reports on the adverse biochemical effects of N_2O in clinical practice, e.g., grave neutropenia after the nonjudicious use of N_2O in a chronically neutropenic patient [4] demonstrate that most clinicians are not fully aware of N_2O use. J. Nunn et al. believe that N_2O-use in clinical anaesthesia should be maintained [5, 6], but that one should solve problems associated with its administration and further improve its services to patients. The debate on N_2O use is not over [7]. Clinicians and researchers should be made aware of the available scientific facts concerning the effects of N_2O when administered for medical purposes. Environmentally related aspects of the exposure to N_2O have been dealt by Halsey [8]. This text will deal with some biochemical aspects of N_2O-use, with the aim to encourage more N_2O-related basic research.

Biochemical, non-anaesthetic effects of N_2O

Cobalamin, vitamin B12 is a rare substance in nature and is essential as a co-enzyme in the functioning of methionine-synthase (MS) which transforms homocysteine to methionine. In vivo, N_2O irreversibly oxidizes the cobalt ion thus rendering B12 inactive as the essential co-enzyme for activity of MS. The enzyme MS enables re-methylation of homocysteine to methionine and de-methylation of methyl-tetrahydrofolate. Tetrahydrofolate renders a methyl-group for conversion of deoxyuridine to deoxythymidine. These biochemical reactions are absolutely essential for DNA replication, and for the proliferation of tissue. The early effects of N_2O can, therefore, be observed in tissues with a very high rate of replication e.g. mucosa, blood-forming tissues, fibrocytes and, surprisingly, less in the male reproductive tissue.

Theoretically, N_2O would be expected to hinder hematopoiesis and wound healing. The earliest measurable effects, however, are noticeable only after breathing of more than 1,1% N_2O for longer than 22 days or 70% for more than 6 hours.

The other known biochemical effect of N_2O is the inhibition of methyl-malonyl CoA mutase which assists in the degradation of fat and amino acids. This effect is also dependent on the N_2O-inhibition of cobalamin but its intensity is so low that no concerns arise in exposure to N_2O of less than 2 days. This N_2O-effect which, not surprisingly, is also dependent on stores of active B12 before exposure to N_2O, will not be further discussed.

Some details of N_2O-induced CH_3-cobalamin inhibition

One molecule of N_2O is needed to oxidize cobalt in cobalamin but the chance for this reaction increases only with time and with a considerable increase of N_2O-partial pressure; high partial pressures of N_2O inactivate cobalamin faster. In healthy humans, it takes six hours or more of exposure to 550 mmHg pressure of N_2O before the methyonine synthase is inhibited to such a degree that signs of postoperative leucopenia become measurable; this is a direct effect of decreased DNA replication. The earliest measurable sign of inactivated cobalamin is an elevated concentration of homocysteine in plasma and urine [9]. Plasma folate and homocysteine levels increase in less than two hours. Changes of serum methionine lag behind, the decrease becoming measurable after 5 to 6 hours of N_2O-anaesthesia [10]. In fit patients all biochemical changes due to N_2O returned to normal within one week postoperatively. The risk that routine nitrous oxide anaesthesia places the patient at a biochemical disadvantage is negligible because the average duration is too short to seriously interfere with the cobalamin-dependent DNA-replication. This scientific evaluation has been supported by J.F. Nunn et al. In this study an incredible safety record of N_2O in clinical anaesthesia on countless millions of anaesthetized patients through fifteen decades was seen.

However, with the advent of remarkably long surgical procedures in the past two decades, an excess of 24 hours is no exception, the biochemical effects of N_2O must be taken into consideration for the conduct of anaesthesia. The simplest answer is to refrain from N_2O use in cases of anaesthesia longer than 5 hours. Unfortunately, this has not always been to the patient's benefit. Moreover, contemporary critical care medicine has provided patients with already compromised nutritional state [11] and with seriously impaired folate metabolism. It has been seen in internal medicine patients that even a short exposure to N$_2$O can be metabolically damaging. Therefore, ways had to be found to compensate for the N$_2$O-effect on cobalamin-dependent metabolism.

Possibilities for compensation of N$_2$O-metabolic effect

Nunn et al. observed [12] that only in very special cases should care the effects of N$_2$O-exposure be either compensated or that N$_2$O should not be used. Cachexic and undernourished patients, multiple exposures to N$_2$O within one week [9] and in cases of already existing pernicious anaemia. One might possibly add cases of patients suffering from rare neurological diseases based on myelin degeneration.

In all these groups of patients one can consider pre-exposure administration of folinic acid (Leucovorin). Metabolically, this substance serves for donation of methyl group in transformation of methionine to thymidine to compensate for the inactivated methyl-cobalamin. In some centres this approach has been put in practice [13], in particular for all N$_2$O-anaesthetics lasting more than 5 hours. Folinic acid should be given at a dose of 1 mg per kilogram body weight, every 8 hours. Care must be taken not to administer this agent in patients treated with cytostatic drugs.

Norwegian researchers evaluated the logical possibility of loading the patient pre-operatively with methionine in order to compensate for blocked methionine production after inactivation of methionine synthase by N$_2$O [14]. It was found that methionine synthase activity is restored more quickly after N$_2$O-exposure. The explanation was that the enzyme becomes inactive during preloading with methionine and is less vulnerable to N$_2$O in this state. No clinical appraisal of this therapeutic approach has been forthcoming although was difficult to introduce preoperative oral intake of methionine. An intravenous preparation of methionine has not been made available for routine use. More investigation is due.

For protection of individuals who are chronically exposed to low concentrations of N$_2$O for example dental and recovering patients, oral intake of folinic acid has been suggested. In this case, too, no practical experience has been reported. During the Dutch Society of Clinical Chemists (1999) it has been suggested to pre-load patients with betaine in order to protect synthesis of methionine from N$_2$O. No elaboration on this idea has been forthcoming although it is known that this agent promotes synthesis of methionine from homocysteine.

Clear-cut contraindications for exposure to N$_2$O

It may be stated in a two-fold way that N$_2$O-anaesthesia is generally safe, in particular for fit patients undergoing anaesthesia for less than 6 hours and, that it has not yet been ascertained which biochemical approach might reliably protect patient's folate-dependent metabolism.

Fortunately, it is absolutely possible to point out those patients in whom N_2O must not be used. Vitamin B12 status preoperatively was a decisive factor for the speed of B12 inactivation during exposure to N_2O. Landon et al. [15] suggested that patients with low preoperative B12 are at disadvantage during N_2O-exposure which should, therefore, be kept very short or N_2O should be avoided.

Fiege [4] published an overview of conditions which lead to severe chronic neutropenia, including infectious states, hematological conditions, immunological reasons and chemotherapy. As in pernicious anaemia, it is wise not to administer N_2O to such patients. Twenty-four disease states were identified by Fiege, some very rare but oncological patients on citostatics very often undergo anaesthesia and surgery. Whatever chemotherapeutic agent is used it is better not to use N_2O in addition because this may cause an over-dose effect of the cell-proliferation-inhibition. Very few surgeons, oncologists and anaesthesiologists are aware of this dangerous synergism. Further training in operative medicine will hopefully make practitioners aware of the existing knowledge in this field and thus decrease iatrogenic complications in oncologic patients who undergo anaesthesia.

Finally it is surprising that the neutropenic effect of N_2O along with its soothing sedative, anaesthetic and analgesic properties has not been introduced in the treatment of some types of myeloid leukemias. This has been suggested several times [16] and substantiated experimentally. It may be that hematologists could collaborate with anaesthesiologists in administering N_2O to critically ill leukemia patients.

References

1. Ramsay DS et al (1992) Acute tolerance to nitrous oxide in humans. Pain 51:367-373
2. Dzoljic M (1996) Nitrous oxide: a study on neurons. Thesis. Foundation for Single Cell Research, Leiden
3. Rupreht J et al (1984) Enkephalinase inhibition prevented tolerance to nitrous oxide analgesia in rats. Acta Anaesthesiol Scand 28:617-620
4. Fiege M et al (1998) Gefährdung von Patienten mit schwerer chronischer Neutropenie durch Lachgasexposition. Anästhesiologie & Intensiv Med 39:347-350
5. Nunn JF, Halsey MJ (1990) Xenon in anaesthesia. Lancet 336:112-113
6. Rupreht J (1990) Nitrous oxide: full rehabilitation of its use in medicine. Giornale di Medicina Critica (Trieste) 2:171-174
7. Shaw ADFS, Morgan M (1998) Nitrous oxide: time to stop laughing? Editorial. Anaesthesia 53:213-215
8. Halsey MJ (1995) Occupational exposure to inhalational anaesthetics. Anaesthesia Rounds. Zeneca Pharmaceuticals (Education), Abingdon
9. Ermens AAM et al (1994) Monitoring cobalamin during nitrous oxide anesthesia by determination of homocysteine in plasma and urine. Clin Pharmacol Therap 49:385-393

10. Kano Y et al (1984) Effect of leucovorin and methylcobalamin with nitrous oxide anesthesia. J Lab Clin Med 104:711-717
11. Amos RJ et al (1982) Incidence and pathogenesis of acute megaloblastic bone marrow change in patients receiving intensive care. Lancet 2:835-839
12. Nunn JF (1987) Clinical aspects of interaction between nitrous oxide and vitamin B12. Br J Anaesth 59:3-13
13. Rupreht J (1989) Lachgas kan vrij van biochemische bijwerkingen. Ned Tijdschr Anesth 4: 14-16
14. Christensen B et al (1994) Preoperative methionine loading enhances restoration of the cobalamin-dependent enzyme methionine synthase after nitrous oxide anaesthesia. Anesthesiology 80:1046-1056
15. Landon MJ et al (1992) Influence of vitamin B12 status on the inactivation of methionine synthase by nitrous oxide. Br J Anaesth 69:81-86
16. Kroes ACM (1987) The inactivation of cobalamin by nitrous oxide. Application in experimental chemotherapy of leukemia. Thesis, Erasmus University Rotterdam, The Netherlands

Anticholinergics: Towards Selective Antimuscarinic Agents?

J. RUPREHT

Molecular pharmacology has identified at least five distinct subtypes of acetylcholinergic receptors in the muscarine-receptor group. These receptors subserve a number of different physiological functions which may become adversely affected by use of non-specific antimuscarinic agents during anaesthesia. To target certain muscarinic receptors by highly selective acetylcholine (ACh) blocking agents have become preferable to classical antimuscarinic agents which may result in a number of unwanted side effects e.g. to protect the heart against neostigmine-induced bradycardia without excessively dry mouth.

A short description of functions dependent on ACh transmission and a review of functions according to specific subtypes of muscarinic receptors will follow. Pharmacological effects of classical antimuscarinic agents will be mentioned and the newer agents, which may gradually replace older antimuscarinic drugs, will be discussed.

Acetylcholinergic transmission

Receptors for ACh occur in various peripheral tissues and in the central nervous system (CNS). They all are stimulated by ACh but differ profoundly in the susceptibility to be blocked. A large group which can be blocked by atropine-like substances are the muscarinic receptors. These have been subdivided into five different types designated as M_1 to M_5 muscarinic receptors. ACh-responsive receptors M_1-M_5 can all be stimulated by muscarine and can be found at the postganglionic endings of parasympathetic nerves, at autonomic ganglia, at chromaffine tissue and chemoreceptors, at motor end plates and motor nerve terminals of striated muscles, and abundantly, in the CNS.

The other group of acetylcholinergic receptor sites are the nicotinic receptors because these sites can be stimulated by low dose nicotine. Nicotinic receptors are found at autonomic ganglia, at motor nerve end plates and diffusely throughout the CNS. Although less is known on nicotinic cholinergic transmission as compared to vast amount of knowledge on muscarine type of cholinergic transmission.

Some of the characteristics of the muscarinic and nicotinic acetylcholinergic transmission are presented in Table 1.

Table 1. Characteristics of acetylcholinergic receptors

Muscarinic	
Agonist	Acetylcholine, muscarine
Antagonist	Atropine, scopolamine
Site	Wide distribution in the central nervous system and periphery
Action	Slow onset, excitatory or inhibitory, second messenger
Subtypes	Five distinct subtypes established
Nicotinic	
Agonist	Acetylcholine, low dose nicotine
Antagonist	Curare, high dose nicotine, A-bungarotoxin
Site	Central nervous system, motor nerve endplates, autonomic ganglia
Action	Rapid onset, excitatory, direct
Subtypes	Pending to be established

Modified from [1]

The reason why so little is known about nicotinic transmission may be the scarcity of naturally occurring exogenous agonists or antagonists. The effect of nicotine with stimulation of nicotinic cholinergic receptors were experimental results on humans until the blocking effect of tubocurare was investigated. However, the curare acts only peripherally and no information was available on behavioural, CNS-effects when nicotinic receptors in the brain are blocked. In contrast, most naturally occurring antimuscarinics easily penetrate into the brain tissue thanks to their tertiary structure which allows for a degree of solubility in lipids. Consequently, a long and rich tradition of knowledge exists about the effects of blocked muscarinic transmission. These are usually a combination of peripheral and central antimuscarinic effects (Table 2). Clinically, one speaks of symptoms and signs which are caused by antimuscarinic agents. Peripheral effects are easy to predict, dryness of the mouth, tachycardia or decreased gastrointestinal motility are all dose-dependent predictable pharmacological actions. Effects of antimuscarinic agents on CNS-functioning are very variable because effects of blocked CNS-muscarinic receptors depend also on the subtype of the blocked receptor and on the interplay of the blocked function with other CNS-transmitters [2].

In short, clinical picture of blocked muscarinic transmission depends on the subtype receptor blocked and on the relative intensity of peripheral versus central signs and symptoms. In anaesthesia and toxicology the well known descriptive *central anticholinergic syndrome* diagnosis is well established [1]. It is important to mention that a specific antagonism of central antimuscarinic effects

Table 2. Symptoms and signs of the antimuscarinic effects in humans

Central	
Agitation	Emotional instability
Amnesia	Muscular incoordination
Ataxia	Nausea, occasionally vomiting
Asynergia	Hyperpyrexia (central origin)
Clouded sensorium	Hyperalgesia
Confusion	Decreased reaction-time performance
Excitement	EEG-behaviour dissociation
Somnolence	Convulsions
Coma	Diminished power of concentration
Apprehension	Stimulation/depression of ventilation
Hallucinations	Fatigue/weakness/sedation
Illusions, delusions	Stereotyped movements
Delirium	Medium-long term mental impairment
Paranoid manifestation	
Peripheral	
Dry mouth	Mydriasis, cycloplegia
Dry skin	Photophobia
Thirst	Disturbed speech
Slight cardiac slowing (low-dose atropine)	Difficulty in micturition
Tachycardia, palpitation (high-dose atropine)	Decreased gastrointestinal motility
Heart dysrhythmias	Flushed skin
Blurred near vision	Hyperpyrexia (peripheral origin)

was established as early as 1864 by successful antagonism of atropine coma with physostigmine [3]. The possibility to manipulate central nervous system transmission by deblocking of blocked synapses has remained rather limited until the present day. Except for physostigmine, which restores ACh-action in the CNS, clinicians can similarly apply opiate antagonists, benzodiazepine antagonists and to some extent dopamine receptor blockers but not much more.

In order to avoid unwanted central effects of antimuscarinic agents clinicians have for some time advocated the use of quaternary antimuscarinics [1]. Nevertheless, the use of familiar atropine sulphate or scopolamine hydrobromide has remained well rooted and indiscriminate also in indications for exclusively peripheral antimuscarinic effects. Only gradually methyl-atropine or glycopyrronium are taking over the place of atropine sulphate in reversal of residual neuromuscular block. In this way, multiple central side effects of antimuscarinics affect patients less in the postoperative period.

Functions subserved by muscarinic transmission

An impressive array of CNS-functions depends on muscarinic transmissions (Table 3) and complete block of all muscarinic receptors leads to coma and death, unless treated. Waking state, complex behaviours, cardiovascular and respiratory control, thermoregulation and learning are just some CNS-functions which can easily be disturbed either by centrally active antimuscarinics or by decreased turn-over of ACh [4]. In several disease states receptors themselves may be afflicted thus also causing a deficit in muscarinic transmission.

Table 3. Functions subserved by the CNS-muscarinic transmission

Auditory input
Olfactory input
Cardiovascular control
Respiratory control
Drinking
Grooming
Affective behaviour
Complex behaviours
Learning (initial stage)
Working (short-time) memory
Transfer to memory store
Attention, alertness
Vigilance
Antinociception
Thermoregulation
Muscle coordination
Reflex coordination
Rapid eye movement sleep
Process of adaptation
Addiction

Modified from [4]

Research will identify CNS-functions which depend on a specific subtype of muscarinic receptors and it will become possible to develop drugs to selectively target these receptors [5]. For the time being a clinician can only avoid non-selective blocking of central muscarinic receptors by using peripherally active antimuscarinics.

Five subtypes of muscarinic receptors have been established for a number of years.

There is indication that a certain subtype of a receptor may behave differently, depending on the type of tissue and on pre- or postsynaptic localization. The drugs which will selectively target muscarinic receptor subtypes will need to be selective in a two-fold manner. One selectivity will concern their action only in the periphery or also in the brain. The other degree of selectivity will enable the clinician to modify a specific function subserved with a certain subtype of the receptor. Some of such drugs have already been introduced and have consider-

Table 4. Overview of muscarinic receptors

Subtype	Prevalence	Aspecific blocker	Specific blocker
M_1	Stomach hippocampus	Atropine	Pirenzepine
M_2	Heart (88%) Brain stem (84%)	Atropine	AF-DX-116
M_3	Glands cortex	Atropine	4-DAMP
M_4	Bronchi c. striatum	Atropine	Ipratropium
M_5	Brain	Atropine	?

Data from [6] and [7].

ably improved the therapeutic effect as compared to classical atropine, an example being ipratropium which selectively relieves bronchospasm (Atrovent).

Areas of improvements by selective antimuscarinic agents

In anaesthesia, a selective M_2-blocker is needed to prevent selective bradycardia of vagal origin. Selective inhibition of salivation by a M_3-blocker would be most useful because it could be administered dose-dependently without causing excessively dry mouth. Both M_2 and M_3 blockers would be free of side effects like decreased intestinal motility, difficulties with micturition or tendency to further increase body temperature in already febrile patients.

Selective muscarinic agonists would also be welcome but there are no perspectives that such agents would soon be forthcoming. A selective muscarinic receptor agonists, other than ACh, are currently being used. Bethanechol is used to increase gastrointestinal motility and urinary bladder contractions [8]. The main advantage of such drugs is longer duration of action because they are eliminated less compared with ACh and are devoid of side-effects on the nicotinic acetylcholinergic receptor.

Some centrally acting muscarinic blockers have been used in treatment of Parkinson's disease. They all produce a degree of unwanted peripheral antimuscarinic effects and also disturb central functions other than tremor. This is due to the fact that despite detailed molecular knowledge about the structure of muscarinic receptors little is known about their function in the CNS. Nevertheless, on theoretical grounds it is now possible to expect advanced antimuscarinic agents which will selectively modify muscarinic functions peripherally, centrally or both.

Note: An impressive compilation of knowledge about classical and experimental antimuscarinics is to be found in the 1998 monograph by Gyermek [7].

References

1. Rupreht J, Dworacek B (1996) The central anticholinergic syndrome in the postoperative period. In: Prys-Roberts C et al (eds) International practice of anaesthesia, vol. 2. Butterworth-
   Heinemann, Oxford 132:1-11
2. Karczmar AG (1990) Physiological cholinergic functions in the CNS. Prog Brain Res 84:
   437-442
3. Kleinwächter I (1864) Beobachtung über die Wirkung des Calabar-Extracts gegen Atropin-
   Vergiftung. Berl Klin Wochenschrift, 1:369-371
4. Van Delft AML et al (1988) Muscarinic receptors in the central nervous system. Prog Pharmacol 7:93-117
5. Subtypes of muscarinic receptors (1984) In: Hischowitz BI et al (ed). Elsevier, Amsterdam,
   Trends Pharmacol Sci[Suppl]
6. Lambert DG, Appadu BL (1995) Muscarinic receptor subtypes: do they have a place in clinical
   anaesthesia? Editorial. Br J Anaesth 74:497-499
7. Gyermek L (1998) Pharmacology of antimuscarinic agents. CRC Press LLC, Boca Raton,
   Florida
8. Staskin DR et al (1990) Urinary incontinence: classification and pharmacological treatment.
   Ciba Foundation Symposium 151:289-306

Evolution of the Use of Anaesthetic Drugs: Neuromuscular Blocking Agents

A. D'HOLLANDER, M. BAURAIN

Recent developments in the use of muscle relaxants can be related to different factors: to several new compounds of medium or short duration – cisatracurium, mivacurium, rocuronium, rapacuronium –, clinical pharmacology, to the spread of peripheral nerve stimulator, or to progressive changes in the clinical activities of the anesthesiologists (by example, the increasing development of day care in our actual practice).

Muscle relaxants loading dose

Usually, muscle relaxant administration is more or less standardized according to the weight of each patient, bolus injection whatever the pathophysiological and pharmacological environments of each patient. Compared to earlier molecules – doxacurium, pancuronium, pipecuronium –, all new compounds have shorter duration of action (Table 1).

Table 1.

Stimulation pattern	Obtaining and maintaining a defined paralysis level		Reversal management	Ref
	Moderate blockade	Intense blockade		
TOF [Count]	▓▓▓▓			1
TOF [Fade]			▓▓▓▓	1
Post-tetanic Count		▓▓▓▓		2
Double Burst Stimulation Fade			▓▓▓▓	3
100Hz Tetanic Fade			▓▓▓▓	4

Onset of paralysis

Recent muscle relaxants as rocuronium or rapacuronium possess shorter onset of action compared to less recent nondepolarizing neuromuscular blocking agents, such as vecuronium, atracurium, pancuronium, etc. Some studies indicate that intubation time after rocuronium – at a high dosage – can be performed after 60 to 90 sec compared to the more or less classical 180 sec proposed for the older relaxants. For such delays, intubation conditions produced by rocuronium are quite comparable to those obtained after succinylcholine administration.

Monitoring the clinical paralysis level

Simple passive clinical observations of patient's movements or listening to surgeon's demand for obtaining deeper paralysis level are poorly sensitive and specific methods for neuromuscular transmission monitoring and are completely inconsistent for a anticipative management of the requested paralysis level. As suggested previously, clinical observations based upon different transcutaneous electrical stimulation patterns are definitively more effective for an on-line active control of the paralysis level during surgery and before the awakening period. These observations are also very easy to obtain with the new generations of compact multifunction peripheral nerve stimulators allowing the delivery of twitch height (TH), train of four (TOF), post-tetanic count (PTC) and tetanic stimulation at 100 Hz. The use of such devices have gained more and more success among anesthesiologists interested in fine tuning of muscle relaxant administration and in obtaining a more objective control of the paralysis level.

Offset of surgical-type paralysis level

In patients with normal renal and hepatic function receiving a single intubation loading dose, the offset of the paralysis level compatible with general surgery – generally defined as the spontaneous return of a twitch height (TH) elicited at 0.1 Hz at 25% – can vary from periods as short as 10 min to a delay of 105 min (Table 2).

Clinical duration of muscle relaxants action

No consensus exists concerning the pharmacological actions of the muscle relaxants even when administered at a single loading dose, but some data referring simply to the return of a 0.1 Hz TH to 0.95 of its initial value resulted in a duration of 15 to 180 min (Table 2). Meanwhile, these data indicate the real clinical

Table 2.

	Routine intubation dose (µg/kg)	Routine intubation delay (sec)	Surgical paralysis duration (min)	Clinical paralysis duration (min)
Atracurium	350	150	45	75
Cisatracurium	200	150	70	90
Doxacurium	50	360	90	145
Mivacurium	150	100	25	35
Pancuronium	90	180	95	150
Pipecuronium	9	150	105	180
Rocuronium	600	90	50	70
Succinylcholine	750	45	10	15
Vecuronium	90	150	55	70

Modified from [5]

duration of action of the muscle relaxants is undoubtedly much more longer than the return to normal of TH. TH normality always precedes substantially the 2 Hz train of four (TOF) recovery. Thereafter, a supplementary delay is still needed to observe the absence of fading or fatigue for tetanic stimulation elicited at 100 Hz [6].

The fact that some muscle relaxants are long duration acting drugs can probably explain why postanaesthesia pulmonary complications are more prone to develop in the patients receiving long versus medium duration nondepolarizing neuromuscular blocking agents (NDNMBA).

Even in normal patients, large variations in interindividual pharmacodynamic response are very well documented for muscle relaxants. In the general population of anaesthetized patients, including quite potentially different pharmacokinetic sub-populations such as neonates, the elderly, renal and/or hepatic failure subjects, variations are undoubtedly substantially greater. In these situations, the clinician will be faced with a larger variation in interindividual pharmacodynamic responses, such as the return to the initial values of the TH or the TOF, e.g. There is evidence that this phenomenon is quite reduced with atracurium and cisatracurium.

Paralysis maintenance methods

In daily practice, two different methods are used: either the administration of a maintenance dose – generally calculated as 20% of the initial loading dose – or an adjustable maintenance infusion. According to this way of administration, the control of the paralysis level can be accomplished with more or less accuracy depending on the monitoring system in use for tracking the paralysis level variations. The visual or tactile assessment of residual muscular activity in response to a TOF or a post-tetanic count (PTC) stimulation are very popular clinical methods. Moreover, as the residual muscular activity depends directly on the muscle relaxant plasma concentration, the clinician can very easily maintain various muscle relaxant plasma concentrations according to the different relative sensitivities of some muscles to the NDNMBAs. So to maintain high muscle relaxant plasma concentrations, the monitoring of a muscle possessing reduced sensitivity to muscle relaxants (Table 3) is more effective than the observation of the *adductor pollicis*. In consequence, adjusting a NDNMBA infusion to obtain a residual posttetanic count of less than 5 responses at the *orbicularis oculi* is probably the most effective way to obtain and to control a very high plasma concentration with any muscle relaxant of intermediate duration of action.

Table 3.

Muscle	Sensitivity to muscle relaxant
Orbicularis oculi	*Reduced*
Orbicularis oris	
Frontalis	
Adductor laryngi	
Diaphragm	
Adductor pollicis	*Medium*
Abductor digiti minimi	
Flexor hallucis brevis	*High*

Modified from [6]

Cardiovascular side-effects

Besides atracurium – producing truncal flush and hypotension when administered in less than 75 sec – and pancuronium – inducing tachycardia and modest systemic hypertension –, all other NDNMBAs produce *per se* quite limited cardiovascular effects. Given after some co-administration of hypnotics and major analgesic drugs increasing the parasympathetic tone, some muscle relaxants – vecuronium, atracurium, e.g. –, could produce marked bradycardia and even cardiac asystoly.

Neuromuscular paralysis reversal

When vecuronium, atracurium, cisatracurium, rocuronium, mivacurium are antagonized at a spontaneous recovery level of four responses at the *adductor pol-*

licis after a TOF stimulation by the use of 40 μg/kg of neostigmine (mixed with 15 μg/kg atropine or 7,5 μg/kg glycopyrrolate), adequate neuromuscular transmission recovery defined as a TOF ratio above .85 and the presence of a slight fatigue (presence of 85% of the maximal force at the end of a 5 sec duration stimulation) at 100 Hz. In case of the pancuronium paralysis reversal, this quite favorable evolution depicted for all medium duration acting NDNMBAs was not observed [7]. These observations underlined the potential greater safety margin represented by all medium duration acting NDNMBAs in comparison to long duration acting compounds.

Anaphylactic and anaphylactoid reactions

Uncorrelated to any unspecific histaminic release, true severe pure anaphylactic reactions are due to NDNMBAs. The clinicians must be aware that cross immune reactions could exist among the different NDNMBAs indicating that careful preanaesthesia investigations are necessary for evidencing the contraindicated molecules in the patients concerned by this type of severe event. The frequency of these reactions appears to be higher for iodine disuccinyl choline than for the NDNMBA family. There is no convincing data regarding a difference in the frequencies of anaphylactic reactions observed between the aminosteroid and benzylisoquinolinium molecules.

References

1. Viby-Mogensen J, Jensen N, Engbaek J et al (1985) Tactile and visual evaluation of the response to train-of-four nerve stimulation. Anesthesiology 63:440-443
2. Viby-Mogensen J, Howardy-Hansen P, Chraemmer-Jorgensen B et al (1981) Posttetanic count (PTC). A new method of evaluating an intense nondepolarizing neuromuscular blockade. Anesthesiology 55:458-465
3. Engbaek J, Ostergaard D, Viby-Mogensen J (1989) Double burst stimulation (DBS): a new pattern of nerve stimulation to identify residual neuromuscular block. Br J Anaesth 62:274-278
4. Baurain M, Hennart D, Godschalx A et al (1998) Visual evaluation of residual curarization in anesthetized patients using one hundred-Hertz, five-second tetanic stimulation at the adductor pollicis muscle. Anesth Analg 87:185-189
5. Pino R, Basta S (1998) Pharmacology of neuromuscular blocking drugs. In: Longnecker D, Tinker J, Morgan G (eds) Principles and practice of anesthesiology. Mosby, pp 765-790
6. Silverman D, Brull S (1994) Monitoring of evoked responses. In: Silverman D (ed) Neuromuscular block in perioperative and intensive care. Lippincott, Philadelphia, pp 51-63
7. Baurain M, Hoton F, d'Hollander A et al (1996) Is recovery of neuromuscular transmission complete after the use of neostigmine to antagonize block produce by rocuronium, vecuronium, atracurium and pancuronium. Brit J Anaesth 77:496-499

Working Mechanisms of Anaesthetic Agents

M. DZOLJIC

Following the suggestion of your president, I have selected as a theme for this evening's lecture a subject which, for a long time, has repeatedly attracted and interested not only pharmacologists, but biologists as well, namely, the relationship between the pharmacologic action of a drug and its recognized chemical or physical properties.

The solution of this problem presents great difficulties.

These words were the opening of Hans Meyer's lecture dealing with the working mechanism of anaesthetic agents, at the Harvey Society on 7th October 1905. The words were, at that time, as relevant as they are now. Many are still attracted by this problem and, indeed, with all the progress that is made in biochemistry, biophysics as well as cell biology this problem still presents a great challenge. Nevertheless, since the formulation of first theories on anaesthetic action in the Middle Ages (or perhaps antiquity), much improvement on theoretical ground has been achieved. This is specially true for the intravenous anaesthetics [1, 2] but less obvious for the volatile anaesthetic drugs. The working mechanism of volatile anaesthetics is still a topic of extensive research that is build upon a long history of thinking about neuronal function.

In 1875 Claude Bernard proposed a hypothesis based on a concept of semicoagulation of the protoplasm of the nerve cell. The idea is that anaesthetic agents can somehow cause a state of greater rigidity of the protoplasm. This hypothesis was later modified by Dubois, according to whom the protoplasm was partially dehydrated during narcosis. The anaesthetic agent was thought to bring the cell in a state comparable to a dehydrated wheat kernel.

While these theories consider the fluids as the crucial components of the interaction between anaesthetics and the brain, others based their theories on the special composition of the brain. Bibra and Harless thought that the anaesthetics extract the fats from the "ganglia cells" which are then transported to the liver where the fat content is assumed to increase.

These and similar theories, some of which were still alive at the end of 19th century, are elegantly reviewed in Overton's monograph "Studien über die Narcose, zugleich ein Beitrag zur allgemeiner Pharmacologie". This work, together with the ideas of Hans Meyer, are a turning point in understanding the actions of anaesthetic agents.

A physical mechanism of general anaesthesia

Meyer and Overton both discovered independently a correlation between the potency of anaesthetics (called general anaesthetics to exclude opioids) and the partition coefficients measured between olive oil and water. The closeness of this correlation implies a unitary molecular site of action and suggests that anaesthesia results when a specific number of anaesthetic molecules occupy a hydrophobic region in the central nervous system.

In spite of the close correlation between the lipid solubility and anaesthetic potency, deviations from this so-called Meyer-Overton rule do exist. The most evident exception was already described by Overton in his monograph. The problem is known in the literature as the "cut-off effect" and describes the phenomenon that large lipid soluble compounds lack anaesthetic properties. Furthermore, minor deviations from the correlation exist, as is the case for enflurane and isoflurane. While these compounds are structural isomers, with approximately the same oil/gas partition coefficient, they have different potencies [3]. The explanation for this difference, which cannot be clarified by the Meyer-Overton rule, requires the acceptance of additional properties of some agents which are able to counteract the predicted anaesthetic effects. For instance, the presence of convulsant properties, as seen with enflurane, may oppose the anaesthetic effects and explain the higher MAC value for this agent.

The major problem is that, although often presented as a theory of narcosis, the data obtained by Meyer and Overton show only a correlation and do not explain how anaesthesia results.

The lipid solubility correlation was taken a step further with the introduction of the volume expansion theory by Mullins [4]. He hypothesized that anaesthesia is a result of an expansion of the hydrophobic part of the membrane beyond a critical volume. Such an expansion, due to an absorption of anaesthetic molecules, will change the properties of different ion-channels or will alter the electrical properties of the membrane itself.

This theory predicts several phenomena which can be tested experimentally. One prediction is that anaesthesia can be reversed by compressing the volume of the membrane and, indeed, high pressures do reverse anaesthetic effects [5]. The theory, however, also implies that since all anaesthetics at 1 MAC cause equal volume expansion, the counter-balancing pressure should be the same for all agents. Experiments exploring the relationship between anaesthetic potency and pressure showed that reversal pressure is not the same for all agents, and that no linear relationship exists between pressure and increase in anaesthetic requirement to produce an anaesthetic condition [6]. The reversal of anaesthetic effects by pressure is probably caused by an increase in the general level of central nervous excitability, since without anaesthetic agents high pressures produce tremors and convulsions [6]. Although different variations on this same theme were proposed, the finding that interaction of general anaesthetics with proteins, which were free of lipids, could result in a change of function, promoted the proteins as the site of anaesthetic action [7]. Many proteins relevant for the signal transduction in neuronal tissue, however, cannot be investigated without the lipid structures surrounding them, thus still allowing for the possibility that changes in the lipid bilayer are the primary site of action and that conformational and functional modulations in the protein are the result of these initial membrane changes. For instance, work has been done supporting the idea that lateral pressure changes of the lipid bilayer caused by anaesthetics may influence the opening of an ion channel [8].

Ion channels

At the cellular level the anaesthetic actions might be found in changes in intrinsic properties of the cell, like membrane potential, currents, resistance, etc., or extrinsic properties like synaptic or humoral communication [9]. It is clear that for most of these properties, voltage gated and ligand gated ion channels play a central role. Research on the effects of anaesthetic agents on different ion channels improved our understanding of to what extent these proteins can be involved in the mechanism of general anaesthesia.

Voltage gated ion channels

Voltage gated ion channels have been extensively studied in relation to different agents. Their importance in stabilizing the membrane potential, as well as generating the action potential, makes them good candidates as modulators of anaesthetic effects.

All anaesthetics that have been investigated have a depressing effect on the sodium channels, as well as on the potassium channels [10]. Voltage gated Ca^{2+} channels, which belong to the same superfamily as K^+ and Na^+ channels, are also affected by anaesthetic agents. Although most studies on this channel were performed on muscle cells, there is evidence that on neurons (which have different types of Ca^{2+} channels) the same depression in function can be observed. While the concentrations of anaesthetic agents required to modulate the K^+ and Na^+ channels exceed the concentrations clinically used, the Ca^{2+} channel proved to be more sensitive [11]. Nonetheless, the most sensitive Ca^{2+} currents measured are inhibited by halothane only at IC_{50} concentrations which are three to four times the predicted EC_{50} concentration for general anaesthesia [12]. Overall, considering the insensitivity of voltage gated ion channels for anaesthetic agents, it is unlikely that they essentially contribute to the state of general anaesthesia [12].

Some of the ligand gated ion channels, on the other hand, proved to be very sensitive to anaesthetic agents.

Glutamate receptors

Since its discovery in the 1950s, L-glutamate is seen as the major excitatory neurotransmitter in the vertebrate central nervous system. Several receptors are sensitive to glutamate and they have been classified according to their selective agonists. The NMDA (N-methyl-D-aspartate) is extensively studied in relation to anaesthetic agents. It was found that NMDA antagonists may exert anxiolytic effects like benzodiazepines and, therefore, may contribute to the anaesthetic state [13]. The dissociative anaesthetic ketamine exerts its effects largely by inhibiting the NMDA receptor [14]. Ethanol at concentrations of 50 mM has been found to reduce NMDA-activated currents [15], while nitrous oxide has been found to inhibit AMPA receptors (α-amino-3-hydroxy-5-methyl-4 isoxazole proprionate; formerly QUIS: quisqualate), another glutamate-gated ion channel [16] and NMDA receptor [17]. Additionally, volatile anaesthetics like halothane, isoflurane, enflurane and diethylether inhibit the NMDA mediated responses in different cell preparations [16, 18]. However, concentrations used to show this modulation of glutamate receptors are usually high (more than three times the EC_{50}) [19]. Nitrous oxide, for instance, showed significant changes in the kinetics of the AMPA receptors only at 1.5 atm 3.

$GABA_A$ receptors

GABA (γ-aminobutyric acid) was established as an inhibitory neurotransmitter in a series of experiments that started in the 1950s. It soon became clear that GABA could bind to two different types of receptors, which became known as $GABA_A$ and $GABA_B$. In the case of the $GABA_A$ receptor, the permeability of the membrane to Cl^- is increased upon interaction with GABA, while the $GABA_B$ receptor is thought to belong to the G-protein coupled receptors, and its stimulation causes closure of Ca^{2+} channels or opening of K^+ channels [10].

After the introduction of the benzodiazepines in the 1960s it became clear that these compounds interact with the GABA-ergic system, and it is now known that they bind to $GABA_A$ receptors and intensify the effect of the endogenous transmitter GABA. As work on these receptors progressed, contradictions appeared, but the $GABA_A$ receptor is still considered to be the prime target for anaesthetic agents.

Ethanol (at a concentration of 0.25-200 mM) potentiates the $GABA_A$ mediated current [20] which is an observation we could confirm, although at a higher dose (400-800 mM). Enhancement of the GABA-ergic system has been shown for enflurane, halothane and isoflurane in hippocampal neurons at clinically relevant concentrations [21]. Additionally, intravenous anaesthetics like propofol and etomidate were all found to interact with this system as well [22, 23].

With the introduction of molecular biology and advancing molecular genetics in the late 1980s, the interest shifted to the composition of the receptors and to the intracellular systems regulating the function of these receptors. It became clear that the "$GABA_A$ receptor", as a term, is hopelessly imprecise. Like other ligand gated channels the $GABA_A$ receptor is now thought to contain five heterologous subunits, and the pharmacological and biophysical properties were found to depend on the subunit composition. The subunit composition determined the possibility of phosphorylation which regulated the $GABA_A$ function [24]. Very soon the effects of different anaesthetics were linked to the subunit composition of the receptor [25] and the possibility of phosphorylation [23, 26-28].

Other ligand gated receptors

It is obvious that GABA and glutamate receptors, although abundantly present in the central nervous system, are not the only possible targets of anaesthetics. Much research has been performed on the nicotinic acetylcholine receptor, but mostly on the neuromuscular junction, making its contribution to the anaesthetic state difficult to assess. Finally, glycine may be of some importance. However, comprehensive anaesthetic studies on this receptor, mostly found in the spinal cord and the brainstem, are lacking.

Conclusions

This review is far from complete and it has been restricted to the most important current topics related to the subject. The hydrate theory, the multisite expansion hypothesis, the microtubular theory as well as many fluidization and phase transition variations have been omitted but are extensively reviewed elsewhere [19, 29]. From the brief review given above it is clear that the field of research considering the working mechanism of anaesthetic agents is a complex one and the site or sites of action of general anaesthetics are yet to be elucidated. Through the years, on the molecular level, the discussion has shifted from the lipid theories to the more specific interaction with the proteins responsible for the signal transduction. Increasing understanding of the regulatory mechanisms that control these membrane proteins (ion channels) prompted us to focus on the intracellular modulation machinery as well [11].

It is not obvious how this type of research will proceed. From the past, however we can learn that the search for the working mechanisms of anaesthetics depends on increasing knowledge of cellular physiology. This is far from enough. Neurons function in networks which are organized in regions. The integration of all these components ranging from molecules to networks is a huge challenge that will profoundly influence our thinking of how the brain functions. There is no valid reason for believing that sufficient knowledge of the brain functions will not explain all that is known about behaviour or its influence through anaesthetic agents. However, with all its connections, possible neurotransmitters, etc., the prospects of an easy and early solution are small.

References

1. Mastronardi P, Cafiero T, Rossi AE (1999) Hypnotics. In: Gullo A (ed) Anaesthesia, Pain, Intensive Care and Emergency Medicine - A.P.I.C.E. Springer, Milano, pp 185-191
2. Dzoljic M, Gelb AW (1997) Intravenous anaesthetics: some cellular sites of action. Eur J Anaesthesiol [Suppl]15:3-7
3. Koblin DD, Eger EII, Johnson BH et al (1981) Minimum alveolar concentration and oil/gas partitition coefficients of four anesthetic isomers. Anesthesiol 54:314-331
4. Mullins LJ (1954) Some physical mechanisms in narcosis. Chem Rev 54:289-323
5. Macdonald AG, Ramsey RL (1995) The effects of nitrous oxide on a glutamate-gated ion channel and their reversal by high pressure; a single channel analysis. Biochim Biophys Acta 1236:135-141
6. Miller KW, Paton WDM, Smith RA, Smith EB (1973) The pressure reversal of general anesthesia and the critical volume hypothesis. Mol Pharmacol 9:131-143
7. Franks NP, Lieb WR (1984) Do general anaesthetics act by competitive binding to specific receptors? Nature 310:599-601
8. Cantor RS (1998) The lateral pressure profile in membranes: a physical mechanism of general anesthesia. Toxicol Lett 100-101:451-458
9. Krnjevic K (1991) Cellular mechanisms of anesthesia. Ann NY Acad Sci 625:1-16
10. Urban BW (1993) Differential effects of gaseous and volatile anaesthetics on sodium and potassium channels. Br J Anaesth 71:25-38
11. Terrar DA (1993) Structure and function of calcium channels and the actions of anaesthetics. Br J Anaesth 71:39-46
12. Franks NP, Lieb WR (1993) Selective actions of volatile general anaesthetics at molecular and cellular levels. Br J Anaesth 71:65-76
13. Xie Z, Commissaris RL (1992) Anxiolytic-like effects of the noncompetitive NMDA antagonist MK801. Pharmacol Biochem Behav 43:471-477
14. Anis NA, Berry SC, Burton NR, Lodge D (1983) The dissociative anaesthetics, ketamine and phencyclidine, selectively reduce excitation of central mammalian neurones by N-methyl-aspartate. Br J Pharmacol 79:565-575
15. Lovinger DM, White G, Weight FF (1989) Ethanol inhibits NMDA-activated ion current in hippocampal neurons. Science 243:1721-1724
16. Yang J, Zorumski CF (1991) Effects of isoflurane on N-methyl-D-aspartate gated ion channels in cultured rat hippocampal neurons. Ann NY Acad Sci 625:287-289
17. Jevtovic-Todorovic V, Todorovic SM, Mennerick S et al (1998) Nitrous oxide (laughing gas) is an NMDA antagonist, neuroprotectant and neurotoxin. Nat Med 4:460-463
18. Daniell LC (1995) Effect of volatile general anesthetics and n-alcohols on glutamate-stimulated increases in calcium ion flux in hippocampal membrane vesicles. Pharmacology 50: 154-161
19. Franks NP, Lieb WR (1994) Molecular and cellular mechanisms of general anaesthesia. Nature 367:607-614

20. Aguayo LG, Pancetti FC (1994) Ethanol modulation of the γ-aminobutyric acidA- and glycine-activated Cl⁻ current in cultured mouse neurons. J Pharmacol Exp Ther 270:61-69
21. Jones MV, Brooks PA, Harrison NL (1992) Enhancement of γ-aminobutyric acid-activated Cl⁻ currents in cultured rat hippocampal neurones by three volatile anaesthetics. J Physiol (London) 449:279-293
22. Hara MM, Kai Y, Ikemoto Y (1994) Enhancement by propofol of the γ-aminobutyric acidA response in dissociated hippocampal pyramidal neurons of the rat. Anesthesiol 81:988-993
23. Uchida I, Kamatchi G, Burt D, Yang J (1995) Etomidate potentiation of GABA$_A$ receptor gated current depends on subunit composition. Neurosci Lett 185:203-206
24. Krishek BJ, Xie X, Blackstone C et al (1994) Regulation of GABA$_A$ receptor function by protein kinase C phosphorylation. Neuron 12:1081-1095
25. Farrant M, Cull-Candy S (1993) GABA receptors, granule cells and genes. Nature 361: 302-303
26. Wafford KA, Whiting PJ (1992) Ethanol potentiation of GABA$_A$ receptors requires phosphorylation of the alternatively spliced variant of the γ2 subunit. FEBS Lett 313:113-117
27. Weiner JL, Zhang L, Carlen PL (1994) Potentiation of GABA$_A$-mediated synaptic current by ethanol in hippocampal CA1 neurons: possible role of protein kinase C. J Pharmacol Exp Ther 268:1388-1395
28. Harris RA, McQuilkin JS, Paylor R et al (1995) Mutant mice lacking the γ isoform of protein kinase C show decreased behavioral actions of ethanol and altered function of γ-aminobutyrate type A receptors. Proc Natl Acad Sci USA 92:3658-3662
29. Koblin DD (1994) Mechanisms of action. In: Miller RD (ed) Anesthesia. 4th edn. Churchill Livingstone, New York, pp 67-99

FAST-TRACK ANAESTHESIA AND POSTOPERATIVE CARE

Fast-Track Anesthesia in Cardiac Surgery and Postoperative Care

J.O.C. Auler Jr, M.J.C. Carmona

The anesthetic objectives for a patient scheduled for cardiac surgery are the provision of an adequate depth of anesthesia with a fine balance of myocardial oxygen supply and demand, thus avoiding ischemia.

A significant evolution of scientific understanding and technical development has occurred in cardiac surgery and anesthesia and in cardiopulmonary bypass techniques over a relatively short time frame. Fast-track anesthesia [1] enables surgical patients to spend less time in the care units and offer both a physiological and economic rationale for the practice[2-5].

Before discussing fast-track anesthesia, it is important to remember that early extubation is only part, although an important part, of the multimodal approach of fast-track cardiac surgery.

Fast-track cardiac surgery

The program of fast-track cardiac surgery involves education, same day admission, early extubation with subsequent early ambulation and aggressive pulmonary care, early ICU and hospital discharge, variance tracking for improved quality assurance and comprehensive follow-up [6].

Education for a successful fast-track surgical program involves patients, families, nurses and physicians [7]. It is essential to recognize from the beginning that most cardiothoracic team members involved with cardiac surgery have been trained learning about the benefits of opioid-based anesthetic techniques, intensive hemodynamic monitoring and the importance of highly trained critical care nursing. The patient education begins in the preoperative period of elective surgeries with information about what to expect in the peroperative period, what they might experience in the postoperative period, how they will be expected to participate in their own recovery and what the course of that convalescence will be [6]. This approach includes preoperative optimization of patients, health status through nutritional supplementation and physical conditioning.

Traditionally, patients used to come to the hospital some days before surgery, for additional team and anesthetic consultation, preoperative blood exams, chest

X-ray, electrocardiogram, and facility tour. Nowadays, most elective patients can come to the hospital just the night before surgery, since all consultations and exams have already been done. Most strict fast-track programs consider that the patients need to come to the hospital only on the day of surgery, and these elective patients have to understand that same day admission is necessary for their planned surgery. In this way, entering the hospital 24 hours before scheduled surgery for preoperative exams, checking and team consultation is not justifiable. To permit same day admission the hospital has to develop a smooth, efficiently-run, reliable method of processing patients in the day(s) before the scheduled operation. This can require plant reorganization and extensive coordination in order for the process to run smoothly for both the patient and hospital staff. This hospital reorganization to permit same day admission will avoid anxious patients and families, the need for pre-admission testing and exams or spending time looking for appropriate staff. This reorganization is essential to avoid delay in beginning operations scheduled for one specific day [6].

During surgery, key aspects of the fast-track approach include minimizing the stress response to surgery and the surgical trauma itself. Specific approaches to accomplish early extubation include expeditious, well-planned, technically superior surgery, efficient surgical team, appropriate patient selection, avoidance of intraoperative complications and residual structural defects, meticulous myocardial protection, reduction of pain and blood loss and management of bleeding, prevention of postoperative hypothermia, appropriate early use of inotropic support and avoidance of stroke and confusional states [8, 9].

Neurological complications have remained among the most feared complications after cardiac surgery because of the significant chronic disability caused. Advances have been made in the understanding and prevention of stroke including ultrasonographic detection of ascending and transverse arch atherosclerosis, detection and avoidance of air emboli, meticulous debridement of aortic valve calcium, and the use of a single aortic cross-clamp or, in some instances, the avoidance of an aortic cross-clamp (porcelain ascending aorta) by using hypothermia techniques. Patients affected by neurological problems are difficult to extubate early [6, 10, 11].

Some adjuvant drugs have been used during surgery in an attempt to improve the fast track, although early extubation does not depend on these adjuncts [9, 12]. Besides vasoactive drugs, perioperative steroids to reduce inflammatory response, metoclopramide to enhance bowel motility and histamine blockers to avoid gastric stress are some of these drugs. These are somewhat controversial adjuncts that are not widely used, but such approaches do have their advocates in the literature. Hemostatic drugs such as antifibrinolytics have been used more frequently in specific situations and can accelerate the stabilization and extubation in the postoperative period [13-15].

It is important to recognize that control of perioperative costs, as part of the fast-track program, must not only include improvement in efficiency, but also no increase in morbidity [16].

Fast-track cardiac anesthesia and postoperative care

This is a perioperative anesthetic management that aims at facilitating and accelerating tracheal extubation in the postoperative period. Early extubation is a major key to the success of the fast-track cardiac surgery pathways. However, there is no consensus regarding when to extubate patients. The length of tracheal intubation in the postoperative period has been continuously decreasing throughout the history of cardiac surgery [6].

The primary considerations justifying high-dose opioid anesthesia and prolonged mechanical ventilation after cardiopulmonary bypass have included the stability of patients relative to new ischemic events and the decrease in myocardial work associated with mechanical ventilation [17]. In addition, if one looks at the distribution of subendocardial blood flow to the left ventricle, the balance between myocardial blood supply and myocardial oxygen demand is optimized with opioid-based anesthetics. Control of heart rate and left ventricular pressure are the most easily treatable determinants of myocardial oxygen consumption. However, with the understanding that perioperative ischemia may be endothelially mediated and not always associated with myocardial blood flow supply/demand imbalance, optimizing endothelial function may be as important as hemodynamic stability to actually lower perioperative ischemic events and thereby improve overall surgical and anesthetic outcome. Nitroglycerin, nitric oxide, calcium channel blocking agents, adenosine regulating agents, and serine protease inhibitors may be equally or more effective in preventing perioperative ischemic events than preload, afterload, or contractility adjustments because of their endothelial regulating effects.

Drugs used in anesthesia must achieve an effective concentration. For volatile anesthetics this has been obtained by specific systems and the ability to measure the concentration of the drug that is in equilibrium with its site of action by means of an end-tidal agent monitor. Intravenous anesthetic drugs can be administered as a single large bolus sufficient to last the entire surgical procedure or for many hours beyond, by intermittent bolus administration resulting in a continuously increasing or decreasing concentration of drug, or in a variable rate continuous infusion that is titrated to match the anesthetic needs of the patient [18]. Nowadays, several studies have clearly demonstrated the superiority of a variable rate infusion over intermittent bolus dosing in providing a more stable anesthetic [6, 19, 20].

In the beginning of cardiac anesthesia, there was a consensus that it was different from the one used in patients subjected to non-cardiac surgery [21]. Nowadays we know that many anesthetic maintenance techniques can be safely used in cardiac patients and numerous protocols are available in the literature [6, 22, 23]:

– use of large doses of fentanyl and midazolam, in substitution for fentanyl and diazepam, but with a long time to extubation in the postoperative period [24-26];

- use of intravenous fentanyl supplemented with isoflurane inhalation, and maintenance of isoflurane administration in the cardiopulmonary bypass machine during this part of surgery;
- substitution of isoflurane for sevoflurane;
- use of short-action opioids and hypnotics, such as sufentanil and propofol [27-31];
- use of other hypnotics, such as thionembutal and etomidate, instead of propofol;
- combination of single peridural with general anesthesia or combination of continuous peridural anesthesia with general anesthesia, inserting the catheter the night before surgery [32];
- combination of single intrathecal anesthesia with general anesthesia [33].

During transportation and in the ICU an infusion of propofol is frequently used while extubation is not possible.

The introduction of drugs that are rapidly metabolized and eliminated was important to permit early extubation in the postoperative period. These new inhaled and intravenous anesthetics cost more, in general, but the expenses in new anesthesia techniques and drugs can be saved in early extubation, as we observed at our institution (Table 1) [34].

Table 1. Anesthesia techniques, cost of anesthetic drugs and time for tracheal extubation

Anesthesia technique and number of patients	Time for extubation (minutes)	Consumption of anesthetic drugs	Cost of anesthetic drugs (US$)
Diazepam-fentanyl ($n = 15$)	592.08 ± 160.39	Diazepam = 28.4 mg Fentanyl = 3061.0 µg	50.84
Midazolam-fentanyl ($n = 15$)	606.00 ± 200.67	Midazolam = 34.0 mg Fentanyl = 3016.5 µg	67.42
Propofol-sufentanil ($n = 12$)	383.33 ± 113.06	Propofol = 1087.5 mg Sufentanil = 549.1 µg	178.59
Midazolam-fentanyl-isoflurane ($n = 15$)	369.70 ± 147.40	Midazolam = 14.4 mg Fentanyl = 1206.0 µg Isoflurane = 36.0 ml	117.44

At our institution, we experiment with different kinds of anesthesia techniques and we are convinced that it is possible to have safe cardiac anesthesia, without risk of ischemia, by using small doses of fentanyl, combined with isoflurane or propofol, and maintenance of isoflurane or propofol during cardiopulmonary bypass. More importantly, we are convinced that large doses of benzodiazepines such as midazolam are critical for prolonging tracheal intubation in the postoperative period. During the induction of anesthesia, small doses of midazolam in combination with propofol or etomidate seem to be a better choice to enable early extubation.

The early extubation protocol is actually quite easy once most staff are already involved with fast-track approach. Short-acting drugs often supplemented with inhaled anesthetic agents could replace long-acting opioid strategies and sedation/analgesia protocols in the postoperative period are also tailored to favor short-acting, easily reversible drugs.

The requirements for postoperative extubation are basically the same in different anesthesia techniques[35-37]:
– awakeness and response to verbal command
– adequate gag reflex and ability to protect the airway
– ability to maintain pH > 7.35 on spontaneous ventilation
– normal temperature
– hemodynamic stability without significant dysrhythmias
– good perfusion with adequate urine output
– no significant mediastinal bleeding, suggesting necessity for reoperation

Most patients can be extubated in the ICU within a few hours of admission from the operating room. As a general starting point, it is believed that there are no absolute contraindications to early extubation. Relative contraindications for early extubation include active bleeding, significant hypoxemia, hypercapnia, hemodynamic instability, ventricular arrhythmias, neurological complications, or low cardiac output syndrome. If a patient comes to the operating room intubated, he will probably require a longer recovery period before extubation. Prophylactic ventilation was usual in the early days of cardiac surgery to reduce the work of breathing, allow adequate postoperative analgesia, and promote better gas exchange. However, studies do not support the use of prophylactic ventilation to prevent atelectasis [38]. The key to maintaining adequate postoperative respiratory function is efficient analgesia, which can be obtained via conventional means, patient-controlled infusions, intrathecal morphine, or thoracic epidural analgesia. Additionally, tracheal intubation and mechanical ventilation, while routinely used in the postoperative period, are not entirely benign, contributing to hemodynamic compromise. Other complications are vocal cord granulomas and ulcerations, depression of tracheal mucus velocity and disruption of the host defenses, contributing to colonization of the tracheobronchial tree. Tracheal intubation contributes to morbidity, which increases with the duration of mechanical ventilation.

It has been suggested that anxiety, agitation and hemodynamic alterations such as hypertension and tachycardia can be reflected by ECG changes. These stress consequences might be controlled with opioid infusions during the postoperative period, perhaps even beyond the traditional extubation routine on the morning of the first postoperative day. It is not clear, however, whether high doses of opioids are capable of completely suppressing the catecholamine responses, because it is impractical to keep patients intubated and receiving high doses of opioid infusions for several days, and at some time the patient needs to be awake and extubated. Early extubation can more efficiently control the stress response than prolonged intubation with its inherent stresses from coughing and suctioning. Additionally, patients who are extubated early require fewer drugs for sedation.

Besides the respiratory, hemodynamic and stress advantages, earlier extubation permits earlier discharge from the ICU, particularly by avoiding oversedation and consequently depression of the respiratory center, representing the economic benefits of fast-track anesthesia. Indirect economic benefits are present in the earlier mobilization of the patient such as less need for sedation, less cardiopulmonary morbidity, reduction of nursing demands and laboratory testing and avoidance of postponing of other cases. However, changing from a routine of overnight ventilation to early extubation may require the cooperation of all the team involved in the patient care.

It is interesting to observe that the first studies of fast-track anesthesia in cardiac surgery were more rigid about the inclusion of patients in the protocols, especially in terms of preoperative status [39, 40]. The ideal candidates for early extubation were those submitted to elective surgery, younger than 70 years of age, with normal renal function, presenting adequate ventricular function, without significant aortic or mitral disease or vascular disease. Nowadays, authors have become more flexible in identifying the candidates for early extubation in terms of preoperative status, and elderly patients are frequently included in early extubation protocols with good results. On the other hand, agreement of surgeons to early extubation is more common today than in the first years of fast-track anesthesia for cardiac surgery. The fast-track approach is not for all patients, but it is useful for many more than we may have believed in the past [41]. Some authors comment that patients need to be early extubated because it makes sense, not because it saves cents [42].

After surgery, the multimodal approach to the fast track includes early ambulation, resumption of a normal diet to ensure adequate nutritional intake and early discharge from the hospital, with a rapid return to normal activities [43].

The goal for the fast-track program is shortening the staying in the ICU [6]. In the fast-track programs, patients frequently stay in the ICU overnight and are transferred to an intermediate unit the morning after. Care maps have been developed specifically for the more common surgeries such as myocardial revascularization, valve replacement and thoracic aneurysm correction. In more aggressive fast-track protocols, patients stand at the bedside the night after surgery, ambulate the next morning, receive liquid nourishing the night after surgery and solid food the next morning. Intensive pulmonary care must be provided soon after the endotracheal tube has been removed. For low risk patients, atrial arrhythmias and respiratory insufficiency are the two most common variances that keep patients in the hospital longer than 5 days. Elderly patients are also very difficult to discharge from the hospital on the 5th postoperative day after major cardiac surgery.

Patients returning home on the 5th postoperative day after cardiac surgery still require significant physical and psychological support, even if they are young and do not present any other problem. The necessity of care and support increases when the patient is older, has concomitant illnesses, or has some sort of perioperative complication. Family understanding, preparation, and support are essential to the success of the fast-track program.

In conclusion, the approach to the patient subjected to cardiac surgery is changing rapidly and the team responsible for the patient care needs to become involved. Although it has recently been demonstrated that early tracheal extubation is safe, cost beneficial, and can improve resource spend in cardiac surgery, questions still remain regarding the significance of early extubation for outcome, the process of care on resource utilization, and the costs of cardiac surgical care [6, 19, 39]. Cardiac surgical and anesthesia programs have been significantly improved, in terms of length of stay, competitiveness and overall quality, but the establishment of a fast-track program requires time, involvement and decisions in every part of the hospital involved with cardiac surgery.

References

1. Kaplan JA (1995) The "fast track". J Cardiothorac Vasc Anesth 9:1
2. Velasco FT, Tarlow LS, Thomas SJ (1995) Economic rationale for early extubation. J Cardiothorac Vasc Anesth 9:2-9
3. Cheng DCH (1998) Fast track cardiac surgery pathways. Early extubation, process of care and cost containment. Anesthesiology 88:29-33
4. Cheng DCH (1995) Early extubation after cardiac surgery decreases intensive care unit stay and cost. Pro: early extubation after cardiac surgery decreases intensive care unit stay and cost. J Cardiothorac Vasc Anesth 9:460-464
5. Kapur PA (1995) Cost containment: at what expense? Anesth Analg 81:897-899
6. Verrier ED, Wright H, Cochran RP et al (1995) Changes in cardiovascular approaches to achieve early extubation. J Cardiothorac Vasc Anesth 9:10-15
7. Coe V (1995) Early extubation: perspective from a community hospital. J Cardiothorac Vasc Anesth 9:37-43
8. Lipowski ZJ (1987) Delirium (acute confusional states). JAMA 258:1789-1792
9. Disesa VJ (1987) The rational selection of inotropic drugs in cardiac surgery. J Card Surg 2:385-406
10. Breur AC, Furlan AJ, Hanson MR et al (1983) Central nervous system complications of coronary artery bypass graft surgery: prospective analysis of 421 patients. Stroke 14:682-687
11. Smith PLC, Treasure T, Nelman SP et al (1986) Cerebral consequences of cardiopulmonary bypass. Lancet 2:823-825
12. Engelman RM, Rousou JA, Flack JE et al (1994) Fast-track recovery of the coronary bypass patient. Ann Thorac Surg 58:1742-1746
13. Alvarez JM, Quiney NF, McMillan D et al (1995) The use of ultra-low-dose aprotinin to reduce blood loss in cardiac surgery. J Cardiothorac Vasc Anesth 9:29-33

14. Arom KV, Emery RW (1994) Decreased postoperative drainage with addition of ε-aminocaproic acid before cardiopulmonary bypass. Ann Thorac Surg 57:1108-1113
15. Laub GW, Riebman JB, Chen C et al (1994) The impact of aprotinin on coronary artery bypass graft patency. Chest 106:1370-1375
16. Cheng DCH (1998) Fast track cardiac surgery: economic implications in postoperative care. J Cardiothorac Vasc Anesth 12:72-79
17. Mangano DT, Siliciano D, Hollenber M et al (1992) Postoperative myocardial ischemia. Therapeutic trials using analgesia following surgery. Anesthesiology 76:342-353
18. Glass PSA (1995) Pharmacokinetic and pharmacodynamic principles in providing "fast-track" recovery. J Cardiothorac Vasc Anesth 9:16-20
19. Higgins TL (1995) Safety issues regarding early extubation after coronary artery bypass surgery. J Cardiothorac Vasc Anesth 9:24-29
20. Mora CT, Dudek C, Torjman MC et al (1995) The effects of anesthetic technique on the hemodynamic response and recovery profile in coronary revascularization patients. Anesth Analg 81:900-910
21. Reves JG, Sladen RN, Newman MF (1995) Cardiac Anesthetic. Is it unique? Anesth Analg 81:895-896
22. Foster GH, Conway WA, Pamulkov N et al (1984) Early extubation after coronary artery bypass: brief report. Crit Care Med 12:994-996
23. Marquez J, Magovern J, Kaplan P et al (1995) Cardiac surgery "fast tracking" in an academic hospital. J Cardiothorac Vasc Anesth 9:34-36
24. Carmona MJC, Menezes VL, Auler Jr JOC et al (1993) Extubação precoce no pós-operatório de cirurgia cardíaca. Rev Bras Anestesiol 43:329-333
25. Caspi J, Klausner JM, Safadi T et al (1988) Delayed respiratory depression following fentanyl anesthesia for cardiac surgery. Crit Care Med 15:238-240
26. Collard E, Delire V, Mayné A et al (1996) Propofol-alfentanil versus fentanyl-midazolam in coronary artery surgery. J Cardiothorac Vasc Anesth 10:869-876
27. Philbin DM, Rosow CE, Schneider RC et al (1990) Fentanyl and sufentanil anesthesia revisited: How much is enough? Anesthesiology 73:5-11
28. Khoury GF (1982) Sufentanil pancuronium versus sufentanil metocurine anaesthesia for coronary artery surgery. Anesthesiology 57:47-51
29. Bovill JG, Warren PJ, Schuller JL et al (1984) Comparison of fentanyl, sufentanil, and alfentanyl in patients undergoing valvular heart surgery. Anesth Analg 63:1081-1086
30. Tuman KJ, McCarthy RJ, el Ganzouri AR et al (1990) Sufentanil midazolam anaesthesia for coronary artery surgery. J Cardiothorac Anesth 4:308
31. Russel GN (1989) Propofol fentanyl anaesthesia for coronary surgery and cardiopulmonary bypass. Anaesthesia 44:205
32. Joachimsson PO, Nyström SO, Tyden H (1989) Early extubation after coronary artery surgery in efficiently reward patients: a postoperative comparison of opioid anesthesia versus inhalational anesthesia and thoracic epidural analgesia. J Cardiothorac Vasc Anesth 3:444-454
33. Chaney MA, Slogoff S (1996) Intrathecal morphine for cardiac surgery and early extubation. Anesth Analg 82:SCA118
34. Carmona MJC, Almeida DJCN, Francheschi RC et al (1997) Tempo de extubação versus custo dos anestésicos utilizados em cirurgia cardíaca. Rev Bras Anestesiol 47:CBA093
35. Karski JM (1995) Practical aspects of early extubation in cardiac surgery. J Cardiothorac Vasc Anesth 9:30-33
36. Michael L, McMichan JC, Rehder K (1979) Measurement of ventilatory reserve as an indication for early extubation after cardiac operation. J Thorac Cardiovasc Surg 78:761-765
37. Michelson EL, Torosian M, Morganroth J et al (1980) Early recogniton of surgically correctable causes of excessive mediastinal bleeding after coronary artery bypass graft surgery. Am J Surg 139:313-317

38. Bendixen HH, Hedley-White J, Laver MB (1963) Impaired oxygenation in surgical patients during general anesthesia with controlled ventilation: a concept of atelectasis. New Engl J Med 269:991-996
39. Higgins TL (1992) Pro: Early extubation is preferable to late extubation in patients following coronary artery surgery. J Cardiothorac Vasc Anesth 6:488-493
40. Siliciano D (1992) Con: Early extubation is not preferable to late extubation in patients undergoing coronary artery surgery. J Cardiothorac Vasc Anesth 6:494-498
41. Kaplan JA (1995) The "fast track". J Cardiothorac Vasc Anesth 9:1
42. Guenther CR (1995) Early extubation after cardiac surgery decreases intensive care unit stay and cost. Con: Early extubation after cardiac surgery does not decrease intensive care unit stay and cost. J Cardiothorac Vasc Anesth 9:465-467
43. Papadakos PJ, Earley MB (1995) Physician and nurse considerations for receiving a "fast-track" patient in the intensive care unit. J Cardiothorac Vasc Anesth 9:21-23

Fast-Track Program for Abdominal Surgery

F. CARLI

Morbidity and mortality associated with abdominal surgery has decreased over the years as a result of preoperative optimization of patient health status and improved anesthetic and surgical techniques. However, postoperative morbidity still occurs even after elective surgical interventions. The key pathogenic factor in postoperative morbidity, excluding failures of surgical and anesthetic techniques, is the surgical stress response with subsequent increased demands on organ function.

These changes in organ function are thought to be mediated by trauma-induced endocrine and metabolic changes, and activation of several biological cascade systems (cytokines, free oxygen radicals, etc.). To understand postoperative morbidity it is therefore necessary to clarify the pathophysiological role of the various components of the surgical stress response and to determine if modification of such responses can improve surgical outcome.

Pathophysiology

Postoperative gastrointestinal tract (GIT) dysfunctions include disturbances of gastric emptying and disturbances of motility resulting in nausea, vomiting and ileus, and other functional deficiencies which reduce the barrier against translocation of endotoxin and bacteria from the intestinal lumen. Altered motility of GIT after anesthesia and surgery is manifested as the inability to tolerate food and fluids and a delay in the return of normal large bowel activity. Motility normally recovers within 4-5 days of major surgery, but more quickly after minor surgery. The causes for postoperative ileus are not entirely clear, but it is thought that a generalized increase in sympathetic tone is a major factor [1]. Postoperative ileus is defined as uncomplicated inhibition of gut motility lasting no more than 3 days. Paralytic ileus, in contrast, is defined as prolonged stasis greater than three days, and is usually caused by factors other than surgical trauma. Generally, bowel surgery is more likely to be followed by ileus than peripheral surgery. However, several studies have shown that postoperative inhibition of bowel function is not related to the degree of intraoperative handling of the bowel. Postoperative ileus delays normal recovery, increases the need for intravenous fluids and drugs and delays postoperative mobilization, thereby increasing the overall cost of hospital stay [2]. Gastric emptying increases the risk of aspiration of gastric content in patients with obtunded protective reflexes in the early postoperative period, delays absorption of oral medicines, and increases the risk of postoperative nausea and vomiting.

The large bowel, especially the descending colon, takes the longest time to recover normal motility after surgery. Colonic ileus is recognized as abdominal distension and failure to pass flatus and stool. It results in third space loss of fluids and electrolytes and may impede respiration by diaphragmatic splinting. Increased intracolonic pressure may decrease colonic blood flow and adversely affect the integrity of bowel anastomosis by decreased perfusion and pressure effects. Impaired mucosal perfusion and ileus are associated with bacterial overgrowth, translocation of endotoxins and development of organ failure [3].

Although the pathophysiological features of postoperative ileus remain ill defined, the most commonly accepted theory is that abdominal pain activates a spinal reflex arc that inhibits intestinal motility. In addition, surgical stress induces sympathetic hyperactivity, and an excessive sympathetic stimulation of the bowel inhibits organized propulsive activity. Thus, both nociceptive afferent and sympathetic efferent nerves are believed to be the key initiators of ileus. Although stimulation of sympathetic nerves inhibits contractile activity, therapeutic intervention with adrenergic blocking drugs does not speed resolution of the ileus. In contrast the lack of efficacy of adrenergic blocking drugs on sympathetic innervation pathways to the GIT can block ileus after abdominal surgery. This observation provides a theoretical framework suggesting that blockade of abdominal nociceptive afferent or sympathetic efferent pathways might abolish inhibition of GIT motility induced by abdominal surgery.

Pharmacological and nutritional modulation of GIT

Many drugs used for anesthesia affect postoperative gastric emptying, but opioids have the most profound action [4]. Even the opioids given by the epidural route cause marked delay in gastric emptying [5]. The mechanism is unclear, although centrally mediated, and spinal sites of action have been suggested from animal studies. The effect of opioids on the large bowel is well known; there is a delay in passage of flatus or feces. The effect of volatile anesthetics is reversible and therefore clinically unimportant. Spinal and epidural local anesthetics have little effect on gastric emptying and improve colonic motility [6]. Epidural local anesthetics improve colonic motility through the blockade of nociceptive afferent pathways, therefore disrupting the afferent limb of the spinal reflex arc that has been postulated to mediate postoperative ileus. Furthermore, epidural local anesthetics can block the efferent limb of the reflex arc by blocking thoracolumbar sympathetic efferent nerves. Segmental neural blockade of thoracic dermatomes with local anesthetics will selectively block nociceptive afferent and sympathetic efferent nerves while leaving parasympathetic innervation (by the vagus and pelvic nerves) intact. The resulting modulation of autonomic balance toward a relative increase in parasympathetic tone during thoracic epidural should increase propulsive activity in the colon. Epidural local anesthetics may also increase GIT function through systemic absorption of local anesthetics and increased blood flow. Epidural opioids may not block transmission of somatic and sympathetic pathways, and therefore may be less effective in reduction of ileus than local anesthetics. This is particularly true on the 3rd and 4th days after surgery. GIT motility can be increased with prokinetic agents such as cisapride and metoclopramide. Although the use of neostigmine has been associated with increased incidence of anastomotic leakage, there is no substantial evidence to support this effect.

Surgical modulation of GIT

The value of antibiotic prophylaxis is well established and the timing of administration, doses and duration of antibiotics have been clarified in recent years. This therapy has contributed to a great reduction in nosocomial infection [7]. The treatment of postoperative wound infections has also changed with the introduction of new suturing material and better understanding of suture techniques. Antithrombotic prophylaxis is well established during the postoperative period with a low-dose heparin regimen. The re-evaluation of postoperative nutritional traditions has shown that early restoration of oral intake is possible, and has beneficial effects in attenuating protein catabolism, controlling the ileus and reducing postoperative septic complications [8]. One of the most impressive changes has been the introduction of minimally invasive (endosopic, laparoscopic) surgery. These developments have also contributed to increased use of ambulatory and semiambulatory settings for surgical procedures.

Upper GIT surgery

The fast-track program for upper GIT surgery aims at reducing the incidence of postoperative complications. Two main complications occur after upper GIT surgery: pulmonary dysfunction and cardiovascular morbidity. The incidence of pulmonary dysfunction (atelectasis and pneumonia) between postoperative day (POD) 1 and 5 was reported to be around 26-35%. Diaphragmatic dysfunction induced by a neural reflex is the leading factor in respiratory changes after upper GI surgery. Myocardial infarction (MI) occurs during the first 3 days after surgery, as recently reported in a large study where serial enzymatic, ECG and pathological indices of MI were conducted in a group of patients with history of ischemic heart disease undergoing major non-cardiac surgery [9].

Anesthetic care

Anesthesiologists can be actively involved in fast-track upper GIT surgery by attempting to reduce postoperative complications. One way is to alleviate pain with epidural blockade. Epidural local anesthetics have been shown to attenuate postoperative pulmonary complications when compared with systemic opioids. However, it is not clear that epidural analgesia per se can provide cardiovascular protection. There is proven evidence that epidural local anesthetics improve GIT motility when compared with systemic opioids. Maintenance of normothermia during surgery and attenuation of the inflammatory and adrenergic response to surgical stress need to be provided. A recent study compared the traditional regimen to a multimodal treatment of thoracic esophageal resection [10]. The multimodal protocol included: 1. Intraoperative combination of general anesthesia and thoracic epidural block with bupivacaine plus sufentanil, block to the fourth thoracic dermatome prior to surgery; 2. Postoperative pain relief with patient-controlled epidural analgesia (PCEA) with low-dose bupivacaine and sufentanil treated to individual needs with VAS scores during rest and during movement; 3. Extubation at the end of surgery and mobilization as quickly as possible; 4. Early oral nutrition. The results of this multimodal approach were a) reduction of ICU stay, b) significant difference in intermediate discharge, c) tendency towards decreased in-hospital mortality.

Surgical care

With regards to the surgical approach, minimally invasive surgery can make upper GIT a fast-track surgery; for example laparoscopic approach without GIT resection compared with the open technique (laparotomy) with resection. The program includes the following: 1. Preoperative optimization of patient health status; 2. Use preoperative test to rule out dismotility; 3. Aggressive antiemetics to avoid disruption of anastomosis. 4. Effective analgesia - a precursor to early extubation and early weaning from respirator; 5. Surgery to be performed as quickly as possible; judicious pre and postoperative administration of i.v. fluids; 6. Avoidance of supine position after surgery and oxygen therapy during the first 2 postoperative nights; 7. Improved peripheral vascular circulation with early mobilization and ambulation.

Lower abdominal surgery

Major colonic surgery is performed for either benign or malignant tumors of the large intestine or for inflammatory bowel disease (IBD). Patients undergoing colonic surgery for tumors are generally over 60 years of age, while those with IBD tend to be in the younger age group. Associated diseases such as respiratory, cardiac, metabolic are frequent in the elderly as well as anemia and loss of muscle mass. Patients with IBD tend to have frequent pain and suffer psychological stress. Preoperative optimization of the patient's health status focuses on correction of anemia, stabilization of cardiopulmonary functions, psychological support and, if time allows, nutritional replenishment. In the preoperative clinic, patients can be informed of the measures taken during the hospital stay by using videotapes or leaflets prepared by the surgical team. The objective of this preparation is to involve patients in the healing process.

Anesthetic care

The role of the anesthesiologist is to minimize the response to surgical stress and therefore choice has to be taken into account. Neural blockade with local anesthetics is strongly recommended as this technique attenuates significantly the metabolic response. The block must be achieved before surgery is initiated, whether the latter is performed by either laparotomy or laparoscopy. Symmetrical sensory block must be extended from T3 to S5 dermatomes. The epidural catheter is introduced at thoracic dermatomes (T8-T10) and analgesia is maintained after surgery for 3-5 days. The requirements for general anesthesia are reduced, and the large doses of opioids are discouraged. Nitrous oxide can be avoided when there is a risk of small and large bowel distension. The excellent quality of muscle relaxation provided by the epidural block can be maintained by a continuous infusion of local anesthetics to which small amount of opioids can be added. As with an extensive sympathetic block, hypotension can occur, and this can be managed with careful administration of i.v. fluids (crystalloids) and use of vasopressors (phenylephrine and epinephrine). Great care must be taken to prevent heat loss from the exposed parts of the body by using active warming devices. At the end of surgery patients must be pain-free and transferred to the recovery room in a semi-reclining position (20-30 degree).

Surgical care

Surgical approach can be achieved by laparotomy or laparoscopy (full or assisted). The surgical incision can be limited to an area where the tumor is present or the bowel has to be resected in order to limit tissue damage. Laparoscopic approach is not favored in presence of tumor for risk of dissemination. Nasogastric tube insertion is discouraged [11]. Heparin s.c. can be administered once the epidural catheter is in place and a successful block is achieved. It is advisable to administer antibiotics before surgery. Bladder catheterization is indicated to monitor fluid balance for a short period of time.

Postoperative care

Great care must be exercised during this period, and often patients are neglected with the risk of developing complications. Aspects of care to be considered in this group of patients are centered around recovery of gut function:

Optimal pain relief

Several retrospective, non-randomized and prospective controlled studies have been conducted on the merit of different methods of pain relief. Although all methods available (parenteral opioids, PCA opioids, epidural opioids and local anesthetics) can provide pain relief of a reasonable quality, it is clear that pain relief measures should also aim to continue the attenuation of surgical stress response and promote recovery. In this context, epidural combination of opioids and local anesthetics has been shown to provide optimal pain relief allowing patients to mobilize rather soon after surgery and achieve rapid recovery of GIT function [12].

Nutrition

There is no reason why patients undergoing elective procedures should fast after surgery for 3-4 days [13]. Incremental feeding can be achieved safely from the first postoperative day to minimize ileus. The use of metoclopromide or cisapride to accelerate gastric emptying is recommended.

Mobilization

Patients should be encouraged to stay out of bed, on a chair or walking. But to achieve this, pain relief must be optimal. Breathing exercises and adoption of semi-reclining posture are simple initiatives that have beneficial effect on recovery. Patients should be discharged with a program of simple daily exercises.

Other measures

Oxygen therapy is advised for 48 hours after surgery, particularly, in patients with cardiopulmonary problems. Keep a semi-sitting (45 degree) position during the postoperative period. Bladder catheter should be removed 48 h after surgery and attention must be made by staff to avoid unnecessary disruption of sleep pattern. Drains and tubes must be removed as soon as possible to allow patient's comfort.

Fast-track surgical procedures

Cholecystectomy

There are no surgical barriers to a fast-track program for laparoscopic cholecystectomy. Anesthetic care includes small doses of opioids, adequate general anesthesia, preoperative infiltration of skin and overlying the peritoneum with bupivacaine 0.5%, control of postoperative emesis with metoclopromide, and postoperative pain relief with a NSAID [14]. From the surgical point of view those patients selected for laparoscopic cholecystectomy should not present with common bile duct stones. In addition those patients in which there is a risk of conversion to open laparotomy, should not be put in the fast-track program as there is a 25% chance of conversion. For example, acute cholecystitis, older than 65 years of age, obesity, male gender and thickened bladder wall on ultrasound [15].

Hernia repair

Hernia repair is a procedure that is increasingly performed on an outpatient basis. Optimal anesthetic techniques associated with the shortest time to discharge include the use of local anesthesia with sedation or peripheral nerve blocks. A fast track program includes a walk-in, walk-out protocol with same-day surgery and open, tension-free mesh repair and one-to-two day recommended convalescence [16]. The local-sedation technique includes: 1. Low-dose midazolan premedication (< 5 mg); 2. Propofol infusion 50 μ/kg/min initially and titrated to maintained patient comfort; 3. Low-dose fentanyl (25-50 μg) given 3 to 4 minutes before local block. An ileoinguinal-hypogastric block with a mixture of bupivacaine 0.5% and lidocaine 2% (30-40 ml). Subfascial administration of the local anesthetic has been shown to significantly reduce pain scores at rest and with coughing and mobilization compared with subcutaneous infiltration. If supplemental analgesia is needed, IV ketorolac is suggested as this is effective in the postoperative period, and does not cause ileus, and facilitates recovery and time to ambulation.

Multimodal approach

A rational approach towards control of the postoperative period is therefore by multimodal intervention. Before surgery, detailed information about the accelerated stay program must be provided, possibly including a videotape program. Such detailed preoperative information has been demonstrated in itself to resulting in less pain and reduction of postoperative days. Stress reduction may be provided by currently available multimodal regimens. Most importantly, pain relief has to be used to facilitate ambulation and nutrition in order to avoid postoperative functional impairment. Several studies, although not controlled and randomized, suggest that a multidisciplinary effort may result in pronounced improvements is surgical outcome and reduction in morbidity and hospital stay [17]. In this context, the combination of minimally invasive surgery, epidural local anesthetics, early nutrition and ambulation and avoidance of opioids can reduce hospital stay and decrease postoperative fatigue and complications. In addition regionalization of major surgical procedures to one center may reduce costs and improve outcome. Finally, the organization of multidisciplinary intervention in rehabilitation units has to be the effort of anesthesiologists, surgeons and surgical nurses.

References

1. Livingston EH, Passaro EP (1990) Postoperative ileus. Dig Dis Sci 35:121-132
2. Moss G, Regal ME, Lichtig LK (1986) Reducing postoperative pain, narcotics and length of hospitalization. Surgery 90:206-210
3. Deitch EA (1990) The role of intestinal barrier failure and bacterial translocation in the development of systemic infection and multiple organ failure. Arch Surg 125:403-404
4. Nimmo WS, Heading RC, Wilson J et al (1975) Inhibition of gastric emptying and drug absorption by narcotic analgesics. Br J Clin Pharmacol 2:121-125
5. Wattwil M (1988) Postoperative pain relief and GI motility. Acta Chir Scand 550[Suppl]: 140-145
6. Liu S, Carpenter RL, Neal JM (1995) Epidural anesthesia and analgesia. Anesthesiology 82: 1474-1506
7. Lau WY, Chu kW, Poon GP et al (1988) Prophylactic antibiotics in elective colorectal surgery. Br J Surg 75:782-785
8. Hessow I (1988) Oral feeding after uncomplicated surgery. Br J Clin Pract 42:275-280
9. Badner N, Knill RL, Brown JE et al (1998) Myocardial infarction after non cardiac surgery. Anesthesiology 88:572-578
10. Brodner G, Pogatzki E, Van Aken H et al (1998) A multimodal approach to control postoperative pathophysiology and rehabilitation in patients undergoing abdominothoracic esophagectomy. Anesth Analg 86:228-234
11. Cheatam ML, Chapman WC, Key SP et al (1995) A meta-analysis of selective versus routine nasogastric decompression after elective laparotomy. Ann Surg 221:469-478
12. Liu S, Carpenter RL, Mackey DC et al (1995) Effects of perioperative analgesic technique on the rate of recovery after colonic surgery. Anesthesiology 83:757-765
13. Stewart BT, Woods RJ, Collopy BT et al (1998) Early feeding after elective open colorectal resection: a prospective randomized trial. Austr N Z J Surg 68:125-128
14. Michaloliakou C, Chung F, Sharma S (1996) Preoperative multimodal analgesia facilitates recovery after ambulatory laparoscopic cholecystectomy. Anesth Analg 82:44-51
15. Fried GM, Barkun JS, Sigman HH et al (1994) Factors determining conversion to laparotomy in patients undergoing laparoscopic cholecystectomy. Am J Surg 167:35-40
16. Callesen T, Beck K, Kehlet H (1998) The feasibility, safety and cost of infiltration anaesthesia for hernia repair. Anaesthesia 53:31-35
17. Bardram L, Funch-Jensen P, Jensen P et al (1995) Recovery after laparoscopic colonic surgery with epidural analgesia, early oral nutrition and enforced mobilization. Lancet 345:763-764

Fast-Track Anaesthesia and Postoperative Care: Orthopaedic Surgery

N.E. SHARROCK

Fast-Track can be accomplished by

- minimizing surgical trauma;
- reducing perioperative complications by providing a minimal physiological trespass.

Surgical factors

Surgical experience and skill is very important. Studies demonstrate that surgeons who perform less operations annually have higher complications (2x) and mortality (3x) rates [1]. Changes in surgical procedures have reduced surgical injury and improved rehabilitation. For example, the shift to arthroscopy-aided anterior cruciate repair has resulted in the majority of these procedures being performed on an ambulatory basis. With the open procedure, patients were in hospital for 3-7 days. The size of incision may reduce trauma. At The Hospital for Special Surgery, total hip replacement (THR) is often performed with an incision less than 10 cm long. This leads to less tissue dissection and improved recovery.

Preoperative education classes facilitate early discharge from hospital by defining what is expected of each patient. Aggressive rehabilitation can be used to maximize the benefits achieved by expeditious surgery and minimal physiological trespass [2].

Minimizing physiological trespass

Reducing blood loss

Intraoperative blood loss

Major orthopaedic procedures are associated with significant blood loss. During THR, intraoperative blood loss is usually reported to be 500-1500 mL [3, 4].

Factors influencing intraoperative blood loss:

– arterial pressure is the major determinant [4, 5];

– venous pressure can be important in certain procedures, e.g. spine surgery;

– cardiac output [6], intraoperative anticoagulation with heparin [7] and hypothermia are minor factors.

Approaches to minimize intraoperative blood loss

– hypotensive anesthesia [8] - epidural [9] or spinal anesthesia [10, 11];

– hypotensive epidural anesthesia (HEA) with an intraoperative blood loss of 100-200 mL [5, 7];

– maintain low/normal venous pressure and normothermia [3].

Postoperative bleeding

Low molecular weight heparin (LMWH) increases postoperative bleeding especially when started within 12-24 hours of surgery; this is dose-related [12]. Therapeutic heparinization increases bleeding within the first 3-4 days following total hip and knee replacement [13]. Hypertension immediately following surgery increases bleeding.

Patients who receive a unit of homologous blood have increased postoperative complications and prolonged hospitalization. Preoperative donation of autologous blood is effective in reducing homologous transfusion [14].

Minimize fluid

Excessive intravenous fluid/crystalloid may lead to fluid overload heart failure in high-risk patients. It is possible that excessive fluid could slow gastrointestinal function or adversely affect wound healing due to edema. Recent studies suggest that delaying fluid resuscitation in major trauma may enhance outcome [15].

How to minimize fluid:

– reduce blood loss with hypotension;

– monitor central venous pressure (CVP) and keeping filling pressure low/normal and NOT elevated as is usual practice.

It is easier to accomplish this goal with regional anesthesia than general anesthesia.

Reduce risk of deep vein thrombosis/pulmonary embolism

Historically, 50% of deaths following THR were from pulmonary embolism (PE). In the 1990s, 30% of deaths are from PE [16, 17].

In THR, epidural or spinal anesthesia can reduce the risk of deep vein thrombosis (DVT). Subset analysis shows that the lowest rates of DVT are with HEA, concurrently using intraoperative heparin. DVT rates with epidural are ≈ 30% [18], 11% with HEA [19] and 7% with HEA and intraoperative heparin [20].

In total knee replacement (TKR), DVT rates are reduced with epidural (from 50% down to 40%) [21, 22] and are reduced further with pneumatic compression devices (from 40% down to 30%) [23]; resulting in an overall reduction rate of 20%. With TKR, epidural anesthesia and analgesia + pneumatic compression boots + aspirin is as effective as LMWH but avoids the risk of bleeding from LMWH (3-8%).

In other orthopaedic surgery, e.g., spine surgery; pneumatic compression is preferred to LMWH to avoid the risk of bleeding.

Pathogenesis of DVT

Thrombogenesis during surgery is association with periods of venous occlusion. During THR, thrombogenesis begins with surgery of the femur [24] and in TKR, with tourniquet inflation [25]. Maneuvers to reduce DVT include shortening periods of venous occlusion, selective anticoagulation during surgery [7], enhancing lower extremity blood flow during surgery [26] and reducing blood loss [27].

If the thrombogenic stimulus during surgery can be minimized, low level anticoagulation with aspirin following surgery is sufficient. By avoiding the need for LMWH, the risk of postoperative bleeding is reduced. This simplifies care and facilitates recovery.

Fat embolization and postoperative lung injury

Reaming the femur and tibia results in release of fat into the venous system [28]. Fat embolization may occur following orthopaedic surgery. The risk is greater following long-stem cemented THR than normal primary THR [29] and the risk is greater for single-staged bilateral total joint replacement than unilateral procedures. Increases in pulmonary vascular resistance occur in TKR during general anesthesia [30], but is not noted with epidural anesthesia [31]. Whether this is due to the anesthetic or other factors is not clear. Minimizing postoperative lung injury is important. Maneuvers include supplemental oxygen, fluid management to avoid excessive fluid, epidural analgesia, and avoidance of airway obstruction. High-risk cases should be kept in a monitored environment for 24-48 hours.

Tourniquet issues

A tourniquet can create an injury at its edge (shear force nerve injury), beneath it (muscle squeezing) and distal to it can cause tissue ischemia. Upon release of the tourniquet, thromboemboli are released which can cause lung injury [30]. Approaches to minimize the sequelae are:

– shortening the duration of surgery;
– lowering the pressure from 300-350 to 200-250 mmHg, which is possible if systolic pressure is maintained at < 100 mmHg.

This should theoretically reduce the risk of neuropraxia and muscle damage. Avoidance of tourniquet results in less muscle injury and enhanced rehabilitation [32].

Postoperative analgesia to enhance recovery

In 3 studies, it has been demonstrated that continuous epidural analgesia results in enhanced rates of rehabilitation following TKA [22, 33-35]. Continuous femoral nerve blockade provides a similar benefit [33, 35]. A similar benefit from local blockade may perhaps be applicable to other surgical procedures.

Avoidance of narcotics

Part of the benefit of local anesthetic techniques is the avoidance of narcotics, which cause nausea, vomiting, constipation and cognitive impairment. Epidural analgesia with a combination of local anesthetic plus narcotics reduces overall narcotic requirements. COX-2 inhibitors may play a role in reducing narcotic dose in orthopaedics.

Other factors

Regional anesthesia does not result in any benefit in rates of confusion or late cognitive disturbances [36]. It is not clear how to reduce the risk of perioperative myocardial infarction and atrial fibrillation [37], which may contribute to adverse cardiac outcome following orthopaedic surgery. Urinary catheters placed during or immediately following surgery and maintained for 24-48 hours do not increase the risk of urinary tract infection [38]. Hypotensive anesthesia does not increase the risk of cognitive disturbances [39], stroke or myocardial infarction [40, 41]. Hypotensive epidural anesthesia can also be used for total knee replacement and lumbar spine fusion.

References

1. Kreder HJ, Deyo RA, Koepsell T et al (1997) Relationship between the volume of total hip replacements performed by providers and the rates of postoperative complications in the state of Washington [see comments]. J Bone Joint Surg [Am] 79:485-494
2. Kehlet H (1997) Multimodal approach to control postoperative pathophysiology and rehabilitation. Br J Anaesth 78:606-617
3. Schmied H, Kurz A, Sessler DI et al (1996) Mild hypothermia increases blood loss and transfusion requirements during total hip arthroplasty. Lancet 347:289-292
4. Sharrock NE, Salvati EA (1996) Hypotensive epidural anesthesia for total hip arthroplasty. Acta Orthop Scand 67:91-107
5. Sharrock NE, Mineo R, Urquhart B et al (1993) The effect of two levels of hypotension on intraoperative blood loss during total hip arthroplasty. Anesth Analg 76:580-584
6. Sharrock NE, Mineo R, Go G (1993) The effect of cardiac output on intraoperative blood loss during total hip arthroplasty. Reg Anesth 18:24-29
7. Sharrock NE, McCabe JP, Go G et al (1999) Dose response of intravenous heparin on markers of thrombosis during primary total hip replacement. Anesthesiology 90:981-987
8. Thompson GE, Miller RD, Stevens WC et al (1978) Hypotensive anesthesia for total hip arthroplasty: A study of blood loss and organ function (brain, heart, liver, and kidney). Anesthesiology 48:91-96
9. Modig J, Maripuu E, Sahlstedt B (1986) Thromboembolism following total hip replacement: A prospective investigation of 94 patients with emphasis on the efficacy of lumbar epidural anesthesia in prophylaxis. Reg Anesth 11:72-79
10. Davis FM, McDermott E, Hickton C et al (1987) Influence of spinal and general anaesthesia on haemostasis during total hip arthroplasty. Br J Anaesth 59:561-571
11. Davis FM, Laurenson VG, Gillespie WJ et al (1989) Deep vein thrombosis after total hip replacement. J Bone Joint Surg [Br] 71-B:181-185
12. Warwick D, Harrison J, Glew D et al (1998) Comparison of the use of a foot pump with the use of low-molecular-weight heparin for the prevention of deep-vein thrombosis after total hip replacement. A prospective, randomized trial. J Bone Joint Surg [Am] 80-A:1158-1166
13. Patterson BM, Marchand R, Ranawat C (1989) Complications of heparin therapy after total joint arthroplasty [see comments]. J Bone Joint Surg [Am] 71:1130-1134
14. Bierbaum BE, Callaghan JJ, Galante JO et al (1999) An analysis of blood management in patients having a total hip or knee arthroplasty. J Bone Joint Surg [Am] 81-A:2-10
15. Bickell WH, Wall MJ Jr, Pepe PE et al (1994) Immediate versus delayed fluid resuscitation for hypotensive patients with penetrating torso injuries. N Engl J Med 331:1105-1109
16. Fender D, Harper WM, Thompson JR et al (1997) Mortality and fatal pulmonary embolism after primary total hip replacement. Results from a regional hip register [see comments]. J Bone Joint Surg [Br] 79:896-899
17. Murray DW, Britton AR, Bulstrode CJK (1996) Thromboprophylaxis and death after total hip replacement. J Bone Joint Surg [Br] 78-B:863-870
18. Eriksson BI, Ekman S, Baur M et al (1997) Regional block anaesthesia versus general anaesthesia. Are different antithrombotic drugs equally effective in patients undergoing hip replacement? Retrospective analysis of 2354 patients undergoing hip replacement receiving either recombinant hirudin, unfractionated heparin or enoxaparin (abstract). Thromb Haemost June[Suppl]:487(PS-1992)
19. Westrich GH, Farrell C, Bono JV et al (1999) The incidence of venous thromboembolism after total hip arthroplasty: A specific hypotensive epidural anesthesia protocol. J Arthroplasty 14:456-463
20. McCabe JP, Sharrock NE, Salvati EA et al (1997) Intraoperative heparin and hypotensive epidural anesthesia in the prevention of thromboembolism following total hip arthroplasty. Orthop Trans 21:124

21. Sharrock NE, Haas SB, Hargett MJ et al (1991) Effects of epidural anesthesia on the incidence of deep-vein thrombosis after total knee arthroplasty. J Bone Joint Surg [Am] 73-A: 502-506
22. Williams-Russo P, Sharrock NE, Haas SB et al (1996) Randomized trial of epidural versus general anesthesia. Outcomes after primary total knee replacement. Clin Orthop 331:199-208
23. Westrich GH, Sculco TP (1996) Prophylaxis against deep venous thrombosis after total knee arthroplasty. Pneumatic plantar compression and aspirin compared with aspirin alone. J Bone Joint Surg [Am] 78-A:826-834
24. Sharrock NE, Go G, Harpel PC et al (1995) Thrombogenesis during total hip replacement. Clin Orthop 319:16-27
25. Sharrock NE, Go G, Williams-Russo P et al (1997) Comparison of extradural and general anaesthesia on the fibrinolytic response to total knee arthroplasty. Br J Anaesth 79:29-34
26. Bading B, Blank S, Sculco TP et al (1994) Augmentation of calf blood flow by epinephrine infusion during lumbar epidural anesthesia. Anesth Analg 78:1119-1124
27. Lieberman JR, Geerts WH (1994) Prevention of venous thromboembolism after total hip and knee arthroplasty. J Bone Joint Surg [Am] 76-A:1239-1250
28. Byrick R, Kay J, Mullen J (1987) Pulmonary marrow embolism: a dog model simulating dual component cemented arthroplasty. Can J Anaesth 34:336-342
29. Patterson BM, Healy JH, Cornell CN et al (1991) Cardiac arrest during hip arthroplasty with a cemented long-stem component. J Bone Joint Surg [Am] 73-A:271-277
30. Berman AT, Parmet JL, Harding SP et al (1998) Emboli observed with use of transesophageal echocardiography immediately after tourniquet release during total knee arthroplasty with cement. J Bone Joint Surg [Am] 80-A:389-396
31. Sharrock NE, Go G, Milman S et al (1999) The influence of tourniquet application on pulmonary vascular resistance and lung shunt during one-stage bilateral total knee arthroplasty. Acta Anaesthesiol Scand[Suppl]43:113
32. Abdel-Salam A, Eyres K (1995) Effects of tourniquet during total knee arthroplasty. A prospective randomised study. J Bone Joint Surg [Br] 77-B:250-253
33. Capdevila X, Barthelet Y, Biboulet P et al (1999) Effects of perioperative analgesic technique on the surgical outcome and duration of rehabilitation after major knee surgery. Anesthesiology 91:8-15
34. Todd MM, Brown DL (1999) Regional anesthesia and postoperative pain management: long-term benefits from a short-term intervention. Anesthesiology 91:1-2
35. Singelyn FJ, Deyaert M, Joris D et al (1998) Effects of intravenous patient-controlled analgesia with morphine, continuous epidural analgesia, and continuous three-in-one block on postoperative pain and knee rehabilitation after unilateral total knee arthroplasty. Anesth Analg 87:88-92
36. Williams-Russo P, Sharrock NE, Mattis S et al (1995) Cognitive effects after epidural vs general anesthesia in older adults. A randomized trial. JAMA 274:44-50
37. Kahn RL, Hargett MJ, Urquhart B et al (1993) Supraventricular tachyarrhythmias during total joint arthroplasty: Incidence and risk. Clin Orthop 296:265-269
38. Michelson JD, Lotke PA, Steinberg ME (1988) Urinary-bladder management after total joint-replacement surgery. N Engl J Med 319:321-326
39. Williams-Russo P, Sharrock NE, Mattis S et al (1999) Randomized trial of hypotensive epidural anesthesia in older adults. Anesthesiology 91:926-935
40. Sharrock NE, Cazan MG, Hargett MJL et al (1995) Changes in mortality after total hip and knee arthroplasty over a ten-year period. Anesth Analg 80:242-248
41. Sharrock NE, Mineo R, Urquhart B (1991) Haemodynamic effects and outcome analysis of hypotensive extradural anaesthesia in controlled hypertensive patients undergoing total hip arthroplasty. Br J Anaesth 67:17-25

Failure to Regain Consciousness After Anesthesia

D.F. ZANDSTRA, M. KUIPER

Failure to regain consciousness after anesthesia/surgery can be due to a wide variety of disorders ranging from delayed anesthetic recovery, postoperative delirium to persistent coma and death.

Postoperative consciousness disorders (POCD) are recognised as potentially severe complications of anesthesia. Patient's fear of not waking up postoperatively has been acknowledged [1]. Although POCD can be considered as an entity of complications it can cause depression of many organ systems inducing subsequent morbidity. The level of consciousness on arrival in the PACU is for instance significantly related to the incidence of respiratory morbidity [2].

POCD is usually the result of a complex interaction between multiple factors. A systematic approach to treatment begins by ensuring cardiac output, oxygenation, ventilation, and supportive metabolic treatment. Potential causes are then considered, ruled out or treated.

Over 95% of the patients will have recovered adequately 3 hours after ambulatory surgery and recovery is usually quite predictable [3]. However it is also recognized that the recovery period is often more difficult to manage safely than induction and maintenance of anesthesia. In severe prolonged POCD intensive care therapy is indicated to treat and prevent further vital organ dysfunction.

Outline

POCD will be analyzed based on electronic data disclosure and clinical experience. POCD will be categorized by epidemiology, etiology, prevention and therapy. In addition, unit derived data will be presented.

Epidemiology

POCD may consist of various disorders, central anticholinergic syndrome (CAS), delirium, acute confusional states, delayed recovery due to various reasons; and unintentional death and coma.

The incidence of POCD is not well known. However for the various sub-entities, some data are available. In relation to specific surgical procedures such as CABG and carotid artery revascularisation the incidence of neurological sequelae has been often studied.

Central anticholinergic syndrome (CAS)

Central anticholinergic syndrome (CAS) occurs often. An average incidence of 2% after general anesthesia in recent studies has been reported although in older studies higher incidences are mentioned [4]. The syndrome is characterised by central signs such as somnolence, confusion, amnesia, agitation, hallucinations, dysarthria, ataxia, delirium, stupor or coma and peripheral signs including dry mouth, dry skin, tachycardia, visual disturbances. Many drugs used in anesthetic practise may cause this syndrome: atropine sulphate, hyoscine (scopalamine), promethazine, benzodiazepines, opioids, halothane, enflurane and ketamine. The differential diagnosis includes, overdose of anesthetics, altered drug metabolism, altered hydration, electrolyte or acid-base disorders, hypercapnia, hypocapnia, hyperthermia, hypothermia and structural damage of the CNS in relation to the procedure, trauma or hemorrhage.

Altered mental status: delirium and confusion

Postoperative delirium (POD) occurs frequently [5]. The incidence of POD in average is 36.8% (range 0-73.5%) [5].

Risk-factors for POD include advanced age and preoperative depression, a preexisting cognitive impairment and a very significant risk-factor for POD. 80% of patients with depression develop POD. Also low endorphin levels and low cortisol levels are associated with POD. Many electrolyte abnormalities are associated with POD (azotemia, hypochloraemia, hypokalaemia, hyponatriaemia). The use of preoperative anticholinergic drugs is significantly associated with POD. In two randomised controlled trials no difference in POD was observed between general and spinal anesthesia. The Relative Risk of delirium from sedatives is 2.5-11.7, narcotics 2.5-2.7, and for drugs with anticholinergic properties the RR is as high as 4.5-11.7.

Prevention of POD: maintainance of adequate tissue oxygenation (hematocrit > 30) and homeostasis of the milieu interieur is of utmost importance. Treatment: timely diagnosis and treatment with haloperidol shortens hospitalisation and further derangements.

Stroke

Estimated occurrences of stroke may vary from 0,2 to 4,8% [6, 7]. The type of surgery and health status of the patient may influence these incidences; for ambulatory surgery the stroke incidence is 0.02%. For general surgery the range varies between 0,2-0.7%, for peripheral vascular surgery up to 3% and for head and neck vascular surgery an incidence of 4.8% has been reported [9]. The incidence of temporary CNS deficit < 12 month varies from 0.02-1.5% as adapted from Sesmu Arbous [8].

Unintentional death

About 10% of the anesthesia related complications occur postoperatively. Perioperative death occurs in 34% of the cases in OR, in the PACU 1.9% dies and in the ICU 52% [8].

Unintentional coma

Unintentional coma after anesthesia occurred in 42 patients from a cohort of 869.483 cases and all these patients died in hospital [9]. In high-risk hip surgery for replacement or fracture the incidence of postoperative unintentional coma was 1.2-2.3 per 10,000 anaesthetics [9]. In our own ICU-patient database ($n = 3571$) over the past 18 months the incidence of a Glasgow Coma Scale (GCS) < 13, 24 hours after surgery (excluding neurosurgery was 1% ($n = 35$).

In cardiac surgery higher incidences of postoperative unintentional coma than in non-cardiac surgery have been reported. This is however not observed in our patients.

Table 1. Data OLVG ICU January 1998-June 1999

Surgical patients primarily admitted to the ICU who have a GCS < 13 24 hours after admission to the ICU and 19 patients had GCS < 8
General surgery (including vascular, $n = 511$) $n = 14$ (2.7%) emerg. surg. $n = 13$
Orthopaedic surgery   ($n = 137$) $n = 2$ (1.5%)
Cardiothoracic surgery   ($n = 2853$) $n = 19$ (0.6%) emerg. surg. $n = 2$

Table 2. Number of patients per GCS cohort 24 hours after surgery

GCS12	GCS11	GCS10	GCS9	GCS8	GCS7	GCS6	GCS3
$n = 2$	$n = 4$	$n = 2$	N = 6	N = 2	N = 3	N = 8	N = 8
2CS	2GS	2CS	4 GS	1 GS	2 GS	6CS	4 GS
	1CS		2CS	1CS	1 CS	1 GS	4 CS
	1OS					1 OS	
2 elec.	2 elec.	2 emerg.	2 elec.	1 elec.	2 elec.	4 elec.	4 elec.
	2 emerg.		4 emerg.	1 emerg.	1 emerg.	4 emerg.	4 emerg.

CS = cardiac surgery, GS = general surgery, OS = orthopaedic surgery, elec. = elective surgery, emerg.= emergency surgery

Of the patients with GCS < 13 ($n = 35$), 18 patients were admitted after elective surgery. The remaining patients were admitted after emergency or urgent surgery ($n = 17$). This implies that after emergency- or urgent surgery the risk for abnormal GCS after 24 hours is considerably higher than after elective surgery (20% of surgical admissions to the ICU are patients after emergency or urgent surgery).

In our series coma (GCS = 3) at 24 hours after surgery is observed in 0,23% of cases admitted to the ICU after surgery including vascular and cardiothoracic surgery.

Summarizing the incidence of POCD varies from 0,012% (coma) – 2% (CAS) of anaesthetic procedures and therefore involves a significant number of patients.

Clinical approach to treatment POCD

If patients remain anaesthetized beyond the expected recovery time the following factors have to be taken into account [9, 10].

1. Has ventilation been sufficient to eliminate the inhaled agents and to prevent severe hypercarbia? Has the patient been hyperventilated for a long time resulting in hypocarbia?
2. Is oxygenation impaired?
3. Is the patient severely acidotic or alkalotic?
4. Has cardiac output been sufficient to deliver drugs from tissue to the lung or liver?
5. Is the patient hypothermic?
6. Potential role of preoperative medication (clonidine, lithium).
7. Impact of premedication.

8. Was combination of inhalation and iv agents given?
9. Adequate reversal of neuro-muscular blocking agents.
10. Impact of advanced age on elimination of drugs.
11. Electrolyte disorders? (Na, K, Mg, phosphate).
12. Blood glucose levels i.e. hypo/hyperglycaemia.
13. Intercurrent central nervous system event occurred?

Residual sedation from anesthetic drugs is the most common cause of postoperative somnolence. Especially the combination of long-acting sedatives used for premedication in combination with supplemental anesthetic drugs.

Therapeutic approach anesthetic overhang

If patients in recovery room or in ICU after anesthesia fail to recover as they should, a structured approach to diagnosis and therapy is advocated. Vital organ functions should be secured and adequately treated in case of malfunction. Specific contribution of anesthetic drugs can be ruled out by initial diagnostic testing with specific antagonists.

The use of antagonists

Opiate antagonists should be used if opiate effects are suspected (low respiratory rate, pin-point pupils). Low dose intravenous naloxon (0.04 mg increments every 2 minutes) can be administered to reverse the sedative effects of intraoperative narcotics.

If effects occur, infusion therapy with naloxon can be started. The half-life time of naloxon is 1 hour.

Flumazenil: Since benzodiazepines are widely used in anesthetic practice as well as in premedication, induction and maintenance of anesthesia inadvertent prolonged recovery may occur due to various reasons as there are interindividual differences in metabolic clearance and interactions with various other drugs used in anesthesia especially the opioids.

Physostigmine: The drug of choice in the diagnosis and treatment of CAS. Initial dosage in adults 1 mg I.V. If repeated administration is needed a continuous infusion can be started.

4-aminopyridine: This drug is known in anesthetic practice for its multimodal effects. It reverses the effects of opioids, benzodiazepines and muscle relaxants. The therapeutic width however is small but dosages of 20 mg iv for an adult can be used to reverse respiratory depression and sedation induced by opioids and benzodiazepines. Overdosing may lead to excitation and epileptic fits.

Use of antagonists in ICU and recovery

In 1995 and 1997 we evaluated the use of fluzamenil, physostigmine, naloxon and 4-aminopyridine in clinical ICU-practice in patients with failure to regain consciousness. The ICU admitted resp.1758 patients and 1904. About 70% of the patients are admitted after surgery including cardiac surgery patients (N = 1224).

Table 3. Number of ampoules used in ICU and costs to treat POCD

| 1995/1997 | No. of ampoules | | Costs | Costs |
	1995	1997	1995	1997
Flumazenil	103	130	Dfl 4200 = $2100	$2600
Physostigmine	135	40	Dfl 85 = $ 42	$ 13
4-aminopyridine	30	40	Dfl 30 = $ 15	$ 16
Naloxon	80	105	Dfl 63 = $ 31	$ 40

A significant percentage of patients (5%) is treated yearly with antagonists because of POCD. The average costs of these drugs is about $1.40 per patient admitted to the ICU. Flumazenil is expensive compared to the other drugs. From cost/effectiveness standpoint of view a test dose with physostigmine and/or naloxon seems to be preferable over flumazenil.

Various causes of anesthetic overhang

Metabolism: Hypothermia postoperatively occurs frequently. The reduced metabolic clearance of drugs in this condition leads to prolonged action. Hypothermia in the recovery phase should be treated actively to prevent further morbidity and mortality.

Hypo- or hyperglycaemia should be checked and corrected.

Recently the ASA has warned of the interaction of herbal medicines on the recovery of anesthesia. Prolonged recovery has been observed after use of St John's Wort.

Neurological evaluation

Perioperative CNS damage usually results from temporary ischaemia due to various reasons including bloodpressure drops during induction of anesthesia, massive bleeding, emboli (air, fluid, thrombi), oxygenation problems in relation to intubation, extubation, and pulmonary edema. Cerebral edema may ensue due to hyponatriaemia, microgravity (position induced edema), anoxia, eclampsia, hypertension, and consequences of brainsurgery or trauma. Furthermore the duration of specific surgical procedures as cardiopulmonary bypass surgery is significantly correlated with increased incidence of neurological complications [11].

If diagnostic testing with antagonists is without any effect, virtually all possible neurological diagnoses should be considered, tested, and ruled out.

Reversible entities should be checked as soon as possible to prevent further delay in treatment and to prevent impaired recovery chances.

Approach to coma after anesthesia is summarised schematically.

There are three principal causes of delayed or absent awakening after anesthesia [12]:

1. prolonged drug action
2. metabolic encephalopathy
3. cerebral injury

This leads to a differential diagnosis of absent or delayed awakening.

Prolonged drug action:
– Overdose
– Increased central sensitivity
– Age
– Biological variation
– Metabolic effects
– Decreased protein binding
– Delayed anesthetic excretion
– Anesthetic redistribution
– Decreased hepatic metabolism, drug interaction, and biotransformation

Metabolic encephalopathy:
– Hepatic, renal, endocrine and neurological disorders
– Hypoxia and hypercapnia
– Acidosis
– Hypoglycemia
– Hyperosmolar syndrome
– Electrolyte disturbance (Na, Ca, Mg)
– Hyperthermia, hypothermia
– Neurotoxic drugs

Neurological injury:
– Cerebral ischemia
– Intracranial hemorrhage

- Cerebral embolus (air, calcium, fibrin, fat)
- Hypoxia and cerebral edema

Trauma: Apart from direct cerebral damage of a headtrauma itself or from cerebral edema after a trauma, intracranial injury has been reported after nasal intubation or after placement of a nasal feeding catheter in the presence of basilar skull fractures.

Apart from causes of delayed or absent awakening directly related to anesthesia and surgery, one must consider other causes: delirium, non-convulsive status epilepticus, postictal state, akinetic mutism, neuroleptic malignant syndrome, functional disorder or other psychiatric disorders as well as locked-in syndrome must be ruled out.

References

1. Shevde K, Panagopoulos G (1991) A survey of 800 patients' knowledge, attitudes, and concerns regarding anesthesia. Anesth Analg 73:190-198
2. Parr SM, Robinson RJ, Glover PW, Galletly DC (1991) Level of consciousness on arrival in the recovery room and the development of early respiratory morbidity. Anaesth Intensive Care 19 (3):369-372
3. Chung F (1995) Recovery pattern and home-readiness after ambulatory surgery. Anesth Analg 80:869-902
4. Link J, Papadopoulos G, Dopjans G et al (1997) Distinct central anticholinergic syndrome following general anesthesia. Eur J Anesthesiol 14:15-21
5. Inouye SK, Schlesinger MJ, Lydon TJ (1999) Delirium: a symptom of how hospital care is failing older persons and a window to improve quality of hospital care. Am J Med 106: 565-573
6. Kam PCA, Calcroft RM (1997) Perioperative stroke in general surgical patients. Anaesthesia 52:879-883
7. Larsen SF, Zaric D, Boysen G (1988) Postoperative cerebrovascular accidents in general surgery. Acta Anesthesiol Scand 32:689-701
8. Sesmu Arbous M (1998) Anesthesia-related risk factors for perioperative severe morbidity and mortality. Thesis University Leiden
9. Curtis D, Stevens WC (1997) Recovery from anesthesia. Int Anesthesiol Clin 29:1-11
10. Mecca RS (1997) Complications during recovery. Int Anesthesiol Clin 29:37-54
11. Wesselink RMJ, de Boer A, Morshuis WJ et al (1997) Cardiopulmonary bypass time has important independent influence on mortality and morbidity. European J Cardiothorac Surg 11:1141-1145
12. Denlinger JK (1983) Prolonged emergence and failure to regain consciousness. In: Orkin FK, Cooperman LH (eds) Complications in anesthesiology. JB Lippincott, Philadelphia, p 369

FOCUS ON PERIOPERATIVE MANAGEMENT IN PAEDIATRICS

New Insights into Mechanical Ventilation During Paediatric Anaesthesia

J.O.C. Auler Jr, D. Fantoni, M.H.C. Pereira

Perioperative ventilation of small children submitted to major surgery has always been a challenge to anaesthesiologists. Most of the difficulties are related to the anaesthetic equipment itself which should be simultaneously able to ventilate the lungs correctly and at the same time deliver inhaled anaesthetics agents. Personal experience and knowledge of the peculiarities of the respiratory system of small children are also important. The natural problems involving superior airway assessment are not the main subject of this chapter. Our purpose is to present a brief review of the main differences between the respiratory system of children and adults, relevant anaesthetic practice, as well as the traditional paediatric breathing circuits employed routinely to administer inhalation agents and promote adequate gas exchange. After that, our discussion will be centred on the real benefit of new ventilatory modalities, available in modern work-station anaesthesia machines, such as pressure-controlled ventilation, low flow anaesthesia, and closed breathing circuits.

Particularities of respiratory system

The target of static and dynamic functions of the respiratory system is simply to ventilate alveoli and to maintain adequate oxygen uptake and carbon dioxide elimination. Thus, the efficiency of gas movement between alveoli and the atmosphere must be assured by some kind of equipment utilised during anaesthesia. In intensive care unit (ICU) patients either the ventilators promote air movement *into* and *out of* the lungs in an open way, or the expiration is passive and totally exhaled to the atmosphere. However, in an anaesthesia machine the expiration process is quite different. The essential features common to modern anaesthesia equipment are the anaesthetic circuits. The main characteristics of modern machines are the re-breathing of gases that go into and out of alveoli, so that air exhaled comes back partially or totally to the lungs. Thus the concept of the removal and prevention of carbon dioxide accumulation in the circuit, as well as of the fresh flow of gas, is of paramount importance in this kind of device. To this end it is desirable that the circuit is simple in design, has a low resistance to the air flow passage and minimal dead space in the apparatus, particularly when it is used for infants and small children.

During growth, changes in the dimensions and numbers of the components of the respiratory tract are comparable with concomitant changes in pulmonary function, especially in lung volumes and the mechanics of respiration. However when we compare the infant or young child to the adult, given parameters of pulmonary function are unchanged when they are related to standard patterns, such as height or surface area.

Diaphragm, rib cage, chest wall muscles, lung function and respiratory mechanics

In spontaneous breathing, the motion of gas into and out of the lung is driven by the movement of the rib cage and diaphragmatic excursion, commanded by the respiratory centre. However, during anaesthesia some physiological differences between the respiratory system of infants and adults may compromise this vital function.

The configuration of the rib cage of infants is quite different from that of adults, resulting in several mechanical disadvantages for the infants. The ribs at birth and during infancy have a circular disposition, consequently the diaphragm muscle is flatter and less efficient than that of adults. Another mechanical disadvantage of the chest wall configuration in infants is the difficulty of thoracic volume gas augmentation. Finally, the high compliance of the infant chest wall makes it more easily deformable during more stronger inspiratory efforts [1]. The elasticity of the thorax plays an important role in determining the resting volume of the lungs. A very compliant chest wall may not maintain an adequate transpulmonary pressure at end expiration, resulting in a decrease of functional residual capacity (FRC), alveolar collapse and hypoxaemia. Anatomically in relaxed state the neonatal diaphragm, compared to that of the adult, is located higher in the thorax, favouring more efficient contraction. This explains why the spontaneous ventilatory efforts of the neonate are critically dependent on the strength and endurance of the diaphragm. So, differently from adults, in the presence of slight insufficient diaphragmatic function, the infant requires ventilatory assistance. In controlled ventilation during anaesthesia this fact seems not to be so important, but in attempts to extubate early after surgery it could be a problem. The composition of diaphragmatic muscle fibres is also different. In contrast to adults, diaphragmatic infant and neonate muscle fibres have a high density of type IIa fast-oxidative, fatigue fibres. This fact explains the marked disposition of infants to diaphragmatic fatigue, particularly when the work of breathing is increased. During anaesthesia increased respiratory work may be necessary in the presence of improper devices and spontaneous breathing [2]. Finally, the infant's diaphragm is attached to a chest wall that is more flexible than that of the adult. Excessive inspiratory efforts, in the presence of spontaneous respiration, which could happen for example if the ventilator provided insufficient gas flow throughout the respiratory circuit, may result in distortion of the lower part of the chest wall. This results in a decrease of diaphragmatic contraction causing ineffective tidal volumes [3].

Characteristically the rib cage of premature babies, neonates at term and infants is very elastic. This chest wall flexibility is responsible for increased compliance, and persists for many months after birth, because it takes some time for the ribs to become totally calcified and rigid. Considering that in normal infants each normal inspiration requires 5 to 10 cm H_2O to expand the lungs, the tonicity of chest wall muscles is critical to augment rib cage rigidity, responsible for fixing the pliable chest wall. The principal function of the rib cage musculature in neonates and infants seems to be the stabilisation of the chest wall during diaphragmatic contraction necessary for lung expansion. During spontaneous ventilation under anaesthesia, the relaxed muscle may permit chest wall distortion during diaphragmatic contraction and consequently the generation of small tidal volumes [4]. The high rib cage flexibility in the infant explains the difficulty that small children and neonates have in maintaining normal levels of functional residual capacity. The maintenance of FRC above the closing volume could be a real problem during anaesthesia, causing hypoxaemia, unless specific strategies are taken, such as application of PEEP and strict surveillance of preset and exhaled tidal volumes.

The infant has a resting oxygen consumption and carbon dioxide output per kilogram of body weight twice that of the adult. As the lung surface area per kg is the same for both, this explains why children and infants have a smaller pulmonary reserve during periods of stress and an increase of metabolic activity characterised by an increase in oxygen consumption demands and CO_2 excretion [5]. Other parameters such as alveolar ventilation • m^{-2} • min^{-1}, respiratory quotient, anatomic dead space • kg^{-1}, dead space • FRC^{-1} • kg^{-1}, and VT • FRC^{-1} are practically unchanged during growth and maturation. The alveolar ventilation to dead space ratio, together with the time constant of mechanical impedance to respiration, set the rate of respiration. Both factors are responsible for a progressive respiratory frequency decrease as body weight increases [6]. The thoracic gas volume has been determined in sedated children from 1 month to 5 years old by means of the body plethysmography method. The mean FRC of healthy newborns measured by helium dilution was 89.9 ± 15 ml. Related to body weight the mean FRC was 29.9 ml • kg^{-1}, i.e. similar values for both neonates and adults [7].

Due to the importance of mechanical ventilation during anaesthesia the specific particularities of respiratory mechanics of infants and children including compliance and resistance, also require some comments. Static mechanical properties of the lung and chest wall are conventionally expressed in volume-pressure curves (VP), so the ratio of ΔV • ΔP^{-1} or compliance gives an index of the relative ease with which the tissue can be altered. In the adult with the respiratory system in a normal resting position, at FRC with relaxed muscle, the force applied to the chest wall from tissue recoil equals the force applied to the lung from intrinsic recoil. These forces are similar but in opposite directions, so the respiratory system may be considered in equilibrium. In short, the lung *in situ* tends to collapse at all volumes, whereas the chest wall provides an increased force to counteract collapse at volumes below the equilibrium position and an inward force to make lung collapse easier at volumes above the point of equilibrium. In contrast the VP curve of neonates and infants is quite different. Due to its marked flexibility, the chest wall of neonates and infants has minimal or no effect on regulating the volume of the respiratory system. So in the small lung volume the opposite force of the chest wall offers finite resistance to total collapse of the system. In a similar way, in lung volumes above equilibrium point at FRC, the opposite force exerted by chest wall against lung expansion is also minimal. Because the chest wall of the newborn is so compliant, total compliance of the respiratory system is essentially equal to the compliance of the lung alone. Gerhadt et al. have measured the compliance of the chest wall [8]. They found a value of 6.4 ml • cm H_2O^{-1} • kg^{-1} in the preterm human neonate, decreasing to 4.2 ml • cm H_2O^{-1} • kg^{-1} in the full term neonate. The chest wall becomes gradually more rigid during growth such that its compliance reaches value of 2.5 ml • cm^{-1} • kg^{-1} by adolescence. The same authors have compared the chest wall compliance in full-term and premature infants. Their findings suggest that during mechanical ventilation the high chest wall compliance and low lung compliance of premature infants prevent a significant rise in pleural pressure which could interfere with central venous return and cardiac output. The transmission of positive airway pressure to the intrapleural space directly depends on lung compliance. The percentage of transmitted pressure which can embarrass cardiac output changes from 17% in normal premature to 25% in normal full-term infants [9]. The compliance of the lung is the measure of the elastic properties opposing a change in volume, that is, the change in lung volume (ml) per unit of pressure (cm H_2O) generating the volume change. Lung compliance depends on the number of open air spaces as well as on the surface tension, tissue elasticity, connective components of the parenchyma, intravascular, extracellular volume and blood vessels. As shown in Fig. 1, the compliance curve of the neonate has markedly low values at the extremes of lung volume. This could be explained by the fact at low lung volumes many alveoli are collapsed and at high lung volumes, a great part of alveoli are distended beyond their elastic limit. Therefore, in a comparative way, between adults and infants compliance is a measure not depending on body weight or height. Compared to the lung volume of FRC, the compliance is termed specific compliance. Although the lung compliance of infants is much lower than that of adults, specific compliance of both is similar [10]. As compliance is a measure of the elastic resistance to respiratory system expansion, resistance is the measure of the resistive forces that act against airflow. As air moves through the lung, resistance to the flow occurs as a result of airway and tissue forces that act in the opposite direction. Airway resistance depends inversely on lung volume. As lung volume increases so does the size of the airways because expansion of alveoli increases at the same time as the airway cross-sectional area. So to compare different subjects it is better to take into account the measures of resistance at FRC. Considering the total re-

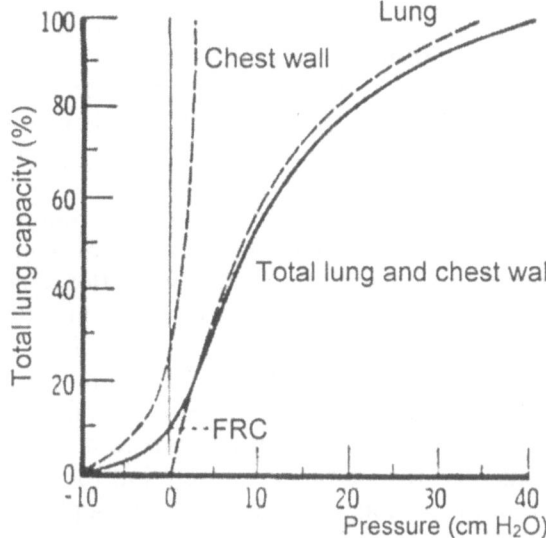

Fig. 1. Compliance curve of the neonate has markedly low values at the extremes of lung volume

sistance of the respiratory system, Doershuk and co-authors found similar values for children and adults [11]. The major challenge during paediatric anaesthesia is related to the resistance offered by the tracheal tube, connections and circuits. Depending on the cross-sectional area of these tubes part of the flow will be wasted during inspiration, decreasing the effective tidal volume. During spontaneous respiratory activity during anaesthesia the work of breathing, necessary to overcome the elastic and resistive properties of the respiratory system, may compromise the effectiveness of gas exchange.

Paediatric breathing circuits

Anaesthetic circuits represents the basis of inhalation anaesthesia. Specific breathing circuits designed for children are a little bit more complicated, since dead space, resistance, and loss of effective volume should always be considered. Characteristically the circuits are designed to offer accurate delivery of oxygen and anaesthetic gases, prevention of CO_2 accumulation, low resistance to air flow, minimal dead space, preserved humidity, and simplicity of management. There are different methods for classifying anaesthetic circuits; the most common is to adopt the movement of flow of gases in the system to define them as open, semi-open or non re-breathing, semi-closed, and closed. However, the classification of breathing systems based on these traditional particulars has brought more confusion than clarity. A more rational approach is to classify them into two systems: 1. those that do not contain the means to absorb carbon dioxide or potentially re-breathing systems, referring the potential to re-inhale expired carbon dioxide; 2. those equipped with means to absorb expired carbon dioxide, presents for instance in the circuit system. The major benefits of a circuit system used with a low flow are economy, heating and humidity conservation of inspiratory moisture, as well as reduction of ambient pollution [12]. The performance of a circuit system is dependent upon the volume of fresh gas flow administered in the circuit. Fresh flows in the order of 4 to more liters differ minimally from inspiratory flow. But when the fresh flows are reduced close to a level of basal body necessities, it is mandatory to monitor the gas composition of the system. The major disadvantage of utilising low flow in a circuit system is the impossibility of safely predicting the composition of inspiratory moisture. At the same time there has recently been a resurgence of interest in the use of low flow techniques with circuit absorber systems to minimise costs of expensive inhalation agents and reduce ambient operating room pollution [13]. The multiplicity of possibilities in inhalation anaesthesia coupled with a safe ventilator, provide a conceptual basis for permanent discussion, and the introduction of new work station anaesthesia machines in our operating room practices, make the question *where are we going*? very pertinent. In this direction much has been written about the benefits and disadvantages of paediatric anaesthetic circuits [14]. Classically the pediatric circuits have been designed to offer minimal resistance to reduce the work of breathing substantially and at the same time to prevent carbonic gas re-inhalation. The principal characteristics of these circuits is the absence of valves to be opened, minimising the work of breathing. Practically the great majority of all non-rebreathing circuits utilised nowadays are derived directly from T-piece tubing. The Ayre T system technique is one of the simplest inhalation anaesthesia technique. As inhaled anaesthetics are delivered directly into airway, and the volume of the non-breathing circuit is much less, the rate of anaesthetic induction should be more rapid. Many modifications of this simple piece, including reservoir bag, different sites of fresh gas flow entry and overflow, have been proposed. These modifications overcome some original disadvantages of the T-piece including lack of a reservoir, high flow anaesthetic delivery, environmental pollution, waste of anaesthetic agents, and poor control of ventilation. Spontaneous breathing is the main feature during anaesthesia utilising a T-piece and its modifications, however, if necessary, the ventilation can be assisted or even manually controlled [15]. Although safe and useful for short surgical procedures, the open or semi-open paediatric simplified circuits are undesirable for prolonged anaesthesia and more complex surgeries. Nevertheless, the production of a machine that combines proper ventilator and a safe breathing circuit to paediatrics has not been an easy task for industry in the recent history of anaesthesia. It is a fact that most paediatric anaesthesiologists have felt more confident manually ventilating their anaesthetised baby patients. Although the superiority of mechanical ventilation may not have reached a consensus among anaesthesiologists, during paediatric anaesthesia manual ventilation may carry some disadvantages. Prolonged manual ventilation mainly utilising T-piece derivatives has so far been far from ideal. High and dry flow, excessive wasting of agents, ambient pollution, irregularity of minute volume, impossibility of correct PEEP application, and requirement of two people during complex surgical procedures are some of the inconveniences. Lung ventilation employing the manual bag system assembled to the anaesthesia machine could be better, but should be considered only for short periods of time. Because of that, enormous efforts have been made by anaesthesia equipment manufacturers to offer a safe, user-friendly machine for anaesthesiologists to use during more complex operations.

Nowadays there is a renewed appeal to utilise standard adult anaesthesia machines in paediatric anaesthesia. The use of adult circle systems, including bellows, and standard CO_2 canister, may be recommended rather than semiclosed partial rebreathing circuits or specially designed paediatric circle systems, with bellows and canister of small size. There are many reasons for this, one of which is the possibility of utilising lower fresh flows or a closed system [16]. The use of an adult circle systems for infant anaesthesia allows lower fresh gas flows than are necessary with partial re-breathing systems. The modern ventilators coupled to an adult anaesthesia machine may also offer small and precise tidal volumes even in case of small infants [17]. Recently, Tobin et al. examined the efficiency of an adult circle system with adult bellows to deliver minute ventilation to an infant test lung model. The results of this laboratory investigation show that when an adult circle system is used during infant anaesthesia, the ventilation delivered depends fundamentally on the respiratory rate, peak inspiratory pressure and the compliance of the lung being ventilated, rather than on the specific mode of ventilator set-up [18]. Considering also the importance of mechanical ventilation during anaesthesia, Lockwood nicely reviewed the techniques of mechanical ventilation in closed and low flow systems. One simple system is to use automatic apparatus to compress a reservoir bag acting as manual ventilation utilising a bag. According to the quantity of fresh gas flow may be considered physically closed. The option is to change the bag with a "trunk", that consists of a long tube with an internal volume larger than the indicated tidal volume. Positive pressure is transmitted along this tube by a ventilator attached to one of these parts. The size of the trunk required is determined by the tidal volume, the rate of fresh gas delivery; the breathing system end of the trunk also acts as a reservoir of the gas system. Any ventilator normally used in an open system may be coupled with the trunk. In another way most of modern working station machines have the possibility of working in a closed reservoir system [19].

Finally before the presentation of part of our research and clinical investigation data, we will comment upon some aspects of the closed system and the pressure controlled ventilation modality used in this study. Closed circle ventilation has never been totally acceptable in infants because of the possibility of large dead space and resistance. Another disadvantage is the reduced ability to predict inspired oxygen, anaesthetic concentrations and the potential for carbon dioxide accumulation in the event of soda lime exhaustion. However modern microprocessor-controlled ventilators coupled to station anaesthesia machines, are capable of delivering very small pre-set tidal volumes, low resistance circuits, compensation for compliance, safety and economy. These concepts make the technique of low flow anaesthesia in children very attractive. Recently, Baker suggested the following classification (Table 1) for flow rates of gases into inhalation anaesthetic circuits. These suggestions are modifications of previous proposals [20, 21].

Table 1.

Metabolic flow	Lower than 250 mL $\cdot$ min^{-1}
Minimal flow	250-500 mL $\cdot$ min^{-1}
Low flow	500-1000 mL $\cdot$min^{-1}
Medium flow	1-2 L $\cdot$ min^{-1}
High flow	2-4 L $\cdot$ min^{-1}
Very high flow	Greater than 4 L $\cdot$ min^{-1}

Closed system anaesthesia is a term reserved for a technique in which significant leaks from system have been eliminated and maintenance of fresh gas flow is just enough to replace the volume of gas and vapour taken up by the organism.

Recently, Igarashi et al. using a Cicero anaesthesia machine (Dräeger, Germany), compared sevoflurane expenditure, inspired gas humidity, soda lime temperature, and compounds A and B in two groups of children during low flow circle and high flow circle anaesthesia. They observed a significant reduction of sevofluorane expenditure, and higher inspired absolute humidity, but not temperature, in the low flow group when compared to the high flow group [22].

Another controversial point in paediatric ventilation is related to the choice of ventilatory modality. In the ICU volume-controlled ventilation (constant inspiratory flow), is used primarily for older children (> 10 kg), simply because appropriate ventilators have been available. The delivered volume is pre-set, although some of this volume will be lost depending on the compliance and resistance of the respiratory system and circuits, as well as leaks around the uncuffed tube. In pressure-controlled ventilation (constant inspiratory pressure), ordinarily used for neonates and small children, tidal volume is not pre-set, alveolar volume depends on respiratory mechanics of lungs as well as the compliance and resistance of circuits. In terms of ventilator settings the pressure gradient is the peak inspiratory pressure (PIP) minus the positive end expiratory pressure (PEEP) if it is applied. There is some discussion as to whether pressure-controlled ventilation of infants and children is superior to volume-controlled ventilation, due to the belief that pressure control may maintain a constant airway pressure and compensate possible losses of tidal volume [23]. In anaesthesia, many of the arguments against circle systems in paediatric anaesthesia disappeared, and by 1980, the use of adult circle systems with controlled or assisted ventilation was considered acceptable and recommended for patients of all ages. Otherwise the question about volume or pressure-controlled modality advantages or disadvantages in anaesthesia has not been sufficiently clarified [24]. The modern micro processed ventilators available for anaesthesia may operate in volume or pressure controlled modality. The discussion of which modality is preferable specifically during anaesthesia is far from being of the same importance as this subject in ICU settings. Due to the scarce literature concerning the use of pressure-controlled ventilation associated with a closed circle system in paediatric anaesthesia, we employed this technique in experimental and clinical research. We present below part of these data.

Research data

In 12 rabbits we investigated the effects of pressure-controlled ventilation (PCV) with a re-breathing anaesthesia closed system compared to volume-controlled time-cycled (TC) with an open or closed system. The rabbits were divided into two groups. Group I - eight animals, mean weight $(2,550 \pm 0.393$ kg); in this group arterial carbon dioxide was maintained near 40 mmHg, by adjusting tidal volume whenever necessary. Group II - eight animals, mean weight $(2,250 \pm 0.206$ kg); in this group carbon dioxide was not corrected during the different ventilatory modalities. The animals were anaesthetised with halothane, tracheostomised and ventilated with a standard adult micro-processed anaesthesia machine. The machines were equipped with adult descendent bellows and a circle system. Conventionally, open systems (OS) were designed to use high fresh flow (1000 ml O_2 min^{-1} mixed with 3000 ml of air) and closed systems (CS), minimal fresh flow (250 to 300 ml of O_2 mixed with 600 to 700 ml of air) to reach a minimal oxygen concentration of 0.4. The established sequence was: 1 - *control* (controlled ventilation 6-8 ml kg^{-1}), without any circle system, exhalation open to the ambient. 2 - TC-OS: volume-controlled, time-cycled, high flow. 3 - *TC-CS*: volume-controlled, time-cycled, minimal flow. 4 - *TC-OS*: volume-controlled, time-cycled, high flow. 5 - *CS*: pressure-controlled $(16.85 \pm 2.85$ cm/H_2O), minimal flow. 6 - *TC-OS*: volume-controlled, time-cycled, high flow. Each programmed ventilatory setting was maintained for 30 minutes. Data were submitted to ANOVA, followed by Tukey's test $(P < 0.05)$. Fig. 2 shows the mean values of PIP (peak inspiratory pressure) in cm H_2O at different ventilatory settings correlated with mean values of arterial pH and carbon dioxide, at two pre-established conditions: corrected and non-corrected carbon dioxide by PIP adjusting. A significant elevation of carbon dioxide and arterial pH decrease was observed when the animals were anaesthetised with a closed system; the

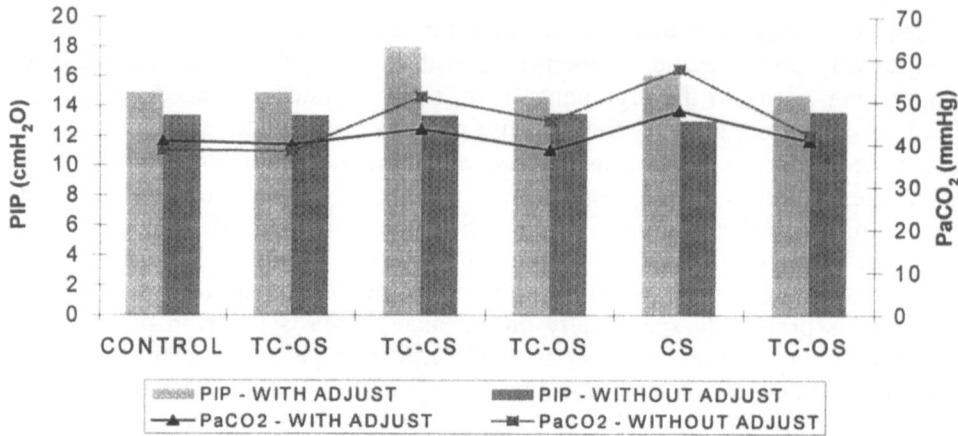

Fig. 2. The mean values of PIP (peak inspiratory pressure) in cm H_2O at different ventilatory settings correlated with mean values of arterial pH and carbon dioxide, at two pre-established conditions: corrected and non corrected carbon dioxide by PIP adjusting

Control: controlled-ventilation, without any circle system, exhalation open to the ambient. *TC-OS*: volume-controlled, time-cycled, high flow. *TC-CS*: volume-controlled, time-cycled, minimal flow. *TC-OS*: volume-controlled, time-cycled, high flow. *CS*: pressure-controlled, minimal flow. TC-OS: volume-controlled, time-cycled, high flow

oxygenation parameters were unaltered. These results showed that when our purpose is to use adult anaesthesia equipment for the low-flow technique in small animals or patients, the circle system apparatus should be carefully checked to the quantity of fresh flow used. Otherwise, the quantity of fresh flow in minimal or low-flow techniques depends closely on the apparatus dead space and resistance. Additional losses caused by uncuffed tubes, or by the respiratory mechanic pattern, should be carefully monitored during anaesthesia. Tidal volume delivered by pressure or volume-controlled ventilation should be adjusted according to airway pressures and arterial and expired gases.

The peak inspiratory pressure (cm H_2O) and arterial pH when tidal volume was or was not adjusted according to carbon dioxide level are presented in Fig. 3.

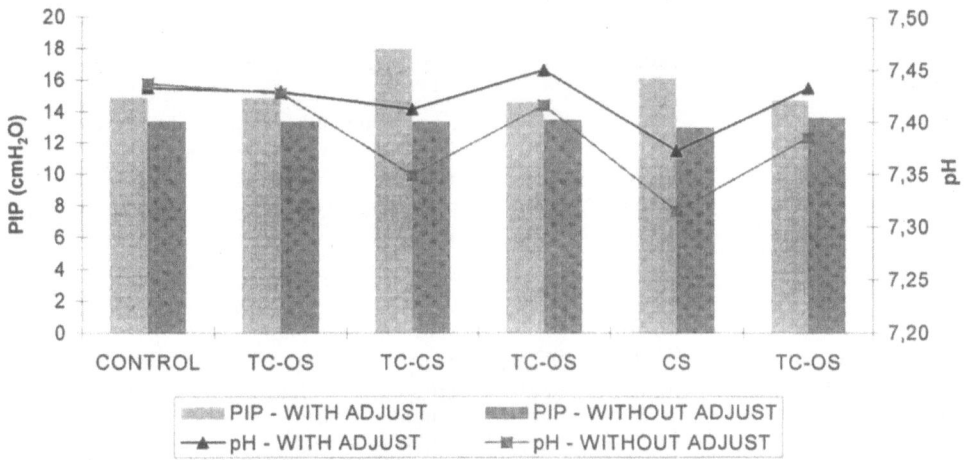

Fig. 3. The peak inspiratory pressure (cm H_2O) and arterial pH when tidal volume was or was not adjusted according to carbon dioxide level are represented

Control: volume-controlled ventilation, without any circle system, exhalation open to the ambient. *TC-OS*: volume-controlled, time-cycled, high flow. *TC-CS*: volume-controlled, time-cycled, minimal flow. *TC-OS*: volume-controlled, time-cycled, high flow. *CS*: pressure-controlled, minimal flow. *TC-OS*: volume-controlled, time-cycled, high flow

Clinical data

In order to evaluate low flow anaesthesia and pressure-controlled ventilation efficacy in paediatric patients we utilised this technique in 15 children submitted to a correction of congenital heart defects under cardiopulmonary bypass in our hospital. We employed an integrated anaesthesia machine (Cicero, Dräeger, Germany). In this equipment the fresh gas flow to the circle is intermittently stopped during inspiration, and flow is directed to a passive reservoir, so tidal volume is not influenced by the fresh gas flow. During expiration the passive reservoir is opened to the system again, and when full, gas is dropped if necessary. At the late phase of expiration the active reservoir, a gas tight piston electrically powered under microprocessor control, draws gas from the bag. The demographic data of the 15 children studied are given in Table 2.

Table 2. Demographic data

Patient	Age	Sex	BW	BS	Operation
1C	2	F	3.12	0.28	Coarctation of the aorta and Rastelli procedure
2	1	M	3.40	0.27	Coarctation of the aorta and VSD
3	2	M	4.70	0.25	TAPVC
4	5	F	4.74	0.31	PDA, PVE, VSD
5	9	M	5.30	0.31	TAPVC
6C	4	M	5.32	0.34	Senning procedure
7C	14	M	6.40	0.35	APVC
8	8	M	6.50	0.34	Ventriculoseptoplasty
9C	12	M	6.95	0.35	Rastelli procedure, VSD, ASD and PVE
10C	13	F	8.85	0.40	Tetralogy of Fallot
11C	12	F	9.06	0.41	Tetralogy of Fallot
12C	23	M	9.20	0.48	Tetralogy of Fallot
13C	17	M	10.00	0.45	VSD
14C	24	M	12.00	0.50	Tetralogy of Fallot
15C	24	F	13.00	0.60	Tetralogy of Fallot
	11.27	5:10	7.24	0.38	
	± 7.70		± 2.27	± 0.07	

Patient C: Cyanogenic disease (10 patients); Age (months); Sex (Female: Male); W: weight (kg), mean ± SD; BS: body surface (m²) mean ± SD; operation (VSD: ventricular septal defect; TAPVC: total anomalous pulmonary venous connection; PDA: persistent ductus arteriosus; PVE: pulmonary valve stenosis; APVR: anomalous pulmonary venous connection; ASD: atrial septal defect)

Tables 3 and 4 present anaesthetics agents and ventilatory data, showing that it is possible to employ workstation machines to anaesthetise and ventilate both adult and children.

Table 3. Anaesthetics agent consumption during anaesthesia (mean ± SD)

Agent	Dosis
Midazolam	0.455 ± 0.293
Pancuronium bromide	10.013 ± 5.471
Fentanyl	0.320 ± 0.141
Sevoflurane	2.207 ± 1.895

Each value is the mean (± SD); midazolam and pancuronium bromide: mg/kg; fentanyl: µg/kg; sevoflurane: mL/h

Table 4. Flow gases, expiratory tidal volume, airway pressure, and blood gases analysis. Each value is the mean (± SD) before and after CPB (cardiopulmonary bypass)

	Before CPB	After CPB
FiO_2	58.91 ± 6.43	60.60 ± 5.24
$\dot{V}O_2$	306.70 ± 37.16	350.00 ± 132.30
Vair	266.70 ± 30.86	276.70 ± 72.87
Ex Vt • kg^{-1}	9.98 ± 1.38	9.87 ± 1.79
P_{aw}max	22.33 ± 3.20	22.67 ± 3.20
P_{aw}plat	17.07 ± 3.47	17.53 ± 4.16
P_{aw}mean	5.00 ± 1.13	5.67 ± 1.23
Ex Sevo	1.31 ± 0.88	0.79 ± 0.37
$ETCO_2$	34.73 ± 4.86	32 70 ± 0.39
$PaCO_2$	38.00 ± 8.13	39.33 ± 6.66
SpO_2	95.73 ± 7.63	98.47 ± 1.77
PaO_2/FiO_2	211.60 ± 129.50	240.80 ± 96.56

FiO_2: inspired oxygen concentration (%); $\dot{V}O_2$: oxygen flow (mL • min^{-1}); Vair: air flow (mL • min^{-1}); Ex Vt • kg^{-1}: expiratory tidal volume (mL • kg^{-1}); P_{aw}max: maximum airway pressure (cm H_2O); P_{aw}plat: plateau airway pressure (cm H_2O); P_{aw}mean: mean airway pressure (cm H_2O); Ex Sevo: expiratory sevoflurane concentration (%); $ETCO_2$: end tidal carbon dioxide (mmHg); $PaCO_2$: arterial carbon dioxide (mmHg); SpO_2: pulse oxygen saturation of haemoglobin (%); PaO_2/FIO_2: arterial oxygen partial pressure/inspired oxygen concentration

In Fig. 4, we can observe that expiratory volume, peak inspiratory pressure, $PaCO_2$, PaO_2/FiO_2 remain unaltered before and after cardiopulmonary bypass.

J.O.C. Auler Jr, D. Fantoni, M.H.C. Pereira

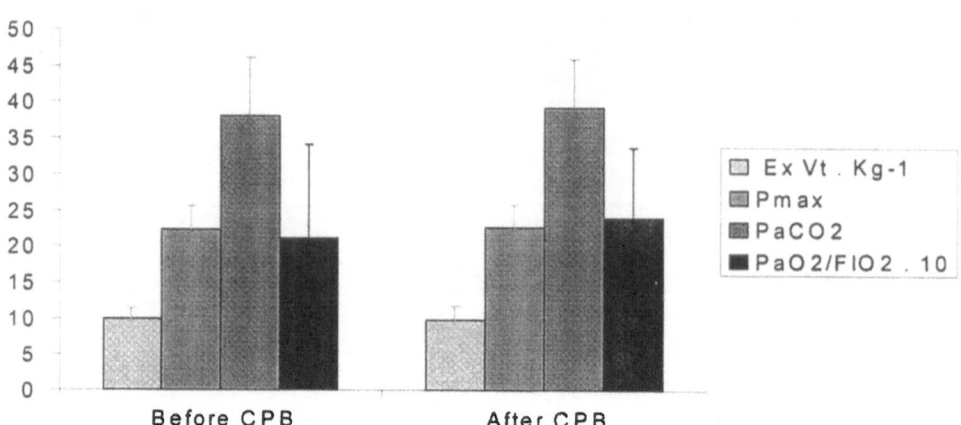

Fig. 4. Expiratory tidal volume, airway maximum pressure value, $PaCO_2$ and PaO_2/FiO_2 before and after cardiopulmonary bypass

Ex Vt $\cdot$ kg^{-1}: expiratory tidal volume (mL $\cdot$ kg^{-1}); Pmax: maximum airway pressure (cm H$_2$O); $PaCO_2$: arterial carbon dioxide (mmHg); PaO_2/FiO_2: arterial oxygen partial pressure/inspired oxygen concentration

Acknowledgements: Erika Miyoshi, MD; Claudia R. Fernandes, MD; Eliana Bonetti, DVM.

References

1. Muller NL, Bryan AC (1979) Chest wall mechanics and respiratory muscles in infants. Pediatric Clin North Am 26(3):503-516
2. Keens TG, Ianuzzo CD (1979) Development of fatigue resistant muscle fibers in human ventilatory musculature. Am Rev Resp Dis[Suppl]119:139-141
3. Lopes J, Muller NL, Bryan MH et al (1981) Importance of inspiratory muscle tone in maintenance of FRC in the newborn. J Appl Physiol 51:830-834
4. Henderson-Smart DJ, Read DJC (1979) Reduced lung volume during behavioral active sleep in the newborn. J Appl Physiol 46:1081-1085
5. Fisher JB, Carlo AW, Doershuk CF (1990) Pulmonary function from infancy through adolescence. In: Scarpelli ME (ed) 2nd edn Pulmonary physiology. Lea & Febiger, Philadelphia New York, pp 421-445
6. Nelson NM (1966) Neonatal pulmonary function. Pediatric Clin North Am 13(3):769-799
7. Klaus MH, Tooley WH, Weaver KH et al (1962) Lung volume in the newborn infant. Pediatrics 30:111-116
8. Gerhardt T, Bancalari E (1981) Maturational changes of reflexes influencing inspiratory timing of newborns. J Appl Physiol 50:1282-1285
9. Gerhardt T, Bancalari E (1980) Chest wall compliance in full-term and premature infants. Acta Paediatric Scand 69:359-364
10. Chu JS, Dawson P, Klaus M et al (1964) Lung compliance and lung volume measured concurrently in normal full term and premature infants. Pediatrics 34:525-532

11. Doershuk CF, Fisher BJ, Matthews LW (1974) Specific airway resistance from the perinatal period into adulthood. Am Ver Resp Dis 109:452-457
12. Conway CM (1985) Anaesthetic breathing systems. Brit J Anaesth 57:649-657
13. Cotter SM, Petros AJ, Dore CJ et al (1991) Low flow-anaesthesia practice, cost implications and acceptability. Anesthesia 46:1009-1012
14. Meakin G, Jennings AD, Beatty PCW et al (1992) Fresh gas requirements of an enclosed afferent reservoir breathing system during controlled ventilation in children. British J Anaesth 68:43-47
15. Mushin WW, Jones PL (eds) (1987) Physics for the anesthetist. 4th edn. Blackwell Scientific, Boston New York, p 375
16. Badgwell JM, Swan J, Foster AC (1996) Volume controlled ventilation made possible in infants by using compliant breathing circuits with large compression volume. Anesth Analg 82: 719-723
17. Stevenson GW, Tobin MJ, Horn BJ et al (1998) The effect of circuit compliance on delivered ventilation with use of an adult system for time cycled controlled ventilation using an infant lung model. Paediatric Anaesth 8(2):139-144
18. Tobin MJ, Stevenson SW, Horn JH et al (1998) Anesth Analg 87:766-771
19. Lockwood GG (1994) Techniques of mechanical ventilation in closed and low flow systems. Anesth Intensive Care 22:419-425
20. Baker AB (1994) Low flow and closed circuits. Anesth Intensive Care 22:341-342
21. Simionescu R (1986) Safety of low flow anesthesia. Circulation 3:7-9
22. Igarashi M, Watanabe H, Iwasaki H et al (1999) Clinical evaluation of low-flow sevofluorane anaesthesia for paediatric patients. Acta Anesth Scand 43:19-23
23. Perez-Fontan JJ, Heldt GP, Gregory GG (1985) The effect of a gas leak around the endotracheal tube on the mean tracheal pressure during mechanical ventilation. Am Rev Respir Dis 132:339-342
24. Smith RM (1980) Anesthesia for infants and children. 4th edn. CV Mosby, St Louis, pp 128-151

Perioperative Management Strategy for Cardiac Surgery in Pediatric Patients

J.O.C. Auler Jr, S. Coppola Gimenez, D. Monteiro Abbelan

Pediatric cardiac postoperative care

The Heart Institute of University of São Paulo Medical School is a center of reference in the treatment of neonatal and pediatric congenital cardiopathies in the state of São Paulo as well as other regions of Brazil that do not have access to specialized centers in this type of care. Over the past five years, 2298 children were operated on; 1592 of these surgeries were carried out using cardiopulmonary bypass (CPB) and 706 without it. In the last 12 months, for example, surgery consisted in connection of inter-atrial communication (52), inter-ventricular communication (59), Tetralogy of Fallot (94), transposition of the great arteries (23), and atrio-ventricular septal defect (38).

Throughout the past years, several protocols have been adopted in our ICU, especially in human resources and intensive care, which have benefited the postoperative results. Progress depends on harmony among several factors such as suspected diagnosis, good planning and scheduling of surgery and postoperative support. The challenge for all of the multi-professional team is to make possible the child's full reintegration into the family with preserved neurological, affective, psychological and social capacity.

Neonatal heart

The neonatal heart presents physiological characteristics that significantly differ from children of other ages or adults, which need to be considered in the perioperative approach [1].

First of all, neonatal contractile force is less than in the adult due to a series of structural alterations. The neonatal heart has a 50% reduction in myofibers and a greater quantity of non-connective tissue, which limits the systolic capacity for example in obstructive cardiopathies. The myofibers are found in a chaotic or non-linear arrangement. Aside from this, the neonatal myocardium has a smaller number of sarcomeres and mitochondria in addition to the sarcoplasmic reticulum being immature for calcium storage. The immature sympathetic nervous system reduces the myocardial storage of catecholamines. Moreover, myocardial contractility during the first week of life occurs due to circulating catecholamines, especially epinephrine, and cardiac output is maintained mainly by the elevated heart rate. Newborns are more dependent on the heart rate due to the action of circulating catecholamines than on preload for maintenance of adequate cardiac output. In contrast, the parasympathetic innervation is similar to that of the adult, making the neonate more susceptible to parasympathetic stimuli.

Secondly, the neonatal myocardial fiber has greater lengthening at baseline conditions, that is, less diastolic reserve to volume overload. In this way, there effectively occurs a reduction in contractility and in ventricular compliance, so the neonatal myocardium is near its functional limit.

Another important point about neonatal and fetal myocardial function is ventricular interdependency [2]. Through this mechanism it is understood that an overload in volume or pressure imposed on one of the ventricles influences the filling characteristics of the other ventricle. Thus, the dilated right ventricle can increase the filling pressure of the left one, and this therefore also generates elevated pressure on the right side in order to maintain trans-atrial flow.

In addition, immature fetal and neonatal myocardium uses metabolism of carbohydrates and amino acids (glycogen, glutamate, pyruvate and lactate) for contraction. Elevated stores of glycogen and a reduced number of mitochondria reflect adaptation to anaerobic conditions, with greater recovery capacity and tolerance to hypoxic and ischemic insults. Therefore, the neonate is more vulnerable to hypoglycemia and reacts to stress situations with rapid alterations in pH, lactic acid, glycemia and temperature. These characteristics are perpetuated not only in the neonatal period. Gradual transformations occur throughout the first year of life, and complete maturity of the myocardium is reached only after two years of age [3, 4].

Cardiopulmonary bypass

Cardiopulmonary bypass (CPB) for cardiac surgery is simple and almost necessary for the majority of congenital cardiopathies. Through it, the blood available in the systemic veins, generally the cavas, is drained by an oxygenator, which provides oxygen, removes carbonic gas and reduces the blood temperature. In the process, the oxygenated blood returns to the ascending aorta by a pump system that generates continuous flow from the CPB to the patient.

The plastic polyvinyl circuits of the CPB system are full of a balanced solution made of colloids and crystalloid, perfusate of which composition varies according to the age and weight of the patient, maintaining pH and electrolyte composition similar to that of the plasma.

To reduce metabolism and for organic protection during CPB, moderate (25 to 32°C) or profound (15 to 20°C) hypothermia is used. Profound hypothermia permits accentuated reduction of flow of CPB and of blood trauma or even total circulatory arrest, mainly during aortic arch repair or in very small children. Hypothermia also preserves the highly energetic phosphate stores and reduces liberation of toxic cerebral neurotransmitters.

Different methods have been proposed in the last several decades for correction of acid-base equilibrium during hypothermia, fundamentally comparing the neurological evolution of patients (stat, alphastat, alkaline). According to du Plessis et al., in 1997, children submitted to surgery using the alphastat method have worse cognitive development in the late postoperative follow-up when compared to those submitted to stat method correction, probably due to the acidification that the stat method provides, favoring vasodilatation and homogeneous hypothermic cerebral protection [5].

In general, CPB alters all physiological processes of the organism, many leading to organ dysfunction of different magnitudes. All is processed simultaneously and inter-relatedly; however, in a didactic manner, we can mention the following alterations: systemic inflammatory reaction, interstitial fluid retention, coagulation factor and platelet consumption, leukocytosis, stress hormone liberation, complement activation, and increase in systemic and pulmonary vascular resistance. Hemodilution to prime the circuits, by contrast, reduces microcirculation resistance while exacerbating interstitial edema.

The formation of edema can be explained by the hemodilution and by the inflammatory process unleashed by the passage of blood and elements through the non-endothelial surfaces of the CPB circuits. Permeability of the capillary vessels is greater in immature individuals than in adults. Potent vasoactive substances are activated, including anaphylatoxins C3a and C5a, tumor necrosis factor, free radicals derived from oxygen and neutrophil activation. Conventional ultrafiltration has been used in an attempt to prevent this edema, however its effectiveness seems limited. Naik and Elliot in 1993 modified the ultrafiltration system, placing the hemoconcentrator between the aorta and the right atrium immediately following CPB. With this modification a reduction in total body water content improved systolic function; increase in diastolic compliance, increase in systemic arterial pressure, hematocrit, fibrinogen and total plasmatic protein elevation, and decrease in endothelial serum, cytokines and C3a and C5a fraction levels of complement compliance were noted [6, 7].

For all these above mentioned factors it remains evident that prolongation of CPB time increases it deleterious effects and imposes systemic cardiocirculatory overload which is often already compromised by the cardiopathy or surgery itself.

Immediate postoperative care and monitoring

Adequate monitoring during the postoperative period involves a combination of clinical or auxiliary methods that can evaluate the surgical correction, myocardial function and the relationship between systemic and pulmonary blood flow [8].

In postoperative care of the pediatric patient it is fundamental that clinical evaluation be complete and systematic. In this way complications can be foreseen and catastrophic situations can be avoided. Care should be initiated while child is still in the operating room, with special attention to rewarming to 36.5°C, control of bleeding, ventilation, acid-base and electrolyte balance. It is very important during this phase to stabilize cardiac function by the adequacy of volemic, heart rate and myocardial contractility.

The main information relating to anesthetic and surgical procedure needs to be transmitted in detail to the multi-professional ICU team: surgical technique, type of anesthesia, perfusion and aortic clamping time, fluid and colloid balance, diuresis, venous and arterial catheter, pacemaker wire and mediastinal or thoracic drainage tube positioning, ventilatory conditions, acid-base balance, heart rate and arrhythmias, coagulation and vasoactive medication in use [9].

Supplementary monitoring is indicated in all children subjected to more serious or complex cardiopathy correction who present: a) significant myocardial dysfunction (left coronary anomaly, transposition of the great arteries, hypoplastic left heart); b) pulmonary arterial hypertension during or prior to the operative period (total anomalous drainage of the pulmonary veins, aortic arch interruption, *truncus arteriosus communis*); c) valvoplasty or correction of atrioventricular septal defect with residual defect of mitral insufficiency. In this way, routine monitoring includes: heart rate, systolic arterial pressure, diastolic and mean arterial pressure, central venous pressure and urinary output, nasogastric tube, mediastinal and/or pleural tubes, rectal temperature, respiratory parameters as well as pulse oximetry. Supplementary monitoring includes: left atrial and pulmonary artery pressure, cardiac output, pulmonary and systemic vascular resistance indexes, bi-dimensional or Doppler echocardiographic evaluation, recatheterization study and myocardial or pulmonary isotopic scintigraphy.

Cardiovascular function

The cardiovascular function of a child can be considered normal in the postoperative period when cardiac output is adequate to supply the demands of cellular oxygen.

As we know, the main determining factors of cardiac output are preload, afterload, contractility, heart rate and diastolic function [1]. Other indirect factors such as anxiety, pain, temperature, hemoglobin level, endogenous and exogenous catecholamines as well as blood biochemical composition can alter the myocardial oxygen supply-demand relationship in addition to affecting the cardiac output [10].

During the postoperative period, cardiovascular dysfunction, represented by low cardiac output, can be caused by a series of reasons: first of all, all pre-operative conditions, from the structural defect itself and the functional cardiac state to general birthing conditions, transfer from hospital to specialized care centers, detailed and careful planning of the surgery as well as associated complications such as respiratory insufficiency, infection, metabolic and electrolyte disturbances. Secondly, the dysfunction is dependent on the surgery performed, degree of myectomies, placement of corrective patches, myocardial protection, CPB time and aortic clamping, level of hypothermia during CPB, use of total circulatory arrest, and the type of anesthesia and intraoperative complications.

Cardiovascular evaluation

Postoperative cardiovascular function can be evaluated by clinical examination, by related tissue oxygen indexes or by echocardiography, or hemodynamic and/or radioisotopic evaluation [10].

Important clinical signals for the evaluation of cardiac output are: perspiration, adequate level of consciousness, coloring and temperature of extremities, thermal gradient between knees and feet, central and peripheral thermal gradient, amplitude of peripheral pulse, capillary filling, arterial pressure and urinary output. In this manner, the cardiac output is considered adequate when there is no cold perspiration or psychomotor agitation, the extremities are warm and colored, the feet are hotter than the knees, the central-peripheral thermal gradient is less than 4°C, the peripheral pulse is easily palpable, capillary filling is satisfactory, arterial pressure is within the normal limits for the age group and urinary output is greater than 1 ml kg^{-1} h^{-1}. It is important to remember that adequate peripheral vasodilatation only occurs after the fourth postoperative hour, with normal re-establishment of tissue perfusion around six hours postoperatively [10].

Among the related tissue oxygen indexes, lactate is a marker of anaerobic metabolism and tissue energy deficit. It reflects hypoxia, ischemia or action of toxic agent tissue aggression. Values for serum lactate above $2.0 - 3.0$ mmol l^{-1} reflect significant evidence of tissue hypoxia. Following total circulatory arrest, profound hypothermia ($< 20°C$) or low cardiac output it is common to find levels above $6\text{-}10$ mmol l^{-1}. Still related to tissue oxygenation, the calculation of the arteriovenous difference, consumption, transport and peripheral extraction of oxygen can be used in evaluation of low cardiac output in newborns, knowing that the prognosis is related to the adequacy of these indexes.

For the evaluation of myocardial injury, according to reports from Taggart and colleagues [11], measurement of troponine is a specific marker during the postoperative period after cardiac surgery employing CPB, with increased levels 6 hours following surgery and remaining elevated for 72 hours. This is contrary to what occurs with CKMB levels that are elevated in patients to surgery not using CPB, and a progressively decrease subjected over 72 hours.

Bi-dimensional or Doppler echocardiography represents a great arsenal in postoperative cardiac functional and structural evaluation. It permits analysis of cardiac chambers, operative results, detection of residual defects, position and function of valvar prostheses, segmental and global myocardial analysis, shortening and ventricular ejection fraction calculation, and estimation of intracavity or transvalvar pressures.

Cardiac catheterization for angiography or manometry of cardiac cavities is a traditional and accepted method that may be used in the postoperative period. The principal indications are: evaluation of systemic-pulmonary shunt permeability (e.g. Blalock-Taussig operation), evaluation of pulmonary vascularization following reunification or centralization of pulmonary arteries, measurement of residual pressure gradients after amplification of the right or left atrium, evaluation of cardiopulmonary anastomosis (e.g. Fontan or modified Glenn operation). During the neonatal period cardiac catheterization is rarely indicated for therapeutic procedures or investigation of residual defects that cannot be clarified using other methods of diagnosis.

Direct measurement of cardiac output can be obtained by invasive and non-invasive methods. The non-invasive method uses a relationship between expected oxygen consumption and the arteriovenous oxygen difference. However, the method is improper when applied in the postoperative period, for the expected consumption, calculated by nomograms, is dependent on heart rate, age, sex and body temperature, factors that are quite variable in the first hours following CPB [12].

Among the invasive methods for determining cardiac output, the most practical one for use in pediatrics is thermodilution and derived cardiac index.

In this method, the cardiac index may be considered normal in children when above $3\ l\ min^{-1}\ m^{-2}$, moderately reduced between 2.0 to $3.0\ l\ min^{-1}\ m^{-2}$ and severely reduced when lower than $2.0\ l\ min^{-1}\ m^{-2}$. In general, cardiac index tends to be lower at the fourth postoperative hour in relation to the immediate postoperative period and increases after the ninth or twelfth hours. Kirklin and colleagues [12] correlated greater number of hospital death with is observed cardiac index below $2.0\ l\ min^{-1}\ m^{-2}$ in a postoperative study of 174 children under the age of three months.

Low cardiac output

Low postoperative cardiac output is mainly caused by a reduction in myocardial contractility due to one of the mechanisms or factors mentioned above. Severe myocardial dysfunction can be observed, for example, in left anomalous coronary re-implant, the Norwood operation for hypoplastic left heart syndrome, the

Jatene operation for transposition of the great arteries, aortic valvoplasty as well as for correction of *truncus arteriosus communis*.

The second cause of hemodynamic instability is inadequate intravascular volume due to a series of factors: endothelial inflammatory process due to CPB that transfers fluids to the interstitial area mainly in the first 24 hours, vasodilatation during the rewarming period, which occurs 4 to 6 hours postoperatively, and urinary output and active blood loss or coagulopathies.

Control of intravascular volume and indirectly of preload should promote more effective systolic volume, according to the Frank-Starling law. In the absence of an atrioventricular valvar lesion, the final diastolic pressure of the ventricles corresponds to the mean pressure of the atrium and therefore volume can be controlled via right and left atrial pressures. During the postoperative period, the atrial pressure should remain around 15 mmHg; it may go up to 18 mmHg in the right atrium and 20 mmHg in the left when there is hypertrophy or hypocontractility, partial obstruction in the ventricular outflow or pulmonary artery hypertension.

Afterload is a third factor of cardiac dysfunction and can be elevated by vasoconstriction secondary to CPB, hypothermia, endogenous stress catecholamines or administration of vasoactive amines. The heart with any degree of myocardial dysfunction can significantly reduce myocardial fiber shortening and consequently its systolic volume when submitted to any increase in afterload.

Heart rate is dependent on factors such as use of digital or betablocker agents in the preoperative period, type of surgery, perioperative rhythm disturbances, volume, temperature, pain, anxiety, anemia, metabolic disturbances and use of vasoactive agents with chronotropic action.

Aside from these factors, postoperative myocardial edema could be responsible for ventricular diastolic restriction.

Treatment

Therapeutic measures for postoperative low cardiac output include three concomitant and related stages: 1) diagnosis; 2) reduction in metabolic demand; 3) adequate tissue perfusion and oxygen transport [1].

The etiological diagnosis of cardiac dysfunction should be suspected and promptly investigated by clinical or subsidiary methods so that specific and effective conduct is adopted. Reduction in metabolic demand uses measures that favor adequate temperature and reduction in respiratory workload. Initial measures, even during diagnostic investigation, can be adopted to maintain body temperature around 36.5°C [10].

Ventilation and respiratory mechanics play a primary role in the hemodynamic state of the postoperative patient, through the use of positive end expiratory pressure and adjustment of $PaCO_2$ and pH. Factors such as general anesthesia, pulmonary retraction and edema due to residual lesion, reduced functional residual capacity, lead to alterations in gas exchange, pulmonary compliance, abnormalities in ventilation-perfusion ratio and intrapulmonary shunts [10].

Mechanical ventilation is maintained until the absence of bleeding, stabilization of hemodynamics, adequate body temperature and absence of metabolic disturbances and acid-base balance. The necessary support for adequate tissue perfusion and oxygen transport is basically related to concomitant employment of inotropic and vasodilator agents.

Catecholamines make up the main therapeutic group in situations of cardiovascular insufficiency or low cardiac output. They can be endogenous such as dopamine and epinephrine or synthetic such as isoproterenol and dobutamine. All act through stimulation of myocardial beta-adrenergic receptors, increasing cyclic adenylate and cyclic adenosine monophosphate (cAMP) [13].

Dopamine increases myocardial contractility through several mechanisms: stimulation of post-synaptic β_1-adrenergic receptors, increase in liberation of norepinephrine in the myocardial pre-synaptic sympathetic storage sites, decrease in enzymatic degradation and reabsorption of norepinephrine. Dopamine also acts as a pulmonary and systemic vasoconstrictor through action in α_1- and $\alpha 1^{-2}$ post-synaptic receptors. Due to its action on dopamine adrenergic receptors it acts as a renal spleen, coronary and cerebral vasodilator. Dopamine, in animal research, has shown to be less efficient in neonates than in adult animals, probably due to the greater clearance, reduced myocardial adrenergic enervation, less density of myocardial β_1-adrenergic receptors, and differing maturation among peripheral α-receptors and myocardial $\beta 1^-$ and dopaminergic receptors. In neonates, dopamine increases cardiac output, heart rate and systemic arterial pressure [10]. Dopamine is indicated in moderately low cardiac output, especially when there is fluid retention from the cardiac insufficiency itself or posts CPB. In doses of 1 to 2 μg kg^{-1} min^{-1}, dopamine acts as vasodilator action on the mesenteric and renal circulation. In doses between 2 and 10 μg kg^{-1} min^{-1} it acts on myocardial β_1-receptors producing increased contractility and coronary flow with consequent improvement in mean arterial pressure and cardiac index. Driscoll and colleagues [14], however, observed that the neonatal myocardium seems less sensitive to the action of dopamine than children and more elevated doses are necessary to obtain the same effects. In another study, Lang and colleagues [15] observed that dopamine increases heart rate, cardiac index and systemic arterial pressure after pediatric cardiac surgery when given in doses 15 μg kg^{-1} min^{-1} but does not have significant action on systemic vascular resistance. In higher doses, dopamine raises pulmonary resistance, which is why it is avoided in cases of previous pulmonary artery hypertension.

Dobutamine is a synthetic sympathomimetic amine, β_1-adrenergic agonist. It differs from dopamine by not liberating endogenous norepinephrine and has little peripheral action. Dobutamine increases cardiac output, reduces systemic vascular resistance and ventricular filling pressure. There is a positive chronotropic effect; its ability to elevate heart rate and tachycardia could be a limiting factor in its use in postoperative cardiac surgery period in children and neonates [12]. Dobutamine is indicated for low cardiac output when not accompanied by severe hypotension. In sepsis without cardiac failure dobutamine is the therapy of choice and when there already exists cardiac compromise it can be indicated when combined with a vasoconstrictor like norepinephrine. Increase in cardiac output and reduction in systemic vascular resistance can be obtained starting dobutamine at low doses like 2.5 μg kg^{-1} min^{-1}. In general, doses of 2 to 20 μg kg^{-1} min^{-1} are effective.

Isoproterenol is a synthetic analogue of norepinephrine, an agonist that stimulates myocardial β_1-receptors, with direct inotropic and chronotropic action, and β_2 peripheral receptors with vasodilatation. It increases cardiac output, systolic arterial pressure, vasodilates renal, spleen and skeletal muscle territory with a reduction in diastolic arterial pressure and systemic vascular resistance [13]. Isoproterenol is indicated mainly in the presence of sinus bradycardia or transitory atrioventricular block. In the neonatal population, it can be indicated for controlling low cardiac output secondary to persistent arterial hypertension in the newborn. Initial dose of isoproterenol is 0.01 – 0.05 μg kg^{-1} min^{-1} for symptomatic bradycardia and 0.05 – 0.1 μg kg^{-1} min^{-1} as a positive inotropic agent. With the increase in heart rate an accentuated increase in myocardial oxygen consumption and transitory myocardial ischemia may occur. Sinus tachycardia ventricular arrhythmias due to compromised coronary flow can appear with more elevated doses.

Epinephrine is an endogenous catecholamine, liberated from the adrenal medulla and derived from norepinephrine. It acts on α, β_1- and β_2-receptors. According to dose it increases heart rate, systolic arterial pressure, decreases diastolic arterial pressure and vasodilates the peripheral vascular bed. In high doses the α-adrenergic effect predominates, compromising cutaneous, splenic and renal perfusion [10]. Epinephrine is indicated for low cardiac output accompanied by severe systemic arterial hypotension, compromising coronary perfusion; especially after cardiac surgery cardiogenic or septic shock do not respond to dopamine and dobutamine. It is also effective in cardiac arrest. In doses between 0.03 – 0.1 μg kg^{-1} min^{-1}, β_1 and β_2 effects are predominant. Between 0.1 to 0.2 μg kg^{-1} min^{-1} there is a mixed α and β effect. In doses above 0.2 until 1 μg kg^{-1} min^{-1} the α response is predominant. Ventricular arrhythmia due to possible subendocardic ischemia and peripheral vasoconstriction may be observed with this agent.

Norepinephrine it is a local adrenergic neurotransmitter. It has β_1 and α action, increasing the systolic arterial pressure as much as the diastolic. Cardiac output can increase or decrease depending on the myocardial reserve. A starting dose of 0.05-0.1 μg kg^{-1} min^{-1} has been recommended. Another possibility of therapy in the control of low cardiac output is the use of phosphodietesrase inhibitors, introduced into clinical practice since 1984.

The phosphodiesterase, amrinone and milrinone inhibitors are non-glycoside non-sympathomimetic agents that selectively inhibit the cyclic phosphodiesterase nucleotide, increasing the myocardial and vascular cAMP, independent of the β-receptors. Elevation of cAMP increases contraction through calcium regulation by two mechanisms: first, by activation of the kinase protein which facilitates the rapid entry of calcium through calcium channels and second, by activation of the calcium stores of the sarcoplasmic reticulum. In this way, the phosphodiesterase inhibitors have three actions: increase in inotropism and contractility, arteriolar and venous vasodilatation as well as increase in ventricular relaxation during diastole. Amrinone increases the cardiac index and decreases left ventricular end diastolic pressure, pulmonary capillary and right atrial pressure in congestive heart failure and in postoperative low cardiac output. Aside from this, when combined with dobutamine, it has greater action of elevation of cardiac index and reduction in systemic vascular resistance, and does not significantly increase heart rate [16].

Milrinone is considered to be 10-30 times more potent than amrinone. It does not elevate myocardial consumption and is a coronary vasodilator. Milrinone is mainly metabolized by the kidneys, so dose correction is necessary in the presence of renal failure. Amrinone is metabolized by the liver and excreted mainly by the kidneys.

Phosphodiesterase inhibitors can be indicated for low cardiac output with myocardial dysfunction and elevated systemic vascular resistance, but without severe arterial hypotension. Pediatric doses of amrinone are variable in the literature but have been cited as: 0.75 mg kg^{-1} bolus dose (at times repeated in 2-3 doses) followed by infusion of 5-10 μg kg^{-1} min^{-1} for maintenance. In neonates: 3 to 4.5 mg kg^{-1} bolus doses, followed by 5 to 15 μg kg^{-1} min^{-1} of continuous infusion. As the half-life of this agent is relatively prolonged (3 to 15 hours), special attention must be given to those children who already have systemic arterial hypotension. In adults with normal renal function, the bolus of milrinone is 50 μg kg^{-1} over 10 min, followed by 0.375 to 0.75 μg kg^{-1} min^{-1} infusion. Hypotension, with the necessity of administration of volume due to vasodilatation, thrombocytopenia, mainly after 7-10 days of its administration, elevation of hepatic enzymes, as described during amrinone infusion.

Vasodilators for low cardiac output are adjuvant to inotropic therapy, reducing systemic arterial resistance and enhancing ventricular ejection. Sodium nitroprusside in doses of 0.5 to 8 μg kg^{-1} min^{-1} acts on vascular relaxation through cGMP, with arteriolar and venous vasodilatation. The start of action after endovenous administration occurs in few minutes. The main metabolites of nitroprusside are tyocyanide and cyanide observed in prolonged infusion [13].

Sodium nitroprusside is the vasodilator most used not only for controlling systemic and pulmonary hypertensive states, but also for reducing afterload in low cardiac output, mainly after cardiac surgery. Nowadays sodium nitroprusside has progressively given place to phosphodiesterase inhibitors, which aside from inotropic are also arteriolar and venous vasodilators, in pediatric postoperative cardiac patients.

Nitroglycerine is a vasodilator in doses of 0.5 to 20 μg kg^{-1} min^{-1} that activates the nitric oxide liberation path. The main hemodynamic effect is vasodilation with reduction in ventricular filling pressures. Nitroglycerine is indicated in situations of increased preload and signs of pulmonary and systemic venous congestion.

The utilization of inhaled nitric oxide in the postoperative period

Nitric oxide produced by the endothelial cells exerts important functions on cardiovascular system. In the lung territory the maintenance of blood vessels in a relaxed status is fundamental, especially in the presence of previous pulmonary hypertension and/or right ventricle dysfunction. Right ventricular dysfunction is frequently observed in infants and children in the postoperative period. Pharmacological and ventilatory manipulations are directed at increasing RV inotropism, utilizing inotropic drugs as above outlined, by optimizing RV preload and controlling pulmonary vascular resistance (PVR). In the presence of RV dysfunction the control of PVR is extremely important, because RV output is very sensitive to the variations of afterload. As discussed, the more common agents utilized to control PVR are sodium nitroprusside, nitroglycerin and phosphodiesterase inhibitors [17]. Prostaglandin E1 (PGE1) and prostacycline (PGI2) both have a pulmonary-vasodilating effect. The problem is that neither drug's effects are limited to the pulmonary circulation. Because of the lack of specificity of vasodilator drugs on the pulmonary bed, newer pharmacological methods of controlling elevated PVR are being recommended. Ultra short acting intravenous vasodilators like adenosine and adenosine triphosphate and inhaled nitric oxide represent nowadays new concepts to treat acute pulmonary hypertension in pediatric postoperative cardiac patients. Although nonselective, NO is rapidly inactivated by hemoglobin; therefore when inhaled the systemic circulation is protected from its vasodilating properties. We administered inhaled NO in a group of patients after cardiac surgery; significant pulmonary vasodilatation and no clinical significant effects on systemic pressure were abserved [18]. These same effects can also been observed in children after cardiac surgery [19]. In more severe situations of RV dysfunction accompanied of pulmonary hypertension, we have used small doses of inhaled NO (3 to 5 parts per million) in our postoperative children. As several studies have demonstrated the vasodilator properties of NO on pulmonary circulation, its recommendation as a routine agent during cardiac surgery in pediatric patients suffering from pulmonary hypertension is still under investigation.

References

1. Feltes T (1998) Postoperative recovery from congenital heart disease. In: Garson A Jr (ed) The science and practice of pediatric cardiology. Williams & Wilkins, Baltimore, pp 2387-2413
2. Kleinman CS (1992) Abnormal fetal cardiovascular physiology. In: Polin RA, Fox WW (eds) Fetal and neonatal physiology. WB Saunders, Philadelphia, pp 666-670
3. Fisher DJ, Heyman MA, Rudolph AM (1980) Myocardial oxygen and carbohydrate consumption in fetal lambs in adult sheep. Am J Physiol 238:H399
4. Fisher DJ, Heyman MA, Rudolph AM (1981) Myocardial consumption of oxygen and carbohydrates in newborn sheep. Pediatr Res 15:843-846
5. Du Plessis AJ, Jonas RA, Wypij D et al (1997) Perioperative effects of alfa-stat versus pH-stat strategies for deep hypothermic cardiopulmonary bypass in infants. J Thorac Cardiovasc Surg 114:990-1001
6. Naik SK, Elliott MJ (1993) Ultrafiltration and pediatric cardiopulmonary bypass. Perfusion 8:101-112
7. Elliott MJ (1993) Ultrafiltration and modified ultrafiltration during pediatric open-heart operations. Ann Thorac Surg 56:1518-1522
8. Stanley TE, Newman MF (1994) Monitoring of the cardiac surgery patient. In: Barash PG, Reves JG (eds) Cardiac anesthesia: principles and clinical practice. Fawzy G. Estafanous, Philadelphia, pp 185-220
9. Reich DL, Kaplan JA (1993) Hemodynamic monitoring. In: Kaplan JÁ (ed) Cardiac anesthesia. WB Saunders, Philadelphia, pp 261-298
10. Wernovsky G, Chang AC, Wessel DL (1995) Intensive care. In: Emmanouilides GC, Allen HD, Reimenschneider TA et al (eds) Heart disease in infants, children and adolescents. 5th ed. Williams & Wilkins, Baltimore, pp 398-439
11. Taggart DP, Hadjinikolas L, Hooper J et al (1997) Effects of age and ischemic time on biochemical evidence of myocardial injury after pediatric cardiac operation. J Thorac Cardiovasc Surg 113:728-735
12. Kirklin JW, Barratt-Boyes BG (1993) Postoperative care. In: Kirklin JW, Barratt-Boyes BG (eds) Cardiac surgery. Churchill Livingstone, New York, pp 195-248
13. Talner NS (1995) Heart failure. In: Emmanouilides GC, Allen HD, Reimenschneider TA et al (eds) Heart disease in infants, children and adolescents. 5th edn. Williams & Wilkins, Baltimore, pp 1746-1773
14. Driscoll DJ, Gilette PC, McNamara DG (1978) The use of dopamine in children. J Pediatr 92:309-314
15. Lang P, Williams RG, Norwood WI et al (1980) The hemodynamic effects of dopamine in infants after corrective cardiac surgery. J Pediatr 96:630-634
16. Wessel DL, Triedman JK, Wernovsky G et al (1989) Pulmonary and systemic hemodynamics of amrinone in neonates following cardiopulmonary bypass. Circulation 80[Suppl II]:II-488
17. Prielipp RC, Butterworth JF, Zaloga GP et al (1991) Effects of amrinone on cardiac index, venous oxygen saturation, and venous admixture in patients recovering from cardiac surgery. Chest 99:820-825
18. Carmona MJC, Auler JOC Jr (1998) Effects of inhaled nitric oxide on respiratory system mechanics, hemodynamics, and gas exchange after cardiac surgery. J Cardiothorac Vasc Anesth 12:157-161
19. Journois D, Puard P, Mauriat P et al (1994) Inhaled nitric oxide as a therapy for pulmonary hypertension after operations for congenital heart defects. J Thorac Cardiovasc Surg 107:1129-1135

MANAGEMENT OF ANAESTHESIA
IN OBSTETRIC PATIENTS

Anaesthetic Management of Obstetric Emergencies

G. Lyons

Emergency anaesthesia is high risk

The most common procedure in obstetrics requiring anaesthesia is caesarean section.

Emergency anaesthesia is a risk factor for maternal deaths. In the most recent Confidential Enquiries into Maternal Deaths [1], of 93 deaths associated with caesarean section, 63 (67%) were in association with emergency operations. In some areas of the United States, some 80% of maternal anaesthetic deaths are in relation to emergency anaesthesia [2].

It is generally accepted that an *emergency* caesarean section is one that requires the delivery of the baby within 30 minutes. Experience shows that there are situations when delivery is required immediately, and there are no accepted definitions for less urgent situations. Of the 30 minutes available, five minutes are for transport to the operating room, five minutes are used in preparing and draping the patient, five to twenty minutes remaining for the anaesthesia. The choice of anaesthetic technique depends on the degree of urgency; the choice of technique has a bearing on risk. Hawkins et al. have calculated that general anaesthesia is 17 times more likely to end with a maternal death than regional blockade [3]. A basis for making the appropriate decision is shown in Table 1.

Table 1.

Time available	Suitable anaesthetic techniques
5-10 minutes	General anaesthesia
10-15 minutes	Spinal anaesthesia, general anaesthesia
> 20 minutes	Existing epidural, spinal, general anaesthesia

The degree of urgency dictates choice of emergency anaesthesia for caesarean section [4]. It is acknowledged that an experienced anaesthetist may require only five to ten minutes to perform spinal anaesthesia, while those with less experience may need longer than 15 minutes.

Indications for emergency caesarean section are shown in Table 2 [4, 5].

Table 2.

Emergency 5-20 minutes	Urgent	Planned emergencies
Foetal *distress*	Meconium stained liquor	Pregnancy induced hypertension
Abruptio placentae with viable foetus	Unfavourable foetal heart rate pattern	Scheduled elective caesarean section in labour
Bleeding placenta praevia	Obstructed labour	
Uterine rupture		
Scar dehiscence		
Cord prolapse		
Delivery of second twin		

Most common emergencies reflect the need to deliver the foetus urgently, and the list above deals with both antepartum and peripartum conditions. Amniotic fluid embolism occurs suddenly and unexpectedly around the time of delivery and is responsible for five deaths annually in the United Kingdom. An Obstetric Anaesthetist is likely to be involved in the resuscitation. A similar number of deaths are due to haemorrhage, which represents a final common pathway for a number of the conditions listed above [1]. Finally, management of the inverted uterus will be discussed.

This review will focus on the problems specific to the obstetric condition, rather than deal with management of anaesthetic problems like difficult intubation, aspiration, or more general problems like coagulopathy and hypertension. Pregnancy induced hypertension is too large a subject to tackle, and good reviews are available elsewhere [6].

Antepartum emergencies

Antepartum haemorrhage

Third trimester bleeding complicates 4% of pregnancies. The two most important causes are placenta praevia and abruptio placentae [7]. Haemorrhage resulting from these conditions kills approximately two women annually in the United Kingdom [1] and is an important cause of admission to the Intensive Care Unit [8].

Placenta praevia

There is little information available on morbidity arising from this condition. A grading system is used to assess risk of haemorrhage with vaginal delivery. Risk decreases as the distance between the placenta and the cervical os increases. The position of the placenta is ascertained by ultrasonography. Because the lower segment enlarges during the third trimester, this distance tends to increase with uterine growth. The grading system is shown in Fig. 1.

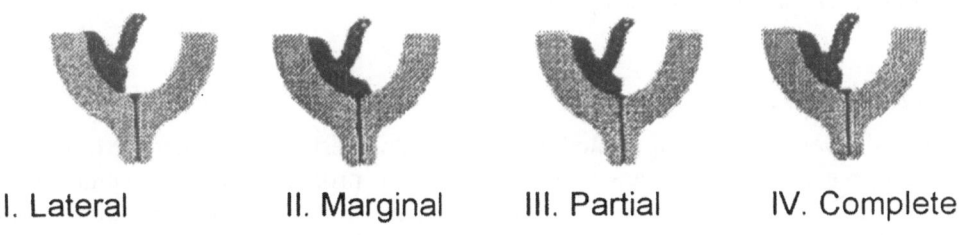

I. Lateral   II. Marginal   III. Partial   IV. Complete

Fig. 1. Placenta praevia

Grades I and II may permit vaginal delivery, but grades III and IV are regarded as an indication for caesarean section. While this may indicate the risk of haemorrhage attached to vaginal delivery, it is of no value in assessing risk of haemorrhage at caesarean delivery. Risk factors for caesarean delivery include age and multiparity, but the most important risk is the presence of a uterine scar. Posterior praevia is of low risk and can be managed with regional blockade, but an anterior praevia in a scarred uterus sometimes proceeds to hysterectomy and intensive care. Many would favour general anaesthesia in this situation. Delivering the baby through the placenta may cause some bleeding, but in a normal uterus this will be rapidly controlled once oxytocin is given. For this reason, anterior praevia in an unscarred uterus is suitable for regional blockade, provided venous access is excellent.

Abruptio placenta

Abruption may be marginal or central. With the former, the foetus may be viable, but this is rarely the case with central abruption. Haemorrhage can be considerable and concealed. The uterus tends to be hard, painful and irritable, and proceeds to expel the dead foetus with a short labour. Severe abruption is associated with disseminated intravascular coagulation, with falling platelet count and fibrinogen levels, and rising titres of fibrin degradation products. The coagulation screen is mandatory, and alternatives to regional blockade should be sought if doubt exists about haemostasis.

Peripartum emergencies

Amniotic fluid embolism

Six women die every year from this condition in the United Kingdom [1]. It is characterised by sudden and unexpected collapse. Risk factors are age, possibly obstetric intervention and uterine overstimulation. It is not generally a complication of an uneventful pregnancy and labour. It can occur during anaesthesia for caesarean section which may be required in an extreme situation. Those that survive the initial collapse develop disseminated intravascular coagulation. Regional blockade has no place.

Foetal distress

When delivery is required immediately, general anaesthesia is often the only option. However the best anaesthetic is one which produces the least acidosis in the foetus. In a large retrospective observational study of premature babies delivered by caesarean section, Rolbin et al. found that after epidural anaesthesia, had fewer Apgar scores below four than after general anaesthesia [9]. Spinal anaesthesia is associated with a small incidence of neonatal acidosis, with pH < 7.2 [10], and one study claims better results with general anaesthesia [11]. Despite this, assessments of neonatal well being are better after regional blockade [12]. Foetal pH reflects both respiratory and tissue acidosis, and it has been suggested that prolonged oxygen debt is better represented by measuring base deficit [13]. This might remove discrepancies between biochemical and clinical assessments, which will favour the use of spinal anaesthesia.

Cord prolapse

The knee elbow position is favoured by many when the cord prolapses, but some compromise is required for induction of anaesthesia. General anaesthesia is often the only option here, but if the foetal head is secure above the cord, and foetal heart rate pattern is steady and reassuring, a confident anaesthetist may attempt spinal anaesthesia.

Uterine dehiscence and rupture

Dehiscence may not be associated with significant changes in mother or baby, and can be managed with spinal anaesthesia. Uterine rupture is more severe and may result in foetal death with sudden maternal abdominal pain; many would favour general anaesthesia in this situation. If uterine rupture occurs during epidural analgesia in labour, peritoneal soiling presents as breakthrough pain. Obstetric concerns are related to the inability to detect prodromal symptoms, increasing tenderness in a uterine scar, in the presence of epidural pain relief. Scar tenderness is assessed by palpation. Presence of a scar is not required for rupture.

Delivery of the second twin

Occasionally, unanticipated difficulties arise delivering the second twin, often because of malpresentation. When good communication has occurred, the anaesthetist is often already in attendance, and epidural anaesthesia in place. If this is not the case, general anaesthesia will be required.

Postpartum emergencies

Postpartum haemorrhage

Postpartum haemorrhage occurs in 4% of pregnancies. The list of risk factors is extensive but uterine atony is generally responsible [14]. Deaths seem more likely when caesarean delivery has been required, and when coagulation is impaired [1]. Placenta accreta is rare and often unanticipated, and complicates management.

Inverted uterus

This does not seem to be a cause of maternal death; it is a rare problem. Hypotension occurs often and sometimes as a result of haemorrhage. General anaesthesia is favoured, but because hypotension tends to be neurogenic, in the absence of bleeding, a theoretical case can be made for spinal anaesthesia, but there are no studies at present.

Prophylactic measures

Obstetric emergencies can generate panic in the unexperienced. As a result, sometimes an anaesthetist is sometimes constrained to expedite delivery. Despite the pressure, the anaesthetist must be the guardian of maternal interests, and adopt sound practices at all times.

Steps can be taken to avoid emergency general anaesthesia. If women at risk can be persuaded to have early epidural analgesia, emergency general anesthesia can be avoided in approximately 75% [15]. The use of a prenatal anaesthetic assessment in clinic can help reduce problems [16]. When the unexpected emergency occurs, good communication, and prepared management protocols are recommended [1]. Drills for managing difficult tracheal intubation and major haemorrhage should be familiar to all staff, and a protocol for the management of pregnancy induced hypertension should be available.

References

1. UK Departments of Health (1998) Why mothers die. Report on confidential enquiries into maternal deaths in the United Kingdom 1994-1996. Her Majesty's Stationery Office, Norwich, pp 2-17
2. Endler GC, Mariona FG, Sokol RJ, Stevenson LB (1988) Anesthesia related maternal mortality in Michigan 1972-1984. Am J Ob Gyn 159:187-193
3. Hawkins JL, Koonin LM, Palmer SK, Gibbs CP (1997) Anesthesia related deaths during obstetric delivery in the United States 1979-1990. Anesthesiology 86:277-284
4. Rout CC (1997) Emergency general anaesthesia. In: Russell IF, Lyons G (eds) Clinical problems in obstetric anaesthesia. Chapman & Hall, London, pp 161-177
5. Medearis AL, Shields JR (1998) Multiple gestation. In: Hacker NF, Moore JG (eds) Essentials of obstetrics and gynecology. Saunders WB, Philadelphia, pp 281-289
6. Dresner M, Walker JJ (1997) Preeclampsia. In: Russell IF, Lyons G (eds) Clinical problems in obstetric anaesthesia. Chapman & Hall, London, pp 11-31
7. Goodman JR (1998) Antepartum hemorrhage. In: Hacker NF, Moore JG (eds) Essentials of obstetrics and gynecology. Saunders WB, Philadelphia, pp 187-195
8. Lewinsohn G, Herman A, Leonov Y, Klinowski E (1994) Critically ill obstetrical patients: Outcome and predictability. Crit Care Med 22:1412-1414
9. Rolbin SH, Cohen MM, Levinton CM (1994) The premature infant: Anesthesia for cesarean delivery. Anesth Analg 78:912-917
10. Noden J, Lyons G (1998) Spinal anaesthesia for caesarean section: good for mother and baby? Int J Obs Anesth 7:200-201
11. Roberts SW, Lucas MJ, Kelly MA et al (1994) Significant fetal acidemia associated with regional anesthesia for elective cesarean section. Am J Obs Gyn 170:167
12. Abboud T, Nagappala S, Murakawa K (1985) Comparison of the effects of general and regional anesthesia for cesarean section on neonatal neurologic and adaptive capacity scores. Anesth Analg 64:996-1000
13. Cheek TG, Lewin S (1999) New developments in fetal monitoring for the anesthesiologist. Curr Op Anaesth 12:289-293
14. Hayashy RH (1998) Postpartum haemorrhage and puerperal sepsis. In: Hacker NF, Moore JG (eds) Essentials of obstetrics and gynecology. Saunders WB, Philadelphia, pp 333-342
15. Morgan BM, Magny V, Goroszeniuk T (1990) Anaesthesia for emergency caesarean section. Br J Obs Gyn 97:420-424
16. Hamza J, Benhamou D, Frizelle H (1997) Antenatal assessment. In: Russell IF, Lyons G (eds) Clinical problems in obstetric anaesthesia. Chapman & Hall, London, pp 249-259

Neonatal Resuscitation

D. Trevisanuto, F. Zacchello

Newborn resuscitation is one of the most frequent procedures carried out in medicine. In fact, approximately 5-6% of all newborn infants and up to 80% of very immature neonates need some degree of resuscitation at birth [1-3]. More than 5 million neonatal deaths occur worldwide each year. It has been estimated that birth asphyxia accounts for 19% of these deaths, suggesting that the outcome might be improved for more than 1 million infants per year through standardisation of clear guidelines and the implementation of simple resuscitative techniques [4].

How to perform neonatal resuscitation

Good interdisciplinary collaboration is essential in the delivery room. In fact, a careful knowledge of the maternal history anticipates the needs of the neonate after birth in approximately 60% of deliveries. For these reasons, several antepartum and intrapartum situations have to be considered before the birth [1-3]. However, perinatal asphyxia, neonatal respiratory failure, and sepsis occur despite prospective low risk assignment early-on in pregnancy, and up to 30-40% of admissions to Neonatal Intensive Care Units are from low risk pregnancies [4].

Equipment for resuscitation should be readily available and in working order at every delivery.

All equipment should be checked on a daily basis by the staff responsible for the delivery room. Prior to each delivery the person responsible for resuscitation should re-check the equipment and ensure the following:

- radiant heater turned on and warm towels available;
- room temperature at 24°C;
- suction apparatus working at 100 mmHg;
- oxygen supply working with blow-off valve set at 30 cm H_2O.

Other preparations such as the drawing up of drugs or preparing appropriate endotracheal tubes should be performed in advance of delivery if resuscitation is anticipated from maternal history.

The goals of neonatal resuscitation are the following: to establish and to maintain a secure airway, to provide effective ventilation and to support the circulation. Additional considerations include the thermal environment and the provision of energy, especially for the low birth weight infant.

The extensive recommendations for neonatal resuscitation at birth are reported in the Textbook of Neonatal Resuscitation 1987, 1990, 1994, endorsed by the American Heart Association and the American Academy of Pediatrics [2].

In a very simple, but didactic way, neonatal resuscitation in the delivery room may be divided in 4 progressive stages with specific times:

Table 1. Stages of neonatal resuscitation in relation to the time

1	2	3	4
Initial step of resuscitation	Ventilation	External cardiac massage (ECM)	Medications
20 seconds	15-30 seconds	30 seconds	

All neonates undergo the 1st step at birth. The goals of this stage consists in avoiding the cold stress, maintaining an open airway and administering tactile stimulation to initiate respiration. This process should take no more than 20 seconds. An evaluation of the newborn must then be performed: respiratory effort, heart rate and color are the 3 clinical signs that will guide the therapeutic intervention. If there is cyanosis, 100% oxygen should be administered by continuous flow holding the tube or the mask as near to the infant's face as possible (1-1.5 cm).

If the infant is apneic, gasping or has a heart rate of less than 80 bpm, it is necessary to pass to the 2nd stage (ventilation) administering positive pressure ventilation (PPV) by face mask or endotracheal tube. The ventilation has to be performed using 100% oxygen, at a respiratory rate of 40-60 bpm. Assisted breaths have to be considered adequate when there are chest wall movements (2.5-5 mm), auscultation of symmetrical breath sounds and contemporary clinical improvement.

Remember: effective ventilation means success of neonatal resuscitation!

The majority of the resuscitated neonates are effectively ventilated using the face mask and about 25% of them will need tracheal intubation [2, 3, 5]. The conditions requiring tracheal intubation are the following: ineffective and prolonged face mask ventilation, meconium aspiration syndrome (thick meconium) and congenital malformations such as congenital diaphragmatic hernia [2].

Only a small number of infants will require the other two resuscitation steps: ECM and medications. In fact, in two large observational studies by Jain [3], and Perlman and Risser [6] only 0.03% and 0.06% needed chest compressions and epinephrine administration, respectively. The indications for ECM are the following: cardiac arrest at birth and heart rate less than 60-80/min despite effective ventilation with 100% oxygen. ECM may be administered by two techniques: the method of the two-thumbs or the two-fingers. The fingers should be placed over the middle third of the sternum. The depth of compressions is 2-3 cm. Assisted ventilation should be continued during ECM with 3 compressions per 1 assisted breath, yelding 120 events in 1 minute (90 compressions, and 30 breaths). For optimal performance two operators are needed.

The indication for using drugs during neonatal resuscitation is bradycardia (< 80 bpm) which persists despite PPV with 100% oxygen and ECM for 30 seconds. At birth, in an emergency situation, the umbilical vein is the route of choice for administration of medications.

Only 4 drugs are considered necessary (useful) at birth: epinephrine, volume expanders, sodium bicarbonate and naloxone.

Table 2. Dosage, mode and route of administration of drugs in neonatal resuscitation

Drug	Dosage	Mode	Route
Epinephrine	0.01-0.03 mg/kg	Bolus	IV or ET
Volume expanders (normal saline, 5% albumine, plasma substitutes, lactate ringers)	10-20 ml/kg	5-10 mins	IV
Sodium bicarbonate	2 mEq/kg	Slowly over 2 mins	IV
Naloxone	0.1 mg/kg	Bolus	IV or ET

The most important pharmacologic effect of epinephrine during the neonatal period is represented by α receptor stimulation, causing a rise in systemic vascular resistance and blood pressure. This peripheral vasoconstriction enhances blood flow to the brain and heart. The improved coronary perfusion increases oxygen delivery to the myocardial cells and, in turn, the heart rate will recover [7-9].

Volume expanders are indicated in the presence of clear signs of hypovolemia such as feto-maternal hemorrhage.

Even if included in neonatal resuscitation recommendations, the administration of alkali (sodium bicarbonate) is controversial. In fact, there are experimental results in dogs showing that the administration of sodium bicarbonate may be detrimental to the cardiovascular system. Moreover, when sodium bicarbonate is given, it is necessary to adequately ventilate the patient as there is a production of CO_2 (Henderson-Hasselbalch equation) [7-9].

Naloxone is not a specific emergency drug in the delivery room, in fact respiratory depression may be resolved by ventilation. The indication for naloxone use is the presence of respiratory depression in an infant whose mother received narcotic medication within 6 hours of delivery. It is important not to give naloxone to neonates of narcotic dependant mothers as acute withdrawal may occur.

Atropine, calcium gluconate and isoprenaline are not recommended for resuscitation of the newborn at birth.

Areas of controversy needing additional research

Until the early 1960s, neonatal resuscitation was based on clinical experience in human newborns. Subsequently, Dawes [10] described the classical changes of perinatal asphyxia in a rhesus monkey experimental model, which probably approximates events in human neonates.

In 1987, standard recommendations for neonatal resuscitation were published in the USA. However, although guidelines and textbooks recommend some specific and clear therapeutic interventions in the delivery room, the scientific background of these has never been established [7-8].

To date, several controversies in neonatal resuscitation exist:
- how to maintain a good temperature?
- what oxygen concentration to use?
- how to ventilate a neonate at birth?
- is there a place for laryngeal mask airway (LMA)?
- is prophylactic surfactant effective?
- what is the efficacy, dosage and route of administration of emergency drugs?

How to maintain a good temperature?

The temperature of the delivery room is frequently set for the comfort of the medical staff rather than of the neonate. Conventional practice consists in drying newborns and putting them under radiant warmers soon after birth [2]. Consequently, high evaporative heat loss is already initiated during the period of early infant stabilization. This may be deleterious for LBW infants, but also for neonates with abdominal wall defects [11].

Recently, Vobra et al. [12] proposed a new method to reduce heat loss in LBW infants at birth. Twenty-seven LBW infants dressed with a polyethylene occlusive skin wrap applied immediately at birth (without drying) were compared with 20 control neonates matched for gestational age and managed in conformity with the protocol described by the Neonatal Resuscitation Program. In the former group, only the head was dried and was left out of the wrap. Airway and vital signs were managed conventionally. Polyethylene wrap applied immediately after birth significantly reduced the postnatal fall in temperature in neonates with gestational age < 28 weeks. Furthermore, a significant reduction in mortality rates in the treated group was found. This method of maintaining temperature seems "easy, cheap, practical, effective and does not interfere with current practice for resuscitation" [12].

What oxygen concentration to use?

The current recommendations of the American Heart Association strongly indicate the use 100% oxygen during neonatal resuscitation [1, 2]. However, recent convincing experimental and clinical studies demonstrate that asphyxiated neonates can be resuscitated with room air as efficiently as with pure oxygen [13-15]. Cerebral blood volume [16] and pulmonary vascular resistances [17] were not different in 21% oxygen and 100% oxygen resuscitated animals. Furthermore, resuscitation with 100% oxygen could depress ventilation and therefore delay the first breath in neonates [15]. As reported by Saugstad, "the optimal O_2 concentration is perhaps 21%, that is, room air. The simplest solution may be also the best one"! Monitoring of arterial O_2 saturation could play a role in improving neonatal resuscitation, particularly in LBW infants [15].

How to ventilate a neonate at birth?

To reduce chronic lung disease (CLD) incidence in VLBW infants, new technologies of ventilation, coming from studies on in adults, have been applied in several limited clinical trials. However, CLD may result from fetal exposure to inflammatory cytokines or to delivery room practice [18]. The guidelines for neonatal resuscitation recommend ventilating the neonate obtaining "good" chest movements and a pink color [1, 2]. Two recent experimental studies demonstrate that, at birth, few inflations with volumes that are probably harmless in other circumstances negatively influence functional and histologic features of the surfactant-deficient lung [19, 20]. In an editorial, Jobe [18] reports that, when the lung is maintained at a reasonable functional residual capacity, a tidal volume of about 5 ml/kg is adequate for the preterm human infant even if "good" chest movements are not obtained. Furthermore, an individualized intubation strategy of ELBW infants was demonstrated to be superior to immediate intubation of all ELBW infants with slight signs of respiratory distress after birth [21]. These findings challenge current neonatal resuscitation practice and suggest that ventilation early after birth needs to be very gentle.

Is there a place for laryngeal mask airway?

The LMA has revolutionized routine airway treatment in anesthetized adults [22]. The device is inserted in the hypopharynx at the interface between the gastrointestinal and respiratory tracts, where it forms a circumferential low pressure seal around the glottis. In neonatal resuscitation, LMA was used as an alternative to face mask ventilation and for difficult airway management [23]. However, there are several significant limitations in the use of the LMA in the resuscitation of the critically ill neonate: as leaks around the LMA usually occur at pressures of 20 mmHg, the distending pressure required to inflate a neonatal lung with low compliance may be impossible to reach. Furthermore, the airway is not protected from regurgitated gastric contents and an access to the lower airway is not secured to permit suctioning. Even if experiences with LMA are reported in neonatal resuscitation, no controlled trials have been published in pediatric literature.

Is prophylactic surfactant effective?

Surfactant replacement therapy significantly improves gas exchange, the severity of the acute respiratory distress and the survival in preterm infants [24]. Surfactant administration at birth (prophylaxis) presents some clinical and economic limitations due to the over-treatment which means exposing some infants (about 50% at gestational age less than 30 weeks) to the risks of the therapy (cyanosis, bradycardia, etc.) and to elevated costs. Experimental and clinical studies demonstrate that prophylactic surfactant administration is more effective than rescue therapy [24, 25].

In a recent meta-analysis a decrease in the incidence of pneumothorax, pulmonary interstitial emphysema, mortality and bronchopulmonary dysplasia or death was associated with prophylactic administration of surfactant. No significant unwanted effects of prophylactic therapy were demonstrated. The authors concluded that "prophylactic surfactant administration to infants at risk of developing respiratory distress syndrome (intubated infants less than 30-32 weeks gestation) has been demonstrated to improve clinical outcome" [25]. However, in a recent European study, early (< 1 hour after birth) surfactant administration was not found to be superior to late treatment (2-6 hours after birth) in terms of relevant outcome variables in preterm infants of 27 to 32 weeks' gestational age [26]. Prophylactic surfactant replacement therapy could be of particular benefit in the subgroup of most immature infants (26 weeks of gestation or less) [24, 25].

What is the efficacy, dosage and route of administration of emergency drug?

The dose and the route of epinephrine is still controversial. The current recommended dose of epinephrine is 0.01 to 0.03 mg/kg of the 1:10.000 concentration. This dose is an extrapolation of the adult dose (0.5 to 1 mg, or 0.007 to 0.014 mg/kg for a 70 kg adult). More recently the debate has centered around the use of high-dose epinephrine. In pediatrics the new guidelines of the Pediatric Advanced Life Support (PALS) group recommend a dose of 0.1 mg/kg if the first standard dose (0.01 mg/kg) is ineffective. The high dose of epinephrine has not been recommended in neonatal resuscitation because of the pathophysiological differences in bradycardia between adults (underperfused cardiac state - ventricular fibrillation) and neonates (perfused cardiac state) and the strong association of hypertension and intraventricular hemorrhage especially in preterm infants [8]. It is possible to administer epinephrine via endotracheal tube but it is necessary to quickly establish an intravenous access. NRP guidelines recommend the same dose be administered endotracheally or intravenously.

Despite the theoretical advantages of the sodium bicarbonate administration (reduction of metabolic acidosis), there are several potential side effects (reduction of intramyocardial pH, hypernatremia, intraventricular hemorrhage) which limit its use. For these reasons, the administration of sodium bicarbonate remains controversial, especially in preterm infants less than 32 weeks' gestation.

Conclusion

Management of neonatal resuscitation is clearly recommended following specific protocols, but several aspects need further research and remain unresolved. Education and formation of the personnel (protocols and courses) have to be included and implemented in every institution where a baby is delivered.

References

1. Emergency Cardiac Care Committee and Subcommittees, American Heart Association (1992) Guidelines for cardiopulmonary resuscitation and emergency cardiac care. VII: Neonatal resuscitation. JAMA 268:2276-2281
2. Bloom RS, Cropley C (1990) Textbook of neonatal resuscitation. In: Chameides L, Dallas (ed) TX: American Heart Association and Elk Grove, IL: American Academy of Pediatrics
3. Jain L, Vidyasagar D (1993) Cardiopulmonary resuscitation of newborns. Pediatr Clin North Am 40:287-303
4. World Health Organisation (1991) Child health and development: health of the newborn. World Health Organisation, Geneva
5. Trevisanuto D, Ferrarese P, Cantarutti F et al (1997) Neonatal resuscitation in delivery room: the experience in 3 Veneto's Centres. Med Surg Ped 19:77-80
6. Perlman JM, Risser R (1995) Cardiopulmonary resuscitation in the delivery room: associated clinical events. Arch Pediatr Adolesc 149:20-25
7. Frand MN, Honig KL, Hageman JR (1998) Neonatal cardiopulmonary resuscitation: the good news and the bad. Pediatr Clin North Am 45:587-598
8. Ginsberg HG, Goldsmith JP (1998) Controversies in neonatal resuscitation. Pediatr Clin North Am 25:1-15

9. Leuthner SR, Jansen RD, Hageman JR (1994) Cardiopulmonary resuscitation of the newborn. An update. Pediatr Clin North Am 41:893-907
10. Dawes G (1968) Fetal and neonatal physiology. Yearbook Medical Publishers, Chicago
11. Narendran V, Hoath SB (1999) Thermal management of the low birth weight infant: a cornerstone of neonatology. J Pediatr 134:529-531
12. Vobra S, Frent G, Campbell V (1999) Effect of polyethylene occlusive skin wrapping on heat loss in very low birth weight infants at delivery: a randomized trial. J Pediatr 134:547-551
13. Ramji S, Ahuja S, Thirupuram S et al (1993) Resuscitation of asphyxic newborn infants with room air or 100% oxygen. Pediatr Res 34:809-812
14. Saugstad OD (1998) Resuscitation with room-air or oxygen supplementation. Clin Perinat 25:741-756
15. Saugstad OD, Rootwelt T, Aalen O (1998) Resuscitation of asphyxiated newborn infants with room air or oxygen: an international controlled trial. The Resair 2 study. Pediatrics 102:E1
16. Feet BA, Bruun NC, Hellstrom-Westas L et al (1998) Early cerebral metabolic and electro-physiological recovery during controlled hypoxemic resuscitation in piglets. J Appl Physiol 84:1208-1211
17. Medbo S, Yu X-Q, Berger KJ et al (1997) Pulmonary circulation and plasma - endothelin-1 (P-ET-1) during hypoxia and reoxygenation with 21% and 100% O_2 in piglets. Pediatr Res 42:307-311
18. Jobe AH (1998) Too many unvalidated new therapies to prevent chronic lung disease in preterm infants. J Pediatr 132:200-202
19. Wada K, Jobe AH, Ikegami M (1997) Tidal volume effects on surfactant treatment responses with the initiation of ventilation in preterm lambs. J Appl Physiol 83:1054-1061
20. Bjorklund LL, Ingimarsson J, Curstedt T et al (1997) Manual ventilation with a few large breaths at birth compromises the therapeutic effect of subsequent surfactant replacement in immature lambs. Pediatr Res 42:348-355
21. Lindner W, Wofsbeck S, Hummler H et al (1999) Delivery room management of extremely low birth weight infants: spontaneous breathing or intubation? Pediatrics 103:961-967
22. Pennant JH, White PF (1993) The laryngeal mask airway. Its uses in anesthesiology. Anesthesiology 79:144-163
23. Brimacombe J, Gandini D (1995) Resuscitation of neonates with the laryngeal mask - a caution. Pediatrics 95:453-454
24. Jobe AH (1993) Pulmonary surfactant therapy. N Engl J Med 328:861-868
25. Soll RF, Morley S (1999) Prophylactic versus selective use of surfactant for prevention of morbidity and mortality in preterm infants. Cochrane Review. In The Cochrane Library, Issue 3. Oxford: Update Software
26. Gortner L, Wauer RR, Hammer H et al (1998) Early versus late surfactant treatment in preterm infants of 27 to 32 week' gestational age: a multicenter controlled clinical trial. Pediatrics 102:1153-1160
27. Trevisanuto D, Ferrarese P, Cavicchioli P et al (1998) Valutazione dell'efficacia di un corso di rianimazione neonatale in sala parto durante il corso di specializzazione in Pediatria. Atti del Congresso della Società Italiana di Neonatologia, 22-24 ottobre 1998, Rimini. Developmental Physiopathology and Clinics 8[Suppl]:219-220

CHALLENGES
IN CARDIOVASCULAR ASSESSMENT,
MONITORING AND MANAGEMENT

Preoperative Cardiovascular Assessment

B. ALLARIA, M. FAVARO, M. DEI POLI

The preparation of a cardiopathic patient for non-cardiac surgery represents a problem of some interest. Perfect awareness of the cardiocirculatory situation, indeed, enables proper preparation (when necessary) and, above all, the correct anaesthesiological conduct to follow.

The information to gather and the strategies to follow are obviously different among various types of patients. Here we will deal with the preparation to surgery of patients with the most frequent cardiovascular problems at the anaesthesiologist's observation: coronaropathic, hypertensive and arrhythmic patients and patients with heart failure.

Preparation to surgery of coronaropathic patients

At rest the heart takes 70% of the O_2 in the arterial blood that perfuses it. Therefore, when requirements increase, a greater supply of O_2 to the cardiac tissue can occur only thanks to an increase of coronary flow. It is consequently fundamental to know which elements control the coronary flow and the influence anaesthesia and the postoperative phase can have on them. There are basically four factors:

1. the perfusion pressure of the coronary circulation;
2. the mechanical events of the cardiac cycle;
3. the extent of the myocardial metabolic activity;
4. the neural control of the coronary vessel caliber [1].

Perfusion pressure of the coronary circulation: whereas the perfusion pressure has poor influence on the overall extent of the coronary flow in a normal subject, it can have a great deal of importance in the case of coronary stenosis. In the case of critical coronary stenosis, indeed, any further requirement of oxygenation can no longer be satisfied with vasodilatation when the resistance vessels (intramyocardial arterioles) are already completely dilated to assure a sufficient trans-stenotic gradient. Only an increased perfusion pressure can assure a gradient able to guarantee an increase of flow.

Mechanical events of the cardiac cycle: during systole, muscular contraction of the left ventricle increases the pressure to a minimum level on the epicardial layers, more so at the level of the intramyocardial layers and even more at the level of the endocardial layers. A considerable reduction of the intramyocardial and subendocardial coronary circulation of the left ventricle thus results during systole. The flow is restored regularly during diastole, up to three times more than the systolic flow. In the right ventricle, where pressures are decidedly lower, the discrepancy between the systolic and diastolic flows is much smaller. It is obvious that in the case of tachycardia, with a reduced diastole time, also the possibility of the heart perfusion is reduced unless the perfusion pressure rises (as in stress). It is therefore just as evident that the tachycardia-hypotension binomial constitutes a risk for all patients, in particular for the coronaropathic patient.

The extent of the myocardial metabolic activity: the myocardial consumption of O_2 (MVO_2) is closely linked to coronary motility. An increase of MVO_2 causes an immediate increase of caliber of the coronary vessels with a flow increase even 5 times higher than normal. Adenosine, produced by the degradation of the cellular AMP (adenosine-5-monophosphate), which is balanced with the ATP (adenosine triphosphate: final energy substrate of the cell metabolism), constantly plays an important role in this flow increase.

Adenosine is produced in relation to cellular metabolism and performs its vasodilatation activity proportionally to the heart energy requirements. Other factors are also involved in the coronary circulation self-regulation (K^+, H^+, pCO_2 and NO).

Neural control of the coronary circulation: it is not that easy to determine the direct effect of sympathetic or vagal stimulation on coronary vessels in man. The indirect effect is so important that it masks and/or nullifies the direct effect.

Indeed, since sympathetic stimulation brings about an increase of frequency and inotropism, it causes a metabolic stimulation followed as we have seen by vasodilatation.

Vagal stimulation, following bradycardia and the subsequent slight drop of inotropism, causes a reduction of coronary flow. Acetylcholine, a parasympathetic mediator, causes vasodilatation if instilled in the healthy coronary circulation but behaves as a vasoconstrictor in the case of alteration of the endothelium. This is true also in the absence of macroscopic alterations of the endothelium. The coronaries of a heavy smoker, for example, can respond to acetylcholine with vasoconstriction even if apparently uninjured. The coronary response directed to the adrenergic stimulus is variable, too. It is well known that the direct coronaroconstrictor effect is decidedly more intense when the endothelium is damaged. The knowledge of these mechanisms is essential in conducting anaesthesia. A light anaesthesia with an abnormal response of both the vagal and sympathetic type can potentially cause harmful coronary vasoconstrictions, as we have seen.

Accordingly, it is fundamental to exactly know the real condition of a patient, in whom a coronary pathology is known or suspected.

An ascertained reduced coronary reserve or a myocardial ischaemia, even at rest, calls for anaesthesiological steps that are a direct consequence of the knowledge of the coronary circulation physiopathology and of the influences some anaesthetics can have on it.

It is obvious that repletion of circulation and anaesthesia level are to be monitored above all to avoid tachycardias and hypotensions; however, even when selecting the anaesthetics, those that do not have negative influences on the coronary circulation are to be preferred.

This latter aspect is not relevant to the subject of our discussion, but it is obvious that awareness of the anti-ischaemic effect of certain halogenates is important in the selection of the anaesthesiological strategy in a coronaropathic patient [2].

Which diagnostic means should we set up in preparing the patient?

The ECG retains its irreplaceable diagnostic value be it at rest, under stress or in response to pharmacological stress (Dipiridamol 0.56 mg/kg IV in 4 mins). In the event of an uncertain response and upon completion of the diagnostic investigations, we can turn to coronary perfusion imaging techniques (e.g. SPECT with Thallium 201 or Technetium 99) that are observed during stress and in the redistribution phase at rest [3].

Which strategies must the anaesthesiologist adhere to once cardiac ischaemia has been ascertained?

We believe it useful to refer to Allaria and colleagues [4], who established the most highly recommended anaesthesiological behaviours following a review of the most recent literature and a comparison of all case histories most common in coronary heart diseases.

1. transmural acute myocardial infarction (AMI): the strategy to be followed is to postpone surgery for a few months, and to stabilize the patient as much as possible;
2. non Q-wave AMI: the approach is the same as in the case of transmural AMI;
3. unstable angina: pharmacological stabilization, in addition to coronarographic investigations and PTCA without thrombolytics;
4. asymptomatic ischaemic ECG picture: diagnostic investigation. If myocardial ischaemia is ascertained, then coronarography and perhaps carefully evaluated revascularization procedures are useful;

5. in emergency cases, or when a patient previously investigated is not amenable to surgical treatment or PTCA, the anaesthesiologist has no choice other than to prepare the patient for surgery.

Preparation of ascertained coronaropathic patients for surgery

In the majority of cases, patients already undergo therapy with nitrates and/or calcium-antagonists and/or beta-blockers, and often with diuretics.

Therapy is not to be interrupted, but the anaesthesiologist must be well aware of the interactions between the drugs and the anaesthetics to be used during surgery.

For example, a patient under nitrates and in chronic therapy with diuretics can be in hypovolaemic conditions, either absolute (diuretics) or relative (nitrates). Deprivation of a compensatory adrenergic response, in addition to further vasodilatation caused by the majority of anaesthetics, can cause significant pressure drops during surgery with a consequent dramatic deterioration of the ischaemia.

Another example is the summation of cardiodepressant effects of verapamil and thiopentone, which can cause highly dangerous haemodynamic imbalances in patients with critical coronary stenoses where the pressure gradient is supported only by the pressure since, as already stated, the possibilities of vasodilatation downstream of stenosis are practically reduced to zero.

In our opinion, evaluation of the circulation filling is a fundamental moment during preparation of the coronaropathic patient for surgery. To this purpose, we use the combined observation of PVC measured at the end of diastole and the time of pre-ejection (PEP: Pre-Ejection Period) measured with the traditional polygraphic technique or with LICAM (Low Invasivity Cardiovascular Monitor) [5] before and after rapid infusion of 250 ml crystalloids. In the event of absolute and/or relative hypovolaemia, we see an evident PEP drop with a slight CVP increase.

If a Swan-Ganz catheter is resorted to, we use the Wedge Pressure (WP) and Stroke Volume (SV) as observation parameters. In the event of hypovolaemia next to slight WP increase, more marked SV increases are seen. We then adjust hypovolaemia in the hours immediately before surgery.

We are convinced that many cases of worsened myocardial ischaemias observed during the intraoperative and postoperative phases are linked to unacknowledged absolute and/or relative hypovolaemias.

Preparation of the hypertensive patient for surgery

A distinction is necessary between well treated hypertensive patients with normal pressure values and patients who are not treated or are treated with poor success and therefore record high pressure values. The first should be considered as normal patients who can undergo surgery without any special preparations. Nevertheless, a perfect knowledge of the action mechanisms of the hypotensive drugs used for hypertensive patients is necessary, thus trying to predict any possible interactions between these drugs and the anaesthetics.

For instance an hypertensive patient treated with diuretic drugs has almost certainly an hypovolaemic intravascular compartment and is more prone to intraoperative hypotension, caused by blood losses or venous return decreases due to a drug-induced increase in the capacitance compartment size (this action being synergistic with mechanical ventilation).

A preoperative filling test can be useful even for these patients, as well as for coronaropathic patients, since the hypertensive patient is often non-apparent or apparent coronaropathic patient.

For example, a hypertensive patient undergoing therapy with a beta-blocker can always have an acute pressure drop upon induction with a barbiturate due to overlapping of the barbiturate and beta-blocker cardiodepressant effects, especially at too high infusion rates and with inadequate reduced dosage.

The second group (i.e. hypertensive patients not treated or treated with poor success) must not undergo surgery if diastolic PA exceeds 110 mmHg, provided the surgical procedure is postponed.

The non treated patient is also hypovolaemic, with a systemic vascular resistance increase and reduced venous district compliance: in acute blood losses or vasodilating anaesthetic drug effects he can even undergo dramatic acute hypotensions, which in turn may activate dangerous decreases in regional blood flow (i.e coronary or cerebral blood flow).

We have already dicussed the mechanisms that cause myocardial ischaemia during hypotension.

As to the cerebral flow, it is worth underlying that self-regulation of the cerebral flow in the hypertensive patient is shifted towards pressure values that are higher than normal, and that therefore pressure drops are less well tolerated compared to non-hypertensive patients [6]. The intensity and frequency of the perioperative hypotensive events are directly proportional to the preoperative pressure values. It is therefore essential to prepare the patient for surgery by normalizing pressure values and the circulation repletion, as previously stressed.

It should, however, be noted that high pressure values immediately prior to surgery in patients with pressure values within normal ranges are generally secondary to an emotional event and are to be interpreted as such. All too often we see patients in good pressure equilibrium who are not operated due to a preoperative hypertensive rise. Proper sedation in a quiet environment (above all without anaesthesiologists and surgeons working hastily) generally permits recovery of normal pressure values and a normal management of anaesthesia.

We have touched upon the hypotensive events that can occur during surgery due to blood losses or to the effect of the anaesthetics, but it is also necessary to remember that the hypertensive patient is more susceptible to hypertensive crises consequent to surgical, emotional or painful stimulation during the post-operative phase. In the perioperative hypertensive crises, alfa2 central stimulants such as *clonidine*, *mivazerol* and *dexmedetomidine* play a role. They carry out a very useful modulating action of the adrenergic responses, thus permitting good perioperative haemodynamic stability without accentuating the influence of the hypotensive events.

It should be noted that the anti-hypertensive effect of clonidine can be antagonized by dehydrobenzoperidol, which must therefore be avoided if clonidine is used. It is just as important to remember that clonidine potentiates the most commonly used anaesthetics, consequently which must be used in reduced doses [7, 8] in patients previously treated with clonidine.

Hypotensive therapies are generally followed up to the time of surgery. Exceptions to the rule are *reserpine* (to be discontinued at least 8 days before surgery) and *ACE-inhibitors*. The short half-life ACE-inhibitors (Captopril) are to be discontinued 18 hours prior to induction and those with a longer half-life (e.g. Enalapril) at least 74 hours before.

Serious hypotensive phenomena can otherwise occur during surgery [7].

Preparation of the arrhythmic patient for surgery

The anaesthesiologist's strategy in preparing patients with ventricular arrhythmia, supraventricular arrhythmia and behavioral disorders is obviously different.

Ventricular arrhythmias: whether we are dealing with isolated, paired or safe PVCs, the anaesthesiologist's first objective will not be to start antiarrhythmic therapy but, rather, to identify the cause of the arrhythmia. Shortages of K^+ or of Mg^{++}, excessive digitalis doses, antiarrhythmic therapies in progress – especially with Group I antiarrhythmic agents (Flecainide, Encainide and Xylocain) – could themselves be the cause of the worsened ventricular arrhythmia.

These antiarrhythmic drugs, which mainly work by slowing down conduction of the stimulus, can cause re-entry phenomena. It must be kept in mind that the same mechanism is referred to to explain arrhythmias from halogenates and that consequently, the simultaneous use of Group I antiarrhythmic drugs and halogenates can cause threatening intraoperative arrhythmias [9].

It is therefore essential to treat any shortages of K^+ and Mg^{++} and to optimize any digitalis therapy, even discontinuing any therapy under way, with Group I antiarrhythmic agents. Even apparently important ventricular arrhythmias rarely worsen during general anaesthesia and that the demonstrated blocking effect of the K^+ channels performed by the halogenates (entirely similar to that of Group III antiarrhythmic agents such as Amiodarone and Sotalol) [10, 11] can explain the antiarrhythmic effect obtained through foranic anaesthesia. This effect, which was attributed only to schedule the anaesthesia in the past, also seems ascribable to an antiarrhythmic effect similar to that of Group III antiarrhythmic drugs [12].

Therefore, the anaesthesiologist faced with ventricular hyperkinetic arrhythmias will set up antiarrhythmic therapy only in exceptional cases (symptomatic arrhythmias and assumed TV) and will do so with Group III antiarrhythmic drugs, such as amiodarone and sotalol. It must not be forgotten that Sotalol on the market is a racemic mixture of d-Sotalol (Group III antiarrhythmic drug) and l-Sotalol (beta-blocker) and therefore using this drug next to an antiarrhythmic effect produces a beta-blocking effect the anaesthesiologist must be aware of, due to its cardiodepressant effect synergistic with anaesthetics.

Ventricular arrhythmias must be kept under close surveillance during the postoperative phase when they generally worsen [13]. The use of antiarrhythmic drugs such as amiodarone is justified during this phase once pain has been sedated, pressure values are normalized, any possible poor oxygenation is normalized and plasmatic K^+ and Mg^{++} levels are adjusted.

Supraventricular arrhythmias: we will overlook isolated or frequent supraventricular arrhythmias, which are of little interest if not correlated to anamnestic paroxysmal tachyarrhythmic events, but we will briefly look at chronic Atrial Fibrillation and Paroxysmal Tachyarrhythmias. Chronic atrial fibrillation does not in itself represent an anaesthesiological problem if ventricular frequency is satisfactory. In the case of a high ventricular frequency, it is worthwhile to postpone surgery (if possible) until the normal frequency has been reached. This is normally obtained with digitalization.

A supraventricular paroxysmal tachyarrhythmia in progress is to be resolved immediately before starting general anesthesia with pharmacological therapy, if time allows, or with electric treatment in case of emergency. The very high frequencies of this arrhythmia do not permit a normal cardiac filling and the overlapping of anaesthetics, as already mentioned, reduces the venous return, worsened also by the artificial ventilation thus leading to disastrous pressure drops.

Upon pharmacological therapy with agents very commonly used in these cases, such as Verapamil and Propafenone, the anaesthesiologist should not underestimate their cardiodepressant effects which can even be marked in patients with a low ejection fraction, especially if the anesthetics cardiodepressant effect is added. Amiodarone is a recommended choice in this case as well.

Conduction disorders: preparation for surgery of patients with non-iatrogenic conduction disorders consists in cardiac endocavitary stimulation, implemented in few cases only. When conduction disorders, even of minor importance, are accompanied by syncopal episodes that can be explained in no other way, cardiac stimulation becomes a precaution to be shared. Thus, events such as sinoatrial blockage, sinusal pauses, bradycardia and atrio-ventricular block (AVB) of any type and bifascicular blockages – which in themselves would not represent an indication for electric stimulation if they are symptomatic – become amenable to stimulation.

Instead, in the case of asymptomatic patients, there are only two absolute indications: the Mobitz type of BAV II and the BAV III.

A dynamic ECG is recommended in all cases of excitoconduction disorder if surgery is not urgent.

Preparation to surgery of the patient with chronic heart failure (CHF)

In general, the patient who is referred to the anaesthesiologist for surgery is already under therapy. However, therapy is not always optimal. Therefore it is to be completed or, in any case, optimized prior to surgery in this case. It is necessary to recall the cornerstones of modern heart failure treatment:

Diuretics: generally, loop diuretics (furosemide and torsemide). Oral furosemide has a completely unpredictable absorption (10 to 80%) and its effectiveness therefore can not be foretold. Furthermore, furosemide has a short half-life (up to 120 minutes). Hence, by using it as is commonly done, during many hours the diuretic is ineffective. On the contrary, since the renal tubule absorbs water and sodium more vigorously in the final phase, the effects can be thwarted with the diuretic in boluses over time.

These problems are common even when the intravenous boluses are given BID or TID. For this reason a bolus, possibly followed by continuous infusion, is advisable where a diuretic therapy is deemed useful for the patient with CHF who is to undergo surgery. In the case of oral administration, torsemide is preferable to furosemide because of a more predictable absorption of 80-90%.

ACE-Inhibitors: these have become irreplaceable agents in CHF therapy.

Initially deemed effective above all for their renin-angiotensin system inhibition mechanism, they are currently also seen as agents able to prevent or slow down the progression of cardiac deterioration by reducing the presence of collagen in the blood. At the University of Navarra School of Medicine recent research discovered that hypertensive patients with CHF had a blood collagen level that was higher when compared to normal subjects, and that the plasma collagen level normalizes following therapy with lisinopril.

This is the first comparison of the ACE-inhibitor's effect on circulating collagen. While it is correct to interrupt the ACE-inhibitor 18-24 hours before surgery in the case of a hypertensive patient without CHF, the drug can be maintained in the case of heart failure, although the possibility of the hypotensive effect strengthening, especially with halogenates must be kept in mind.

Nitrates: these are obviously used both in the most acute phases of pulmonary edema (EPA) and in the maintenance phase due to their effect in reducing pre-load and afterload. It is still debated whether use of low doses of furosemide (40 mg IV in single bolus) with high doses of nitrates (isosorbide dinatrate 3 mg IV in 5 min.) or the use of high doses of furosemide (80 mg IV in 15 min.) with low doses of nitrates (1 mg/h) is more effective in the acute phase. A recent study by Cotter and colleagues published in *Lancet* seems to demonstrate that the former strategy is the most effective [14].

Therefore, in the case of a patient with CHF in a worsening phase possibly leading to pulmonary oedema, we will turn to the combined use of a loop diuretic with the provisos mentioned previously (bolus + continuous infusion) plus a nitrocompound at high doses. Once the most acute phase is over, an oral ACE-inhibitor will be added, and only after satisfactory compensation has been reached can we proceed with the scheduled surgery.

It is naturally necessary to underline that next to the anaesthetics particularly indicated for patients with CHF during anaesthesia, such as the opioids, there are others with a depressant effect on the myocardium, such as the halogenates.

Anaesthesia with opioids (morphine, fentanyl and sufentanyl), supplemented by low concentrations of halogenates, can therefore be scheduled for these patients.

Proper monitoring of the cardiovascular functions is in any case essential in patients with CHF. This topic is discussed in another section of this volume.

We have not mentioned Digitalis among the cornerstones of CHF therapy. Indeed, this agent, which has been the only possible one for this pathology for many years, is today considered with less interest for such indication. We still use it.

References

1. Agnati LF (1966) Fisiologia cardiovascolare. Piccin, Padova
2. Cope DK, Impastato WK, Cohen MV, Downey JM (1997) Volatile anaesthetics protect the ischaemic rabbit myocardium from infarction. Anaesthesiology 86:699-709
3. Marvick TH, Shaw LJ, Laner MS et al (1999) The non invasive prediction of cardiac mortality in men and women with known or suspected coronary artery disease. Am J Med 106:172-178
4. Allaria B, Favaro M, Dei Poli M (1997) Therapy of perioperative myocardial ischaemia. Crit Care Med Springer - APICE 12th, pp 211-221
5. Allaria B, Dei Poli M, Brunetti B, Trivellato A (1994) Computerized analysis of biologic cardiovascular signals: prospectives monitoring. 9th Eur Congress of Anaesthesia - Jerusalem (ABS)
6. Serpellon M, Zaffiro G, Decastello M (1997) Malattia ipertensiva cardiovascolare e anestesia. Anestesia e malattie concomitanti. Springer, Italia, pp 106-137
7. Lehot JJ, Girard C, Filley S et al (1997) Why are hypertensive patients at risk in the perioperative period? Crit Care Med Springer - APICE 12th, pp 31-40
8. Helbo Hansen S, Fletcher R, Lundberg D et al (1986) Clonidine and the symphatics adrenal response to coronary artery by-pass surgery. Acta Anaesthesiol Scand 30:235-240

9. Atlee JC, Horner LD, Tolley RE (1975) Diphenylidantoine and lidocaine modifications of A-V conduction in Halotane anaesthetized dogs. Anaesthesiology 43:49
10. Supan F, Buljnbasic N, Marjic J et al (1991) Effects of halotane and enfluorane on K current in canine cardiac Purkinje cells. Anaesth Analg 72:S286
11. Supan F, Buljnbasic N, Marjic J et al (1991) Effects of volatile anaesthetics on transient outward potassium current in Purkinje fibers. (ABS) Anaesthesiology 75:1368
12. Allaria B (1998) Aritmia nel periodo perioperatorio. Anestesia e malattie concomitanti. Springer, Italia, pp 88-105
13. O'Kelley B, Browner WS, Massic B et al (1992) Ventricular arrhythmias in patients undergoing non cardiac surgery. JAMA 268:217-221
14. Cotter G, Metzkor E, Kaluski E et al (1998) Randomized trial of high-dose isosorbide dinitrate plus low-dose furosemide versus high-dose furosemide plus low-dose isosorbide dinitrate in severe pulmonary oedema. Lancet 351:389-393

Perioperative Hemodynamic Monitoring: Invasive Vs. Non-Invasive

B. Allaria, M. Dei Poli, D. Culotta

General and locoregional anesthesia and/or the surgical procedure could be viewed as conditions in which the physiologic mechanisms regulating the body omeostasis are altered, although for a limited span of time.

Monitoring in the perioperative period is thus traditionally performed both as a warning for life-threatening abnormalities and to allow the maintenance of a stable physiological condition.

Modern devices not only protect the anesthesiologist from possible errors – the "sentinel" function – but also favor better knowledge about patients undergoing surgery and of the anesthesiologic culture in general.

Cardiovascular monitoring is part of any anesthesiologic safety standard and a guideline in the operating theatre: different levels of complexity vary from locoregional anesthesia or sedation (for ASA 1 or 2 patients) in which clinical observation, 3/5 leads electrocardiogram (EKG), non invasive blood pressure (NIBP) are required, to major surgery or patients at risk in whom invasive blood pressure must replace NIBP, and hourly recorded diuresis, central venous pressure (CVP) and pulmonary artery catheter (PAC) could be added (the – intermediate – recommendations for general anesthesia with tracheal intubation are: clinics, EKG, NIBP – or invasive BP –, diuresis).

When considering the perioperative period as a whole, these indications may appear somewhat restrictive: much information about the patient's cardiocirculatory status and performance must be obtained preoperatively – usually once – in order to assess and stratify the risk. These procedures – echo 2D, myocardial scintigraphy, coronarography, etc. – could be viewed as part of a cardiovascular/anesthesiologic staging. Continuity from intraoperative to postoperative period is otherwise suggested for other data and parameters (filling pressures, ST segment elevation, diuresis, oxygen transport and utilization).

The timing of application (pre-, intra-, and postoperative period), the level of complexity – including invasivity –, the feature of continuous monitoring vs. spot determination, the parameters studied (pressures, volumes, flow, function, etc.), all contribute to define an array of different tipologies of devices and clinical situations.

The concept of invasivity has traditionally been associated to the monitoring of cardiac output (and the cascade of calculated data) and more specifically to the PAC: thus invasive vs. non-invasive hemodynamic monitoring is often viewed as a debate on the usefulness of a set of data that includes the cardiac index (CI), the wedge pressure (WP), the systemic vascular resistances (SVR) and others measured or calculated data.

Pulmonary artery catheter

The PAC has been widely used, in the three decades since Swan and colleagues described it, to monitor cardiac function and to manage patients both in operating room and in the Intensive Care.

For many years PAC has meant cardiac output and has represented the invasive way to explore hemodynamics.

The potential benefits of the device are its ability to measure important hemodynamic indices (cardiac output, pulmonary artery occlusion pressure, mixed venous oxygen saturation): the cardiocirculatory status of the critically ill or at risk patient could be more accurately determined than by clinical assessment alone.

Preoperative PAC insertion could be helpful in determining the safety – for high risk patients – to select surgery. A lower mortality rate (a) or reduced intraoperative complications [1] were demonstrated in patients preoperatively monitored rather than in patients first monitored after surgery [2].

During surgery, PAC data often help evaluate serious perioperative complications from hemodynamic changes.

Perioperative PAC should be considered in patients with an increased risk of complications from hemodynamic changes: the risk must be assessed as a function of the health status of the patient, the type of surgical procedure and the characteristics of the setting.

An important subset of perioperative risk is represented by patients with ischemic heart disease (CAD, coronary artery disease).

In order to identify patient groups (known CAD, at risk for CAD, low risk of CAD) many different diagnostic tests have been evaluated (exercise EKG, exercise thallium imaging, dipyridamole thallium imaging, stress echocardiography). Dobutamine stress echocardiography allows a dynamic assessment of ventricular function, and shows the best positive and negative predictive value [3].

The relationship between the development of intraoperative myocardial ischemia and a rise in PA occlusion pressure (WP) is well demonstrated [4]. Although any improvement in clinical outcome has never been proved with controlled studies, the use of invasive hemodynamic monitoring – mainly through PAC – has been strongly suggested in noncardiac surgery for CAD patients.

The cardiac risk stratification for noncardiac surgery has been well described by 3 groups:

1. high risk: major surgery, particularly in the elderly; aortic and other major vascular surgery; peripheral vascular surgery; anticipated prolonged procedures or large fluid shifts or blood loss;

2. intermediate risk: carotid endoarteriectomy; head and neck surgery; intraperitoneal and intrathoracic surgery; orthopedic surgery; prostatic surgery;

3. low risk: endoscopic procedures; superficial procedures; cataract removal; breast surgery.

PAC insertion may be part of a standard monitoring set in group1-high risk procedures for patients who recently suffered from myocardial infarction complicated by congestive heart failure, those with CAD symptomatic for unstable angina and those with systolic or diastolic left ventricular dysfunction and those with cardiomyopathy [5].

Among the absolute indications for PAC insertion Weil, in a recent review [6], indicates the perioperative monitoring of every surgical procedure in patients suffering from severe mitral stenosis. In the same work the author discusses other indications as preoperative hemodynamic optimization and non complicated cardiac, vascular and thoracopulmonary surgery.

In 1997 a Consensus Conference debated on the usefulness and the indication of PAC in different clinical and surgical settings [7] (American College of Chest Physicians, American Thoracic Society, European Society of Intensive Care Medicine, Society of Critical Care Medicine, American Association of Critical Care Nurses): among the different topics discussed, questions about the adequacy of PAC in different surgical settings could find an answer.

– reduction of complications and mortality in cardiac surgery: not useful in low risk patients; possibly useful in patients with severe left ventricular dysfunction; further studies required to define improved outcome;

– reduction of complications and mortality in peripheral vascular surgery: yes, with uncertain data about mortality;

– reduction of complications and mortality in geriatric surgery: no;

– reduction of complications and mortality in neurosurgery: no;

– application of a strategy aimed at DO_2 supranormal values in high risk surgery setting: controlled studies not available; $\dot{V}O_2$ should be measured but not calculated.

One of the conclusions of the Conference is that "... the clinician's knowledge about the use of PAC and its complications must be improved...".

Indeed many authors had questioned, in past and recent years, the positive risk-benefit ratio and the effect on outcome of utilizing PAC [8-10].

In these studies the settings of PAC use were mainly the Intensive Care Units (rarely the Operating Rooms), often in their "open" version, i.e. where any physician of the medical staff could accept and care for critically ill patients. The different level of skill in handling PAC and different cultural levels in interpreting data for treatment (see also Iberti et al. [11] and Gnaegi et al. [12]) could have heavily biased the results of these studies.

Several studies suggest that the presence of a trained physician improves patient management and outcome [13, 14].

Trans-esophageal echocardiography

The introduction of epicardial echocardiography (EE) in the operating room dates back to the early 1970s, while the use of transesophageal echocardiography (TEE) was first described in 1980 and became commonplace since high frequency transducers and color Doppler imaging became available in 1985.

TEE universally seen as a quasi non-invasive method of hemodynamic evaluation, offers important advantages over other diagnostic monitoring techniques.

TEE provides information not just about cardiac function, since it also explores the anatomy, the size and the regional wall motion of the atria and ventricles, the structure and function of the septum, the presence of abnormal structures and gives information about the pericardium and the pulmonary arterial circulation.

In a recent review McLean has underscored the importance of the availability of these data to anesthesiologists and critical care physicians in the perioperative period [15].

TEE can monitor interventions throughout the operative course without disturbing the surgeon's work (unlike transthoracic – TTE – or epicardial – EE – echocardiography).

Not only is PAC much more invasive and exposes patients to a greater risk of complications (arrhythmias, pulmonary artery ruptures and pulmonary infarction, infections, etc.), but it provides a consistently reduced set of functional information about cardiac performance, wall motion and valvular disturbances.

Limitations to TEE consist in a scarce visualization of some regions of the heart (i.e. right chambers), potential traumatisms of pharynx, larynx, teeth, esophagus, the need of a skilled operator, its inapplicability to the awakened patient.

The inaccurate interpretation of TEE images can lead to an improper clinical decision.

The new generation of TEE devices involves a considerable improvement in automated measures, as acoustic quantification of LV area and volume, or multiplane analysis of ultrasound signals and the extensive use of Color Doppler in valvular studies.

Non-invasive alternatives

The 1990s have witnessed major advances in computer technology that have led to further advances in medical devices technology. A very promising growth of non invasive monitoring took place in recent years, offering new opportunities to replace PAC to anesthesiologists and critical care physicians.

Impedance cardiography is a totally non-invasive method of cardiac output measurement based on measuring impedance changes within the thorax, cardiac output being estimated from variables derived from the impedance waveform.

Biological impedance, or bioimpedance, could be expressed as the fall of the electrical potential of a low intensity alternating current during its passage through the thoracic segment. Impedance is the opposite of conductance, and may be defined as an analogue of the resistance, and thus measured in Ohm.

Water in the human body is a good conductor, owing to its ionized molecules content: the composition of the thoracic segment (defined by two horizontal plans, one passing through the base of the neck and one at the level of the sternal xiphoid prominence), in terms of water, fat, bones, muscles and viscera, shows a peculiar individual impedance (base impedance or Z_0). Base impedance many explore the thoracic fluids, in terms of excess or pulmonary edema: this condition usually invalidates further hemodynamic measurements, by altering the impedance waveform.

The cyclic variations of thoracic impedance are respectively due to respiratory and cardiac cycles: only the latter is studied, by recording and mathematically treating the impedance waveform, both in temporal (ΔZ) and in instantaneous (dZ/dt) pattern.

Cardiac (aortic) impedance cyclic variations are probably due to the volumetric modifications of the large thoracic vessels (mainly descending aorta) during systole, and to the synchronous orientation of red cells during the ejective phase of systole.

The dZ/dt is a waveform very similar in shape to the Doppler aortic flow velocity, and in some respect to aortic pressure waveform: it is easily possible to define the beginning and ending of ventricular ejection (cardiac systole), and therefore to measure the systolic time intervals (STI) (pre-ejection time, PEP and left ventricular ejection time, LVET) and their ratio (systolic time ratio, STR or Weissler index, PEP/ET).

Systolic volume (and cardiac output, SVR, left ventricular systolic work, by computation) is then calculated from the STR, the morphologic thoracic data (input by the physician) and the dZ/dt itself.

Impedance cardiography was originally studied by NASA for remote and non-invasive control of the astronauts: it is a very powerful tool for studing an healthy subject.

On the contrary many studies showed a correlation instability when TEB was applied to the very critically ill patient (septic, tachyarrhythmic, shocked, heavily edematous).

Its use in the operating room is limited to the surgery of the neck, of the thorax, of the upper abdomen: otherwise bioimpedance is very simple to install, completely safe, absolutely cheap (only 4 pairs of electrodes are needed for the test), user friendly. Its application could represent a true continuous, beat to beat monitoring that can follow the patient from the operating theatre to the ICU bedside.

A wide use of challenge test (filling test, inotropic drugs, diuretics) is strongly recommended, to better understand and appreciate intrapatient hemodynamic variations.

Developed by Kubicek in 1966 [16], impedance cardiography has been considerably improved by coupling it with computer technology and software advances: the new generation of cardioimpedance devices permits sophisticated signal processing, analog visual displays, powerful signal filtering capabilities, with a better reliability of data and a good correlation with other monitoring standards.

The STI constitutes a set of measures based on cardiac electromechanic activity (the cardiac cycle). They are strongly related to the cardiac chambers filling (fibers diastolic length) and to the heart contractile force, and relatively independent of the intrathoracic pressures and other noncardiac events.

Thus, some other devices that utilize these measurements have been developed.

Among these, the Low Invasivity Cardiovascular Monitor (LICAM) described by Allaria [17], that upon peripheral (radial) arterial pressure waveform measures EKG and CVP tracings, beat-to-beat STI, systolic volume by arterial ejective profile and right ventricular end diastolic pressure (RVEDP, by identifying the CVP value corresponding to EKG Q wave).

The Dynemo 3000 of Sometec, a Belgian Company, has been studied and developed by the group of Muchada in Lyon.

It measures descending aortic blood flow with a specially designed intraesophageal Doppler echo probe. First, an A scan system measures the diameter of the vessel, then a continuous wave velocimeter determines the spatial mean velocity of the blood. An output calculator determines the descending aortic blood flow [18].

The grade of invasivity of this device is similar to TEE: when compared to other aortic Doppler flowmeters (ODM1, Abbott), the Dynemo 3000 provides a more stable Doppler signals and more accurate flow recordings, owing to the sharp definition of the vessel walls and to the optimal targetting of the Doppler beam.

The Dynemo 3000 integrates the flow data with the STI (measured on the aortic flow profile) to structure a data set of flow, filling and cardiac performance.

If PAC may be considered as representative of the invasive way to monitor the hemodynamic status of the patient, and the TEE the standard of non invasive (or quasi non-invasive) monitoring, then the new horizon in the perioperative evaluation is the so called "therapeutic monitoring".

Monitoring becomes therapeutic when its results can be used to guide changes in clinical treatment: to date the commonest categories of therapeutic monitoring devices are those which provide the quantification of flow (cardiac index) and oxygen delivery to tissues and those studying regional tissue perfusion [19].

Right heart catheterization (PAC), Doppler aortic flow (ODM 1, Dynemo 3000) and TEB allow the anesthesiologist to study the tissues oxygen metabolism at a different level of sensitivity and accordance.

Gastric tonometry is becoming the standard in the evaluation of splanchnic perfusion.

In the contest of low flow the gut is the organ that suffers from the most severe vasoconstriction, thus increasing the risk of mucosal ischemia, disturbance of its physiological barrier function, increase of membrane permeability, bacterial traslocation.

Gastric tonometry allows the physician to monitor the mucosal pH (pHi) decrease or the variation of the $PrCO_2$-$PaCO_2$ ratio, and to observe this data as a feedback as to the effects of therapeutic interventions.

A number of studies have used the pHi result to influence treatment [20].

Further randomised controlled studies are needed before a widespread use in the clinical setting is recommended.

In recent years the study of the heart performance and of the hemodynamic status of the vascular system (hemodynamic invasive monitoring, PAC) has shifted to the monitoring of tissues and organ oxygen metabolism (SvO_2, gastric tonometry, capnometry or flow capnography).

This leads to the "core" of the hemodynamic problem and forces the anesthesiologists and critical are physicians to a more "etiologic" and modern approach.

The pro/con about hemodynamic monitoring cannot ignore a new interesting insight on the unsolved problem of the body water balance and composition.

As previously seen about thoracic impedance, the bioelectric properties of the human body can be used to study the resistive and capacitive characteristics of the body, considered as a whole or segmented in trunk and limbs.

Body impedance analysis (BIA) is a promising device that allows the physician, with a simple, quick and inexpensive measure [21], to know the body water content, its distribution in compartments (mainly intra- and extracellular spaces), the cellular mass and the fat tissue content.

During and after major surgery it is not uncommon to observe major fluid shift, third space sequestration, massive organ edema that disturb the precise recording of I/O balance and leave doubts about the volemic and hydration status of the patient.

The NICO (non invasive cardiac output) is a completely non invasive cardiac output measurement device. Its use is currently limited to artificially ventilated patients with stable tidal volume.

During short periods of rebreathing the device automatically provides at fix intervals, the $PetCO_2$ and the VCO_2 are monitored by volumetric capnography.

The increases of $PetCO_2$ and the decreases of VCO_2 during the rebreathing phase allow to evaluate the amount of cardiac output which participates in gas exchange (pulmonary capillary blood flow, PCBF).

PCBF is computed with an alternative form of the Fick equation defined as "the differential Fick partial rebreathing method" [22].

The device then adds PCBF and the amount of shunted flow (Qs/Qt), which is calculated by the Nunn nomogram to obtain the cardiac output.

Two monitoring and clinical plus are thus obtained: 1) a cardiac output non invasive measurement 2) VCO_2 monitoring, a useful parameter for the evaluation of the patient matabolic status.

References

1. Shoemaker WC (1990) The efficacy of central venous and pulmonary artery catheters and therapy based upon them in reducing mortality and morbidity. Arch Surg 125:1332-1338
2. Del Guercio LRM, Cohn JD (1980) Monitoring operative risk in the elderly. JAMA 243: 1350-1355
3. Lane RT, Sawada SG, Segar DS et al (1991) Dobutamine stress echocardiography for assessment of cardiac risk before noncardiac surgery. Anesth Analg 74:586-598
4. Kaplan JA, Wells PH (1981) Early diagnosis of myocardial ischemia using the pulmonary arterial catheter. Anesth Analg 60:789-793
5. ACC/AHA Task Force Report (1996) Guidelines for perioperative cardiovascular evaluation for noncardiac surgery. J Cardiothor Vasc Anesth 10:540-552
6. Weil (1988) The assault on the Swan Ganz catheter. P Chest 113:1379-1386
7. Pulmonary Artery Catheter Consensus Conference (1997) Crit Care Med 25:910
8. Robin ED (1985) The cult of the Swan Ganz catheter: overuse and abuse of pulmonary flow catheters. Ann Intern Med 103:445-449
9. Gore JM, Goldberg RJ, Spodick DH et al (1987) A community-wide assessment of the use of pulmonary artery catheters in patients with acute myocardial infarction. Chest 92:721-727
10. Connors AF, Speroff T, Dawson NV et al (1996) The effectiveness of right heart catheterization in the initial care of critically ill patients. JAMA 276:889-897
11. Iberti TJ, Fischer EP, Leibowitz AB et al (1990) A multicenter study of physician's knowledge of the pulmonary artery catheter. JAMA 264:2928-2932
12. Gnaegi A, Feihl F, Perret C (1997) Insufficient knowledge of intensive care physicians concerning right heart catheterization at the bedside: time to act? Crit Care Med 25:213-220
13. Reynolds HN, Haupt MT, Thill-Baharozian MC et al (1988) Impact of critical care physician staffing on patients with septic shock in a university hospital medical intensive care unit. JAMA 260:3446-3450

14. Knaus WA, Wagner DP, Loirat P et al (1982) A comparison of intensive care in the USA and France. Lancet ii:642-646
15. Mc Lean AS (1998) Transesophageal echocardiography in the intensive care unit. Anesth Intensive Care 26:22-25
16. Kubicek WG, Karnegis JN, Patterson RP (1966) Development and evaluation of an impedance cardiac output system. Aerospace Medicine 37:1208-1212
17. Allaria B, Dei Poli M, Brunetti B et al (1994) Computerized analysis of biological cardiovascular signals: prospective monitoring. Abs 9th European Congress of Anesthesiology, pp 373
18. Cathignol D, Lavandier B, Muchada R (1985) Debitmetrie aortique par effet Doppler transesophagien. Ann Fr Anesth Reanim 4:438-443
19. Boyd O, Rhodes A (1998) Therapeutic monitoring in the perioperative period. Apice - Critical Care Medicine, Springer, pp 314-319
20. Gutierrez G, Palizas F, Doglio G et al (1992) Gastric intramucosal pH as a therapeutic index of tissue oxygenation in critically ill patients. Lancet 339:195-199
21. Dei Poli M (1999) L'acqua e la sua compartimentazione nel malato critico: nuovi orizzonti nella complessa diagnostica e nel monitoraggio della terapia. Minerva Anest 65[Suppl 1]: 313-316
22. Jaffe MB (1998) Partial rebreathing cardiac output. Overview. Technical report 9806 Rev. 00 Novametrix Med. Systems Inc, pp 1-10

Extracorporeal Circulation: Prevention and Management of Complications

J.O.C. AULER JR

The development of extracorporeal circulation (ECC) has indubitably been extremely important in the progress of cardiac surgery. The possibility of bypassing blood outside the heart and lungs, pumping oxygenated blood from the venous system directly to the arterial system, has permitted all types of cardiac surgery. Extracorporeal circulation has also allowed surgical approaches to complex diseases, such as correction of thoracic aortic aneurysms, resection of renal cell carcinoma, treatment of neurobasilar aneurysms, lung transplantation, and thrombo-endarterectomy of pulmonary arteries. Others uses of ECC include veno-venous bypass in liver transplantation, in acute respiratory failure as part of a "lung protective strategy", in acute pulmonary hypertension of newborn, in high-risk angioplasty patients and ventricular assistance. Ideally, to replace the functions of the heart and lungs cardiopulmonary bypass (CPB) should achieve several aims, with minimal risks and interferences to normal physiology. The main purpose of CPB is to maintain systemic perfusion with adequate oxygen transport and carbon dioxide elimination, preserving homeostasis while the heart and lungs are not providing these functions. All extracorporeal circuits that return blood to the patient require the incorporation of some kind of pumping device. This pumping mechanism may occur by various basic principles of fluid movement which include positive displacement, centrifugal vortexing and pneumatic and electrical pulsation. Positive displacement pumps have been largely used in ECC since it was proposed by Gibbon [1]. The second type of pump device used in ECC is the centrifugal pump or resistance-dependent pump. This system works by the addition of kinetic energy to the fluid through the forced rotation of an impeller or cone. A centrifugal pump was proposed for clinical use in 1976, and since then its acceptance in CPB has increased progressively. The other components of cardiopulmonary circuitry are the oxygenators, heat exchangers, cannulae and tubing, and the cardioplegia delivery system. The oxygenators have the main function of gas transfer, and, at the same time, they should have a low rate of bioreactivity. Oxygenators utilized in CPB are currently divided into two classes based on the method of gas exchange: bubble and membrane oxygenators. Although more complex in design, membrane oxygenators are much more used nowadays in routine CPB, mainly because this is thought to be a much safer system than bubble oxygenators, which cause gaseous microemboli and induce hematologic damage to the formed elements of blood [2, 3]. As described below, it has been known for several years that CPB triggers an inflammatory response that can lead to the development of postoperative organ dysfunction. This response may occur with both oxygenators, bubble and membrane [4], but the use of bubble oxygenators has been shown to be able to induce a greater inflammatory response when compared to membrane oxygenators. Bubble oxygenators seem to be responsible for greater complement activation and lung leukocyte sequestration when compared to membrane [5]. Another study demonstrated higher levels of intercellular adhesion molecule-1 (sICAM-1) in the blood during use of bubble oxygenators when compared to membrane [6].

However, as it is a very invasive procedure, CPB may trigger several undesirable effects, some predictable and preventable, but some unpredictable, that can promote cellular or organ lesions of different magnitude and outcome.

Our aim in this chapter is to talk about complications and prevention of extracorporeal circulation. We will divide this matter in three parts:
– Complications related to aorta or femoral cannulation, organ perfusion and others related to the technique;
– Inflammation and other complications related to the exposition of the blood to non endothelial surface of extracorporeal circuits;
– Measures to reduce the systemic inflammation related to CPB and others complications.

Complications related to arterial cannulation

To bypass the pump function of the heart and the gas exchange of the lungs, extracorporeal circulation requires venous drainage through one or two cannulae inserted in a large vein system, like the cava vein or femoral. After gas exchange in the oxygenator the blood is pumped away to the arterial system. The blood is returned to the arterial system through a major artery, in general via a cannula positioned in the ascending aorta or femoral artery. In the ascending aorta the cannula insertion may cause some problems that need prompt recognition and correction.
– Arterial cannula malposition inside the aorta: In this situation the flow may be directed to the innominate artery or to the left common carotid artery. The immediate consequences of cannula malposition are excessive brain flow and systemic hypoperfusion. Sometimes the cannula tip may be inserted in the aorta intima or toward the aortic valve. Any cannula malposition may be suspected in the presence of an unexplained fall in arterial pressure, or high pressure in the line connected to the bypass pump system. In any case of perfusion into the innominate artery it is possible to observe unilateral changes of color in the face. In general a malpositioned aortic cannula provokes persist-

ent low arterial pressure that is unresponsive to usual treatments such as vaso-constrictors and pump flow increase [7, 8].

- Arterial dissection: This is a catastrophic event that may occur at any time during bypass. Unexplained hypotension during CPB that is unresponsive to usual maneuvers and is accompanied by a decrease of venous return to the reservoir should be a signal of acute dissection. Sometimes the surgeon can see the sign of dissection if it involves the anterior wall of the aorta, but depending on the place this is sometimes not possible [9]. Once the dissection is diagnosed during CPB, it requires immediate treatment. In general the patient is cooled to profound levels to protect vital organs, while the surgeon tries to repair the site of disruption. A different arterial cannulation site is prepared under hypothermia and, sometimes, CPB arrest.

- Arterial gas embolism: Not necessarily related to correct insertion of the cannula in a major arterial vessel, gas embolism can happen at a relatively significant incidence during bypass. Sometimes, if present in small amounts, gas embolism may not be recognized and treated promptly. Macroscopic massive gas embolism is a catastrophic and sometimes fatal event during CPB. The survivors may be at high risk of permanent neurologic deficits. The principal causes are related to inattention to low levels of blood in the oxygenator, reversal of left ventricular or aortic vent flow, unexpected cardiac contraction of opened heart in the presence of unclamped aorta, and inadequate air removal from cardiac chambers before re-establishment of circulation. The treatment for massive air embolism during CPB demands immediate stop of the machine pumped flow in an attempt to locate the origin of the air, and, at the same time, trying to aspirate the gas. The Trendelenburg position has also been recommended. After that, CPB should be re-installed, deepening the hypothermia level. Air bubbles promote mechanical blockage of blood vessels in the brain, producing different degrees of ischemia or even infarction. Glucocorticoids and phenytoin have been proposed as part of the treatment [10]. Considerable recovery from neurologic injury has been reported when hyperbaric oxygen in appropriate chambers is used for treatment of arterial gas embolism, when suspected or diagnosed during cardiac surgery [11].

Inflammatory response and other complications related to the exposure of the blood to the nonendothelial surface of extracorporeal circuits

Cardiac surgery with the use of CPB has been associated with systemic inflammatory activation leading to an acute phase response, sometimes resembling severe infection, during the immediate postoperative period [12]. The clinical manifestations are quite complex and include bleeding, ischemia/reperfusion injury in different organs, leading to a multi-organ failure, fever, infection, hypotension, and vasodilatation. The damaging effects of CPB are probably related to the blood exposure to nonendothelial surfaces, shear stresses, and incorporation of abnormal substances during bypass. An integral part of this whole body inflammatory response involves the so-called humoral amplification system. This involves a variable and individual response including the coagulation cascade, the kallikrein cascade, the fibrinolytic system, and the complement system. The coagulation cascade is activated immediately after the onset of CPB by contact of blood with nonendothelial surfaces of extracorporeal components. Activation of Hageman factor (XII) leads to activation of the kallikrein system and kininogen to begin coagulation via the intrinsic coagulation pathway. The extrinsic coagulation pathway is activated by the expression of tissue factor by tissue injury and monocytes. The activation of the Hageman factor also leads to the production of bradykinin, which produces alterations in vascular permeability, initiates smooth muscle contraction, and dilates precapillary arterioles. High levels of bradykinin have been demonstrated during CPB [13]. Complement consumption during CPB was demonstrated by Parker and colleagues in 1972 [14]. Since then several studies have tried to demonstrate the correlation between inflammatory response after CPB and complement system activation. Although complement activation has been demonstrated during cardiac surgery without CPB, the magnitude of activation seems to be higher in procedures accompanied by CPB. It is interesting to note the relation between morbidity after CPB and complement activation since the anaphylatoxins C5a and C3a have physiologic effects similar to those observed in many patients after major surgery with and without CPB [15, 16].

Neutrophils are activated by other agonists during CPB and are responsible for much of the inflammatory reaction associated with cardiac surgery causing organ dysfunction. Neutrophil endothelial cell adhesion has a central role in post-ischemic reperfusion seen after CPB. Initially, oxygen free radicals are released from neutrophils in reperfused organs, such as lung and heart, leading to alterations in endothelial cells, which promote neutrophil entrapment, activation of serum complement and induction of cytokine synthesis. The neutrophil displays three primary surface adhesive receptors or integrins. One of these integrins, CD11b, has a specific adhesive endothelial receptor, termed intercellular adhesion molecule (ICAM). This specific receptor permits the neutrophil to bind to and adhere to endothelium at a site of injury or inflammation as the initiating step in neutrophil transvascular immigration [17]. Specific integrins have been described as responsible for lung and myocardial reperfusion injury following CPB [18, 19].

Monocytes are also activated in the CPB-induced inflammatory response. Monocytes express tumor necrosis factor (TNF), both in the surgical wound and in the perfusion circuit. TNF is strongly procoagulant and ignites the extrinsic coagulation pathway. Monocytes also produce several proinflammatory and antiinflammatory cytokines during surgery. Plasma concentrations of almost all cytokines peak several hours after CPB [20]. Cytokines are small proteins that resemble hormones, in that after they are produced by and released from their cells of origin, they are transported to distant parts of the body and affect the function of cells in these places. Many cytokines have been identified so far and include TNF, the interleukins, the interferons, and several growth factors. The interleukins have a significant function in facilitating communications among leukocytes, and work as regulatory proteins to control many aspects of the body's inflammatory activity.

Recently several studies have hypothesized the importance of the L-arginine-nitric oxide pathway in the inflammatory reactions observed with CPB [21]. Matheis and colleagues have suggested that endogenously produced nitric oxide (NO) may be involved in myocardial reperfusion injury during CPB [22]. It is consistent that CPB induced bronchial epithelial cell inflammation and injury. The role of NO in lung injury after bypass is still under hypothesis. Delgado and colleagues showed a significant increase in calcium independent nitric oxide synthase activity in human lung after cardiopulmonary bypass [23].

Release of endotoxin during CPB is associated with reductions in mesenteric blood flow. Systemic endotoxemia occurs on the onset of CPB, with a secondary increase after aortic cross-clamp release [24]. Once released during CPB, endotoxin is a powerful potential generator of the inflammatory reaction, being related to the production of cytokines, complement and neutrophil activation.

Once established, the systemic inflammatory response after CPB may persist in the postoperative period with different degrees of clinical expression for hours or days. Several organs may present clinical signals of dysfunction caused by ischemia/reperfusion injury aggravated by inflammatory reaction. Although the lungs, the brain, and, to a lesser extent, the kidney have long been considered as the primary targets of inflammatory mediators released during CPB, it is now increasingly recognized that these compounds can also adversely affect myocardial function. In an experimental study, Shandelya and colleagues, utilizing a model of isolated rat heart, showed severe deterioration of post-ischemic myocardial function. The pathogenic role of complement and neutrophils in mediating this contractile failure was elegantly demonstrated by these authors [25]. The inflammatory cascade may be perpetuated by several factors including cytokine production (TNF, interleukins, interferons), endothelial activation expressed by neutrophil activation, increased production and release of nitric oxide via independent calcium synthase enzyme, under the influence of endotoxin and cytokines [26, 27].

Although most of the studies have ascribed the inflammatory reaction observed in the postoperative period due to blood exposure to nonendothelial surfaces during CPB, it may be part of the cascade of events. Recently Fransen and colleagues compared the inflammatory response after cardiac surgery in two groups of patients who underwent operation with and without CPB. They showed that the acute inflammatory phase response found in coronary bypass grafting patients is a result of the surgical trauma and/or anesthetics, rather than of the CPB procedure by itself. However, in the same study they showed that neutrophil activation markedly increases only in the CPB group [28].

Measures to reduce the systemic inflammation related to CPB and other complications

Despite progress in the safety of CPB, its use is still associated with significant morbidity and mortality. Among them, the inflammatory reaction is the most important, since it can lead to the development of postoperative organ dysfunction [29]. Once triggered, the inflammatory response to CPB may sometimes be self limited by an internal reaction against pro-inflammatory substances. Sometimes a high magnitude inflammatory reaction may occur, characterized by acute organ dysfunction, mainly in the respiratory system, accompanied by intense clinical manifestations. Several attempts have been made to reduce the inflammatory reaction and consequently the magnitude of organ dysfunction. Among the protective measures to minimize the inflammatory activation are: attenuating complement activation, reducing neutrophil activation, leukocyte depletion, heparin coating of CPB circuits, and preoperative gut sterilization [30-32].

Pharmacological agents

Glucocorticoids: Nowadays most groups active in cardiac surgery still employ glucocorticoids routinely, in the thought that these agents may attenuate the inflammatory activation due to CPB. Almost twenty years ago, in a controlled study in patients submitted to cardiac surgery with CPB, Niazi and colleagues demonstrated a better postoperative hemodynamic performance in a group pretreated with methylprednisolone [33]. Later studies have demonstrated that glucocorticoids administered before CPB will not prevent the increase in plasma levels of endotoxin, but will attenuate complement and neutrophil activation [34].

Aprotinin: Considerable research is under way on the antiinflammatory effects of protease inhibitors during CPB. Protease inhibitors have been employed in many patients to reduce the magnitude of bleeding due to excessive fibrinolysis seen in CPB. Substantial reduction of blood loss has been described in several studies involving aprotinin. Aprotinin inhibits both plasmin and kallikrein, but the inhibitor doses for kallikrein are much greater than those for plasmin. Thus it is reasonable to suppose that high doses of aprotinin could exert antiinflammatory activity including inhibition of complement activation and subsequent reduction in cytokine release and serum protease activation [35].

Heparin: The artificial surface of the CPB circuit and the surgical trauma offers a huge substrate for procoagulant agent stimulation in cardiac surgery. To prevent clot formation on the CPB circuit, high doses of heparin are used. Heparin acts by increasing the action of antithrombin III on thrombin, to prevent clotting formation during CPB, but it does not completely stop the thrombin generation. Thrombin generation during bypass is undesirable because excess of thrombin may predispose to some degree of clotting formation. This sub-clinical coagulation may enhance the consumption of coagulation proteins causing postoperative bleeding. The development of thrombi during CPB may be important in the development of postoperative stroke and subtle neurological injuries. Thrombin is also involved in the activation of platelets, neutrophils, and monocytes, participating in the inflammatory activation in CPB [36]. Another point related to the protective effect of heparin is related to the production of tissue factor pathway inhibitor (TFPI). TFPI appears to be the main agent in controlling tissue factor mediated coagulation, and TFPI release by heparin seems to be dose-dependent [37]. In view of the central role of heparin to control thrombin formation and to induce the release of TFPI from the endothelium during CPB, the use of other types of anticoagulants and heparin-bonded circuits to replace the action of heparin should be discussed [38].

Hypothermia

Body temperature during CPB is another important point to discuss. Traditionally the groups that work with cardiac surgery have used hypothermia (28 to 30°C) in an attempt to adjust the metabolism and oxygen consumption to the lower blood flow generated during CPB. Recently some groups have proposed advantages in using normothermia during CPB. In two groups of patients, both submitted to cardiac surgery, Menasché and colleagues compared the effects of CPB with normothermia and hypothermia on neutrophil activation and cytokine production. Hypothermia during CPB results in lower ICAM, interleukin I receptor antagonist, a marker of cytokine production, and plasma elastase, a marker for neutrophil degranulation, when compared to normothermia [39].

Hemofiltration

Hemofiltration has been widely used in cardiac surgery to reduce the volume of fluid added in oxygenators, mainly in children and in patients with renal dysfunction, during and at the end of CPB. Recently several studies have demonstrated the improvement of hemodynamics, coagulation parameters and time to extubation in children submitted to hemofiltration at the end of CPB [40]. Lower levels of inflammatory mediators after CPB in patients submitted to hemofiltration compared to a control group have also been reported [41].

Conclusion

It is well known that CPB provokes a generalized inflammatory response that is mediated by the activation of neutrophils, their adhesion to endothelial cells, and subsequent release of cytotoxic products. It has been known that this inflammatory response may cause organ dysfunctions of different magnitudes. Lung injury was for years considered the principal target of cytotoxic mediators. Nowadays the harmful consequences of the inflammatory reaction on myocardial function have become more evident. Protective measures to minimize the harmful effects provoked by the wide spectrum of compounds have been proposed in the literature. Although most of these protective measures may be considered still speculative, some interventions are used routinely or are under investigation. As discussed above, glucocorticoids, aprotinin, hypothermia, hemofiltration, heparin coated circuits, and membrane oxygenators have been recommended in the literature. Future strategies should also encompass those designed specifically to control compounds classified as triggers: complement-derived anaphylatoxins; mediators: cytokines, adhesion molecules; and effectors: thrombin, nitric oxide, leukotrienes, and proteolytic enzymes.

References

1. Gibbon JH (1937) Artificial maintenance of circulation during experimental occlusion of pulmonary artery. Arch Surg 34:1105-1131
2. Pearson DT (1990) Gas exchange: bubble and membrane oxygenators. Semin Thorac Cardiovasc Surg 2:313-319
3. Boers M, Van den Dungen JM, Karliczeck GF et al (1983) Two membrane oxygenators and bubble. A clinical comparison. Ann Thorac Surg 35:455-462
4. Moat NE, Shore DF, Evans TW (1993) Organ dysfunction and cardiopulmonary bypass: the role of complement and complement regulatory proteins. Eur J Cardiothorac Surg 7:563-573
5. Cavarochi NC, Pluth JR, Schaff HV et al (1986) Complement activation during cardiopulmonary bypass. J Thorac Cardiovasc Surg 91:252-258
6. Gillinov AM, Bator JM, Zehr KJ et al (1993) Neutrophil adhesion molecule expression during cardiopulmonary bypass with bubble and membrane oxygenators. Ann Thorac Surg 56: 847-853
7. Sudhaman DA (1991) Accidental hyperperfusion of the left carotid artery during CPB (letter). J Cardiothorac Vasc Anesth 5:100-101
8. Watson BG (1983) Unilateral cold neck. A new sign of misplacement of the aortic cannula during cardiopulmonary bypass. Anaesthesia 38:659-661
9. Murphy DA, Craver JM, Jones EL et al (1983) Recognition and management of ascending aortic dissection complicating cardiac surgical operations. J Thorac Cardiovasc Surg 85: 247-256
10. Bayindir O, Paker T, Akpinar B et al (1991) Case 6 - 1991: A 58-year-old man had a massive air embolism during cardiopulmonary bypass [clinical conference]. J Cardiothorac Vasc Anesth 5:627-634
11. Armon C, Deschamps C, Adkinson C et al (1991) Hyperbaric treatment of cerebral air embolism sustained during an open heart surgical procedure. Mayo Clin Proc 66:565-571
12. Butler J, Rocker GM, Westaby S (1993) Inflammatory response to cardiopulmonary bypass. Ann Thorac Surg 55:552-559

13. Ellison N, Behar M, MacVaugh H III, Marshall BE (1980) Bradykinin, plasma protein fraction and hypotension. Ann Thorac Surg 29:15-19
14. Parker DJ, Cantrell JW, Karp RB et al (1972) Changes in serum complement and immunoglobulins following cardiopulmonary bypass. Surgery 71:824-827
15. Kirklin JK, Westaby S, Blackstone EH et al (1983) Complement and the damaging effects of cardiopulmonary bypass. J Thorac Cardiovasc Surg 86:845-857
16. Fosse E, Mollnes TE, Ingvaldsen B (1986) Complement activation during major operations without cardiopulmonary bypass. J Thorac Cardiovasc Surg 93:860-866
17. Carlos TM, Harlan JM (1990) Membrane proteins involved in phagocyte adherence to endothelium. Immunol Rev 114:5-28
18. Dreyer WJ, Michael LH, Nguyen T et al (1992) Neutrophil-mediated pulmonary injury in a canine model of cardiopulmonary bypass: evidence for a CD18-dependent mechanism. Circulation 86[Suppl I]:I629
19. Wilson I, Gillinov AM, Curtis WE et al (1993) Inhibition of neutrophil adherence improves post-ischemic ventricular performance of the neonatal heart. Circulation 88:372-379
20. Downing SW, Edmunds LH Jr (1992) Release of vasoactive substances during cardiopulmonary bypass. Ann Thorac Surg 54:1236-1243
21. Ruvuolo G, Greco E, Speziale G et al (1994) Nitric oxide formation during cardiopulmonary bypass. Ann Thorac Surg 57:1055-1056
22. Matheis G, Sherman MP, Buckberg GD et al (1992) Role of l-arginine-nitric oxide pathway in myocardial re-oxygenation injury. Am J Physiol 262:H616-H620
23. Delgado R, Rojas A, Glaria LA et al (1995) Calcium-independent nitric oxide synthase activity in human lung after cardiopulmonary bypass. Thorax 50:403-404
24. Jansen NJG, van Oeveren W, Gu YJ et al (1992) Endotoxin release and tumor necrosis factor formation during cardiopulmonary bypass. Ann Thorac Surg 54:744-748
25. Shandelya SML, Kuppusamy P, Weisfeldt ML et al (1993) Evaluation of the role of polymorphonuclear leukocytes on contractile function in myocardial reperfusion injury: evidence for plasma-mediated leukocyte activation. Circulation 87:536-546
26. Boyle EM Jr, Pohlman TH, Johnson MC et al (1997) Endothelial cell injury in cardiovascular surgery: the systemic inflammatory response. Ann Thorac Surg 63:277-294
27. Hall RI, Smith SM, Graeme R (1997) The systemic inflammatory response to cardiopulmonary bypass: pathophysiological, therapeutic and pharmacological considerations. Anesth Analg 85:766-782
28. Fransen E, Maessen J, Dentener M et al (1998) Systemic inflammation present in patients undergoing CABG without extracorporeal circulation. Chest 113:1290-1295
29. Moat NE, Shore DF, Evans TW (1993) Organ dysfunction and cardiopulmonary bypass: the role of complement and complement regulatory proteins. Eur J Cardiothorac Surg 7:563-573
30. Johnson D, Thompson D, Hurst T et al (1994) Neutrophil mediated acute lung injury after extracorporeal circulation. J Thorac Cardiovasc Surg 107:1193-1202
31. Redmond JM, Gillinov AM, Sturat RS et al (1993) Heparin-coated bypass circuits reduce pulmonary injury. Ann Thorac Surg 56:474-479
32. Martinez-Pellus AE, Merino P, Bru M et al (1993) Can selective digestive decontamination avoid the endotoxemia, and cytokine activation promoted by cardiopulmonary bypass? Crit Care Med 21:1684-1691
33. Niazi Z, Flodin P, Joyce L et al (1979) Effects of glucocorticoids in patients undergoing coronary artery bypass surgery. Chest 76:262-268
34. Andersen LW, Baek L, Thomsen BS et al (1989) The effect of methylprednisolone on endotoxemia and complement activation during cardiac surgery. J Cardiothorac Anesth 3:544-549
35. Boldt J, Osmer C, Schindler E et al (1995) Circulating adhesion molecules in cardiac operations: influence of high dose aprotinin. Ann Thorac Surg 59:100-105
36. Edmunds LH (1995) Why cardiopulmonary bypass makes patients sick: Strategies to control the blood-synthetic surface interface. Adv Card Surg 6:131-167
37. Broze GJ (1995) Tissue factor pathway inhibitor and the current concept of blood coagulation. Blood Coagul Fibrinolysis 6[Suppl I]:S7-S13

38. Cardigan AR, Mackie IJ, Machin SJ (1997) Hemostatic endothelial interactions: a potential anticoagulant role of the endothelium in the pulmonary circulation during cardiac surgery. J Cardiothorac Vasc Anesth 11:329-336
39. Menasché P, Peynet J, Lariviere J et al (1994) Does normothermia during cardiopulmonary bypass increase neutrophil-endothelium interactions? Circulation 90:I1275-I1279
40. Elliot MJ (1993) Ultrafiltration and modified ultrafiltration in pediatric open heart operations. Ann Thorac Surg 56:1518-1522
41. Journois D, Pouard P, Greeley WJ et al (1994) Hemofiltration during cardiopulmonary bypass in pediatric cardiac surgery. Anesthesiology 81:1181-1189

Beta Blockers and General Anesthesia: Prevention of Myocardial Ischemia

R. MUCHADA

The prevention of myocardial ischemia should be one of the main objectives during anesthesia [1]. If we define the myocardial ischemia as the rupture of the balance between the transport of O_2 (DO_2) and the local metabolic needs, two different types can be identified:

- absolute ischemia, following the total absence of perfusion. This situation leads to irreversible cellular alterations. All preventive actions are, in this case, impracticable;
- relative ischemia, for DO_2 that is inadequate but sufficient to maintain temporary cellular viability. It is a high-risk situation which must be recognized and treated very fast. The causative mechanism frequently involved is tachycardia, generally determined by an adrenergic discharge with beta-1 positive effects.

When the diagnosis of relative ischemia is made, beta blockers may be used even in a preventive aim. Beta blockers may be used during general anesthesia if some imperatives are respected:

1. the beta blocker should be injected intravenously (IV), in bolus or in a continuous perfusion manner;
2. the dosage should be modulated and adapted to the sensitivity of each patient;
3. the half-life of the product should be short and its action quickly reversible, spontaneously or by drug competition;
4. the action should be characterized by specificity on the wanted effect.

Choice of product

Respect of the previously listed imperatives guides the selection towards one specific product: esmolol [2]. Esmolol is a beta blocker used intravenously, with a half-life of 9 min and a total duration of action of 15-25 min. It is beta-1 specific at the standard therapeutic doses. Continuous IV perfusion is possible. The dose may be adjustable over objective parameters, according to each patient's individual reaction.

Esmolol is not irritating to the venous walls; therefore it can be perfused in a peripheral vein, without risks of local damage. Its plasmatic metabolism induces the production of degradation products 1500-times less effective in beta-1 blockade. Degradation into methanol does not implicate a risk for the patient since, with the maximum therapeutic doses used, the concentrations of by-product are only 2% of the minimum toxic level. Renal elimination of the degradation products is not affected by moderate renal failure. In this case it is necessary to avoid the maximum dose recommended, for more than 72 h [3].

Myocardial depression appears when esmolol is used. The chronotropic, bathmotropic, dromotropic and inotropic functions are affected negatively [4]. The product has a positive lusiotropic action on ischemic myocardial areas [5].

If the risk of myocardial ischemia is determined fundamentally by tachycardia [6], a patient could be protected by a planned therapy with a product having a negative chronotropic effect. A decrease in heart rate (HR) increases the diastolic period [7], and increases the diastolic time of coronary filling [8]. At the same time, the positive lusiotropic action diminishes the diastolic myocardial tonus, collaborating to the improvement of coronary filling.

However, the negative inotropic effect of the beta blocker has some inconveniences that should be considered. Coronary filling does not depend only on the above-mentioned diastolic conditions, but also on the blood flow and on the diastolic arterial blood pressure (DAP). A depression in contractility can decrease the blood flow and the arterial pressure.

When a specific beta blocker is used, a persisting peripheral adrenergic action could maintain the vascular resistance, thereby compensating the fall in arterial pressure due to the reduced blood flow [9]. As a consequence, all decreases of arterial pressure caused by esmolol correspond to a decrease in blood flow, without a decrease, or better yet, with an increase of the afterload.

Fortunately, under these conditions, the DAP is little affected. DAP-dependent coronary hypoperfusion is then little modified by this fact. Coronary perfusion could be preserved if blood flow is sufficient in volume and in distribution.

Monitoring

The tachycardia observed during general anesthesia does not necessitate the systematic use of a beta blocker. The therapeutic decision should be based on evaluation of the risk factors, clinical and physiopathologic elements, and cardiovascular monitoring data [10].

From the clinical point of view, knowledge of a patient's history, the preanesthetic evaluation and the hemodynamic modifications occurring during anesthesia can guide the therapeutic decision:

– *standard* monitoring (electrocardiography, HR and arterial pressure, AP) does not always provide sufficient information for deciding upon beta blocker use.

Even so, a very interesting index can be derived from this basic monitoring;

- the *relationship between DAP and HR* is an interesting element in evaluating the risk of myocardial ischemia. A DAP/HR ratio between 0.7 and 1 or superior to 1 is considered to be indicative of absence of risk, when HR is 55-90 beats/min and DAP is 40-90 mmHg. A ratio between 0.5 and 0.7 needs particular attention, while a ratio inferior to 0.5 indicates the need for therapeutic correction. This index varies in function of both DAP and HR. When the value is modified for an increase in HR, the use of a beta blocker has to be considered;

- *surveillance of the ST segment* contributes to the detection of ischemic alterations during anesthesia;

- *transesophageal echography* also helps in the diagnosis in that it detects dyskinetic ventricular areas and shows changes in ventricle volume by following modifications in its diameter.

One last type of monitoring, less used nowadays, is the continuous surveillance of the *systolic time intervals (STI)*, integrated in a hemodynamic profile. The pre-ejection period (PEP) is the most interesting parameter to detect beta stimulation or beta blocking actions [11]. The normal value of this parameter indexed to the HR is 130 ± 5 ms. A value under 128 ms, together with an HR over 85 beats/min, can be considered to be a direct sign of beta stimulation.

Therapy decision

When clinical evaluation and monitoring lead to the diagnosis of a risk for myocardial ischemia, it becomes necessary to choose a therapy. The endogenous beta stimulation occurring during anesthesia can have diverse origins, e.g. algid adrenergic discharges, insufficient narcosis, uninhibited vascular or visceral reflexes, vasoplegia, arterial hypotension, hypovolemia, and individual reactions. Blockage of the endogenous beta stimulation can be done when suspected tachycardia, modified DAP/HR ratio, altered ST segment, varied PEP, or kinetic or morphologic myocardial modifications are observed. It is necessary to treat all the other possible causes of cardiovascular modifications. Only in this manner can the use of esmolol be evoked.

Dosage

The recommended bolus dose is 0.5 mg/kg, although 0.25 mg/kg should be enough, in my experience. The bolus is followed by an IV perfusion, starting at 5 μg/kg min and increasing, every 5 min, by steps of 5-10 μg/kg min until 100 μg/kg min. The objective is to diminish the HR to a "normal value".

However, it is important to remember that cardiac output (CO) is the result of the HR multiplied by the stroke volume (SV). In some patients, mainly in the elderly presenting with myocardial "rigidity", the SV is dramatically stable. The only way that these patients have to maintain an appropriate CO or to compensate a decrease in CO during anesthesia, is to increase HR, until the maximum tolerated within the range of normality (85-90 beats/min). Therefore, in certain circumstances the increase in HR should be evaluated and sometimes accepted.

When following cardiovascular evolution with a reduced monitoring system, it is possible to decide upon the use of esmolol by observing the combined variation of HR and AP. The decrease in AP under the action of esmolol is flow-dependent [12]. A decrease in HR due to esmolol can be beneficial while it does not introduce a significant decrease in AP. Remember that an acute drop in AP implies a fall in blood flow in the absence of any action of a beta blocker on the vascular resistance.

Monitoring the other hemodynamic parameters, such as evolution of the ST segment, modification of hypokinetic areas, and recovery of the contraction synergy, should allow a narrow regulation of the beta blocker dose. When beta blocker therapy is applied with the noninvasive cardiovascular monitoring of blood flow, left ventricle systolic performances, preload, afterload, HR and other parameters relative to tissue perfusion ($PetCO_2$ trends, for example) [10], the dosage will be adapted to obtain a PEP under 160 ms and tolerating a decrease of blood flow, without modification of tissue perfusion.

Indications

The main indications for the use of esmolol during anesthesia are the following [12-15]:

1. control of tachycardia caused by endogenous beta-1 stimulation in patients with myocardial ischemic risks or leading to an alteration of myocardial perfusion;
2. control of blood flow-dependent arterial hypertension (hyperkinetic syndrome with normal or low vascular resistance);
3. reduction of supraventricular arrhythmias;
4. prevention of some specific causes of heart failure. This last condition may be a new indication for esmolol use, taking into account its negative chronotropic and positive lusiotropic actions. However, for the moment it is not one to be applied during general anesthesia. In contrast, the use of esmolol for "near vegetative protection", to avoid acute hypertensive [16-18] during intubation, is at the moment extremely debatable, given the absence of physiopathologic evidence and the recently described accidents.

Considering that esmolol has beta-1 cardiospecific action, supratherapeutic doses and special reactivities in certain patients require extreme wisdom in its use, especially regarding asthmatics, psychotics, diabetics, pregnant women, and patients with electrical conduction heart blockades.

Conclusions

The use of a beta blocker during general anesthesia should be based on clinical evidence and objective data obtained from cardiovascular monitoring. Esmolol, for its beta-1 cardiospecific actions, for its short half-life, for the possibility of being administered as an IV bolus and in continuous perfusion, appears nowadays as product of choice for general anesthesia.

Indications for esmolol use during general anesthesia should be limited to the control of tachycardia in patients with a myocardial ischemic risk, and to the treatment of blood flow-dependent hypertension and supraventricular rhythm dysfunctions. Esmolol and other beta blockers are contraindicated whenever their secondary actions may produce complications in direct opposition to the desired effect.

References

1. Lehot JJ, Foex P, Durand PG (1990) Bêta-bloquants et anesthésie. Ann Fr Anesth Réanim 9: 137-152
2. Reves JG, Flezzani P (1985) Perioperative use of esmolol. Ann J Cardiol 56:5-62
3. Alexander R, Binns J, Hetred M (1994) A controlled trial of the effects of esmolol on cardiac functions. Br J Anaesth 72:594-595
4. Zannad F (1987) Les bêta-bloquants. In: Gilgenkrantz JM, Roger RJ, Zannad F (eds) Thérapeutique en Pathologie Cardio-Vasculaire. Flammarion, Paris, pp 33-47
5. Vatner SF, Baig H, Manders WT et al (1977) Effects of propanolol on regional myocardial function, electrograms and blood flow in conscious dog with myocardial ischemia. J Clin Invest 60:353-360
6. Slogoff S, Keats AS (1985) Does perioperative myocardial ischemia lead to postoperative myocardial infarction? Anesthesiology 62:107-114
7. Dagnino J, Prys-Roberts C (1985) Assessment of beta-adrenoreceptor blockade during anesthesia in humans: Use of isoproterenol dose-response curves. Anesth Analg 64:305-311
8. Guth BD, Heusch G, Seitelberger R, Ross J Jr (1987) Elimination of exercise-induced regional myocardial dysfunction by a bradycardic agent in dogs with chronic coronary stenosis. Circulation 75:661-669
9. Holtzman JL, Finley D, Johnson B et al (1986) The effects of single dose of atenolol, labetalol and propranolol on cardiac and vascular function. Clin Pharmacol Ther 40:268-273
10. Muchada R (1988) Continuous and noninvasive hemodynamic monitoring including aortic blood flow, systolic time intervals and PetCO$_2$ measurements. In: Kazuyuki Matsuyuk D, Toieni K (eds) State of the art technology in anesthesia and intensive care. Elsevier, Amsterdam, pp 75-85
11. Boudoulas H (1990) Systolic time intervals. Eur Heart J 11[Suppl 1]:93-104
12. Gray RJ (1988) Postcardiac surgical hypertension. J Cardiothorac Anesth 2:678-682
13. Balser JR, Martinez EA, Winters BD et al (1998) Beta-adrenergic blockade accelerates conversion of postoperative supraventricular tachyarrhythmias. Anesthesiology 89:1052-1059

14. Raby KE, Brull SJ, Timimi F et al (1999) The effect of heart rate control on myocardial is-
    chemia among high-risk patients after vascular surgery. Anesth Analg 88:477-482
15. Bold MI, Sacks DJ, Grosnoff DB et al (1989) Use of esmolol during anesthesia to treat tachy-
    cardia and hypertension. Anesth Analg 68:101-104
16. Gold MI, Brown M, Caveman S, Merrington C. (1986) Heart rate and blood pressure effects
    of esmolol after ketamine induction and intubation. Anesthesiology 64:718-723
17. Liu PL, Gatt S, Gugino LD et al (1986) Esmolol for control of increases in heart rate and
    blood pressure during tracheal intubation after thiopentone and succinylcholine. Can Anaesth
    Soc J 33:556-562
18. Cucchiara RF, Benefiel DJ, Matteo AS et al (1986) Evaluation of esmolol in controlling in-
    creases in heart rate and blood pressure during endotracheal intubation in patients undergoing
    carotid endarterectomy. Anesthesiology 65:528-531

Heart and Electrolytes

F. Schiraldi, P. Ferraro, B. Maglione

Critically ill patients often have electrical instability of the heart, either due to intrinsic cardiac diseases or to electrolyte and acid-base imbalance. In addition, they are submitted to aggressive drug therapies (inotropic drugs, amines, antiarrhythmics, etc.), which may badly influence myocardial excitability, provoking eventually a proarrhythmic effect [1-3]. In order to improve the therapeutic strategies in such patients, it could be perhaps useful to recall some basic principles about the electrolyte mediated physiologic properties of the heart. Moreover, this reevaluation will hopefully offer a deeper insight on the real cellular mechanisms underlying the antiarrhythmic action of different drugs [4].

Basic electrophysiology

1. Membrane conductance or ionic conductance (g) is expressed by the velocity (cm/sec) of any electrolyte passing through the cell membrane; as opposed to the membrane resistance (R), i.e.: $g = 1/R$, it is also expressed as the electrical current (I) divided by the potential difference (E), i.e.: $g = I/E$. Almost every antiarrhythmic drug, some inotropes and hormones, and the plasmatic electrolyte concentrations, by theirselves, can modify g, therefore influencing the resting and action myocardial potentials.

2. Resting potential is mainly dependent on the external/internal cellular concentrations of potassium. The transmembrane voltage at which the electrical gradient is equal and opposite to the concentration gradient is the K electrochemical equilibrium potential Ek, as described by the Nernst equation $Ek = RT/F \log [K]o/[K]i$. Solving the equation predicts a transmembrane voltage of about -96 mV in cardiac muscle, which is very similar to the observed voltage ($\cong -90$ mV). Hyperkalemia acts on this resting potential, reducing the electronegativity, while hypokalemia at the same time increases the electronegativity, and reduces the specific conductance (gK), which is a substrate of the QT dispersion (long QT, prominent U wave) [5, 6].

3. Action potential starts by means of a sudden increase of the membrane conductance to Na ($g Na$); this is closely related to the difference (Δ) between the threshold and resting potentials. The larger the difference (Δ), the higher the 0 phase upstroke.

4. Impulse conduction is very homogeneously and quickly transmitted over the different tissues in the heart only when the 0 phase upstroke is normal; when hyperkalemia, hypermagnesemia or hypocalcemia reduce the resting-threshold voltage difference, the impulse conduction is slowed down (QRS enlargement, A-V blocks, atrial paralysis) [7].

5. Repolarization is closely linked to the previous depolarization: the former should last an "optimal" time. Too fast/too slow repolarizations could provoke refractoriness and inhomogeneity, which implies an increased likeliness of microreentry arrhythmias [8]. Blood pH derangements, hypoxia, ischemia, and K, Mg or Ca disorders can modify the specific g immediately after depolarization: this is supposed to be the main electrophysiological substrate of triggered activity linked either to early afterdepolarizations (EADs) or to delayed afterdepolarizations (DADs) [9, 10].

6. Early afterdepolarizations are potentially life-threatening impulses, sometimes responsible for hyperkinetic triggered arrhythmias; it is useful to remember that class Ia, Ic, and III antiarrhythmic drugs could have proarrhythmic effects by their interfering in some electrolyte conductances (g) [11].

7. Delayed afterdepolarizations are Ca-linked oscillatory currents immediately following the ventricular repolarization; they are mainly caused by the "ischemia-reperfusion" syndrome, adrenergic hyperactivity or digitalis toxicity. As the intracellular Ca-overload is probably responsible for any DADs-dependent arrhythmias, it is also the "vulnerable parameter" to be corrected by the therapy [12, 13].

8. Proarrhythmia is defined as the development of a new or more dangerous arrhythmia after treatment with antiarrhythmic drugs [14, 15]; primary proarrhythmia is provoked or worsened by a drug at a subtherapeutic or therapeutic level; secondary proarrhythmia is due to an adjunctive factor (electrolyte imbalance, ischemia, drugs), which reduces the therapeutic index of the specific drug [16].

The clinical connection

Whenever an electrolyte imbalance happens acutely, some electrophysiological effects should be expected. As depicted in Figs. 1, 2, 3, 4, 5, 6, the resting and action potentials of myocytes and Purkinje tissue are modified in such a predictable way sometimes as to allow a diagnostic hypothesis (about any underlying dyselectrolytemia) just by evaluating the EKG recordings.

Moreover:

– electrolyte-based arrhythmias are likely to be cured by electrolytes;
– most antiarrhytmic drugs act on electrolyte transmembrane fluxes;
– some antiarrhythmic toxicities can be corrected by electrolytes [17].

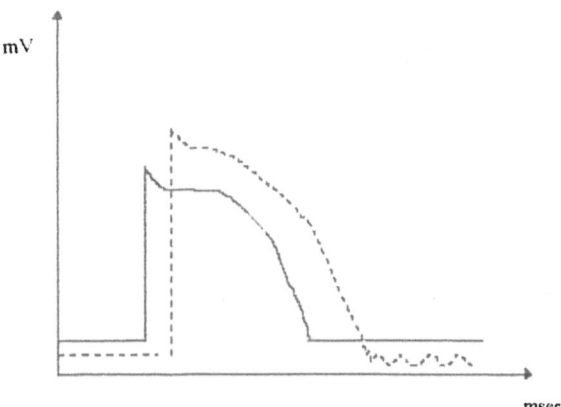

Fig. 1. Hypokalemia

– ↑ electronegativity .... → QRS narrowing
– ↑ conduction velocity .... →   „   „
– ↑ upstroke .... → high voltage QRS
– ↓ g K .... → long QT
– phase 3 prolongation .... → triggered activity (EVB)

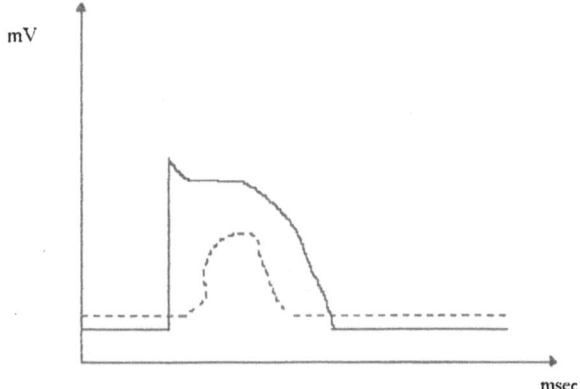

Fig. 2. Hyperkalemia

– ↓ electronegativity .... → QRS enlargement
– ↓ upstroke .... ↓ voltage
– ↓ conduction velocity .... → atrial paralysis, AV delay
– phase 3 shortening .... peaked T wave

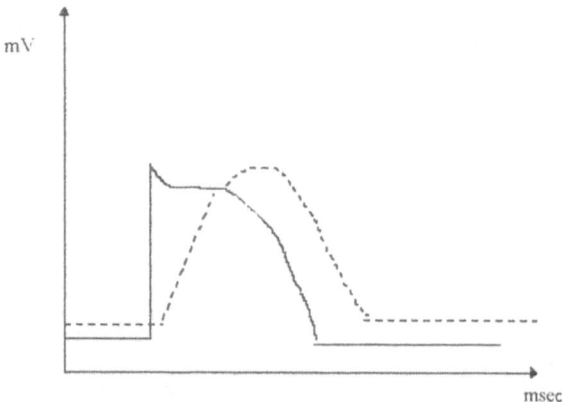

Fig. 3. Hypocalcemia

– ↓ electronegativity
– ↓ upstroke
– ↓ conduction velocity... → intraventricular delay?
– phase 3 delay .... → long JT

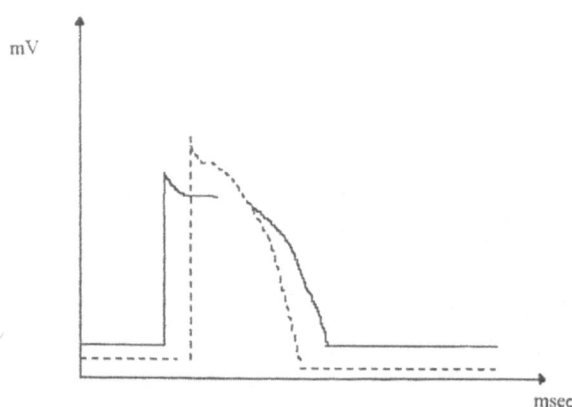

Fig. 4. Hypercalcemia

– ↓ inward Na... slow conduction............................. AVB I, II
– ↓ plateau.. short J-T
– ↑ myocardial contractility
– ↑ digitalis toxicity

- ↑ ectopic beats

- ↓↑ S-T , ↓ T

- long QT

- TdP, VT

- ↑ digitalis toxicity

Fig. 5. Hypomagnesemia-related EKG changes

- A-V blocks

- intraventricular blocks

- ↓ ventricular rate in hyperkinetic
  arrhythmias

Fig. 6. Hypermagnesemia-related EKG changes

A classical example of an electrolyte-based therapy of an electrolyte-based life-threatening arrhythmia is the positive effect of i.v. calcium administration in hyperkalemia. The electrophysiological basis of this is linked to the calcium effect on the myocardial threshold, exactly opposed to the hyperkalemic effect on the resting potential (Fig. 7).

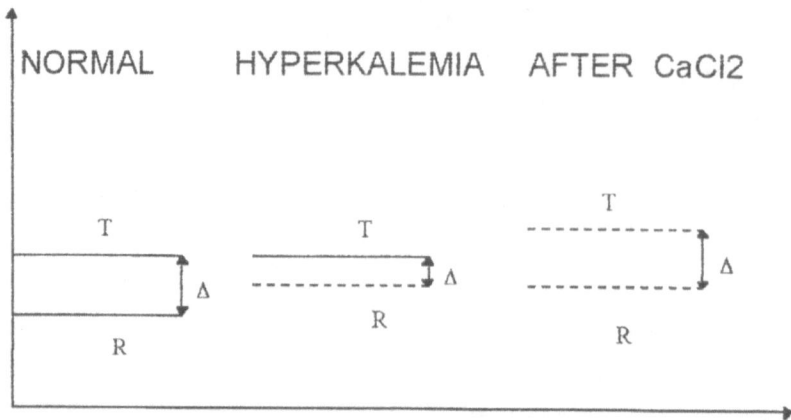

Fig. 7. Calcium correction of hyperkalemic effects. (R = Resting potential, T = Threshold potential, Δ = Difference)

Moreover such an electrophysiologic antagonism has an optimal time-onset, as compared to the other more common approaches (Table 1) [18].

Table 1. Time scheduled approach to hyperkalemia

Substance	Time onset	Lasting
Calcium chloride	1-2'	15-20'
Sodium bicarbonate	10-15'	60-120'
Insulin + glucose	20-30'	2-4 hours

Antiarrhythmics and electrolytes

As a practical rule, it could be better in critically ill patients to firstly correct any possible electrolyte disorders, before approaching any arrhythmia by drugs. Moreover it could be useful to recall which specific ionic conductances are modified by the specific classes of antiarrhythmic drugs [19, 20]. As reported in Fig. 8, the main pharmacodynamic effect is mostly mediated by a "conductance-targeted" action. From this point of view, it is easy to see how, e.g., hypertonic Na-Cl could antagonize some propafenon side effects [21], or how hypokalemia and hypomagnesemia could worsen the therapeutic index of amiodarone and sotalol. It also underlines how dangerous it could be to add a second antiarrhythmic drug when the first choice has been unsuccessful, particularly if both could interact with the same g.

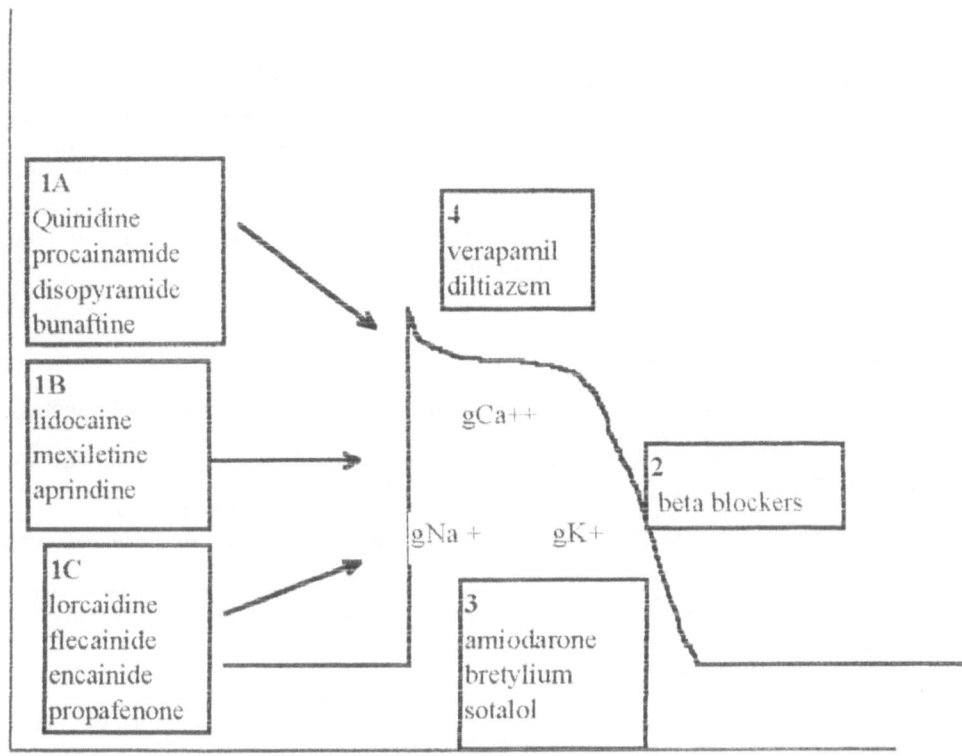

Fig. 8. Ionic conductances and antiarrhythmic drug effect

Practical electrophysiology of antiarrhythmic drugs

A clinical subdivision of antiarrhythmic drugs could help the intensivist to match a therapeutic choice with the underlying substrate and ionic balance. In Table 2 the main "expected" effects of the different antiarrhythmic classes are reported [22].

Table 2. MAIN g - mediated effects of antiarrhythmic drugs

Antiarrhythmic drug	HR	QRS	A-V cond.	ERP	J-T
Class I A	↓	↑	Slowed	↑	↑
I B	=	=	=	↑	↓
I C	= ↓	↑	Slowed	=	=
Class II	↓	=	Slowed	= ↑	=
Class III	↓	↑	Slowed	↑	↑
Class IV	↓	=	Slowed	↑	=

Conclusions

The electrolyte pattern is one of the main determinants of normal cardiac electrophysiological behavior; in the critically ill some acid-base and electrolyte derangement is common, and it could influence the outcome for the worse, inducing life-threatening arrhythmias [23]. As a matter of fact, the main therapeutic mechanism of antiarrhythmic drugs relies on some influence on electrolyte conductances. It seems safer to first correct any such underlying disorders, instead of always approaching arrhythmia treatment with drugs.

References

1. Task Force of the Working Group on Arrhythmias of the European Society of Cardiology (1991) The Sicilian Gambit. Circulation 84:1831-1851
2. Morganroth J (1992) Proarrhythmic effects of antiarrhythmic drugs: evolving concepts. Am Heart J 128:575-586
3. Atlee JL (1997) Perioperative cardiac dysrhythmias. Anesthesiology 86:1397-1424
4. Kerin N, Somberg J (1994) Proarrhythmia: definition, risk factors, causes, treatment, and controversies. Am Heart J 128:575-586
5. Tsuji H, Venditti FJ et al (1994) The association of levels of serum potassium and magnesium with ventricular premature complexes (the Framingham Heart Study). Am J Cardiol 74: 232-235
6. Gettes L (1994) Electrolyte abnormalities as triggers for lethal ventricular arrhythmias. In: Akhtar (ed) Sudden cardiac death. Williams and Wilkins, Philadelphia, pp 327-340
7. Curran ME, Splawsky I et al (1995) Amolecular basis for cardiac arrhytmias: HERG mutations cause long QT syndrome. Cell 80:795-803
8. Oreto G (1997) I disordini del ritmo cardiaco. Centro Scientifico Editore, Torino
9. Singh BN (1993) Controlling cardiac arrhythmias by lengthening repolarization: emerging perspectives. Am J Card 72;16:1F-124 F
10. Sanguinetti MC, Jiang C et al (1995) A mechanistic link between an inherited and an acquired cardiac arrhythmia: HERG encodes the Ik potassium channel. Cell 81:299-307
11. Hondeghem LM (1987) Antiarrhythmic agents. Modulated receptors applications. Circulation 75:514-520
12. Roden DM (1994) Risks and benefits of antiarrhythmic therapy. N Engl J Med 331:785-791
13. Seller RH (1971) The role of magnesium in digitalis toxicity. Am Heart J 82:551-556
14. Atlee JL (1998) New concepts of antiarrhythmic strategies. In: Gullo A (ed) APICE Proceedings. Springer Verlag, pp 291-297
15. Kowey PR, Marinchak RA et al (1997) Intravenous amiodarone. J Am Coll Cardiol 29:1190-1198
16. Daoud EG, Strickberger SA et al (1997) Preoperative amiodarone as prophylaxis against atrial fibrillation after heart surgery
17. Tzivoni D, Banai S et al (1988) Treatment of torsade de pointes with magnesium sulfate. Circulation 77:392-397
18. Schiraldi F (1993) Acqua, elettroliti, equilibrio acido-base: l'essenziale. Ed. Idelson, Napoli
19. The CAST Investigators (1989) Preliminary report: Effect of encainide and flecainide on mortality in a randomized trial of arrhythmia suppression after myocardial infarction. N Engl J Med 321:406-412
20. Mason JW (1987) Amiodarone. N Engl J Med 316:455-458
21. Funck-Brentano C, Kroemer HK et al (1990) Propafenone. N Engl J Med 322:518-525
22. The Sicilian Gambit (1994) Antiarrhythmic therapy: a pathophysiologic approach. Futura, Armonk, pp 3-337
23. Steinbach KK, Merl O et al (1994) Hemodynamics during ventricular tachyarrhytmias. Am Heart J 127:1102-1106

RECOMMENDATIONS
ON PERIOPERATIVE MANAGEMENT

Patient-Assessment in the Postanaesthesia Care Unit (PACU)

H. V. SCHALK

For most patients, recovery from anaesthesia is a smooth, uneventful emergence from an uncomplicated anaesthetic and operation. But due to increasing age and multimorbidity in surgical patients, responsibility not only for the anaesthetic regimen but also for comorbidity in the post-operative period must be taken by anaesthesiologists. Therefore, patient assessment during the premedication visit is the first step in planning post-anaesthesia care unit PACU treatment. The scope of work of the PACU includes complications similar to those encountered in intensive care units (ICU). Therefore, facilities and staff must be sufficient and competent to deal with emergencies. While the size of a PACU is determined by the surgical workload, intensity of nursing and needed, medical care depends on case mix and number of accessible ICU beds [1-3].

Recovery from anaesthesia

In most cases the recovery process from anaesthesia actually begins in the operating room. With the use of short-acting intravenous anaesthetics even after long procedures awakening after termination of the perfusion is prompt. Since the time of recovery from inhaled anaestheties is a function of the solubility coefficient and the alveolar ventilation, monitoring of spontaneously exhaled minute volume (MV) and the concentration of the volatile agent used is mandatory before extubation. Recovery from morphine-based anaesthetics is not only dose dependent but also influenced by kidney function. Pharmacokinetics of reversing agents and re-uptake phenomena must be taken into account. With the use of short-acting opioids rapid awakening from anaesthesia is feasible, but sufficient pain therapy in the postoperative period may be a problem. Neuromuscular blockade with short-acting substances is now possible and car monitored with reliable methods. Reversing agents for benzodiazepines, opioids and muscle-relaxants are now seldom needed, since short-acting substances are in use.

Recovery from regional anaesthesia

The type of nerve blockade, the local anaesthetic used and amount of sedation define the course of recovery from regional anaesthesia. A patient discharged from a PACU with still present palsy of the legs must be considered at risk on a ward where there are fewer personnel available. In patients breathing room air, arterial hypoxaemia is most readily detected with a pulse oximeter. This also holds true to a lesser extent for upper limb nerve block.

Postoperative ventilatory support

In most cases, the patient is transferred from the operating room to the PACU without ventilatory support when short-acting substances have been used for anaesthesia. Only patients undergoing major surgery for many hours remain intubated for PACU follow-up treatment or, if indicated, for transfer to ICU. The use of laryngeal masks has made tracheal intubation necessary in fewer operations while providing a safe airway for the immediate postoperative period with minimal discomfort to the patient. It is recommended to keep the patient on his or her side side during the postoperative period in order to prevent airway obstruction or aspiration of gastric contents. Since in most PACUs patients routinely receive oxygen therapy via a face mask, nurses and physicians should be aware that there might be discrepancies between arterial oxygen saturation (SaO_2) and pulse oximetry (SpO_2) values [4]. Hyperventilation, hypertension and deterioration of alertness are most often the signs of hypoxia and hypercarbia. Arterial blood gas measurement will be the first step in diagnosing the problem. *Airway obstruction* is detected clinically and treated accordingly. *Aspiration* is another problem and a *pneumothorax* may become clinically relevant, sometimes with hours of delay after attempts to puncture the subclavian vein. In patients with COPD coughing may be insufficient and the assistence of pulmonary therapists may be necessary. Special attention must be paid to the ventilatory pattern of patients with known sleep apnoea or after neurosurgery.

Pulmonary oedema is known to be associated with left ventricular failure. Accordingly, fluid therapy should be balanced with special care in patients with heart disease or kidney failure [9]. In rare circumstances anaphylaxis is the reason for pulmonary oedema [5]. Postoperative *pulmonary embolism* was a frequent complication before the routine perioperative use of heparin. Despite this regimen, this serious complication has not been completely eliminated. Radiological diagnosis without delay after the first clinical signs will guide therapy.

The treatment of hypoxaemia in the PACU consists of treatment of the underlying cause and oxygen therapy or ventilatory support. CPAP by face mask is routinely used postoperatively in many patients to increase the functional residual capacity. If initiated in time, in a still co-operative patient, tracheal intubation may often be avoided. In patients with preoperatively anticipated ventilatory problems, training might be helpful [6].

Hypoventilation during the postoperative period occurs as a result of poor respiratory drive as seen after neurosurgery or narcotic depression, muscle dysfunction after abdominal surgery, a high rate of carbon dioxide production as in sepsis, or as the direct result of acute or chronic lung disease. Measurements of the maximum inspiratory force and vital capacity are used for weaning the patient from ventilatory support. Vital capacity should be at least 10 ml/kg LBW, inspiratory force should be more than 20 cm H_2O.

Postoperative cardio-circulatory therapy

Hypotension in the postoperative period is a pathophysiologic sign of decreased ventricular preload, reduced myocardial contractility or reduced systemic vascular resistance. Blood loss due to surgery or a coagulation disorder as well as third space fluid loss are common reasons for hypotension and tachycardia. Perioperative myocardial infarction or ongoing sepsis may be the cause of heart failure. In hypovolaemic, cardiogenic and septic shock the standard of intensive care medicine is necessary in the PACU. Hypertension due to pain, hypercarbia, hypoxaemia or fluid overload is to be treated according to the underlying cause. Severe hypertension may lead to arrhythmia, myocardial infarction and left ventricular failure due to insufficient myocardial oxygen provision. In patients preoperative medication with long-acting antihypertensive substances is not interrupted because of the scheduled operation. If necessary, hypertension is additionally treated with short-acting substances while adequate pain therapy must be guaranteed [7, 8].

Renal complications

Postoperative renal failure very often results from hypovolaemia or circulatory failure. Monitored fluid therapy and diuretics may be necessary. Post-renal oliguria is caused by obstruction of the urinary collecting system. Diagnosis by ultrasound, followed by insertion of a nephrostomy tube or ureteral catheter should prevent damage to the kidneys. Acute tubular necrosis may ultimately need dialysis [9].

Postoperative pain therapy

Pain is the most common problem requiring treatment in the PACU. Pre-emptive analgesia, continuous intravenous application of narcotics and analgesics, patient-controlled analgesia and regional anaesthesia are all used for the relief of postoperative pain. With the use of epidural catheters and continuous infusion pumps patient comfort with minimal doses of medication is possible [10].

Postoperative nausea and vomiting

Patients undergoing laparoscopic surgery or strabismus surgery are especially susceptible to suffering nausea and vomiting. Obviously, the type of surgery has more influence than the anaesthetic technique. Antiemetics can be given at the end of the procedure to patients with a history of vomiting in previous surgery. Droperidol may also be effective.

Conclusion

While hospital plans define PACU use according to statistical needs, in daily routine there is no limit to the variety of patients to be cared for even in a well defined PACU:

ASA class I patients scheduled for minor surgery may by treated according to the rules of day case surgery and thereby need hours of PACU stay before they are sufficiently safe for ambulation. Other ASA class I patients may be transferred to the regular ward for further treatment very shortly after emergence from anaesthesia. ASA class IV patients will probably need several hours of postoperative treatment to balance their organ functions. In many cases qualified ICU treatment may be necessary when ICU beds are occupied. Continuous assessment of patients in the PACU should not only evaluate the patients' acute physical status but also determine their prognosis for further treatment from the viewpoint of an intensive care specialist.

References

1. Feeley TW (1999) The postanesthesia care unit. In: Miller RD (ed) Anesthesia. Churchill Livingstone, New York, pp 2113-2133
2. Hines R, Barash P, Watrous G et al (1992) Complications occurring in the postoperative care unit: a survey. Anesthesia Analg 74:503-509
3. Kalish RI et al (1995) Costs of potential complications of care for major surgery. Am Journal of Medical Quality 10:48-54
4. Temper KK, Barker SJ (1989) Pulse oximetry. Anesthesiology 70:89-93
5. Crandall ED, Staub NE, Goldberg HS et al (1983) Recent developments in pulmonary edema. Ann Intern Med 99:808
6. Smith RA, Kirby RR, Gooding JM et al(1980) Continuous positive airway pressure (CPAP) by face mask. Crit Care Med 8:483
7. Mangano DT (1990) Perioperative cardiac morbidity. Anesthesiology 72:153-184
8. Rose DK, Cohen MM, DeBoer DP (1996) Cardiovascular events in the postanesthesia care unit. Anesthesiology 84:772-781
9. Prough DS, Foreman AS (1992) Anesthesia and the renal system. In: Barasch PG, Cullen BF, Stoelting RK (eds) Clinical anesthesia. Lippincott, Philadelphia, pp 1125-1156
10. Practice guidelines for acute pain management in the peripoperative setting (1995) A report by the ASA Task Force on Pain Management Acute Pain Section. Anesthesiology 82:1071-1081

HOW TO SET UP AN ACUTE PAIN SERVICE

How to Set Up Acute Pain Services

N. Rawal, R. Allvin, C. Zetterberg

Recent years have seen the development of new analgesic drugs and sophisticated drug delivery systems. Pain management modalities such as patient controlled analgesia (PCA), epidural analgesia with opioids and/or local anaesthetic drugs and regional blocks are being increasingly used. However, in general the obstacles to bringing research to the bedside have not been overcome. The most common technique for providing postoperative analgesia has been and still is the use of i.m. opioids prescribed by surgeons and administered by ward nurses on an as-needed basis. The inadequacies of this method of pain management are well recognized.

Newer analgesia techniques such as PCA, spinal opioids and regional analgesia techniques provide superior pain relief as compared to intermittent i.m. opioids but such techniques have their own risks and therefore require special monitoring. Traditional methods of analgesia are not risk-free either but the risks have rarely been quantified. It is becoming increasingly clear that the solution to the problems of postoperative pain management lies not so much in the development of new techniques as in development of an organization to exploit existing expertise. This is one of the main conclusions of interdisciplinary expert committee reports by the National Health and Medical Research Council of Australia, Royal College of Surgeons of England and the College of Anaesthetists, US Department of Health and Human Services and the International Association for the Study of Pain (IASP). These reports also published guidelines which recommend actions such as using pain assessment tools, frequent pain assessment and evaluation of treatment efficacy, and bedside pain documentation systems. One of the most important recommendations of these reports is that there is a need for effective organization for postoperative pain service which is based on a team approach.

In the United States 24-h acute pain services provide good quality analgesia by using PCA and epidural techniques in increasing numbers of surgical patients [7]. Almost all major institutions in the USA have acute pain services (APS). Such comprehensive pain management teams usually consist of staff anaesthesiologists, resident anaesthesiologists, specially trained nurses and pharmacists. Sometimes physiotherapists are also included. Patients under the care of APS are visited and assessed regularly by one or more members of the team. A pain fellow or anaesthesiology resident is on-call for emergencies and "non-regular" working hours.

Problems with anaesthesiologist-based APS (USA-style)

Anaesthesiologist-based APS organization models usually provide "high tech" pain management services. This is not surprising because anaesthesiologists have special expertise in the field of advanced analgesic techniques such as epidural and PCA. Therefore most APS in the USA are essentially PCA and/or epidural services only.

Although the implementation of anaesthesiologist-based APS has had a considerable impact on pain management on surgical wards only a small percentage of patients receive the benefits of such APS. A good APS organization is one which ensures optimal pain management for every patient who undergoes surgery including children and those undergoing surgery on ambulatory basis. Furthermore, the record of USA-style APS in implementing hospital-wide quality assurance measures such as frequent recording of pain intensity ("make pain visible") and recording of treatment efficacy (visual analogue scales (VAS) before and after treatment) has been generally unimpressive so far. Additionally, the costs of USA-style APS are very high ($100-$300 per patient). It is not surprising that such costs are being increasingly questioned by payers. A downsizing of many APS is taking place in the USA, and further reductions are predicted by many. A more important issue with anaesthesiologist-based APS is one of professional satisfaction.

APS in Europe

Few European hospitals have organized APS. The USA model is not transferable to most European hospitals because of state-run health services and cost issues. Except for the work of a few enthusiasts the situation in Europe is generally unsatisfactory. Models for APS have been proposed from Germany [4], UK [2, 3, 9], Switzerland, Norway [1], Sweden [6]. However, these models are from individual institutions and their impact on pain management on a country-wide basis is unclear. After the publication of the report by a joint working party of the Royal College of Surgeons and College of Anaesthetists in 1990 there has been considerable interest in improving postoperative pain relief in the UK. This has centred around development of high dependency units (HDU), acute pain teams and expansion in the use of techniques such as PCA. It has been estimated that less than 30% of British hospitals have a HDU; therefore if complex analgesia techniques such as epidural, PCA, and regional blocks are restricted to HDUs there would be little improvement in the quality of pain relief for the majority of patients undergoing surgery [9]. A few nurse-based APS have been successfully implemented in the UK. The lack of organized APS at most institutions is mainly due to administrative difficulties and financial restrictions. Even when resources are available it may be difficult to introduce new analgesia techniques on surgical wards due to practical constraints, communication problems and perhaps most importantly, nursing policies [2].

Development of a low-cost model

It is becoming increasingly clear that simpler and less expensive models have to be developed if the aim is to improve the quality of postoperative analgesia for every patient who undergoes surgery. The organization should also include patients who undergo day-care surgery. Furthermore, in countries with state-financed health services and current budgetary restraints the USA-style anaesthesiology-based comprehensive, multidisciplinary postoperative pain control teams appear unrealistic for most institutions. It is generally recognized that effective analgesia alone will not improve postoperative outcome. Improved pain relief allows more postoperative activity and has to be exploited in an aggressive postoperative rehabilitation program which includes physiotherapy, active mobilization routines and early enteral feeding. If an institution does not have an organization to implement such rehabilitation programs, it is doubtful if "high-tech" epidural combination techniques should be used at all since less invasive and simpler techniques can provide comparable analgesia.

At Örebro Medical Centre Hospital a nurse-based anaesthesiologist-supervised acute pain service was introduced in February 1991. Our APS is based on the concept that postoperative pain relief can be greatly improved by provision of in-service training for medical and nursing staff, regular recording of pain intensity and treatment efficacy, optimal use of systemic opioids (including use of PCA) and peripherally acting analgesics and use of epidural technique and regional blocks in appropriate patients.

It is emphasized that the majority of patients undergoing surgery do not require PCA or epidural analgesia. The role of simple analgesic techniques should not be overlooked or underestimated. With attentive nursing, greater flexibility of administration, better understanding of the pharmacokinetics of prescribed analgesics and regular pain scoring, i.m. or i.v. opioids and/or non-opioids can provide excellent analgesia. Furthermore, quality assurance measures such as frequent recording of pain intensity can no longer be ignored.

At the time of preoperative evaluation patients are informed about pain assessment by VAS and about pain management techniques that are available and the rationale underlying their use. Every patient who has undergone surgery (under general or regional anaesthesia) is asked to grade his or her pain severity on VAS. This is done every 3 h and recorded on a specially reserved place on the vital sign chart. The idea is to emphasize that routine pain scoring is as important as recording of temperature, heart rate and blood pressure. To evaluate the effect of prescribed treatment pain intensity is also scored before and about 45 min after treatment. Pain intensity is recorded more frequently (every hour) in the following categories of patients: a) patients on ICU, b) patients on PACU, c) patients undergoing day-care surgery and d) patients receiving PCA or epidural opioids.

Appropriate protocols, pain management guidelines, standard orders and monitoring routines have been developed in co-operation with surgeons for each surgical section. A specially trained acute pain nurse (APN) makes daily rounds of all surgery departments. Her duties are described in Table 1. In this organization the treatment of individual patients is based on standard orders and protocols developed jointly by the section anaesthesiologist, surgeon and ward nurse. This gives nurses the flexibility to administer the analgesics when necessary. In Sweden nurses are allowed to inject drugs i.v. and in epidural catheters. The duties of the section anaesthesiologist consist of providing anaesthesia services as well as acute pain services (Table 1). He selects patients for special pain therapies such as PCA, epidural, peripheral nerve blocks. During regular working hours this anaesthesiologist is available for consultation or any emergency; later the anaesthesiologist on-call has the same function.

In the organization described above the only additional cost is that of the APNs. At our hospital about 20,000 surgical procedures are performed annually; all of these patients can be expected to benefit from this organization. The cost of 1.5 APNs is about US $ 45,000 or less than US $ 3 per patient (excluding drug and equipment costs). The acute pain services were introduced gradually on a department-by-department basis. The implementation of the services for the whole hospital took about 18 months. The routine recording of VAS on surgical wards as described above has demonstrated for surgeons and ward nurses that even repeated injections of i.m. opioids may be unable to maintain VAS scores that are considered acceptable (VAS < 3) for the department; this is particularly valid in patients with severe pain such as those undergoing upper abdominal, thoracic or knee surgery. This has resulted in increased requests for and better acceptance of techniques such as PCA and epidural techniques on the surgical wards. The development of a structured program with readily available assistance is appreciated by nurses and surgeons on the ward. Since surgeons are active members in this organization it is easier to implement aggressive postoperative rehabilitation programmes to exploit the full potential of improved analgesia. Although all anaesthesiologists are involved with postoperative pain management of their patients, the section anaesthesiologists (Table 1) are responsible for developing protocols and standard orders for their section. This system is professionally more stimulating because the anaesthesiologist provides continuity of patient care since he or she is routinely involved in preoperative assessment, intraoperative management and postoperative follow-up.

Table 1. Organization of acute pain services at Örebro Medical Centre Hospital, Örebro, Sweden

Health care member "pain representatives" (named)	Responsibility
– Section anaesthesiologist	Responsible for pre-, peri- and postoperative care (including postop pain) for his/her surgical section
– "Pain representative" ward surgeon	Responsible for pain management on his/her ward and for implementing active postop rehab program
– "Pain representative" day nurse and "Pain representative" night nurse	Responsible for implementation of pain management guidelines and monitoring routines on the ward [a]
– Acute pain nurse (nurse anaesthetist)	– Daily rounds of all surgical wards – Check VAS recording on charts (every patient VAS < 3) – "Trouble-shoot" technical problems (PCA, epidural) – Refer problem patients to section anaesthesiologist (liaison between surgical ward and anaesthesiologist)
– Acute pain anaesthesiologist	Responsible for co-ordinating hospital-wide acute pain services and in-service teaching

[a] Patients are treated on the basis of standard orders and protocols developed jointly by chiefs of anaesthesiology, surgery and nursing sections. Pain representatives (named) meet every three months to discuss and implement improvements in pain management routines. This organization benefits about 20,000 patients a year (VAS < 3); it has been functioning satisfactorily since 1991

Postoperative pain - surgeons' views

The views of the surgeon are clearly related to pain management during and after surgery. There are many different aspects of pain and its management. I will concentrate my views on the practical issues. I shall also take up some controversial questions. Our main concern is to improve recovery in as many patients as possible. For that to happen various components of hospital organization and individuals have to work as a team. This co-operation is sub-optimal in many institutions and situations.

Possibility to operate

All surgeons, irrespective of their speciality, like to operate. Indeed some surgeons feel unwell if they do not get to operate. A basic requirement is good anaesthesia service during the per- and postoperative period including adequate postoperative pain relief. It is therefore important for the surgeon to be supportive of administration efforts to recruit and train good anaesthesiologists and nurse anaesthetists. Presumably, at most places "turf" thinking and professional jealousies prevent appropriate staff distribution amongst different specialities. In Sweden ageing factors and cost reductions in the health care budget have led to a shortage of anaesthesiologists and nurse anaesthetists. In such a situation it is difficult to expect anaesthesiologists to devote much time to the development and quality assurance of certain areas such as postoperative pain management; however, failure to do so can be expensive in the long run due to unnecessarily prolonged hospitalizations.

Competence

The training and competence level of anaesthesia staff has to be high to allow the surgeon to provide safe and effective service during and after surgery. Shortage of trained staff increases the risk of ineffective per- and postoperative pain management. If the shortage leads to a decrease in general competence it can result in negative feelings in the patient both as regards pain experience and recovery. Thus, the surgeon in her own interest should be involved in the recruitment of anaesthesia staff.

Different roles

What are our roles towards patients as anaesthesiologists, nurse anaesthetists, surgeons and ward staff? Are we aware of our roles and how we are perceived by patients? As a surgeon responsible for a ward I have total responsibility for patient care. The anaesthesiologist's role in patient care is not perceived as being responsible for the patient, but rather as a person who puts the patient to sleep and wakes the patient up after surgery. This may appear unfair but is a reality in my organization. The anaesthesiologist is together with each patient for a relatively short time, a short conversation before surgery and often no contact at all postoperatively. He appears on charts as a name which prescribes medication and does not really exist for the patient. It is I as surgeon and the staff on the ward who symbolize health care for the patient. We are the ones who are at the receiving end of the patient's displeasure due to poor pain relief. As a surgeon I am responsible for medication and total patient care, however I cannot influence all medication, some medication is prescribed by anaesthesiologists. Sometimes I do not have appropriate knowledge to have views on such prescriptions. This division of responsibility may be necessary but can create problems which influence patient care. A recent example: Our standard premedication is tablet Stesolid 10-15 mg and any change has to be justified and documented. During the last month 17 different premedications have been prescribed, no justification has been given, five drug combinations included drugs which we do not and never have had in our departmental pharmacy and two of these drugs are not even available in Sweden (prescription was done by Swedish doctors). During this month it took the nurses 7 hours to find the prescribed medication. This month is not unique. The reason for this divergence is not organizational but presumably due to the fact that doctors often ignore care guidelines and have individual strategies. This does not mean that it is medically incorrect or less effective, but it creates so many practical problems that in the final analysis it reverses any medical benefits. Middle aged Swedish doctors seem to have a great need to demonstrate their independence to an extent which surprises other specialities in health care. In addition to practical problems this is a regular source of conflicts, and much times is wasted in discussing "your or my" treatment rather than the patient's treatment. Clearly this also leads to unnecessary costs. Similar problems can be seen in many parts of health care. Within different staff categories we are quite clear regarding our roles but the patient's perception about this is rather vague. In spite of everything it is the patient's perception which is most important. Do they feel comfortable safe and in the organization we provide? Have we asked them? If so did we do it the right way? In any case should we be the ones asking those questions? That the patient feels comfortable and safe is most important for reducing hospitalization. The way we take care of our patients and also our own inter-relationships are crucial for this. Good communication between different staff categories is extremely important.

Communication between surgeon and anaesthesiologist is a definite safety feature both for the professional and the patient. The patient must feel that co-operation exists. If the patient gets different information from different staff members regarding this care she will become fearful, which in an already anxious patient can cause chaos. Good communication is crucial in all sections of health care, it should be coordinated; however, there are many problems in this area today. The reasons are difficult to explain, but many factors may contribute. Some important factors are:

– physician attitude and sometimes reluctance to co-operate across specialities
– lack of time

Most of these problems can be solved without additional costs and it is possible that even measurable gains can be achieved. Perhaps hospital organizations should enforce co-operation across specialities and provide the basis for unproved surgical stay programmes which the units will be required to follow. This may lead physicians to see this as limitation of their professional freedom; however, if the physicians cannot manage it themselves perhaps that is the only way for the patient to receive overall good care. It is not enough that every physician provides what he considers medically correct treatment if the total experience of the care is negative for the patient. It is easy to forget that simple and less expensive things can make a difference between a good experience of patient care and a terrifying experience. Unfortunately, these issues are often difficult to agree upon.

In this connection several questions should be considered. Why do all patients experience postoperative nausea on certain days? Why does the post anaesthesia care unit report that on certain days all patients have severe pain on recovery? On other days everything appear to be peaceful and the patients are satisfied. Why? Usually we say "well, it was one of those days" but can we accept that? What is the reason for this? I have a feeling that it depends on the particular nurse anaesthetist. This is to such an extent that one could arrange the staff of the surgical ward depending on which nurse anaesthetist is working. Why? Did they not all get the same training, does it depend on their professional roles, or is it the communication between the anaesthesiologist and nurse anaesthetist? Anaesthesiologist and surgeon? Are there minor variations that cannot be systematically examined? Or perhaps it is not interesting enough for the anaesthesiologist to examine. In any case someone should be interested in these questions. The increasingly individual planning of patient care should be for the patient, not for staff - this should be remembered. Everything changes; perhaps it is not more today than in earlier times, but it does feel that the changes now are very fast. We are at the threshold of big changes which affects our work and make us insecure. One is "the new patient". She is born in the late 1970s and 1980s. She has been raised by us, she did not turn out as we had expected. She is independent, does not respect authority, is rarely impressed by anything and has the knowledge or access to knowledge whenever she desires. She lives in the information and communication society and has the world at her feet and wants complete control over herself and her body. She is a nightmare for most physicians and has instruments we do not understand.

Are we at a disadvantage? Can we handle this without going into an aggressive-defensive position? Can we manage our professional role when we are questioned? How much should the patient decide? Many questions with no real answers.

The answer to the last question is nevertheless quite simple and does not require much thought. The patient should have complete control and it is the health care professional's job to provide such information that the decision is made on the basis of scientific evidence and established clinical experience. Most of what we do can be done in many different ways and one method may not be more correct than the other. With patience and flexibility we will get a satisfied patient who probably will recover faster.

One of the new patients' mottos is "I want control".

In a gynaecology department there are many relatively young patients with minor ailments. We get to experience new patient demands before other specialities. Naturally they have practical consequences for patient care. Already we have had to solve several problems when patients do not accept our normal routines.

- Patient does not want premedication, wants to stay awake and wants to see and communicate with the staff members who are involved with her care in the operating room. Our justification for premedication is not accepted and we have to change our routine and take care of the patient without premedication. We have asked ourselves the question: For whom is the premedication? The answer is not self-evident. It is possible that a premedicated patient is easier to "handle" for anaesthesia staff? Surely there must be technical and pharmacological solutions which provide similar medical safety as the traditional premedication.

- Patient does not want a bladder catheter, an enema, does not want to fast, etc. Again we have to ask why we need to do this. Is it medically necessary? Is it good for the patient? Or is it an old tradition which is not questioned?
- Patient does not want to be sedated. She would rather experience some pain. Difficult to accept since we have decided that patient should have good postoperative analgesia. Why?
- Patient has no time to stay in the hospital. This is of course a problem since some time is clearly needed. However, hospitalization can be quite short with appropriate patient expectations and modern surgical techniques. Access to the world outside the hospital from her bed in the ward by using modern technology is another way of satisfying the demands of the modern patient. The latter can clearly be argued, but it is important to remember that tomorrow's patient is different from our times in terms of life style and values. To discuss what is right or wrong is not relevant.

Care philosophy

At our department we have developed a "care philosophy" with great effort. The patient is involved in her own care and takes responsibility for her recovery. For far too many years the staff has told the patient how she is doing and what she is allowed to do, etc., this has led to patient insecurity and the patient has been scared to leave the security of the ward. We have had standard hospitalization times for different procedures (operations). This has been strictly followed and the patient who wanted to go home earlier has had to state in writing that she is doing it at her own risk.

We have now left this to the patient's own decision in situations where it is possible.

The patient decides when she is ready to go home. Clearly we provide medical advice when necessary. She decides when she wants to eat and drink unless the nature of surgery contraindicates early oral intake. We have shown that most patients want to eat on the day of surgery. We have not seen any problems with this. The body has many functions which it self-regulates which we in health care have worked hard to suppress. These functions are now our instruments instead. It seems also that perhaps expectations affect recovery most, and when we inform our patients in detail about our routines and they themselves decide when, hospitalization times have been reduced considerably.

The most important part of pain control is postoperative pain relief. In the past we administered an injection every 4 hours, neither more nor less, irrespective of the type of surgery. We then went through a period with VAS where the scale decided when pain should be tréated and now we have reached a stage of patient controlled analgesia (PCA) after surgery. Pain and pain experience are probably the most individual experience of mankind; it is therefore natural that the treatment is as individual as technology and pharmacology allow. We now have PCA pumps with preferably Ketogan (ketobemidone - a synthetic opioid which is equipotent with morphine) as our standard technique after abdominal surgery. Patients are informed preoperatively about the method and about the importance of pain relief. They are informed that we expect them to take amounts of analgesia that allow them to breathe adequately without hurting and that they should be able to get out of bed. This has been very effective and the postoperative opioid consumption has gone down drastically. Patients are very satisfied with PCA. Occasional patients may require other analgesia methods as a complement but that is surprisingly rare. The patient feels safe when she is in control. This leads to decreased need for drugs. We all know about the patient who sleeps well with the sleeping pill on the bedside table. This type of analgesia is clearly also appropriate for "the new patient".

Leaving more responsibility to the patients has not been easy. The role of staff in the ward has changed from caregiver to adviser and this has not been problemfree. The result has been very good with independent, secure and rapidly mobilized patients (even after major abdominal surgery) who are satisfied with their care. A small group of elderly patients may feel confused initially about deciding themselves about their care, but they soon adapt to the new routines.

In summary, as a surgeon (with my staff) I would like to have the following wish list about peri- and postoperative pain management:
- As little sedation as possible. The patient wants to be awake and in control.
- Elimination of nausea without sedation.
- Early oral intake.
- Short preoperative fasting (what is really necessary?).
- Totally individual and patient controlled analgesia postoperatively (PCA).
- Standard routines for individual patient categories, which are *always* followed by *all* anaesthesiologists, unless required for medical reasons.

Most patients do not expect *complete* pain relief and do not need it for satisfaction or early recovery. What they do need is security in care, which can only be achieved if all involved with patient care give the same information and advice.

Clearly all patients cannot take their own responsibility, some are too sick, but there are always some parts of care where they can decide themselves.

In all honesty how would you want it if you were in the patient's position?

The role of the nurse

Ward nurses have a central role in postoperative pain management. They coordinate nursing care and, compared with other healthcare professionals, they spend more time with patients. In addition, pain medication is prescribed by surgeons or anesthetists, but it is ward nurses who have the responsibility for assessing patients' pain intensity, for administering some prescribed analgesic treatments and for monitoring their efficacy. It is therefore clear that the ward nurse is well placed to exert a positive influence on individual patients' pain management.

There is increasing interest in establishing dedicated acute pain services in hospitals, and the close cooperation and participation of ward nurses in such schemes is vital for their success, both with regard to effective day-to-day management of pain and also for the effective implementation of long term programmes for pain management. The acute pain nurse provides an important link between the ward nurse and the anaesthesiologist, who often has only limited understanding of ward policies.

The importance of education

A critical element in improving the contribution of ward nurses to postoperative patient care and in implementing the findings of research is the continuing education of ward staff. This should include an element of formal teaching, including the pathophysiology of pain and basic pharmacology of analgesics. Nurses' knowledge should be regularly assessed and discussion groups held, where news can be disseminated and misconceptions remedied. Such educational initiatives should be ongoing, providing explanations for any changes in pain management methods. Often, staff do not understand the rationale for change. In this regard, it is important that new research data are presented in a clear and systematic fashion so that resultant changes in pain management approaches can be readily put into practice. New guidelines and monitoring protocols should be developed in such way as to facilitate independent work by nursing staff. The education of nursing staff is also important to avoid the possibility that anxiety in nurses is transmitted to their patients. Those who are unfamiliar with new techniques of pain management may lack confidence and this issue must be addressed. The aim is not only to achieve but also to maintain high standards of pain management.

The education of patients represents another important initiative as this may help to reduce their anxiety and stress. Patient information material should be developed as a multidisciplinary project that is coordinated by the nurse. The importance of education for both staff and patients, and the key role that nurses can play in such initiatives, are illustrated by the results of an audit performed at the Freeman Hospital, Newcastle, UK [11]. This audit showed that the appointment of a specialist pain nurse who was subsequently involved in the frequent review of patients, and the implementation of regular education of surgical ward staff, resulted in a substantial improvement in the efficacy of analgesic regimens.

Making pain visible

Unless the response to pain therapy is regularly evaluated, there is no basis for rational, individualized therapy. Regular and reliable monitoring of patients' pain intensity by ward nurses is important in assessing the standard of care provided. Indeed, implementation of routines for pain assessment could be regarded as the first step towards high quality postoperative pain management. New analgesic techniques such as epidural analgesia and PCA require extensive, systematic monitoring by nursing staff. Establishment of pain monitoring protocols helps to focus the attention of carers on postoperative pain, heightening "pain awareness" in staff. It is also worth remembering that in the absence of formal documented pain assessment, many nurses will continue to believe that patients who do not report pain do not feel pain. Finally, use of multimodal patient monitoring protocols allows early detection of treatment side effects. New monitoring protocols should be developed in such a way as to be simple enough for routine implementation on general wards.

The importance of audit

APS organizations that educate and update their staff and patients raise the standard of pain management and provide a platform for research and review. A regular audit of patients' pain intensity and of any side effects of analgesic therapy is vital for quality assurance. Gathering of data allows APS staff to identify problems with postoperative pain management and to assess the success of measures implemented in the attempt to solve such problems. Presentation of audit data also proves useful in maintaining the interest and involvement of staff in their work and in implementing new procedures, as they see the overall results of their efforts.

Conclusion

Ward nurses are well placed to exert a positive influence on patients' postoperative pain management and should be considered as important members of APS teams, receiving continued education and support from other APS staff. The quality of care provided by ward nurses is an important determinant of the overall quality of patients' postoperative care, and nursing staff should be given the accurate education and support they need to effectively treat pain.

References

1. Breivik H, Högström H, Niemi G et al (1995) Safe and effective post-operative pain relief: introduction and continuous quality improvement of comprehensive post-operative pain management programmes. Ballieres Clin Anaesth 9:423-460
2. Cartwright PD, Helfinger RG, Howell JJ, Siepmann KK (1991) Introducing an acute pain service. Anaesthesia 46:188-191
3. Gould TH, Crosby DL, Harmer M et al (1992) Policy for controlling pain after surgery: effect of sequential changes in management. Br Med J 305:1187-1193
4. Maier C, Kibbel K, Mercher S, Wulf H (1994) Postoperative Schmerztherapie auf Allgemeinen Krankenflegestationen - Analyse der achtjährigen Tätigkeit eines Anästhesiologischen, Akut-Schmerzdienstes (Postoperative pain therapy on normal wards. Eight years experience with an Acute Pain Service). Anästhesist 43:385-397
5. Rawal N (1995) Acute Pain Services in Europe - A 17-nation survey. Reg Anaesth 20:S85
6. Rawal N (1994) Organization of Acute Pain Services - a low-cost model. Pain 57:117-123
7. Ready LB, Oden Rollin Chadwick HS, Benedetti C et al (1988) Development of an anesthesiology-based postoperative pain management service. Anesthesiology 68:100-106
8. Semple P, Jackson IJB (1991) Postoperative pain control. A survey of current practice. Anaesthesia 46:1074-1076
9. Wheatley RG, Madej TH, Jackson IJB, Hunter D (1991) The first years experience of an acute pain service. Br J Anaesth 67:353-359
10. Zimmermann DL, Stewart J (1993) Postoperative pain mangement and Acute Pain Services activity in Canada. Can J Anaesth 40:568-575
11. Coleman SA, Booker-Milburn J (1996) Audit of postoperative pain control. Influence of a dedicated pain nurse. Anaesthesia 51:1093-1096

CENTRAL NERVOUS SYSTEM

DEVELOPMENT, DAMAGE AND REPAIR
IN THE CENTRAL NERVOUS SYSTEM

Neural Development in the CNS: Biochemical Mechanisms of Cell Fate Determination

A. Cestelli, G. Savettieri, I. Di Liegro

Neural induction

Ever since the 1930s, when Spenmann and Mangold showed that the prospective dorsal side of the amphibian embryo is conveniently marked by the *blastopore lip*, a site where endoderm and mesoderm invaginate at the start of gastrulation [1], developmental biologists have been fascinated by the search for endogenous inducing molecules. When these two scientists transplanted a small piece of tissue including the blastopore lip from one embryo to the ventral side of another, the host embryo responded to the grafted tissue by forming a complete secondary dorsal axis. In the following years, other researchers found that transplanting tissue around the anterior end of the primitive streak in avian and mammalian embryos, called *Hensen's node*, also duplicates the dorsal axis and induces a secondary nervous system [1]. Thus, in all vertebrate embryos there is a region, called *Spenmann's organizer*, that initiates the formation of neural tissue by inducing dorsal ectoderm to form a neurogenic epithelium rather than undergoing epithelial differentiation.

For decades, the identification of the *neural inducer* has been the focus of several generations of neuroscientists: unfortunately, this search proved to be more problematic and elusive than expected, because embryonal ectoderm could be easily neuralized when exposed to a wide variety of differentiated tissues, tissue extracts, purified molecules, many of which were clearly non-physiological. Undoubtedly, the pivotal concept that emerged from these early experiments was that neural inducers are not instructional but permissive [2], in other words, they function by neutralizing neural inhibitors: in this new view, ectoderm is epidermalized by an endogenously produced factor, suggesting that ectoderm needs an active mechanism to become epidermal rather than neural. *Noggin, follistatin*, and *chordin*, three factors recently identified in frogs as candidate neural inducers released by Spenmann's organizer, share two common characteristics [reviewed in 3 and 4]. First, these factors can neuralize the ectoderm and dorsalize the mesoderm (thus they have two distinct activities, depending on the type of tissue they act on). Second, these molecules bind to and inactivate bone morphogenetic protein (BMP) factors in the extracellular space, and this inactivation seems to account for both the neuralizing and dorsalizing activities.

Early neural morphogenesis

The process through which an embryo forms a *neural tube*, the rudiment of the central nervous system (CNS) is called *neurulation*. At the cellular level, the ectoderm loses the morphology associated with a simple embryonic epithelium and acquires the morphology of of the pseudostratified *neuroepithelium* of the neural plate and tube. At the tissue level, the neuroepithelium undergoes complex morphogenetic movements to form the neural tube, pinches off from the surrounding ectoderm, and segregates into the embryo as a separate tissue anlage (Fig. 1).

As the neural plate rolls up and closes into a tube, a series of constrictions appear in its wall, subdividing the rostral end of the neuraxis into a series of expanded vesicles representing the anlagen of forebrain (*prosencephalon*), midbrain (*mesencephalon*) and hindbrain (*rhombencephalon*); caudal to the hindbrain, the tube forms a long and uniformely narrow cylinder that is the precursor of the *spinal cord* (Fig. 2). By the time the posterior end of the neural tube closes, secondary bulges, the *optic vesicles*, have extended laterally from each side of the developing forebrain. The forebrain goes on to become subdivided into the anterior *telencephalon* (which will eventually form the *cerebral hemispheres*) and the more caudal *diencephalon* (which will give rise to *thalamus* and *hypothalamus*, and the region that receives neural input from the *retina*, which indeed is a derivative of the diencephalon). The midbrain does not become subdivided, and its lumen eventually becomes the *cerebral aqueduct*. The hindbrain becomes subdivided into an anterior *metencephalon* (which will give rise to the *cerebellum)* and a posterior *myelencephalon* (which will become the *medulla oblongata*) [reviewed in 5].

Since its neural induction commencement, the nervous system is organized along two principal axes: the rostrocaudal (or anteroposterior, A/P) axis (*neuraxis*), which corresponds to the main body axis, and the dorsoventral (D/V) axis. During gastrulation, the organizer tissues come to underlie the neural plate along the A/P axis of the embryo: in particular, the *notochord* and the *prechordal plate* underlie respectively the portion of the neural plate that will eventually form the midbrain, hindbrain and spinal cord on one hand, and the forebrain on the other. The experiments of Mangold in which strips of different mesoderm segments along the A/P axis were inserted into the blastocoele provided the main support in favor of *vertical* (or *radial*) *interactions* that establish the initial A/P polarity along the neuraxis (Fig. 3). On the other hand, Spenmann demonstrated that the same A/P polarity could be imposed via a *planar interaction* between the organizer tissue and the adjacent dorsal ectoderm (Fig. 4). The main difference between planar and vertical signaling resides in timing: planar signaling is likely to be effective at early gastrula stage, when the presumptive neural plate still abuts the organizer tissue. In contrast, by late gastrula, the shortest distance between the organizer tissue and the dorsal ectoderm is by a vertical interaction.

As described in the previous section, isolated ectoderm can be neuralized by treatment with a panoply of artificial inducers called activators. Both the activa-

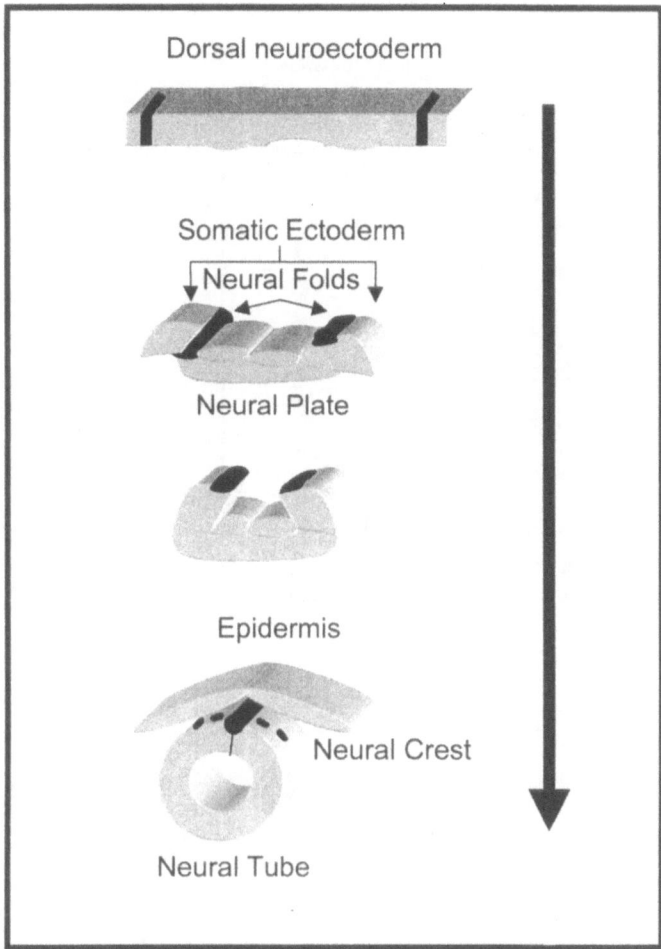

Fig. 1. Neurulation in amphibians and amniotes. The ectodermal cells are represented either as precursors of the neural crest cells (black) or as precursors of the epidermis (gray). The ectoderm folds in at the most dorsal point, forming an outer epidermis and an inner neural tube connected by neural crest cells

tors and *bona fide* neural inducers (such as chordin, noggin, and follistatin) induce forebrain-like neural tissue, based on the fact that it expresses gene markers that are normally found in the anterior neural plate [reviewed in 6]. These three proteins antagonize the action of BMP factors, suggesting that the induction of anterior neural plate differentiation involves the inhibition of BMP signals that repress neural development. The type of neural tissue induced by activators was proposed to be the ground state, which could be induced to be more posterior by treatment with *transforming signals*, incapable, on their own, of neuralizing the ectoderm.

A. Cestelli, G. Savettieri, I. Di Liegro

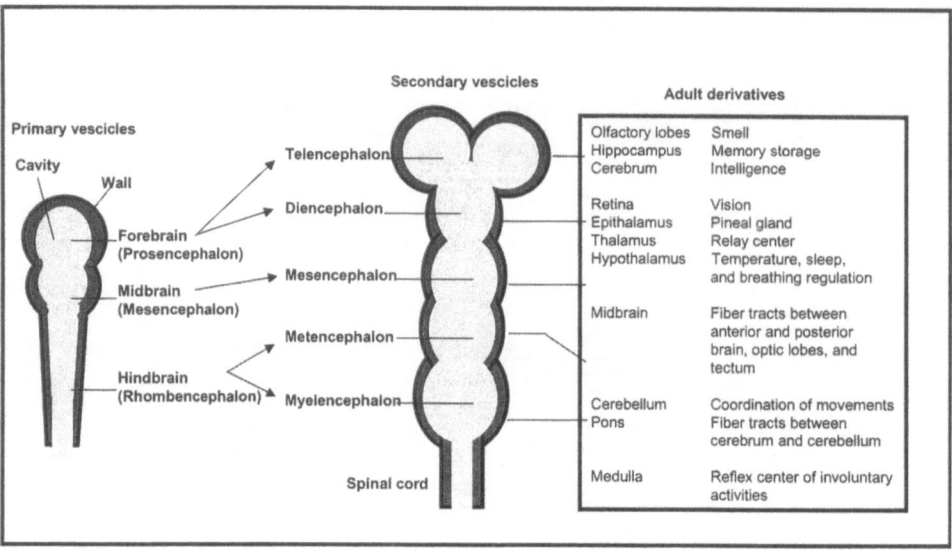

Fig. 2. Early human brain development. The three primary brain vesicles continue to subdivide as development goes on. In the right table are indicated the adult derivatives formed by the walls and cavities of the brain

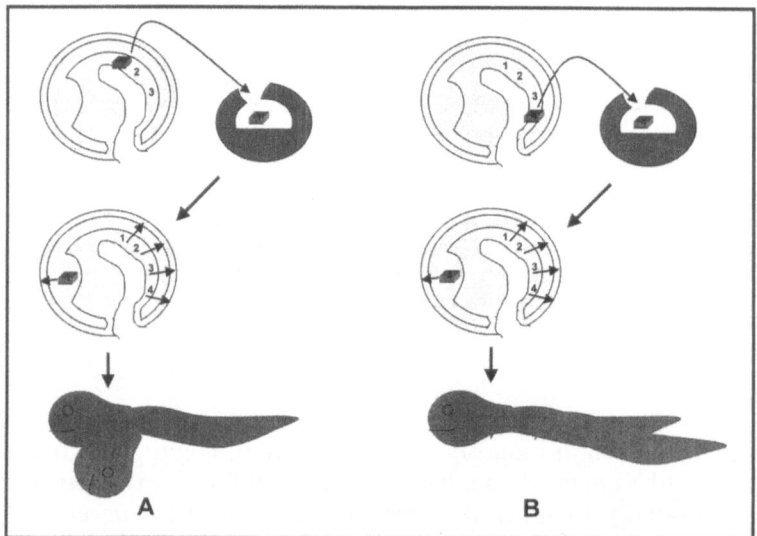

Fig. 3. The contribution of vertical signaling to neural induction can be experimentally tested. A piece of dorsal mesoderm, dissected out from gastrula and transplanted into the blastocoele of a host embryo, at the time of gastrulation of the second embryo is pressed up against the ventral mesoderm. When this experiment is performed with prechordal (head) mesoderm, the explant induces a secondary head, containing a brain. Conversely, when this experiment is performed with posterior mesoderm, the explant induces a tail containing a spinal chord

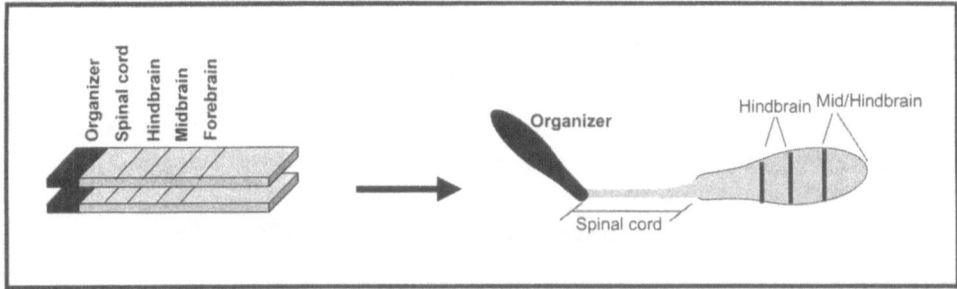

Fig. 4. The contribution of planar signaling to neural induction can be experimentally tested by excising the organizer tissue with adjacent dorsal ectoderm from two embryos and placing them together with the insides facing each other, In this way the explant remains flat, so that the mesoderm and presumptive neural tissue extend in opposite directions. Even though the only contact between the organizer tissue and ectoderm lies across the boundary they share at blastula stage, the neural tissue that forms is properly patterned along the A/P axis

Formation of brain regions

Once the overall polarity along the A/P axis has been established, subsequent patterning events further subdivide the neural tube into smaller organizational units. Subdivisions by *segmentation* (metamerism) is a developmental theme common to many animal phyla: this phenomenon involves the allocation of blocks of precursor cells into an axially repeated set of similar modules. In this way developmental fields remain small and specializations of cell type and pattern can be generated as local variations on the repetitive theme. Although it has long been acknowledged that embryonal mesoderm is segmented, only recently has segmentation also been recognized to play a substantial role in CNS development. In particular, developing hindbrain shows a segmental pattern that specifies the places where certain nerves originate. Eight swellings called *rhombomeres* divide the rhombencephalon into smaller compartments. Within these structures, neuronal differentiation and axonogenesis start at the border of alternate even-number rhombomeres, forming a *two-segment repeat pattern* that involves all of the early forming neural systems [7]. Moreover, six or seven neuromeres have been identified also in the forebrain, but their significance remains unclear.

Of the utmost importance in understanding CNS pattern formation is the discovery that *developmental control genes*, related to genes with a known patterning role in *Drosophila* embryo, are also expressed in spatially restricted domains of vertebrate neural plate and tube. These genes fall into two main categories: those encoding transcription factors, and those encoding cell surface or secreted signaling molecules (Fig. 5). The *kreisler* gene, that encodes a leucine zipper transcription factor, is expressed in r5 and r6 and participates in the establishment of the initial parasegmental subdivision, probably via the regulation of the

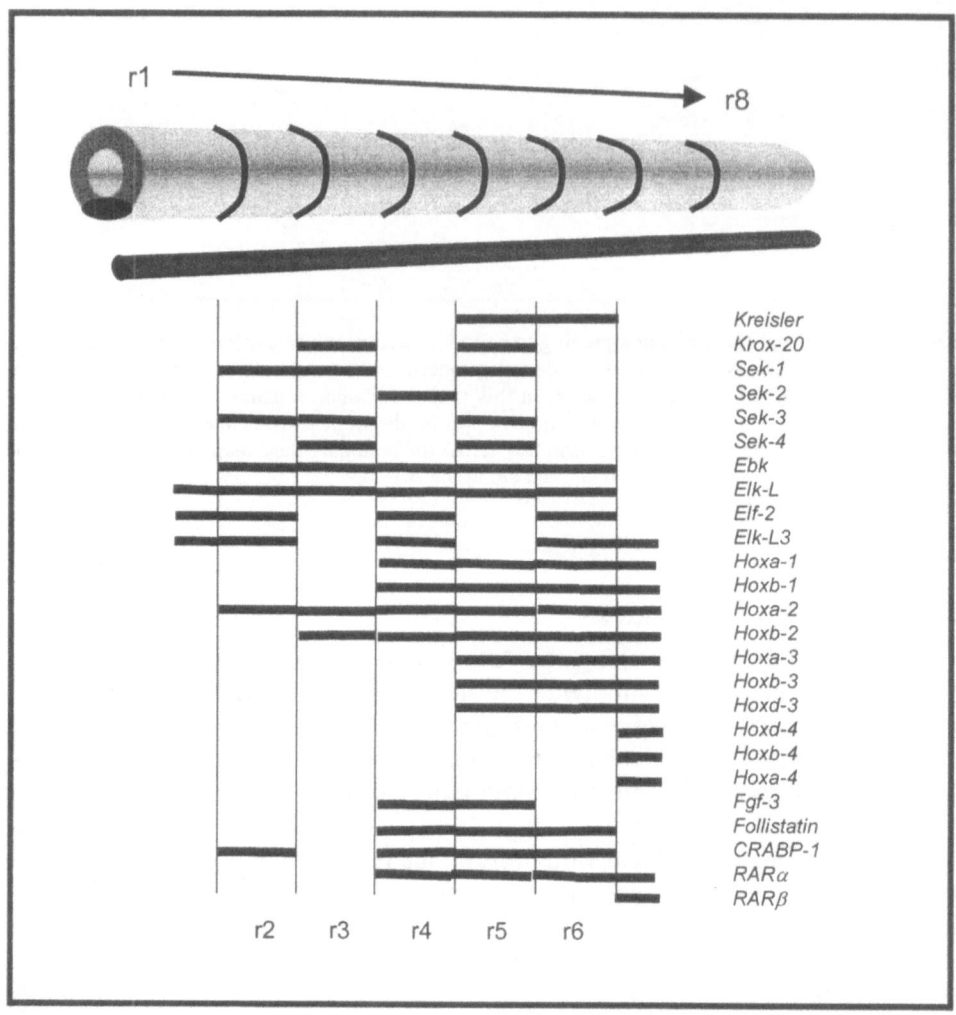

Fig. 5. Diagram showing the correlation between gene expression and specific rhombomeres in vertebrate embryos. Notochord and overlying floorplate are indicated in black. Boundaries between rhombomeres are indicated in white. The intensity of gray correlates to the level of gene expression

zinc finger transcription factor *Krox-20*, which, in turn, may be responsible for generating periodicity along the A/P axis by controlling *Hox* genes, the vertebrate homologs of the homeotic selector genes (*Hom* genes), which in *Drosophila* coordinate the development of structures appropriate to axial positioning of the epidermal segments. Consistent with their probable function in ancestral deuterostomes, *Hox family* of homeobox genes retain a clustered chromosomal organization in which the relative position of every single gene reflects its boundary of expression along the A/P axis (*principle of colinearity*). Duplication during evolution of the vertebrate genome brought an increase in the number of *Hox* genes (mammals may have up to four copies of genes that are singly represented in *Drosophila*), and this divergence, in turn, brought a tremendous refinement in pattern resolution. The overlapping distribution of *Hox* gene transcripts in vertebrate hindbrain suggests that their proteins probably act in a combinatorial manner to set positional value of individual rhombomeres and hence control their identity and phenotypic specializations. Genes encoding molecules that control cell interactions represent another class of genes involved in hindbrain segmentation: these include members of the Eph family of receptor tyrosine kinase-transmembrane proteins (*Sek1-4*) and their ligands (*Elk-L, Elf-2, Elk-L-3*).

In addition to the role of *kreisler* and *Krox-20* in locally regulating *Hox* expression, *retinoic acid* (*RA*) emerges as a strong candidate for overall mediator of nested *Hox* expression. Hensen's node, in fact, is a rich source of retinoids [8], and *RA* may act as a morphogen conferring positional information on cells at different A/P positions by differentially regulating *Hox* expression in a manner consistent with the principle of colinearity (i.e., there is a direct correspondence between the location of a *Hox* gene in the genetic cluster and its responsiveness to *RA*: 3′ genes respond more rapidly and at lower RA concentrations than 5′ genes) [9].

In the midbrain, beyond the anterior limit of *Hox* gene expression, local A/P pattern is generated through the activity of a long range signaling region, the *isthmic constriction*, at the junction of mesencephalic and rhombencephalic vesicles. This region is marked by the most posterior expression of the *Otx-2* gene (homolog to *orthodenticle*, *otd*, which is expressed in the anteriormost neuromere of *Drosophila*). When mid-to-anterior mesencephalon is transplanted to the diencephalon or rhombencephalon, it induces the cells surrounding to develop mesencephalic fates (in the diencephalon) or cerebellar fates (in the rhombencephalon): this mes/met-inducing region appears to be controlled by *fibroblast growth factor 8* (*FGF8*) [10]. Indeed, it has been recently found that isthmus-forming region does secrete *FGF8* (Fig. 6). Moreover, *FGF8*-containing beads transplanted into diencephalon or rhombencephalon are responsible for midbrain duplication. At the molecular level, *FGF8* induces the expression of *Wnt1*, *Engrailed-2*, and *FGF8* itself in the surrounding tissues. *Wnt1* and *Engrailed-2* are known to be important for the formation of cerebellum. Even though this region does not express *Wnt1* gene, mice deficient in *Wnt1* lack midbrain regions and cerebellum [11]: it has been established, in fact, that *Wnt1* stimulates *Engrailed* gene expression in the cerebellar precursor cells, enabling them to proliferate [12].

It has been demonstrated that the forebrain is also composed of six neuromeric regions called the *prosomers* [13]. *Prosomers p1-p3* comprise the diencephalon, whereas *prosomers p4-p6* comprise the hypothalamus (ventrally) and the telencephalon (dorsally). The prosomeric boundaries coincide with the expression boundaries of genes that are thought both to play a key role in neural

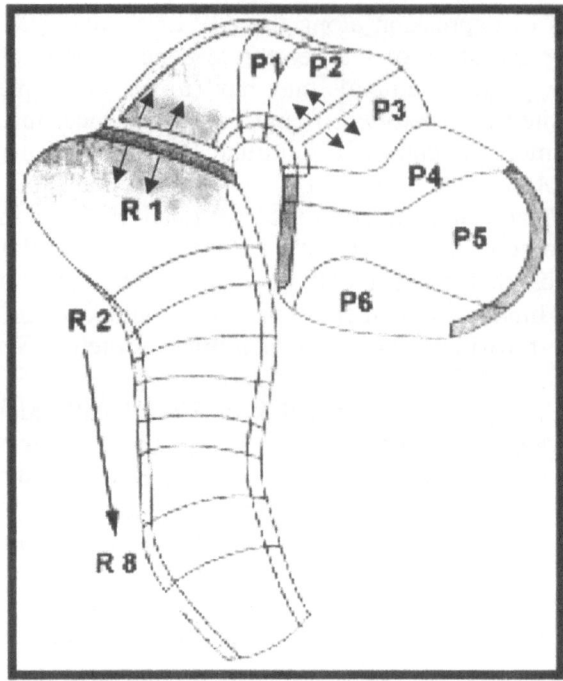

Fig. 6. Neuromers of the brain with inductive events superimposed on them. The mesencephalon/metencephalon boundary coincides with FGF8 and *Wnt1* gene expression. The p2/p3 border is thought to be the source of hedgehog protein

specification and to limit the responses to pivotal external stimuli (Fig. 6). In particular, the p2/p3 boundary seems critical in patterning the whole forebrain: this boundary corresponds to the *zona limitans* and is the source of *Sonic hedgehog (Shh)*, a diffusible protein known to induce patterning during gastrulation and limb formation [14].

As already mentioned, CNS exhibits a characteristic D/V zonation, particularly evident in the hindbrain and spinal cord. Specialized glia, the *floor plate cells*, form a narrow strip at the ventral midline, *motor neurons* develop in the ventral third of the neuroepithelium on both sides of the floor plate, *relay neurons* in the middle third, and *small interneurons* in the dorsal third. The most dorsal region, represented by the early *neural folds* that mark the transition between tissues with neural and epithelial fates, produces the migratory *neural crest cells*, that give rise to the glia and the majority of neurons in the peripheral nervous system. Later, after the neural crest has departed, the dorsal midline is formed by a nonneurogenic *roof plate* [5]. During these processes, the ventral neural tube is patterned by the *Shh* protein, coming from the underlying notochord and floor plate [reviewed in 14]. This protein induces the ventrolateral cells to express genes that allow them to differentiate into motor neurons, and inhibits in the same cells the expression of other genes, such as *dorsalin*, *Pax 3*, and *msx1* (Fig. 7). These latter genes, stimulated by *BMP4* and *BMP7*, secreted by the presumptive dorsal epidermis, promote commitment of dorsally specific neural fates [15].

Neurogenesis and migration

In the developing CNS neurons are generated at sites far from the positions they will occupy in adulthood. The key features of neurogenesis derive from the geometry of the system: the original neural tube is composed of a germinal neuroepithelium that is one cell thick, and each individual of this rapidly dividing cell population is continuous from the luminal edge of the neural tube to the ouside edge. In the mid 1930s Sauer showed that the nuclei of these cells are at different heights, thereby giving the wrong impression that the wall of the neural tube is composed of numerous cell layers [16]. DNA synthesis (S phase) occurs while the nucleus is in proximity to the external edge of the neural tube, then, as mitosis approaches, the nucleus migrates luminally, and mitosis occurs close to the ventricular zone (Fig. 8). During early development, 100% of the neural tube cells incorporate radioactive thymidine into DNA. Shortly thereafter, certain cells stop incorporating DNA precursors, thereby indicating that they have definitely come out from their last cell cycle. In this review we summarize the basic principles that govern the formation of cortical structures. Other main districts of the developing CNS are covered by other reviews: see [17] for cerebellum, [18] for olfactory bulb, [19] for retina, and [20] for spinal cord.

In the ventricular zone, one of the first cells to express markers of differentiation is a specialized form of glial cell, called the *radial glial cell*. These cells extend long processes perpendicular to the luminal surface toward the overlying *cerebral wall*.

These radial processes continue to grow as the lamina thickens, extending several millimeters in the cortex of primates [22]. In developing cortex young neurons migrate along these radial glial cells in the route of their migration from the germinal zone to their final destinations (Fig. 9).

The geometry of the emerging brain cortices, with cells crowded in the tubular neuroepithelium, is unique: as rapid cell division thickens the proliferative zone, from a simple neuroepithelial sheet the developing cortical structure emerges into a complex multilaminar structure (Fig. 10): as a consequence of continuous cell proliferation, the migrating cells form a second layer external to the luminal surface, called the *intermediate zone*, which separates the germinal luminal epithelium (now called the *ventricular zone*, and, later, the *ependyma*) from the *preplate*. As the pace of neural production goes on, from the ventricular zone arise neurons destined for the different layers of the cortex. These cells migrate through the intermediate zone and form the *cortical plate*, a structure that splits the embryonic preplate into two regions: the *marginal region*, or future *layer I* (which consists of tangential fibers and the first generated neurons),

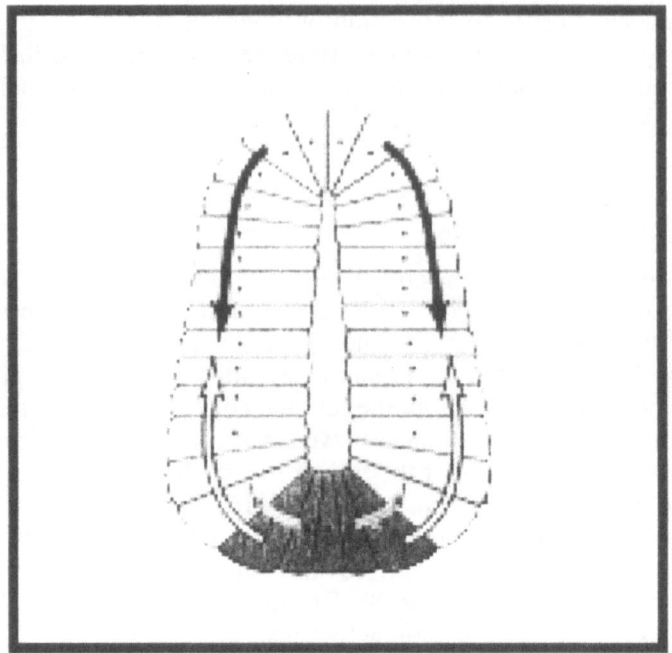

Fig. 7. Summary of interactions whereby *Shh* promotes motor neuron differentiation while inhibiting dorsalization signals

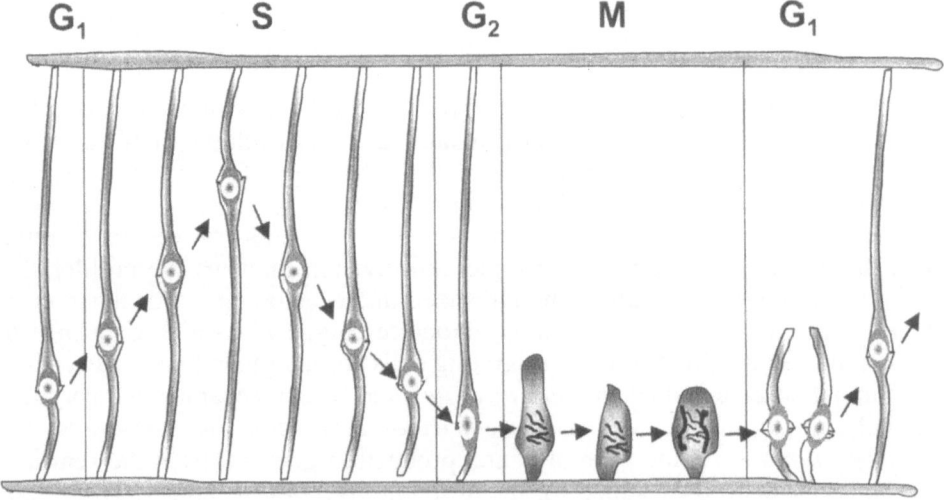

Fig. 8. Schematic representation of early developing neural tube, showing the position of the nucleus in a typical neuroepithelial cell in relation to the cell cycle. Mitotic cells are only found adjacent to the luminal side of the neural tube

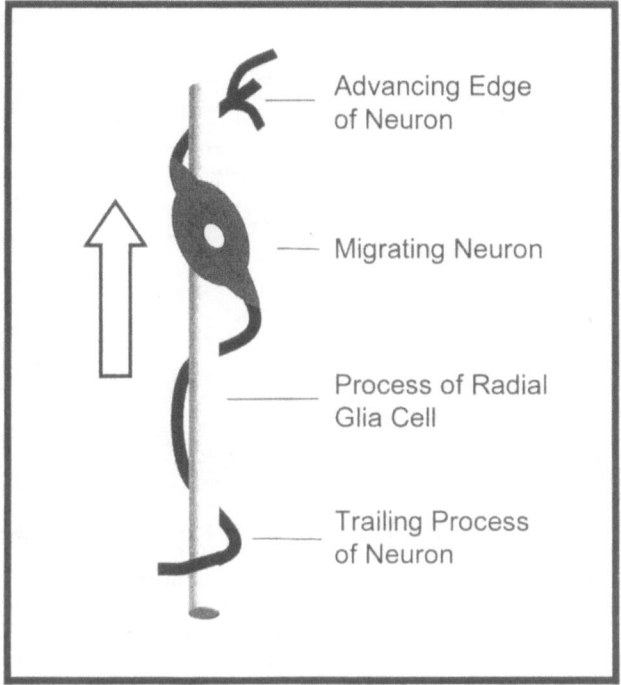

Advancing Edge
of Neuron

Migrating Neuron

Process of Radial
Glia Cell

Trailing Process
of Neuron

Fig. 9. Relationship between a migrating young neuron and a radial glial fiber in developing mammalian cortex

and the *subplate*, a transient population of neurons, destined to disappear by programmed cell death early in postnatal life. Neurons of the cortical plate are generated continuously by germinal cells in the ventricular zone. The first neurons to be generated migrate outward to contact layer I. Once arrived near the surface of the cortical plate, neurons are displaced to deeper levels by those that arrive later. Thus, with the exception of layer I, layers II-VI are generated in an insideout sequence. Finally, during the middle and latter stages of neurogenesis, a second germinative zone arises between the ventricular and the intermediate zones: the *subventricular zone*. This specialized secondary germinal layer apparently arose in higher vertebrates to generate extremely abundant neuronal populations late during development of the CNS [22]. In the forebrain, the subventricular zone gives rise to neurons destined to the olfactory bulb, cortical glial cells, and granule cells of the hippocampus.

Radial migration does not account for the significant tangential migration which is undertaken by many neurons in developing cortex. It has been recently demonstrated in fact, that substantial neural populations move tangentially along axonal tracts within the intermediate zone [23]: this phenomenon provides an important contribution to the complex cytoarchitecture of mammalian cortex.

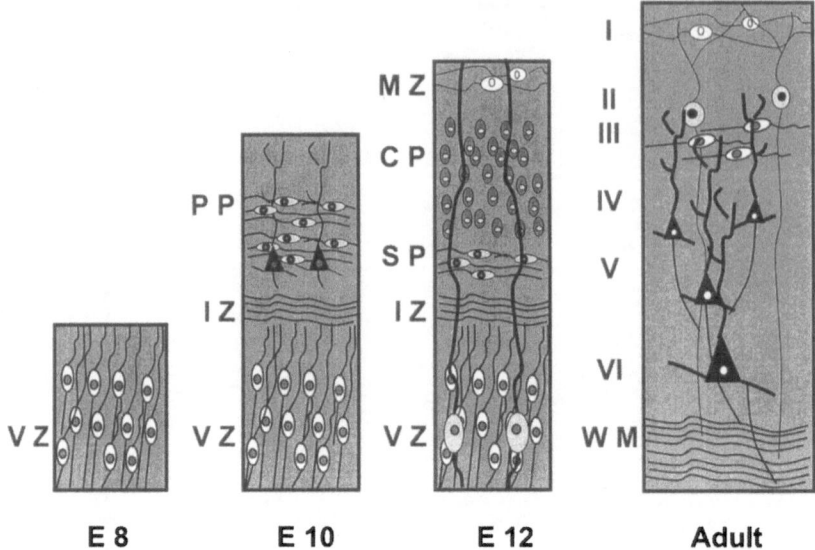

Fig. 10. Development of mammalian cerebral cortex. The ventricular zone (VZ) harbors the progenitors of neurons and glia. The first generated neurons colonize and establish the preplate (PP). Their axons, as well as axons coming from developing thalamus, make up the intermediate zone (IZ). As new generations of neurons move from VZ, the first neurons of preplate are pushed to the marginal zone (MZ), the future layer I. The new cohorts of neurons, that will form layers II-VI, establish the cortical plate, which splits the preplate into MZ and the subplate (SP), a population of neurons destined to die. After the completion of neuronal migration and differentiation, six cortical layers overlie the white matter (WM)

Establishment of nerve cell polarity

The principles of neural development, some aspects of which have been discussed in the previous sections, could be summarized as follows: a) the main features of the anatomical and functional organization of the nervous system, like that of the entire organism, are maintained through generations and are due to the expression, at the right places and times, of a hierarchy of genes, the functions of which are highly conserved in evolution; these genes constitute the 'program' for the emergence, division, migration and differentiation of nerve cells and fix the rules for the molecular assembly of neural connections; b) in spite of this conservation of the program, high phenotypic variation does exist even among isogenetic individuals; and this variation increases with increasing brain complexity, in the course of vertebrate evolution; c) in the developing brain, postmitotic neurons leave the proliferative layer and start migration to their definitive position [5], from which they will begin forming connections. This phase is redundant: a high proportion of the neurons initially formed will perish through an active process known as programmed cell death or apoptosis [24]. Moreover a high proportion of the synapses, initially formed by each differentiating neuron, will be also eliminated later [25]; d) since the first stages of formation of the neural networks, spontaneous waves of neural activity have been recorded in the developing brain [for review, see 26]. It is not yet clear, however, whether spontaneous activity is permissive or instructive; but in any case, activity seems to be essential for the formation of a mature system of neural connections [27]. In other words, development of single neurons is regulated by the activity of the developing neural network, which controls the process of selective stabilization of specific groups of synapses among the totality of those initially formed. As the final stabilization of synaptic connections does not depend any more on genes but on function, it has been called 'epigenetic'. Interestingly, the same mechanisms that underlie morphogenesis and terminal differentiation of the nervous system probably form the functional basis for learning and memory; it seems indeed that higher brain functions rely on repeated use of specific neural networks and on both anterograde and retrograde transmission of signals among neurons [reviewed in 28-30].

When we consider neural development from the point of view of single neurons, two processes are of the greatest importance: i) the establishment of cell polarity and ii) the specification of cell type with respect to neurotransmitter production.

The concept of neuronal polarity derives from the idea that signals (i.e. neurotransmitters) are released from the axon terminals of presynaptic neurons and received by dendrites on postsynaptic neurons. Although it is now clear that retrograde messages from postsynaptic to presynaptic neurons also exist, this schematic view suggests correctly that axons and dendrites are different in many ways [discussed in 31]. Major differences between the two neuronal districts include shape (axons are long and thin, run very long distances and branch extensively only in the vicinity of their targets, while dendrites are highly branched and, in general, short and thick), and organelle complement (dendrites contain almost all of the organelles found in the cell body, including ribosomes, whereas these latter organelles are virtually absent in the axons). The absence of ribosomes in axons implies that nerve terminals depend on mechanisms able to transport proteins, and even cytoskeletal preformed elements for long distances. Once presumed to be relatively uniform, the cytoskeleton of the axon shows wide variation both in size and composition along its entire length [for review, see 32, 33]. For example, neurofilaments are sixfold more numerous at distal levels of mouse optic axons than at proximal levels, while microtubule number actually decreases slightly [33]. These differences in the cytoskeletal architecture are achieved even if the mentioned cytoskeletal components (neurofilaments and tubulins, respectively) travel at the same rate along the axon, with the so called slow axonal transport system. It is likely that some cytoskeletal elements in transit stop moving and accumulate locally, causing regional specializations of the axon [33]. Local formation of specialized cytoskeletal network could be also enhanced by selective protein degradation. It has been recently suggested indeed that specific localization of tau and microtubule-associated protein (MAP)-2 to axons and dendrites, respectively, might be due to selective stabilization of the two proteins in the two compartments [34]. At the molecular level, axons and dendrites also differ in the proteins present on their plasma membranes; this implies that some mechanism must exist that ensures differential addressing of Golgi-derived vesicles to one or the other of the two compartments. In accord with this hypothesis it was found that specific classes of the small Ras-like GTPases (Rabs), involved in membrane trafficking, are present in either the axonal or dendritic compartment [31]. Moreover, there is an interesting equivalence (not absolute, however) between apical and baso-lateral domains of epithelial cell membranes and axonal and dendritic membranes of neurons, respectively. As an example of this similarity, we can cite the selective enrichment of proteins, anchored through a glycosyl-phosphatidyl-inositol (GPI) moiety, in both apical membrane of epithelial cells and axons [31, 35].

But, how is polarity established and maintained? As mentioned above, the mechanisms that permit the establishment of distinct axons and dendrites involve an interplay between the genetic program of a neuron and environmental cues [discussed in ref. 35]. In 1994, Banker and collaborators obtained almost well-polarized hippocampal pyramidal neurons, by culturing them in close proximity with astrocytes, in a defined medium which inhibits overgrowing of the glial cells [cited in ref. 31]. By using this experimental system the authors were able to demonstrate that the process of polarization comprises several intermediate stages: initially, neurons develop a series of thin neurites that are equivalent until one of them starts elongating faster; this particular neurite will become the axon and only after its appearance will the other neurites be given the opportunity to develop dendritic branches [31] (Fig. 11). Interestingly, at the ultrastructural level, all the immature, thin neurites look like immature axons; they show, for instance, an axon-like array of microtubules oriented with their minus ends toward the cell body. A second very useful experimental model for studying establishment of neuronal polarity was developed by Higgins and collaborators [35]. These authors cultured rat sympathetic neurons in a defined medium, in the absence of glial cells, but in the presence of nerve growth factor (NGF). They found that, in these conditions, neurons formed only axons; however, local addition of either glial cells or serum induced rapid appearance of dendrites as if a positive signal was given or a negative one removed [cited in 31]. These findings suggested that the process of developing axons is somehow a "default pathway", while specific signals are required for developing dendrites. Among the latter signals, differential substrate adhesivity seems to be of outstanding importance [36-38]. Signals from the extracellular matrix (ECM) activate in turn specific intracellular pathways of signal transduction, leading to regulation of the expression of specific genes [38]. In addition to ECM effects, soluble factors can also influence neural development. Among these factors, thyroid hormones (TH) have well known effects on brain maturation [39]. It has been recently demonstrated that TH and specific ECM molecules (e.g. laminin) play synergistic roles in regulating the establishment of cell polarity in rat fetal cortical neurons, cultured in a synthetic medium [40]. In particular, it was shown that the cooperative effects of laminin and TH affect the distribution of

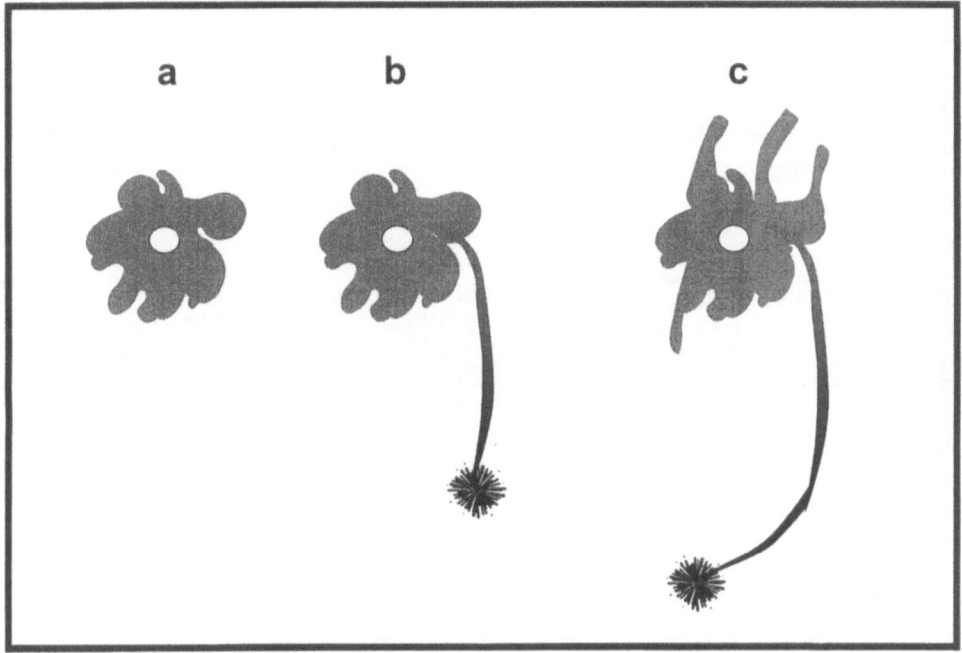

Fig. 11. Hippocampal pyramidal neurons, cultured in the presence of astrocytes, develop initially a series of equivalent, thin, axon-like neurites (a); then, one of these neurites starts elongating faster and becomes a the axon (b); after that, the other neurites will assume dendritic phenotypes (c)

specific proteins, such as components of the cytoskeleton and its associated molecules [40]. It is likely that the asymmetrical distribution of cytoskeletal proteins might induce, in turn, further asymmetry, by influencing localization of other proteins.

Asymmetric distribution of proteins can be achieved, in principle, by at least two different mechanisms: i) proteins can be synthesized in the soma and then transported to specific final destinations; ii) mRNAs can be targeted to specific cell subdomains and then translated locally into the corresponding proteins [41]. In the second case, the possibility exists that translation efficiency might be regulated at the level of specific synapses by incoming signals [41, 42] (Fig. 12). A prerequisite for this mechanism is that specific subsets of mRNAs, among them those encoding neurotransmitter receptors, are recognized and transported to dendrite terminals. Recognition and transport are mediated by cis-acting regulatory sequence elements, often present in the 3′-untranslated region (UTR) – but sometimes involving the 5′-UTR or even the coding region – of the message [for reviews, see 42, 43]. The fact that consensus sequences have not yet been recognized in the cis-acting elements suggests that secondary/tertiary elements of the nucleic acid structure may be of importance in regulating mRNA target-

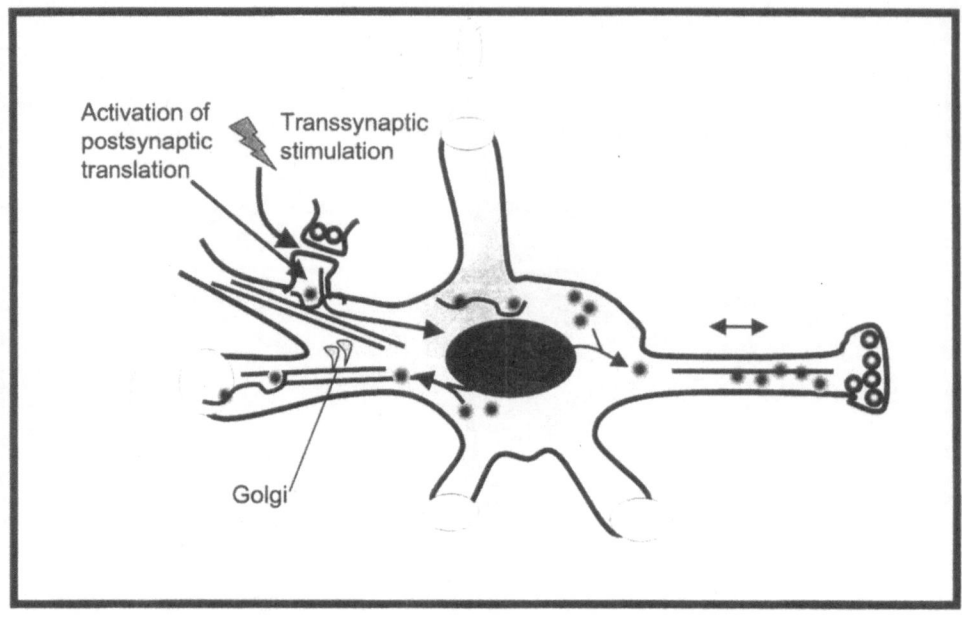

Fig. 12. Schematic drawing of the somato-dendritic and axonal domains of a neuron. Synapse-specific modification of the translation rate of given mRNAs, induced by trans-synaptic signaling, might cause local accumulation of the corresponding proteins and modification of the synaptic strength. The question mark at the axon terminal indicate that no clear function has been attributed up to now to mRNAs localized to axons

ing [42]. On the other hand, cis-acting sequence elements are bound by RNA-binding proteins which form part of the complex that mediates mRNA transport along the microtubules [reviewed in 43]. It is likely that mRNA-protein complexes (mRNP) interact with one or more courier proteins which in turn interact with microtubule-dependent motors such as kinesin. Drugs that depolymerize microtubules are indeed able to abolish mRNA localization [43]. In spite of several efforts, so far little is known about the proteins involved in recognizing, transporting and anchoring polyadenylated mRNA within dendrites. However, a few RNA-binding, sometimes neuron-specific proteins, have been described [see, for example, 44-46] and it is likely that many others will be discovered in the near future. What about axons? In general, axonal RNA transport seems to be a rare, very specific and highly regulated event [reviewed in 42]; moreover, at least in some cases, mRNA transport occurs after releasing from ribosomes. The message could be stably stored in particles at axon terminal but it is not clear if it can be translated locally. One intriguing possibility is that axon-localized mRNA can be sequestered in a silent form and carried back to the cell body for translation as an effect of retrograde trans-synaptic signals.

Specification of neurotransmitter phenotype

An important feature of the mature phenotype of a neuron is the type (or the combination of types) of neurotransmitter that it produces and secretes. From the biochemical point of view, production of neurotransmitters depends on the presence of a large set of proteins; not only the specific enzymes involved in the synthesis of a given neurotransmitter are required but the nerve cell must produce also all of those proteins required for packaging the signal molecule into synaptic vesicles (sometimes specific), transporting, anchoring and releasing it. All of these proteins need to be synthesized in a coordinated manner. How is this goal realized? In the case of cholinergic neurons, for instance, the genes encoding choline acetyltransferase and vesicular acetylcholine transporter contains identical cis-acting regulatory elements 5′ to the start site of transcription. The latter, however, seems to be a unique case [discussed in ref. 47]. Interestingly, the expression of most neurotransmitters and their receptors is specified before formation of synaptic connections, thus suggesting that the process is coordinated with axonal pathfinding and synaptogenesis [47]; it is, however, not yet clear if the neurotransmitter choice represents an independent subprogram of these processes. In any case, it is likely that extracellular signals somehow activate expression of specific transcriptional regulators which in turn activate expression of the proteins that specify one particular phenotype. One of the first transcriptional regulators identified was UNC-30, a homeodomain protein, expressed in the GABAergic type-D neurons of *Caenorhabditis elegans*. This protein has been recently shown to regulate the genes for GABA-synthesizing, glutamic acid decarboxylase and the GABA vesicular transporter [47]. In *Drosophila melanogaster*, two out of the four neurons derived from the 7-3 neuroblast (NB7-3) will become serotonergic. This latter choice depends on the products of at least four genes: *engrailed*, *islet*, *huckebein* and *eagle*. Many efforts have been devoted to identifying transcriptional regulators of neurotransmitter phenotype also in vertebrates. It has been reported, for instance, that the inactivation of the gene encoding the orphan nuclear receptor Nurr 1 causes disappearance of dopamine and the enzymes (tyrosine hydroxylase and aromatic amino acid decarboxylase) involved in its synthesis in the midbrain and the substantia nigra [47]. On the other hand, determination of noradrenergic phenotype seems to depend on the expression of a group of proteins, among them transcription factor Mash1 (a mammalian homolog of the *Drosophila* proneural genes).

At the end of this very brief and partial catalogue of factors involved in neurotransmitter specification, we can say that it is likely that neurotransmitter choice results from a complex interplay between extracellular signals, able to be transduced up to the nucleus, and modifications of gene expression, induced by the extracellular stimuli but then able to modify cell behavior and signal transmission by the neuron.

Neurotransmitters may be also specifically targeted to specific subsets of synaptic sites and this targeting is vital in controlling the polarized flux of information through the nervous system. For example, it has been recently demonstrated that metabotropic glutamate receptors are differentially targeted when expressed in cultured hippocampal neurons: mGluR1a and mGluR2 are transported to dendrites and excluded from axons, whereas mGluR7 is targeted to both dendrites and axons [48]. Selective targeting of metabotropic glutamate receptors depends on their C-terminal cytoplasmic domains [48].

As a concluding remark, it is important to keep in mind that the neurotransmitter choice it is not necessarily irreversible, at least at its first appearance, and that switches from a given neuronal phenotype to another one have been also described during neural development.

References

1. Spenmann H (1938) Embryonic development and induction. Hafner, New York
2. Holtfreter J (1947) Neural induction in explants which have passed through a sublethal cytolisis. J Exp Zool 106:197-222
3. Sasai Y (1998) Identifying the missing links: genes that connect neural induction and primary neurogenesis in vertebrate embryos. Neuron 21:455-458
4. Chitnis AB (1999) Control of neurogenesis - lessons from frogs, fish and flies. Curr Opin Neurobiol 9:18-25
5. Jacobson M (1991) Developmental neurobiology, 3rd ed. Plenum Press, New York
6. Rubenstein JLR, Beachy PA (1998) Patterning of the embryonic forebrain. Curr Opin Neurobiol 8:18-26
7. Lumsden A, Krumlauf R (1996) Patterning of the vertebrate neuraxis. Science 274:1109-1115
8. Chen YP, Huang L, Russo AF et al (1992) Retinoic acid is enriched in Hensen's node and is developmentally regulated in the early chick embryo. Proc Natl Acad Sci USA 89:10056-10059
9. Simeone A, Acampora D, Nigro V et al (1991) Differential regulation by retinoic acid of the homeobox genes of the four HOX loci in human embryonal carcinoma cells. Mech Dev 33:215-228
10. Crossley PH, Martinez S, Martin G (1996) Midbrain development induced by FGF8 in the chick embryo. Nature 380:66-68
11. McMahon AP, Bradley A (1990) The Wnt-1 (int-1) proto-oncogene is required for the development of a large region of the mouse brain. Cell 62:1073-1085
12. Danielian PS, McMahon AP (1996) Engrailed as a target of Wnt-1 signaling pathway in vertebrate brain development. Nature 383:332-334
13. Rubinstein JLR, Puelles L (1994) Homeobox gene expression during development of vertebrate brain. Curr Top Dev Biol 29:1-63
14. Goodrich LV, Scott MP (1998) Hedgehog and Patched in neural development and disease. Neuron 21:1243-1257
15. Liem KF, Tremml G, Roelink K et al (1995) Dorsal differentiation of neural plate cells induced by BMP-mediated signals,from epidermal ectoderm. Cell 82:969-979
16. Sauer FC (1935) Mitosis in the neural tube. J Comp Neurol 62:377-405
17. Hatten ME, Heintz N (1995) Mechanisms of neural patterning and specification in the developing cerebellum. Annu Rev Neurosci 18:385-408
18. Lin DM, Ngai J (1999) Development of the vertebrate main olfactory bulb. Curr Opin Neurobiol 9:74-78
19. Altshuler DM, Turner DL, Cepko CL (1991) Specification of cell type in the vertebrate retina. Dev Visual System 3:37-58

20. Leber SM, Sanes JR (1992) Migratory paths and phenotypic choices of clonally related cells in the avian optic tectum. Neuron 6:211-225
21. Schmechel DE, Rakic P (1979) A Golgi study of radial glial cells in developing monkey telencephalon: morphogenesis and transformation into astrocytes. Anat Embryol 156:116-152
22. Marin-Padilla M (1998) Cajal-Retsius cells and the development of the neocortex. Trends Neurosci 21:64-71
23. Pearlman AL, Faust PL, Hatten ME et al (1998) New directions for neuronal migration. Curr Opin Neurobiol 8:45-54
24. Bergeron L, Yuan J (1998) Sealing one's fate: control of cell death in neurons. Curr Opin Neurobiol 8:55-63
25. Innocenti GM (1981) Growth and reshaping of axons in the establishment of visual callosal connections. Science 212:824-827
26. O'Donovan MJ (1999) The origin of spontaneous activity in developing networks of the vertebrate nervous system. Curr Opin Neurobiol 9:94-104
27. Crair MC (1999) Neural activity during development: permissive or instructive? Curr Opin Neurobiol 9:88-93
28. Savettieri G, Cestelli A, Di Liegro I (1996) Biochemistry of neurotransmission: an update. In: Gullo A (ed) Anesthesia, Pain, Intensive Care and Emergency Medicine. Springer-Verlag, Milan, pp 43-73
29. Cestelli A, Savettieri G, Di Liegro I (1999) Integrated axon-synapse unit in the CNS. In: Tiengo M, Paladini VA, Rawal N (eds) Regional Anaesthesia, Analgesia and Pain Management. Springer-Verlag, Milan, Berlin, pp 3-22
30. Miller S, Mayford M (1999) Cellular and molecular mechanisms of memory: the LTP connection. Curr Opin Neurobiol 9:333-337
31. Prochiantz A (1995) Neural polarity: giving neurons heads and tails. Neuron 15:743-746
32. Bray D (1997) The riddle of slow transport - an introduction. Trends Cell Biol 7:379
33. Nixon RA (1998) The slow axonal transport of cytoskeletal proteins. Curr Opin Cell Biol 10:87-92
34. Hirokawa N, Funakoski T, Sato-Harada R et al (1996) Selective stabilization of tau in axons and microtubule-associated protein 2C in cell bodies and dendrites contributes to polarized localization of cytoskeletal proteins in mature neurons. J Cell Biol 132:667-679
35. Higgins D, Burack M, Lein P et al (1997) Mechanisms of neuronal polarity. Curr Opin Neurobiol 7:599-604
36. Bradke F, Dotti CG (1997) Neural polarity: vectorial cytoplasmic flow precedes axon formation. Neuron 19:1175-1186
37. Jareb M, Banker G (1998) The polarized sorting of membrane proteins expressed in cultured hippocampal neurons using viral vectors. Neuron 20:855-867
38. Savettieri G, Mazzola GA, Rodriguez-Sanchez MB et al (1998) Modulation of synapsin gene expression in rat cortical neurons by extracellular matrix. Cell Mol Neurobiol 18:369-378
39. Bernal J, Nunez J (1995) Thyroid hormones and brain development. Eur J Endocrinol 33:390-398
40. Savettieri G, Licata L, Catania C et al (1999) Synergistic effects of laminin and thyroid hormones on neuron polarity in culture. NeuroReport 10:1269-1272
41. Kuhl D, Skehel P (1998) Dendritic location of mRNAs. Curr Opin Neurobiol 8:600-606
42. Tiedge H, Bloom FE, Richter D (1999) RNA, whither goest thou? Science 283:186-187
43. Gao FB (1998) Messenger RNAs in dendrites: localization, stability, and implications for neural function. Bio Essays 20:70-78
44. Gao FB, Keene JD (1996) Hel-N1/Hel-N2 proteins are bound to poly(A) + messenger-RNA in granular RNP structures and are implicated in neuronal differentiation. J Cell Sci 109:579-589
45. Scaturro M, Nastasi T, Raimondi L et al (1998) H1° RNA-binding proteins specifically expressed in the rat brain. J Biol Chem 273:22788-22791

46. Nastasi T, Scaturro M, Bellafiore M et al (1999) PIPPin is a brain-specific protein that contains a cold-shock domain and binds specifically to H1° and H3.3 mRNAs. J Biol Chem 274 (in press)
47. Goridis C, Brunet JF (1999) Transcriptional control of neurotransmitter phenotype. Curr Opin Neurobiol 9:47-53
48. Nash Stowell J, Craig AM (1999) Axon/dendrite targeting of metabotropic glutamate receptors by their cytoplasmic carboxy-terminal domains. Neuron 22:525-536

Cellular Mechanisms of Brain Damage

G. Savettieri, I. Di Liegro, A. Cestelli

In recent years, the great advance in the area of genetics and cellular and molecular neurobiology has led neuroscientists to attempt to discover the cellular and molecular basis of neurological diseases. A neurological disease can be caused by a defective gene, an environmental insult, or by the interaction between environmental factors and preexisting genetic abnormalities. The mechanisms by which cell damage or dysfunction occurs in the nervous system are multiple and related to the nature of the pathological agents. Nevertheless some general mechanisms leading to cell death can be activated independently of the pathological agents. In this review some cellular and molecular mechanisms of brain damage will be focused on, looking at the unifying routes of neuronal cell death.

Ischemia and hypoxia

Insults to the brain that interrupt blood (ischemia) or oxygen (hypoxia) supply immediately cause cell dysfunction and, as a consequence, cell death. No aspect of metabolism is spared in severe hypoxic or ischemic injury. There are several lines of research which focus on animal models of ischemia; complementary approaches concern insult limitation by the use of appropriate treatment schedules. The possibility to reduce the intrinsic vulnerability of brain parenchyma has been approached in recent years, starting from data suggesting that toxic overactivation of neuronal glutamate receptors (excitotoxicity) may contribute to the pathogenesis of hypoxic-ischemic neuronal death [1].

In this section this latter mechanism of brain-related ischemic damage will be examined.

Under normal conditions glutamate is stored inside synaptic vesicles at nerve terminals; when it is released, an energy-dependent cellular uptake rapidly removes glutamate from the extracellular space. Under conditions of ischemia or hypoxia, cellular energy reserves fall, and consequently function of ion pumps decreases. This dysfunction causes membrane depolarization, opening of voltage-sensitive ion channels, and is followed by a cascade of events that ultimately lead to cell death. Depolarization-induced entry of Ca^{2+} stimulates release of neurotransmitters stored inside synaptic vesicles, including glutamate. At the same time Na^+-dependent uptake of glutamate is impaired. Thus, impaired glutamate uptake together with enhanced glutamate release determine a sustained elevation of glutamate concentration in the extracellular fluids of ischemic brain and, as a consequence, an overstimulation of glutamate receptors. This overstimulation in turn determines ionic imbalance, with an overload of intracellular Na^+ and Ca^{2+}. Sustained elevation of intracellular Ca^{2+} can activate the "toxic" mechanism responsible for cell death [2]. Of the four major families of glutamate receptors, N-methyl-d-aspartate (NMDA), and α-amino-3-hydroxy-5-methylisoxazole-4-propionate (AMPA)/kainate subtypes are involved in excitotoxicity. The toxic cascade that ultimately led to cell death involves many steps linked to each other (Fig. 1).

Firstly, elevated intracellular calcium concentration activates catabolic enzymes, such as phospholipases and endonucleases; secondly, the rise of intracellular calcium leads to the initiation of protein-kinase and lipid-kinase cascades, and generation of reactive oxygen species (ROS) [3]. Cytoskeleton may undergo disruption because of the activation of the Ca^{2+} dependent cysteine protease calpain. Activation of endonucleases leads to DNA breakdown. The important role of the "glutamate hypothesis" in hypoxic-ischemic brain damage is further supported by the protective effect of NMDA and AMPA/kainate antagonists in an experimental model of focal brain ischemia [4]. This protective action has probably the most important effect in penumbra ischemia. The penumbra is the area which surrounds the ischemic region. In this area insult severity is submaximal, but glutamate receptors may be briskly activated. Although glutamate receptor antagonists have shown their effects in several in vitro and in vivo models of ischemic brain damage, clinical tests are at present not encouraging. Many factors can explain this discrepancy; the most intriguing speculation on this issue concerns the possibility that attenuation of calcium entry into neurons may actually continue to exert apoptosis-promoting consequences [5]. The fact is that the precise relationship between cellular calcium homeostasis and programmed cell death cascades has not been well characterized. On the other hand, there is growing evidence that not only exocitotoxicity, but also apoptosis is involved in brain cell death after hypoxic-ischemic insult [5]. In agreement with this view, transgenic mice overexpressing the anti-apoptotic gene bcl-2 have smaller infarcts than their littermates after hypoxia-ischemia insult.

Cell damage in neurogenetic disorders

Several human neurogenetic disorders that lead to aberrant cell death result from genetic alterations in the cell death pathway.

The current model for the cell death pathway (apoptosis) includes several different steps [6]. In the course of each phase, genetic and biochemical events

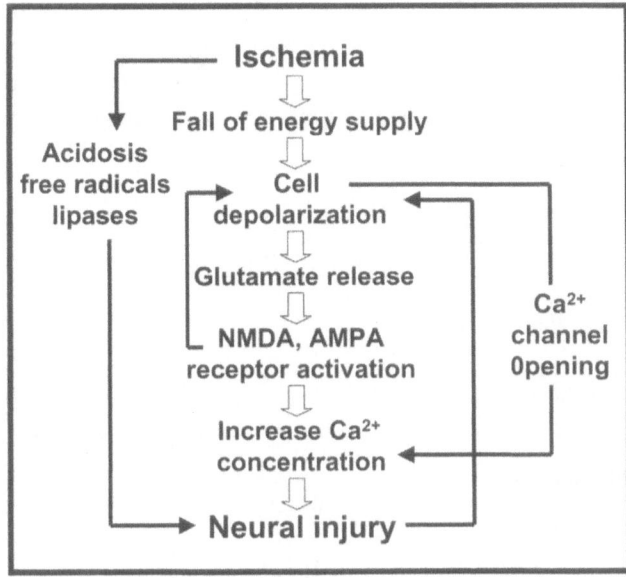

Fig. 1. Path leading to neural injury from ischemia

occur in a well-defined sequence. The cell death pathway includes (Fig. 2) a latent phase during which a preexisting cellular abnormality leads to the accumulation of compounds that, at a critical threshold, activate the program for cell death. The activation phase is characterized by the withdrawal of trophic factor support and the accumulation of reactive oxygen species. The activation phase is followed by a propagation phase that consists in deep changes in the metabolic pathways and in the expression of genes involved in apoptosis. Some of these genes encode proteins that, under normal physiologic conditions, regulate progression through the cell cycle (cyclin D1 and c-jun). During the following step (commitment phase) additional genes are expressed, among which is c-fos. Among others, there are two important proteins that function during the commitment phase: bcl-2 and bax proteins. Unlike bcl-2, which is an anti-apoptotic protein, bax promotes cell death. The equilibrium between bcl-2 and bax determines the balance between cell death and survival. In addition, during the end of the commitment phase, cysteinyl aspartic acid-specific proteases (caspases) are activated (Fig. 2).

As shown in Fig. 2, the programmed cell death pathway is constituted by very delicate well-defined sequences of events. A dysregulation of this machine has been found in several inherited disorders of the nervous system.

Herein we will discuss two representative disorders of nervous system just to typify some alterations in the programmed cell death pathway.

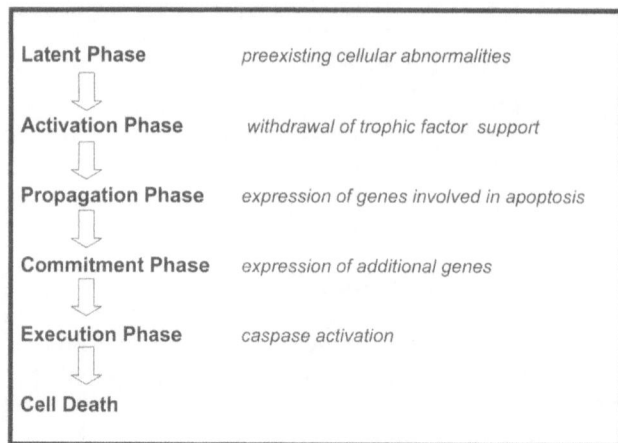

Fig. 2. Programmed cell death patway

Huntington's disease (HD)

HD is an autosomal dominant disorder with high penetrance, in which affected individuals, in adulthood, present psychiatric symptoms, cognitive decline, and dystonia and choreiform movements. HD is characterized by selective and severe neuronal loss in neostriatum and in cerebral cortex [7]. HD is linked to chromosome 4p16.3 [8]. In this chromosomal region one gene (IT15, now called the HD gene) contains an expansion of a repeated sequence of CAG nucleotides within the coding region [9]. Normal subjects have 11 to 34 repeats, whereas HD patients have more than 40 repeats [10]. The HD gene encodes a large 350 KDa cytoplasmic protein of unknown function called huntingtin.

Mice lacking huntingtin expression die during embryonic development [11], while mice expressing a huntingtin gene with an expanded trinucleotide repeat show impaired performances on neurobehavioral tests. Furthermore, in these mice a specific neuronal loss was demonstrated in the globus pallidus and subthalamic nuclei. These neurons show cellular and biochemical features of apoptosis [12]. At least 4 different proteins interact with abnormal huntingtin [13]. Two of these proteins can be involved in apoptotic processes. HIP3 (huntingtin interacting protein 3) binds to huntingtin and its expression is higher in areas affected in HD. HIP3 is a ubiquitin conjugating enzyme target of proteasomal degradation. Activation of HIP3 during programmed cell death could specifically increase cleavage of proteins involved in cell survival, while stimulating the programmed cell death pathway. Another interesting molecule that interacts with huntingtin is glyceraldehyde-3'-phosphate dehydrogenase (GAPDH). GAPDH is involved both in energy metabolism and in DNA repair and replication. Thus, loss of GAPDH function leads to energy depletion and aberrant

DNA repair and replication with consequent activation of programmed cell death.

Another proposed mechanism of huntingtin-induced death of neuronal cells concerns aberrant processing of abnormal huntingtin. The mutant protein is in fact cleaved in fragments containing an increased amount of glutamine residues. These fragments, conjugated with ubiquitin, are carried to the proteasome complex to be enzymatically cleaved, but incomplete cleavage leads to the formation of molecules (huntingtin, ubiquitin, and other proteasome components) that are transported to the nucleus where aggregates form. Over time, this process leads to cell death [14].

Amyotrophic lateral sclerosis (ALS)

The motor neuron diseases, an etiologically heterogeneous group of disorders, are manifested by weakness/muscle atrophy and/or spastic paralysis, reflecting the involvement of lower motor and/or upper motor neurons, respectively.

Amyotrophic lateral sclerosis (ALS) is the most common degenerative motor neuron disorder. ALS is clinically characterized by signs and symptoms due to the involvement of both upper and lower motor neurons. The disease is usually sporadic, but in 5 to 10 percent of cases it is familial and inheritance exhibits an autosomal dominant pattern [15, 16]. The familial form shows clinical features not different from the sporadic one. The prognosis and the natural history of the two forms of the disease are identical. This strongly suggests that these diseases are due to similar pathogenic mechanisms. The mechanisms that account for "selective" neuronal degeneration are still unknown. However, the identification of specific genes that are mutated or deleted in the inherited forms of the disease allowed investigators to create in vivo and in vitro model systems.

In a subgroup of patients affected by the familial form, a mutation at chromosome 21 has been demonstrated. This mutation occurs in the gene which encodes the superoxide dismutase type I (SOD1) that is involved in the regulation of intracellular free radicals [17]. Superoxides are unstable and highly active molecules that cause oxidation of cell constituents either directly or through toxic and stable derivatives.

In familial ALS, intracytoplasmic inclusions contain SOD1, ubiquitin, and neurofilament immunoreactivities [18]; and a huge amount of neurofilaments accumulate in cell bodies and neuronal processes. The role of these inclusions is unclear. The presence of ubiquitin immunoreactivity suggests that these inclusions contain proteins destined for degradation, presumably in part via the proteasome.

Activation of apoptosis by mutant SOD1 protein has been documented in primary neurons in culture [19, 20]. In transgenic mice expressing a Cu/Zn superoxide dismutase mutation there is motor neuron degeneration. In these transgenic mice, overexpression of bcl-2 (an inhibitor of apoptosis) prolongs motor neuron survival [21]. There is a large consensus that SOD1 mutation determines a "gain of function" that is lethal to motor neurons [22].

Neurotrophic factors and neurological dysfunction

Neurotrophic factors (NTFs) are polypeptides that support growth, differentiation, and survival of neurons [23].

Nerve growth factor (NGF), which belongs to the neurotrophin family, was the first NTF discovered and the best characterized. The discovery of NGF and the understanding of its mechanisn of action led to the formulation of the "neurotrophic factor hypothesis". According to this hypothesis, when a developing neuron reaches, through its processes, its target, it competes with many other developing neurons for a limited supply of NTF provided by the target cells. Fortunate competitors survive, unsuccessful ones die. NTFs act on specific receptors located on the surface of the processes of innervating neurons. Their concentration is lower than that necessary to maintain the viability of all innervating neurons. Local infusion of NGF antibodies into the rat footpad produced in fact a reduction in axonal diameter and neurofilament level [24]. Other lines of evidence suggested that NGF produced in hippocampus and neocortex is a target-derived NTF for developing basal forebrain cholinergic neurons (BFCNs) [25]. NGF also acts on developing caudate-putamen cholinergic neurons, which have a role in the control of movements. Experimental studies demonstrated that failed NGF signaling in adults may correlate with dysfunction and death of BFCNs [26]. In recent years, animal models of human neurological disorders have been employed to test the therapeutic potential of NTFs. NGF has been shown to prevent or reverse biochemical and clinical abnormalities in several models of peripheral neuropathy (i.e. diabetic neuropathy; HIV-associated sensory neuropathy) [27, 28].

Moreover, brain derived neurotrophic factor (BDNF), a NTF belonging to the neurotrophin family, is under investigation, to evaluate its potential beneficial effect for amyotrophic lateral sclerosis (ALS), a degenerative motor neuron disease.

Concluding remarks

In this review we focused on some mechanisms of cell damage responsible for neurological disorders. The unifying feature of the described diseases is a pathogenetic mechanism in which apoptotic events play a leading role. It is emerging in fact that the balance between apoptotic and anti-apoptotic genes is of the greatest importance in determining a normal life of cells and that disruption of the balance give rise to cellular and molecular abnormalities that determine the appearance of diseases. The agents able to interact with the apoptotic machinary are more than one, but the final effect, from a biological point of view, is similar for many neurological disorders. The clinical characteristics of each disease depend ultimately on the site of the damage.

References

1. Choi DW (1996) Ischemia-induced neuronal apoptosis. Curr Opin Neurobiol 6:667-672
2. Greene JG, Greenamyre JT (1996) Bioenergetics and glutamate toxicity. Progr Neurobiol 48: 613-634
3. Dingledine R, McBain CJ (1999) Glutamate and aspartate. In: Siegel GJ, Agranoff BW, Albers WR et al (ed) Basic neurochemistry. Lippincott-Raven, Philadelphia New York, pp 315-333
4. Choi DW, Rothman SM (1990) The role of glutamate neurotoxicity in hypoxic-ischemic neuronal death. Ann Rev Neurosci 13:171-182
5. Choi DW (1996) Ischemia-induced neuronal apoptosis. Curr Opin Neurobiol 6:1261-1276
6. Li H, Yuan J (1999) Deciphering the pathways of life and death. Curr Opin Cell Biol 11: 261-266
7. Kowall NW, Ferrante RJ, Martin JB (1987) Patterns of cell loss in Huntington's disease. Trends Neurosci 10:24-29
8. Gusella JF, Wexler NS, Conneally PM et al (1983) A polymorphic DNA marker genetically linked to Huntington's disease. Nature 306:234-238
9. The Huntington Disease Collaborative Research Group (1993) A novel gene containing a trinucleotide repeat that is expanded and unstable on Huntington's disease chromosomes. Cell 72:971-983
10. Martin JB (1996) Pathogenesis of neurodegenerative disorders: the role of dynamic mutations. Neuroreport 8:1-7
11. Duyao MP, Auebarch AB, Ryan A et al (1995) Inactivation of the mouse Huntington's disease gene homolog Hdh. Science 269:407-410
12. Davis SW, Turmaine M, Cozens BA et al (1997) Formation of neuronal intranuclear inclusions underlies the neurological dysfunction in mice transgenic for the HD mutation Cell 90:537-548
13. Gusella JF, McDonald ME (1998) Huntington: a single bait hooks many species. Curr Opin Neurobiol 8:425-430
14. Alves-Rodrigues A, Gregori L, Figueiredo L, Figueiredo-Pereira ME (1998) Ubiquitin, cellular inclusions and their role in neurodegeneration. Trends Neurosci 21:516-520
15. Mulder DW, Kurland LT, Offord KP, Beard CM (1986) Familial adult motor neuron disease: Amyotrophic lateral sclerosis. Neurology 36:511-517
16. Brown RH Jr (1997) Amyotrophic lateral sclerosis. Insights from genetics. Arch Neurol 54:1246-1250
17. Rosen DR, Siddique T, Patterson D et al (1993) Mutation in Cu/Zn superoxide dismutase gene are associated with familial amyotrophic lateral sclerosis. Nature 364:362
18. Kato T, Katagiri T, Hirano A et al (1989) Lewy body-like hyaline inclusions in sporadic motor neuron disease are ubiquitinated. Acta Neuropathol 77:391-396
19. Rabizadeh S, Gralla EB, Borchelt DR et al (1995) Mutations associated with amyotrophic lateral sclerosis convert superoxide dismutase from an antiapoptotic gene to a proapoptotic gene: studies in yeast and neural cells. Proc Natl Acad Sci 92:3024-3028
20. Ghadge G, Lee JP, Bindokas VP et al (1997) Mutant superoxide dismutase-1-linked familial amyotrophic lateral sclerosis: molecular mechanisms of neuronal death and protection. J Neurosci 17:8756-8766

21. Kostic V, Jackson-lewis V, de Bilbao F et al (1997) Bcl-2: prolonging life in a transgenic mouse model of familial amyotrophic lateral sclerosis. Science 277:559-562
22. Martin JB (1999) Molecular basis of the neurodegenerative disorders. N Engl J Med 340: 1970-1980
23. Yuen EC, Howe CL, Yiwen Li et al (1996) Nerve Growth Factor and the neurotrophic factor hypothesis. Brain Dev 18:362-368
24. Gold BG, Mobley WC, Matheson SF (1991) Regulation of axonal caliber, neurofilament content, and nuclear localization in mature sensory neurons by nerve growth factor. J Neurosci 11:943-955
25. Holtzman DM, Kilbridge J, Li Y et al (1995) TrkA expression in the CNS: evidence for the existence of several novel NGF-responsive CNS neurons. J Neurosci 15:1567-1576
26. Holtzman DM, Santucci D, Kilbridge J et al (1996) Developmental abnormalities and age-related neurodegeneration in a mouse model of Down syndrome. Proc Natl Acad Sci USA 93: 13333-13338
27. Diemel LT, Brewster WJ, Fernyhough P, Tomlinson DR (1994) Expression of neuropeptides in experimental diabetes; effects of treatment with nerve growth factor or brain-derived neurotrophic factor. Brain Res Mol Brain Res 21:171-175
28. Apfel SC, Arezzo JC, Brownlee M et al (1994) Nerve growth factor administration protects against experimental diabetic sensory neuropathy. Brain Res 634:7-12

Repair Mechanisms in the CNS

D.A. Siegel, M. Huang, S. Walkley

As our knowledge of the specific genetic lesions responsible for many neurological disorders increases, we are finding that this information does not necessarily lead to therapeutic advances nor to a better understanding of disease processes. More often than not questions arise asking: What is the relationship between an isolated gene and the pathology and clinical presentation of the disease in question? This is true not only for the most recent genetic discoveries associated with specific neurological disorders, such as SOD and amyotrophic lateral sclerosis, apolipoprotein E and certain types of familial Alzheimer's disease, and NCP1 and Niemann-Pick disease type C, but also for those inborn errors of metabolism whose causes have been long known, such as Tay-Sachs and other lysosomal storage diseases.

Moreover, even when treatments are apparent and possible (the CNS presents unique obstacles for both drug and gene therapies) another question arises: Can such treatments reverse existing pathologies or are they limited to preventing further CNS deterioration? If limited, are there other means available for reversing damage already done?

This report focuses on lysosomal storage diseases, an ideal paradigm in examining many of these questions. This group of disorders has clearly identifiable CNS pathologies, is amenable to drug, enzyme and gene replacement therapies, and is available for study in several species. Further, a pathognomonic feature unique to several of these diseases, i.e. the initiation of extensive ectopic dendrite growth at the axon hillock of cortical pyramidal cells, not only provides an assay system for evaluating CNS repair following therapy, but also, offers a window into normal developmental processes. In addition, the study of ectopic dendritogenesis, as discussed below, may provide new therapeutic approaches for a variety of unrelated diseases in which dendritic pathology is associated with clinical symptoms (e.g. the neurodegenerative diseases, several types of mental retardation as well as CNS injury).

The lysosomal storage diseases
A model of primary dendritogenesis

The lysosomal storage diseases are a family of disorders most commonly result-ing from a deficiency of a specific lysosomal hydrolase and characterized by the accumulation of large amounts of undigested materials within the cell. Most of these disorders have CNS involvement; symptoms range from moderate to se-vere mental retardation. Death in early childhood is not uncommon. A subset of this group of diseases, typified by, but not restricted to, Tay-Sachs disease, is characterized by the presence of ectopic dendrite growth at the axon hillock of cortical pyramidal cells (see Fig. 1) [1-8]. The initiation of these new, primary dendrites on mature, CNS neurons is a highly unusual event. Primary dendrito-genesis, i.e. the initiation of dendrites directly from the cell's soma, normally occurs only during early CNS development. In diseased animals, ectopic dendri-togenesis begins after a neuron has already established its normal dendritic ar-bor and continues throughout the animal's lifetime. Although unusual in both location and time of initiation, ectopic dendrites establish normal appearing synapses (9,10). Thus, ectopic dendritogenesis seems to be a recapitulation of a normal developmental process temporally displaced [11, 12].

Extensive work by our laboratory has demonstrated a strong correlation be-tween the storage of the sialylated glycosphingolipid GM2 ganglioside and the

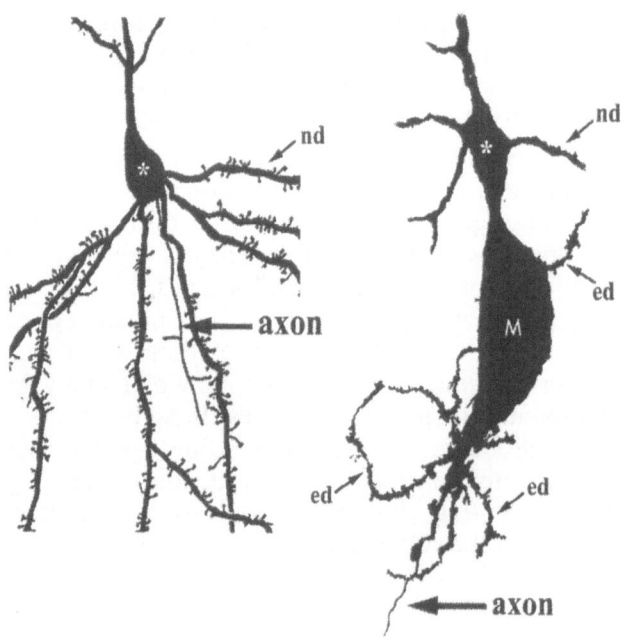

Fig. 1. Camera lucida of normal and Tay-Sachs cortical pyramidal cells. nd = normal dendrite, ed = ectopic dendrite, * = cell soma, M = meganeurite

presence of ectopic dendrite growth [11-13]. The greater the amount of GM2 stored the more extensive the amount of ectopic dendrite growth observed. GM2 gangliosidosis and Niemann-Pick disease type C, which store the largest amounts of GM2, exhibit the most prolific levels of ectopic dendrite growth. By contrast, α-mannosidosis, which stores significantly less GM2 has significantly fewer ectopic dendrites. Storage diseases which do not accumulate GM2 do not have ectopic dendrites.

GM2 ganglioside accumulates in the GM2 gangliosidoses as a direct result of lesions in the catabolic pathway of GM2. It is not known why GM2 accumulates in some of the other lysosomal storage diseases, while in still others it does not accumulate at all. Nor is it clear how storage of this relatively simple lipid leads to the reactivation of the complex machinery necessary for the initiation of dendrites. As already mentioned, knowing the genetic lesion of a disease does not necessarily lead to an understanding of the pathogenesis of that disease.

Therapy

The course of action for treating the lysosomal storage diseases is clear, at least in theory. Replace the deficient lysosomal enzyme and cell metabolism should return to normal. In practice, however, this has not been easy to accomplish. In visceral tissue, enzyme replacement therapy has had some success, e.g. β-glucosidase treatment in Gaucher's disease does reduce the storage load in non-CNS tissues. However, when the CNS is involved enzyme and gene replacement therapies have been less effective.

Cell mediated enzyme replacement therapy, through, for example, bone morrow transplantation (BMT), has had limited success. Our laboratory has demonstrated successful treatment of a feline model of α-mannosidosis through BMT [14, 15]. Normally, affected α-mannosidosis animals do not survive more than six to eight months. Following transplantation one animal has remained relatively healthy for more than eight years. Normal α-mannosidosis cDNA is easily detected in blood, and the animal has experienced relatively little neurological deterioration since transplantation. However, similar experiments in a feline model of Sandhoff's GM2 gangliosidosis have demonstrated little clinical benefit.

The effects of BMT appears to be due to microglial colonization of the brain [16, 17]. The difference in therapeutic outcomes between α-mannosidosis and GM2 gangliosidosis BMT experiments appears to be the ability of the colonizing microglia to secret the necessary enzymes. In vitro experiments using cultured cat microglia have shown that α-mannosidase is secreted in relatively large quantities, while Hex A β-hexosaminidase, the enzyme that catabolizes GM2 ganglioside, is not [18]. The reasons for these differences are unknown, nor is it clear if microglia over secreting Hex A could ameliorate symptoms in

GM2 gangliosidosis as the stability of the secreted enzyme and neuronal uptake are, as yet, unknown.

Our experience with the α-mannosidosis cat model raises the question posed initially. Can successful treatment of a neurological disease reverse damage already done or will it at best merely halt further deterioration? Our experience with another model of α-mannosidosis sheds some light on this question.

Swainsonine and ectopic neurite growth

In addition to work on the inherited model of feline α-mannosidosis our laboratory has also developed an inducible model of this disease using the indolizadine alkaloid swainsonine, a potent and reversible inhibitor of lysosomal α-mannosidase [10, 19, 20]. Animals treated with swainsonine develop a clinical, biochemical and morphological disease similar to the inherited disorder. When treatment is stopped enzyme levels return to normal and most stored materials are eliminated, yet one of the morphological hallmarks of this disease, the presence of ectopic dendrites at the axon hillock of the cell, remains after the "disease" has been "cured" i.e. after the removal of swainsonine [20]. This finding suggests that even if severe neurological disease is successfully treated, reversal and repair of all neurological ailments may not occur.

This observation has led us to consider the following: What is the mechanism responsible for initiating dendrites and can this mechanism be turned on and off at will? If this process can be controlled, then it might be possible to inhibit ectopic dendritogenesis and, perhaps more significantly, stabilize existing or even initiate new dendrite growth in neurodegenerative diseases characterized by dendritic atrophy. Exploiting the feline model of GM2 gangliosidosis we have begun experiments aimed at identifying the initiating signals and other components of the pathway responsible for primary dendritogenesis in CNS neurons.

Genetic analysis of dendritogenesis

Overall rationale

Ectopic dendritogenesis in Tay-Sachs disease appears to recapitulate the process of normal dendritogenesis that occurs during development. This complex developmental mechanism is likely to require changes in gene expression, both up and down. By comparing patterns of gene expression in the cerebral cortex of normal newborn kittens, and mature GM2 gangliosidosis cats (both states of extensive primary dendrite growth), against normal mature cat cortex (where primary dendritogenesis does not occur) it should be possible to isolate genes specifically involved in the process of primary dendrite initiation. We have chosen the differential display methodology to identify these genes.

Design

The technique of differential display was designed to detect minimal differences in gene expression between nearly identical samples [21, 22]. Thus, even modest changes in gene expression within the same tissue at different ages, or between normal and diseased tissues may be detected.

The method used is primarily that of Pardee et al. [21, 22], with modifications by Shen (personal communication), as well as some changes made in our laboratory. In general, mRNA from each sample is reverse transcribed and the cDNAs PCR amplified with one random 10mer primer and a second series of primers anchored at the 3' end of the gene. PCR products are resolved on a sequencing-like acrylamide gel. The size of the random primers and PCR condition were chosen to give the maximum number of discernable bands in each lane of the gel. In order to reach a 0.95 confidence level for detecting any message as a cDNA fragment, Bauer et al. [23] have calculated that a minimum of 25 upstream random 10mer primers are required.

Results

The initial differential display screening using all 25 random 10mers has been completed. Over 80 differentially expressed "bands" have been isolated based on the stringent requirement that the newborn and GM2 samples must share bands that are absent (or significantly reduced in intensity) in the normal mature cat, or vise versa, that the newborn and GM2 samples must lack bands (or they must be significantly reduced in intensity) that are present in the normal mature cat. Isolated bands have ranged in size from about 120 to over 500 base pairs in length.

To date, 35 of the 89 differentially displayed "bands" have been used as probes on northern blots. Ten of these (~ 29%) have been confirmed by northern analysis to be differentially expressed genes, three of these have been cloned and sequenced. Two, numbers 15 and 34 (see Table 1), show greatest expression in normal mature cortex, less in age matched GM2 gangliosidosis cortex, and little or no expression in the new born cortex, suggesting that up regulation of these genes may be involved in turning off the process of dendritogenesis. A BLASTN search of DNA data bases shows clone number 15 to have a 67% homology to a segment of human chromosome 2, of, as yet, unknown function. Clone 34 shows no significant homology to any sequences in the data bases.

Clone 24 exhibits greatest expression in the new-born and GM2 gangliosidosis cats brains, suggesting that this gene is up regulated during dendritogenesis.

Table 1. Differential gene expression between animals undergoing active dendritogenesis and controls

Dif Dis Band No.	Size (bp) Approximate[1]	Northern Blot Analysis[2] K G A	Message Size[3] (Approximate)	Cloned	Vector	Sequenced	Known Homologies
2	280	+ + –	< 1800	–			
4	180	+ + –	1) < 1800 2) < 4700	–			
15	294	– ± +	> 4700	+	pCR II	+	67% Hu BAC 1D9 (hum. ch. 2) Function unknown
24	149	+ + –	> 4700	+	pCR Script	+	87% Human HMG CoA reductase
34	203	– ± +	> 4700	+	pCR Script	+	No known homologies
56	300	+ + –	1) < 1800 2) > 4700	–			
70	115	+ + –	> 4700	–			
76	480	+ + –	> 4700	–			
85	220	+ + –	1) < 1800 2) < 1800	–			
86	130	+ + –	> 4700	–			

1. Approximate sizes based on band position on acrylamide sequencing-like gels run with size standards. Sizes of cloned DNAs are exact
2. Northern Blot Analysis describes the strength of the signal in each animal tested. K = 3-Day-Old Kitten; G = GM2 Gangliosidosis Cat; A = Adult Normal (Note: Adult normal is age matched to GM2 gangliosidosis cat.)
3. Approximate message size is based on the position of the band of interest relative to 28S (4718 bp) and 18S (1874 bp) ribosomal subunits. Note: Three probes (4, 56, and 85) gave two bands on northern blots, these may be alternative splice variants

A BLASTN search of the sequence of clone 24 shows it to have significant homology to human (87%) and hamster (85%) 3-hydroxy-3-methylglutaryl coenzyme A (HMG CoA) reductase. HMG CoA reductase synthesizes mevalonic acid, an important precursor involved in the de novo synthesis of cholesterol and isoprenoids. HMG CoA reductase activity is elevated during early brain development, and it has been hypothesized that this may reflect the brain's need for increased levels of cholesterol to match the increased levels of new membrane biosynthesis occurring at this time. However, mevalonic acid has also been shown to be of critical importance in stimulating cell division in a variety of cell types including neurons, and this property of mevalonate appears to be mediated not through the cholesterol biosynthetic pathway, but through the formation of isoprenoids and their subsequent incorporation into regulatory proteins by prenylation [24-26]. A classic example of this is farnesylated-Ras [27]. There is also evidence that mevalonic acid, through this same pathway, can inhibit cell division and initiate differentiation [28]. The role of mevalonate in this regard appears to be cell type specific, analogous to many second messenger systems.

Discussion and significance

Using a feline model of GM2 gangliosidosis we have begun to examine the pathogenesis of a disease process that goes beyond the apparently simple metabolic disorder caused by the loss of activity of β-hexosaminidase. Similarities between the normal developmental process of dendritogenesis and ectopic dendritogenesis have led us to look for common patterns of gene expression that might shed light on both processes. Preliminary results are encouraging. Of the 35 candidate bands examined so far, ten have been shown to be differentially expressed genes. Three of the ten have been cloned and sequenced, two are unknown genes, the third appears to be HMG-CoA reductase. Albeit tempting, it is premature to envision the up-regulation of HMG CoA reductase as part of a developmental program specific to dendritogenesis. More work with this clone needs to be done. First, the clone is only 149 bp in length (see Table 1), and although it shows 87% homology to human HMG CoA reductase, more sequence is required to confirm this homology. Second, it is necessary to demonstrate, either by in situ hybridization or immunohistochemical techniques with antibodies against HMG CoA reductase, that only those neurons undergoing normal and ectopic dendritogenesis have increased levels of expression of this enzyme. Once these two criteria are met further characterizations will be done. Remaining candidates are currently being cloned and sequenced.

In conclusion, the lysosomal storage diseases offer an excellent model for studying the pathogenesis and treatment of CNS disorders and repair mechanisms. However, they are also a cautionary tale for those in pursuit of the genetic causes and treatments for neurological disorders. Tay-Sachs is a quintessential example of how knowledge of the genetic basis of a disease does not necessarily offer insights into the disease process, or result in immediate treatment. The metabolic lesion of Tay-Sachs disease has been known for a generation, but the pathobiology of the disease is as remote today as it was when first recognized over 100 years ago. Enzyme replacement and gene therapy are years away, and may, at best, merely halt the disease process, not repair damage already done. Yet, in the long run, much may be gained form studies focusing on the pathogenesis of Tay-Sachs disease, including insights into many other CNS disorders, and possibly unique cures.

Supported in part by Research Grant No. 12-FY99-274 from the March of Dimes Birth Defects Foundation.

References

1. Purpura DP, Suzuki K (1976) Distortion of neuronal geometry and formation of aberrant synapses in neuronal storage disease. Brain Res 116:1-21
2. Purpura DP (1978) Ectopic dendrite growth in mature pyramidal neurones in human ganglioside storage disease. Nature 276:520-521
3. Purpura DP, Walkley SU (1981) Aberrant neurite and spine generation in mature neurons in the gangliosidoses. In: Rapport M, Gorio A (eds) Gangliosides in neurological and neuromuscular function, development and repair. Raven Press, New York, pp 1-16
4. Walkley SU (1987) Further studies on ectopic dendrite growth and other geometrical distortions of neurons in feline GM1 gangliosidosis. Neuroscience 21:313-331
5. Walkley SU (1988) Pathobiology of neuronal storage disease. International Reviews of Neurobiology 29:191-244
6. Walkley SU, Wurzelmann S, Rattazzi MC et al (1990) Distribution of ectopic neurite growth and other geometrical distortions of neurons in feline GM2 gangliosidosis. Brain Res 510: 63-73
7. Goodman LA, Livingston PO, Walkley SU (1991) Ectopic dendrites occur only on cortical pyramidal cells containing elevated GM2 ganglioside in α-mannosidosis. Proc Natl Acad Sci USA 88:11330-11334
8. Walkley SU, Siegel DA, Dobrenis K (1995) GM2 ganglioside and pyramidal neuron dendritogenesis. Neurochemical Research 20:1287-1299
9. Walkley SU, Wurzelmann S, Purpura D (1981) Ultrastructure of neurites and meganeurites of cortical pyramidal neurons in feline gangliosidosis as revealed by the combined Golgi-EM technique. Brain Res 211:393-398
10. Walkley SU, Siegel DA, Wurzelmann S (1988) Ectopic dendritogenesis and associated synapse formation in swainsonine-induced neuronal storage disease. J Neuroscience 8:445-457
11. Walkley SU, Siegel DA, Dobrenis K (1998) GM2 Ganglioside as a regulator of pyramidal neuron dendritogenesis. In: Hakomori S, Ledeen R, Schneider J et al (eds) Sphingolipids as signalling modulators in the nervous system. Annals of the New York Academy of Sciences 845:188-199
12. Walkley SU, Siegel DA, Dobrenis K (1995) GM2 Ganglioside and pyramidal neuron dendritogenesis. Neurochemical Research 20:1287-1299
13. Siegel DA, Walkley SU (1994) Growth of ectopic dendrites on cortical pyramidal neurons in non-ganglioside storage diseases correlates with abnormal accumulation of GM2 ganglioside. J Neurochem 62:1852-1862
14. Walkley SU, Thrall MA, Dobrenis K et al (1994) Evidence for correction of enzymatic defect in CNS neurons in α-mannosidosis following bone marrow transplant. Proc Natl Acad Sci (USA) 91:2970-2974
15. Walkley SU, Thrall MA, Dobrenis K et al (1992) Evidence for correction of enzyme defect in CNS neurons in a lysosomal storage disease following bone marrow transplant. Proc Soc Inherited Metabolic Diseases
16. Walkley SU, Thrall MA, Dobrenis K (1996) Targeting gene products to the brain and neurons using bone marrow transplantation: a cell-mediated delivery system for therapy of inherited metabolic human disease. In: Lowenstein P, Enquist L (eds) Gene transfer into neurons: Towards gene therapy of neurological disorders. Wiley, New York, pp 275-302
17. Dobrenis K (1998) Microglia in cell culture and in transplantation therapy for CNS disease. In: Rosental R, Chiu FC (eds) Methods: A companion to methods in enzymology: Techniques for purification, functional evaluation and transplantation of brain cells. Academic Press, New York, Vol 16, pp 320-344
18. Dobrenis K, Finamore PS, Masui R et al (1996) Secretion of lysosomal glycosidases by microglia in culture. Molec Biol Cell 7[Suppl]:325a
19. Siegel DA, Walkley SU, Suzuki K (1982) Characterization of specific α-mannosidase inhibitor from locoweed. Trans Am Soc Neurochem 13:159

20. Walkley SU, Wurzelmann S, Siegel DA (1987) Ectopic axon hillock-associated neurite growth is maintained in metabolically reversed swainsonine-induced neuronal storage disease. Brain Res 410:89-96
21. Liang P, Pardee AB (1992) Differential display of eukaryotic messenger RNA by means of the polymerase chain reaction. Science 257:967-971
22. Liang P, Averboukh L, Pardee AB (1993) Distribution and cloning of eukaryotic mRNAs by means of differential display: refinements and optimization. Nucleic Acids Res 21:3269-3275
23. Bauer D, Muller H, Reich J et al (1993) Identification of differentially expressed mRNA species by an improved display technique (DDRT-PCR). Nucleic Acids Research 21:4272-4280
24. Carlberg M, Dricu A, Blegen H et al (1996) Mevalonic acid is limiting for N-linked glycosylation and translocation of the insulin-like growth factor-1 receptor to the cell surface. Evidence for a new link between 3-hydroxy-3-methylglutaryl-coenzyme A reductase and cell growth. J Biol Chem 271:17453-17462
25. Perez-Sala D, Mollinedo F (1994) Inhibition of isoprenoid biosynthesis induces apoptosis in human promyelocytic HL-60 cells. Biochem Biophys Res Com 199:1209-1215
26. Goalstone ML, Draznin B (1996) Effect of insulin on farnesyltransferase activity in 3T3-L1 adipocytes. J Biol Chem 271:27585-27589
27. Cuthbert JA, Lipsky PE (1995) Suppression of the proliferation of Ras-transformed cells by fluormevalonate, an inhibitor of mevalonate metabolism. Cancer Research 55:1732-1740
28. Larsson O, Blegen H (1994) Inhibitory effect of mevalonate on the EGF mitogenic signaling pathway in human breast cancer cells in culture. Cancer Biochem Biophys 14:193-200

STROKE IN THE YOUNG

Stroke in the Young: Epidemiology

G. SAVETTIERI, G. CUCCIA, G. SALEMI

For long time the attention of epidemiologists focused mainly on the distribution, analysis of risk factors, and prognosis of stroke in old patients [1, 2]. This was because of the progressive increase of stroke frequency with advancing age and the high disability and mortality that follow a stroke episode. In recent years, growing knowledge of the distribution and clinical features of stroke in adults, and evidence of a progressive decrease of its frequency [1, 2], have progressively shifted the interest of epidemiologists towards stroke affecting young patients. This topic has revealing peculiar features. The frequency of the various subtypes and the principal causes of stroke, and also prognosis and preventive measures, appear in part different in younger patients compared to older patients [3]. An exhaustive knowledge of these peculiarities is of the utmost importance because of the long life expectancy for a young patient, who needs information on the possibility of recovering from a physical handicap, on the recurrence risk, and, particularly, on the likelihood of regaining the ability to work.

Descriptive epidemiology

Information on the distribution of stroke in the young originates mainly from incidence studies more than prevalence ones. This is due to various reasons: the need for incidence data in order to provide an adequate number of stroke units, the possibility of better characterizing patients from a clinical point of view, and the likelihood of obtaining reliable information about case fatality ratio after a stroke. Moreover, considering the relatively low frequency of stroke in the young, a very large population is required to obtain stable rates.

Figure 1 and Table 1a summarize crude and age-specific *incidence* ratios *of stroke in the young* reported in the principal surveys conducted in the last two decades [4-13]. A high variability of incidence is evident. Methodological issues, including the diversity in the age groups under investigation (i.e.: 0-44, 15-44, 15-55), and the different sizes of populations under study, partly explain this discrepancy. The two principal studies conducted in Italy [7, 11] found incidence ratios similar to that reported for Western countries.

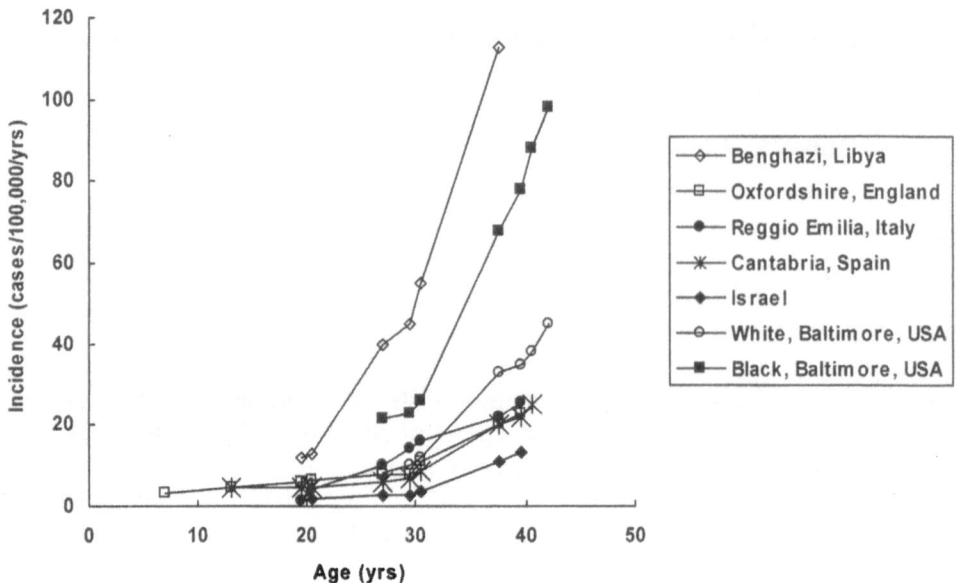

Fig. 1. Age-specific incidence of stroke in the young. An international comparison

Prevalence of stroke in the young was evaluated mainly during door-to-door two-phase surveys carried out to determine the frequency of stroke in the entire population. The prevalence ratios obtained through this approach in the few studied performed [14-16] are homogeneous (Table 1b).

A study performed in the biracial community of Copiah County, Mississippi, USA [14], and another one in Baltimore County, USA [10] indicate that American blacks suffer stroke more frequently than other ethnic groups. This feature occurs irrespective of the age at onset and contrasts with the apparently low prevalence of stroke among blacks living in Africa. Well-structured studies on the frequency of stroke in young black Africans are necessary to clarify this topic. The excess of risk among black Americans is not associated with a higher prevalence of hypertension, diabetes, obesity, cigarette smoking, homocysteine elevation, or coagulation disorders [17-19].

Prospective population-based incidence studies provide the best source of information to evaluate the frequency of stroke subtypes in the young. According to the studies performed [6, 7, 11, 12], ischemic stroke appears the more frequent form among young patients (Table 2). Subarachnoid hemorrhage (SH) and intracerebral hemorrhage (IH) account for more than 30% of cases, with a slightly higher frequency of SH [7, 11, 12]. This pattern differs from that in the elderly for a higher frequency of SH and IH [1].

Tables 3 and 4 list the causes of stroke in the young. Recent population-based studies [20, 21] confirmed findings from the referral centers [22] that

Table 1. Incidence (cases/100,000 population/years) and prevalence (cases/100,000) ratios of first-ever stroke

A. Incidence

Population source	Study design	Incidence
Stockholm, Sweden, 1973-1977, N = 733 [4]	NA	16
Hiroshima & Nagasaki, Japan, 1950-1974 [5]	NA	24
Benghazi, Libya, 1983-1984, N = 63 [6]	Prospective	39.8
Florence, Italy, 1983-1985, N = 47 [7]	Prospective	8.8
Oxfordshire, England, 1981-1986, N = 27 [8]	Prospective	9.0
Poznan, Poland, 1985 [9]	NA	34.8
Baltimore, USA, 1988, white, no SH, N = 53 [10]	Retrospective	13.6
Baltimore, USA, 1988, black, no SH, N = 84 [10]	Retrospective	30.1
Baltimore, USA, 1988, total, no SH, N = 137 [10]	Retrospective	20.7
Reggio Emilia, Italy, 1987-1989, N = 29 [11]	Retrospective	13.6
Cantabria, Spain, 1986-1988, N = 58 [12]	Prospective	10.9
Israel, 1992-1993, N = 125 [13]	Prospective	5.8

B. Prevalence

Population source	Study design	Prevalence (age groups)		
		0-34	15-39	0-39
Copiah County, USA 01.01.1978 [14]	Door to door two phase survey	36.8	NA	NA
Rural Kashmir, India 01.11.1986 [15]	Door to door two phase survey	NA	41	NA
Three Sicilian municipalities, Italy 01.11.1987 [16]	Door to door two phase survey	NA	NA	40.4

NA, not available; SH, subarachnoid hemorrhage

nonatherosclerotic vasculopathies, specifically cervical arterial dissection, patent foramen ovale, atrial septal aneurysm, and vasculitis, are more common than atherothrombotic vasculopathies in young adults. The percentages of ischemic stroke attributed to IgG anticardiolipin antibodies, oral contraceptive use, and migraine account for a limited part of ischemic stroke in the young [20, 21]. The different etiologic causes underlying ischemic stroke in young and old people [1, 2] must be taken into account in the choice of the diagnostic flowchart. Intracerebral hemorrhage is mainly lobar in location and results from vascular malformation. Hypertension is the other common cause of IH [23].

Information on *prognostic factors of stroke in the young* is limited. The 30 day case-fatality ratio indicates a higher survival compared to stroke in the elderly, with lower mortality mainly for the ischemic type (Table 2). The few data available on long term prognosis concern ischemic stroke and are all obtained from referral centers [24-26]. The results of these studies indicate that the young with ischemic stroke have lower mortality and fewer recurrences than adults [24, 25]; however survivors will have residual emotional, social or physical impairments that hamper employment and lower the quality of life [26]. Negative

Table 2. Annual incidence rates of first-ever stroke per 100,000 population by clinical type and case fatality ratio (%)

Population source	Study design	Age groups	Ischemia	Intra-parenchymal hemorrhage	Subarachnoid hemorrhage	Case fatality ratio (30 d)
Stockholm, Sweden 1973-1977, N = 283 [4]	NA	15-44	5.0	5.0	NA	NA
Benghazi, Libya 1983-1984 [6]	Prospective	15-40	36.4	5.8	4.8	NA
Florence, Italy 1983-1985 [7]	Prospective	15-44	3.4	1.9	3.2	NA
Reggio Emilia, Italy 1987-1989 [11]	Retrospective	15-44	8.0	2.8	2.8	17%
Baltimore, USA 1988, white, N = 53 [10]	Retrospective	15-44	10.5	3.1	NA	NA
Baltimore, USA 1988, black, N = 84 [10]	Retrospective	15-44	21.7	9.2	NA	NA
Baltimore, USA 1988, total, N = 137 [10]	Retrospective	15-44	12.1	5.6	NA	NA
Cantabria, Spain 1986-1988 [12]	Prospective	11-50	6.5	3.8	3.4	22%
Northern Sweden 1991-1994 [20]	Prospective	15-44	11.3	NA	NA	NA

NA, not available

prognostic factors are occlusions within the internal carotid and middle cerebral arteries and severity of stroke.

Table 3. Ischemic stroke in the young: a list of principal causes

Atherosclerotic cerebrovascular disease
    Cigarette smoking
    Advanced age
    Male gender
    Diabetes mellitus
    Systolic blood pressure
    Serum lipids and lipoprotein
    Obesity
    Hyperhomocysteinemia
Non-atherosclerotic cerebral vasculopathies
    Cervicocephalic arterial dissections
        Idiopathic
        Blunt or penetrating trauma
        Marfan's syndrome
        Ehlers-Danlos Syndrome type IV

      Coarctation of the aorta
      Cystic medial necrosis
      Extreme vessel tortuosity
      Pharyngeal infections
      Luetic arteritis
      Alpha-1-antitrypsin deficiency
      Sympathomimetic drug abuse
      Lentiginosis
Moyamoya
      Idiopathic
      Neonatal anoxia
      Trauma
      Basilar meningitis or tuberculosis meningitis
      Leptospirosis
      Cranial radiation therapy
      Neurofibromatosis or tuberous sclerosis
      Brain tumors
      Polyarteritis nodosa
      Marfan's syndrome
      Pseudoxanthoma elasticum
      Cerebral dissection and saccular aneurysm
      Sickle cell anemia or Fanconi's anemia
      Apert's syndrome
      Factor XII deficiency
      Type-I glycogenosis
      NADH-Coenzyme Q reductase deficiency
      Renal stenosis
      Down's syndrome
      Coarctation of the aorta
Fibromuscular dysplasia
Vasculitis
Migraine
Cardiac embolism
Hematological (hypercoagulable) disorders
      Antithrombin III deficiency or protein C or protein S deficiency
      Activated protein C resistance
      Antiphospholipid antibodies
      Increase of homocysteine
      Increase of tissue plasminogen activator or fibrinogen levels
      Oral contraceptive intake
Metabolic
      MELAS (mitochondrial myopathy, encephalopathy, lactic acidosis and stroke-like episodes)

Analytic epidemiology

The earliest case-control studies performed to identify *risk and protective factors of stroke in the young* focused on the typical risk factors of ischemic stroke [27, 28]. These studies confirmed that traditional risk factors play a role also in young people. An Italian multicenter study performed on 308 young patients with ischemic stroke and 616 matched controls showed the significance of mi-

Table 4. Non-ischemic stroke in the young: a list of principal causes

---

Intracerebral hemorrhage
   Vascular malformation
   Aneurysms
   Hypertension
   Bleeding diathesis
   Cerebral amyloid angiopathy
   Vasculitis
   Illicit drug abuse
   Intracranial tumours
      Glioblastoma multiforme
      Oligodendroglioma
      Medulloblastoma
      Ependymoma
      Pituitary adenoma
      Meningioma
      Intraparenchymal brain plasmocytoma
      Von Hippel-Lindau disease
      Metastatic tumours
   Others
Cerebral venous occlusive disease
   Septic
   Aseptic
      Thrombophilia
      Antithrombin III deficiency
      Protein C or protein S deficiency
      Activated protein C resistance
      Sickle cell anemia
      Thrombocythemia
      Paroxysmal nocturnal hemoglobinuria
      Inflammatory bowel disease
      Behcet's disease
Subarachnoid hemorrhage

---

graine with aura, cigarette smoking, alcohol abuse, elevated serum triglycerides, arrhythmias, mitral stenosis, coronary heart disease and carotid stenosis or occlusion as independent risk factors of ischemic stroke [27]. Another interesting study performed in Baltimore and Washington, USA, compared the occurrence of some traditional risk factors in black and white young people [28]. The authors concluded that hypertension, diabetes mellitus and current cigarette smoking were important risk factors in this biracial population, and that cigarette smoking and hypertension played an important role particularly among black young patients. Various case-control studies showed the relevance of other risk factors proposed as specific of young people [3]. However, a discrepancy exists between indications coming from case-control studies and the low frequency of some of these causes observed in the population-based surveys. This discrepancy is of practical importance in the establishment of a diagnostic flowchart for a young patient affected by stroke. Some issues will be analyzed in detail, some others have been extensively investigated in a recent review [3].

The association between increased total homocysteine concentration in the blood (tHcy) and ischemic stroke has been demonstrated in case-control studies [29]. The meaning of this association is uncertain and the existence of various potential biases has been reported [29]. A recent study has partially clarified the significance of this association [30]. The fasting and post-methionine load level of tHcy, the genotype frequency of the C677CT mutation in the methylenetetrahydrofolate reductase gene (MTHFR), and the concentration of various factors of the fibrinolytic system were evaluated in 80 young patients with ischemic stroke and compared with 41 healthy control subjects. The post-methionine load level of tHcy was associated with a 4.8 fold increased risk of ischemic stroke, while no difference in the polymorphism of MTHFR gene was observed between cases and controls. Abnormal response to methionine loading seems to be associated with higher tissue plasminogen activator (tPA) mass concentration levels, suggesting an interaction between the fibrinolytic system and the Hcy metabolism [30]. In addition, two recent case-control studies, aimed to evaluate the variation of the carotid wall thickening, showed an association between hyperhomocysteinemia and atherosclerosis [31, 32].

Alterations of the fibrinolytic system and disorders of the coagulation are infrequently associated with ischemic stroke [33-35]. Recent clinical series and case-control studies indicate a more frequent association with tPA mass concentration level [30, 36, 37].

The importance of measuring immunoglobulin G (IgG) anticardiolipin (ACLA) antibodies as a marker of coagulation disorder is controversial. The discovery of an association between these antibodies and the risk of ischemic stroke [38] stimulated various surveys [39]. Most of these studies are concordant in considering this as a slight association [20, 21]. Recently, an Italian group criticized the methods used to titrate ACLA and proposed measuring antiphosphatidylinositol antibodies together with ACLA [40]. They reported, in their sample of 77 young patients affected by ischemic stroke, a high prevalence of these antibodies (44.1%). Disappointingly, this interesting study lacks a control group.

An important association is that between ischemic stroke and oral contraceptive intake. Women who had taken oral high-estrogen or progestogen contraceptive pills had a higher risk of ischemic stroke [41, 42]. Recent large case-control studies reported a marked reduction of this risk among women who use low-estrogen contraceptives or minipills (progestogen-only pills) [43-48]. However, the risk increases in a multiplicative way when another risk factor is present (e.g. a women with diabetes using an oral low-estrogen contraceptive would have an odds for ischemic stroke of 9.9 [5.4, odds for diabetes, 1.8, odds for contraceptives]) [44].

That pregnancy is associated with stroke in the young is an assumption of great interest, but supported by scant data. The few studies performed on this topic are in line with the idea that pregnant women are not at risk for stroke [49, 50]. A recent study carried out in central Maryland and Washington DC in the period 1988-1991 on 140,167 pregnancies confirms the lack of association between delivery and stroke. In the same study an evident association between the six weeks after delivery and stroke is, however, present (relative risk: 8.7 for IS; 28.3 for IH) [50]. The conclusions of this large study, even if of the main importance, need further confirmation.

The association between migraine and stroke has been extensively studied. It is of particular importance because migraine is quite frequent among young women [51]. A recent review discussed extensively the increased risk of stroke for young women affected by migraine and the multiplicative increase of risk for women who take a low-estrogen contraceptive [3]. In the same review it is underlined that "*the absolute risk of ischemic stroke in young women is quite low, on the order of 10-20 per 100,000. Thus, recommendations regarding oral contraceptive use in migraneurs need to take into account the benefits of oral contraceptive use versus the risks*". In the present year a study performed in the Dijon stroke registry on 2,389 patients, was published; the data reported confirm that migraine history is uncommon among young patients with stroke (2%) and that such a history is more common among women (2.8% versus 1.1% men) [52]. A hospital-based case-control study by a collaborative European study group, performed on 291 women affected by stroke and 736 age and hospital matched controls, reported a higher risk of ischemic stroke in women affected by migraine (OR 3.54) [53]. The coexistence of oral contraceptive use, high blood pressure, or cigarette smoking, exerts a greater than multiplicative effect on the association between ischemic stroke and migraine [53].

Conclusions

In conclusion, various interesting topics arose from recent epidemiological papers on stroke in the young. The high frequency of nonatherosclerotic vasculopathies among the causes of ischemic stroke is definitely acquired. The risk of oral contraceptive use when another risk factor is present is a definite acquisition that must influence all the programs of prevention for stroke.

The role of numerous alterations of the fibrinolytic and coagulative systems and of the presence of various autoantibodies, sometimes detected, remains to be further clarified. Illumination of these topics could allow a better understanding of suggested role of inflammatory mechanisms during stroke and could indicate new therapeutic or preventive approaches [54].

Finally, issues little studied at present, but in need of investigation, are the role of genetics in stroke predisposition, and the interaction between genetic and environmental factors in the risk of stroke. This area of investigation seems one of the most promising in understanding stroke in the young.

References

1. Davis PH, Hachinski V (1991) Epidemiology of cerebrovascular disease. In: Anderson DW, (ed) Neuroepidemiology: A tribute to Bruce Schoenberg. Boca Raton, FL: CRC Press, pp 27-53
2. Warlow CP (1998) Epidemiology of stroke. Lancet 352[Suppl III]:1-4
3. Kittner SJ (1998) Stroke in young adults: progress and opportunities. Neuroepidemiology 17: 174-178
4. Mettinger KL, Söderström CE, Allander E (1984) Epidemiology of acute cerebrovascular disease before the age of 55 in the Stockholm County 1973-77: I. Incidence and mortality rates. Stroke 15:795-801
5. Lin CH, Shimizu Y, Kato H et al (1984) Cerebrovascular diseases in a fixed population of Hiroshima and Nagasaki, with special reference to relationship between type and risk factors. Stroke 15:653-660
6. Radhakrishnan K, Ashok PP, Sridharan R et al (1986) Stroke in the young: incidence and pattern in Benghazi, Libya. Acta Neurol Scand 73:434-438
7. Nencini P, Inzitari D, Baruffi MC et al (1988) Incidence of stroke in young adults in Florence, Italy. Stroke 19:977-981
8. Bamford J, Sandercock P, Dennis M et al (1988) A prospective study of acute cerebrovascular disease in the community: The Oxfordshire community stroke project 1981-86: 1. Methodology, demography, and incident cases of first-ever stroke. J Neurol Neurosurg Psychiatry 51: 1373-1380
9. Wender M, Lenart-Jankowska D, Pruchnuik D et al (1990) Epidemiology of stroke in the Poznan District of Poland. Stroke 21:390-393
10. Kittner SJ, McCarter RJ, Sherwin RW et al (1993) Black-white differences in stroke risk among young adults. Stroke 24:113-115
11. Guidetti D, Baratti M, Zucco RG et al (1993) Incidence of stroke in young adults in the Reggio Emilia area, northern Italy. Neuroepidemiology 12:82-87
12. Leno C, Berciano J, Combarros O et al (1993) A prospective study of stroke in young adults in Cantabria, Spain. Stroke 24:792-795
13. Rozenthul-Sorokin N, Ronen R, Tamir A et al (1996) Stroke in the young in Israel. Incidence and outcomes. Stroke 27:838-841
14. Schoenberg BS, Anderson DW, Haerer AF (1986) Racial differentials in the prevalence of stroke: Copiah County, Mississippi. Arch Neurol 43:565-568
15. Razdan S, Koul RL, Motta A et al (1989) Cerebrovascular disease in rural Kashmir, India. Stroke 20:1691-1693
16. Patti F, Failla G, Reggio A et al (1998) Stroke in the young in Sicily: prevalence and clinical features. J Stroke Cerebrovasc Dis 7:196-199
17. Giles WH, Kittner SJ, Hebel JR et al (1995) Determinants of black-white differences in the risk of cerebral infarction. The National Health and Nutrition Examination Survey epidemiologic follow-up study. Arch Intern Med 155:1319-1324
18. Kittner SJ, Giles WH, Macko RF et al (1999) Homocyst(e)ine and risk of cerebral infarction in a biracial population: the stroke prevention in young women study. Stroke 30:1554-1560
19. Chaturvedi S, Joshi N, Dzieczkowski J (1999) Activated protein C resistance in young African American patients with ischemic stroke. J Neurol Sci 163:137-139
20. Kristensen B, Malm J, Carlberg B et al (1997) Epidemiology and etiology of ischemic stroke in young adults aged 18 to 44 years in northern Sweden. Stroke 28:1702-1709
21. Kittner SJ, Stern BJ, Wozniak M et al (1998) Cerebral infarction in young adults: the Baltimore-Washington Cooperative young stroke study. Neurology 50:890-894
22. Adams HP Jr, Kappelle LJ, Biller J et al (1995) Ischemic stroke in young adults. Experience in 329 patients enrolled in the Iowa registry of stroke in young adults. Arch Neurol 52:491-495
23. Ruiz-Sandoval JL, Cantu C, Barinagarrementeria F (1999) Intracerebral hemorrhage in young people: analysis of risk factors, location, causes, and prognosis. Stroke 30:537-541

24. Hindfelt B, Nilsson O (1992) Long-term prognosis of ischemic stroke in young adults. Acta Neurol Scand 86:440-445
25. Ferro JM, Crespo M (1994) Prognosis after transient ischemic attack and ischemic stroke in young adults. Stroke 25:1611-1616
26. Kappelle LJ, Adams HP Jr, Heffner ML (1994) Prognosis of young adults with ischemic stroke. A long-term follow-up study assessing recurrent vascular events and functional outcome in the Iowa Registry of stroke in young adults. Stroke 25:1360-1365
27. Marini C, Carolei A, Roberts RS et al (1993) Focal cerebral ischemia in young adults: a collaborative case-control study: Neuroepidemiology 12:70-81
28. Rohr J, Kittner S, Feeser B et al (1996) Traditional risk factors and ischemic stroke in young adults: the Baltimore-Washington cooperative young stroke study. Arch Neurol 53:603-607
29. Sacco RL, Roberts JK, Jacobs BS (1998) Homocysteine as a risk factor for ischemic stroke: an epidemiological story in evolution. Neuroepidemiology 17:167-173
30. Kristensen B, Malm J, Nilsson TK et al (1999) Hyperhomocysteinemia and hypofibrinolysis in young adults with ischemic stroke. Stroke 30:974-980
31. Spence JD, Malinow MR, Barnett PA et al (1999) Plasma homocyst(e)ine concentration, but not MTHFR genotype, is associated with variation in carotid plaque area. Stroke 30:969-973
32. McQuillan BM, Beilby JP, Nidorf M et al (1999) Hyperhomocysteinemia but not the C677T mutation of methylenetetrahydrofolate reductase is an independent risk determinant of carotid wall thickening. The Perth carotid ultrasound disease assessment study. Circulation 99:2383-2388
33. Munts AG, van Genderen PJ, Dippel DW et al (1998) Coagulation disorders in young adults with acute cerebral ischemia. J Neurol 245:21-25
34. Nabavi DG, Junker R, Wolff E et al (1998) Prevalence of factor V Leiden mutation in young adults with cerebral ischaemia: a case-control study on 225 patients. J Neurol 245:653-658
35. Douay X, Lucas C, Caron C et al (1998) Antithrombin, protein C and protein S level in 127 consecutive young adults with ischemic stroke. Acta Neurol Scand 98:124-127
36. Kristensen B, Malm J, Nilsson TK et al (1998) Increased fibrinogen levels and acquired hypofibrinolysis in young adults with ischemic stroke. Stroke 29:2261-2267
37. Macko RF, Kittner SJ, Epstein A et al (1999) Elevated tissue plasminogen activator antigen and stroke risk: The stroke prevention in young women study. Stroke 30:7-11
38. Kushner M, Simonian M (1989) Lupus anticoagulants, anticardiolipin antibodies, and cerebral ischemia. Stroke 20:225
39. Tanne D, Triplett DA, Levine SR (1998) Antiphospholipid-protein antibodies and ischemic stroke. Not just cardiolipin any more. Stroke 29:1755-1758
40. Toschi V, Motta A, Castelli C et al (1998) High prevalence of antiphosphatidylinositol antibodies in young patients with cerebral ischemia of undetermined cause. Stroke 29:1759-1764
41. Thorogood M, Mann J, Murphy M et al (1992) Fatal stroke and use of oral contraceptives: findings from a case-control study. Am J Epidemiol 136:35-45
42. Hannaford PC, Croft PR, Kay CR (1994) Oral contraception and stroke. Evidence from the Royal College of General Practitioners' oral contraception study. Stroke 25:935-942
43. Lidegaard O (1993) Oral contraception and risk of a cerebral thromboembolic attack: results of a case-control study. BMJ 306:956-963
44. Lidegaard O (1995) Oral contraceptives, pregnancy, and the risk of cerebral thromboembolism: the influence of diabetes, hypertension, migraine, and previous thrombotic disease. Br J Obstet Gynaecol 102:153-159
45. WHO Collaborative Study of Cardiovascular Disease and Steroid Hormone Contraception (1996) Ischaemic stroke and combined oral contraceptives: results of an international, multicentre, case-control study. Lancet 348:498-505
46. Petitti DB, Sidney S, Bernstein A (1996) Stroke in users of low-dose oral contraceptives. N Engl J Med 335:8-15
47. Schwartz SM, Petitti DB, Siscovick DS et al (1998) Stroke and use of low-dose oral contraceptives in young women: a pooled analysis of two US studies. Stroke 28:2277-2284

48. Lidegaard O (1998) Thrombotic diseases in young women and the influence of oral contraceptives. Am J Obstet Gynaecol 179:S62-S67
49. Wiebers DO, Whisnant JP (1985) The incidence of stroke among pregnant women in Rochester, Minnesota, 1955 through 1979. JAMA 254:3055-3057
50. Kittner SJ, Stern BJ, Feeser BR et al (1996) Pregnancy and the risk of stroke. N Engl J Med 335:768-774
51. Rasmussen BK (1995) Epidemiology of headache. Cephalalgia 17:685-701
52. Sochurkova D, Moreau T, Lemesle M et al (1999) Migraine history and migraine-induced stroke in the Dijon stroke registry. Neuroepidemiology 18:85-91
53. Chang CL, Donaughy M, Poulter N (1999) Migraine and stroke in young women: case-control study. The World Health Organization Collaborative Study of Cardiovascular Disease and Steroid Hormone Contraception. BMJ 318:13-18
54. DeGraba TJ (1998) The role of inflammation after acute stroke: utility of pursuing anti-adhesion molecule therapy. Neurology 51[Suppl 3]:S62-S68

Pathogenesis of Stroke in Young Adults

A. ANZINI, M. RASURA, C. FIESCHI

The lower and upper limits of age that define a young adult with stroke are rather arbitrary. By convention the age span in this situation is usually set in the range of 15-18 years up to 45-50 years of age. The definition of this range is useful and justified by differences in etiologies, evaluation and prognosis in this younger population as compared with stroke in the elderly. Defining the diagnosis and cause of stroke in the young is often a challenging task. The causes of stroke among young adults are more diverse than in the elderly and require an extensive diagnostic workup. Bogousslavsky and Pierre [1] listed up to 120 causes of stroke in the young and some authors [2, 3] also provided guidelines for clinical management of both commonly and rarely encountered cerebrovascular disorders in young adults. Hower, it is difficult to give an accurate hierarchy of causes of stroke based on their frequency because most studies come from secondary or tertiary care centers so that the results are invariably biased toward uncommon causes. Yet, the etiology or the underlying disorder of approximately one third of ischemic stroke remains undetermined. Table 1 shows the potential causes of ischemic stroke in young adults.

Atherosclerosis has been considered to be the cause of stroke in about 25% of patients younger than 50 years. Patients with atherosclerosis usually have the classical risk factors such as arterial hypertension, diabetes mellitus, dyslipidemia, smoking habit or a family history of premature disease.

An atherothrombotic etiology was considered if angiography or Doppler sonography of the symptomatic cerebral artery territory show > 50% stenosis or occlusion or an ulcerated plaque of the internal carotid artery or intracranial occlusion without evidence of cardiac abnormalities. An atherosclerotic pathogenesis was also presumed if the patient had two or more atherogenic risk factors, in the absence of other identifiable causes [4, 5]. Case-control studies have shown that increased levels of homocysteine are associated with an increased risk for atherothrombosis. Atherosclerotic etiology is rare in the first decades (about 5%). At this age the cardioembolic mechanisms are more frequent: 15-45% according to different diagnostic criteria for cardioembolism and the extent of investigations [6]. A classification of cardiac abnormalities, based on transesophageal echocardiography (TEE), has been proposed by Labovitz and Pearson [7] (Table 2).

Table 1. Potential causes of ischemic stroke in young adults

Atherosclerotic large artery disease (9-48%)
> 50-60% stenosis or ulcerated plaques or two or more atherosclerotic risk factors
Non-atherosclerotic disease (10-33%)
Carotid or vertebral dissection (3-25%), fibromuscular dysplasia, angiitis
Cardioembolism (7-35%)
Congenital heart disease, infective endocarditis, valvular disease, patent foramen ovale (PFO),
interatrial septal aneurysm (ASA)
Prothrombotic states (8-15%)
Antiphospholipid antibody syndrome, antithrombin III, protein C/S deficiencies,
activated protein C resistance (factor V mutation), factor II mutation
Miscellaneous (1-20%)
Migraine (2-15%), MELAS, CADASIL hyperhomocysteinemia
Undetermined (7-40%)

Table 2. Cardiac embologenic sources identified by TEE

Definite
Left atrium thrombus
Left ventricle thrombus
Tumors
Complicated aortic plaques
Probable
Patent foramen ovale (PFO)
Spontaneous echocontrast
Atrium septal aneurysm with or without PFO
Possible
Degenerative valvulopathy
Redundant cordae tendinae
Left ventricle wall motion abnormalities
Mitral valve prolapse

Patent foramen ovale (PFO) has been found in 40-50% of young adults with cryptogenic cerebral ischemia and in about 10% of controls [8]. The mechanism for stroke in patients with PFO is paradoxical embolism, defined as embolic material originating in the venous circulation or right cardiac chamber, migrating into the systemic circulation through vascular shunts that bypass the pulmonary capillary bed. In patients with PFO there is not a sustained right-to-left interatrial shunt, but paradoxical embolism could be induced by transient shunting particularly during elevation of right atrial pressure (provoked by cough or Valsalva's maneuver). The pathogenetic importance of PFO is debated. Its role is more likely when the following conditions are present: no evidence of other sources of embolism, coexistence of deep venous thrombosis or pulmonary embolism, large PFO or larger amounts of interatrial shunting or both, association of PFO with atrial septal aneurysm (ASA) (25%) or with mitral valve prolapse (MVP), both potential cardioembolic sources [9]. ASA is another occult embolic cardiac source of cerebral ischemia, especially those with a greater than 10 mm excursion [10]. Cerebral ischemia in patients with ASA could be secondary to embolism from thrombi in the aneurysmal sac or to paradoxical embolism through a PFO.

Cervicocephalic arterial dissection is a leading cause of stroke in young subjects and the most common nonatherosclerotic vasculopathy. Arterial dissection is classically associated with flexion or extension injuries to the neck, although many cases do not record any history of neck injury. Coughing, nose blowing, chiropractic manipulation, sports activities, motor vehicle accidents are some of the most common activities associated with arterial dissection. In dissection, as the false lumen fills with blood, it expands and can result in significant narrowing of the vessel lumen or lead to local thrombus formation with secondary embolization. Clinically, dissection may cause transient retinal, hemispheric or posterior fossa ischemia, Horner's syndrome, pain, or cranial nerve palsies [11]. The diagnosis usually requires standard or MR angiography, which should be performed soon after the event because the features of arterial dissection may rapidly change, either towards a normalization of the lumen or into a "classic" atherothrombotic appearance [12]. Some diseases appear to be associated with an increased tendency for arterial dissection, such as fibromuscular dysplasia, Marfan's syndrome and cystic degeneration.

Other nonatherosclerotic vasculopathies are represented by vasculitis, an heterogeneous group of disorders characterized by inflammation and necrosis of blood vessel walls and ultimately occlusion of inflamed vessels. Cerebral vasculitis is an uncommon etiology of stroke in young adults.

Vasculitis should be considered when the stroke is recurrent, associated with encephalopathic manifestations, fever, weight loss, fatigue, arthralgias, myalgias, skin lesions, or multifocal neurological signs. A vasculitic process in young patients can be secondary to HIV infection. In these patients, stroke can also be caused by embolism from infective endocarditis and from coagulation abnormalities (disseminated intravasal coagulation, presence of lupus anticoagulant, blood hyperviscosity). Immune-mediated endothelial damage can also be induced by *Chlamydia pneumoniae* infection. Recent studies [13] have suggested a pathogenetic association between chronic infection and atherosclerosis, showing high IgG and/or IgA antibody titers in patients with myocardial infarction, coronary disease and carotid atherosclerosis.

Hematological and immunological conditions should be considered in patients with a personal or family history of venous or arterial thromboses and in patients with an intraluminal carotid or vertebrobasilar clot without underlying occlusive disease or a potential cardioembolic source. Hematological and coagulation disorders have been described in about 10% of young stroke patients [14]. This is probably a low estimate as a few studies have screened for the full spectrum of disorders. The number of abnormalities reported with ischemic stroke is growing rapidly. The most commonly reported disorders are deficiencies of coagulation inhibitors (antithrombin III, protein C, protein S). Reduction in their activity of 20-30% is probably associated with an increased risk. Mutation in the 3' untranslated region of the prothrombin gene is a recently identified congenital risk factor for venous thrombosis; it is associated with high levels of prothrombin. The factor II mutated allele was demonstrated to be associated with an increased risk for myocardial infarction in young women, especially if they are smokers. De Stefano et al. [15] found that 12.5% of patients with ischemic stroke younger than 50 years of age are carriers of the factor II G20210A gene mutation; in the control group, the prevalence of the carriers was 2.5%. Another new pathological condition termed "activated protein C (APC) resistance" has recently been reported to be the most common hereditary blood coagulation disorder associated with familial thrombosis. APC resistance is characterized by a poor anticoagulant response to APC in the plasma of patients and is due to a mutation 1691G to A in the factor V gene. Its role in arterial thrombosis is controversial, whereas it is associated with a 7-fold increased risk for venous thrombosis [16]. The "antiphospholipid syndrome" is a well-known cause of ischemic stroke. The presence of antiphospholipid antibodies, i.e. the lupus anticoagulant or anticardiolipin antibodies is associated with recurrent venous thromboses and cerebral arterial occlusion. Other manifestations of the syndrome include skin lesions, recurrent miscarriages, severe preeclampsia and fetal death. The pathogenesis of thrombosis in this syndrome is unknown [17].

Rarer causes of stroke also exist. Mitochondrial disease may present with stroke in patients under 45 years of age. The diagnosis of mitochondrial encephalopathy, lactate acidosis and strokelike episodes (MELAS) should be considered in young stroke cases after other more usual causes have been excluded, in particular in patients suffering occipital stroke. Features such as raised blood and CSF lactate, clinical features (hearing impairment, epilepsy, short stature) and a maternal family history of neurological disease may support a mitochondrial etiology [18]. CADASIL, a newly coined acronym for cerebral autosomal dominant subcortical arteriopathy with ischemic leukencephalopathy, is recognized as a cause of hereditary multi-infarct dementia. In the earlier stages of the disease, affected individuals may experience stroke before the age of 45 years. CADASIL should be suspected in patients with unexplained subcortical ischemic strokes, whenever they are associated with MRI signal abnormalities in white matter and basal ganglia. These findings should prompt a genealogical study including all first- and second-degree relatives [19].

There are some conditions whose pathogenetic correlation with stroke are not clear. They include: migraine, oral contraceptive use, pregnancy, postpartum condition, alcohol and drug abuse, and hyperhomocysteinemia. Migraine may increase the risk of stroke especially in young women, if they have other risk factors such as smoking and use of oral contraceptives [20]. Migrainous stroke is a rare event considering the high prevalence among migraine in the general population (about 5% of ischemic stroke in the young) [21]. The diagnosis of migraine stroke is primarily based on exclusion of other conditions and it is essential to use strict criteria, otherwise a diagnosis of migraine stroke will be made in every migraineur who suffers a stroke [22]. The diagnosis of migraine stroke can be made reliably only in known migraineurs who develop a cerebral infarct during a typical attack of migraine.

Ischemic stroke occurs primarily in the second and third trimesters and during the first postpartum week [23]. The pregnancy-specific causes of strokes include: amniotic embolism, choriocarcinoma, hypercoagulability, and pulmonary emboli from the site of a peripheral phlebothrombosis when a PFO coexists (during delivery, which leads to a repeated Valsalva maneuver). Changes occur in the coagulation and fibrinolytic system during pregnancy, especially in the last trimester and in the first few weeks after delivery. They include an increase of fibrinogen, plasminogen factors VII, VIII, IX and X and a decrease of antithrombin III, protein C and S levels [24]. Hyperhomocysteinemia can be due to the inhibition of one or more of the homocysteine metabolizing pathways for enzymatic defects (mutation in the methylentetrahydrofolate reductase (MTHFR) gene) or vitamin deficiencies (B6, B12). The mechanisms by which hyperhomocysteinemia contributes to atherogenesis are incompletely understood. Increase level of homocysteine has been found to be damaging to endothelial cells, impairing endothelial vasodilatation. A variety of negative effects on the homeostasis has been shown, such as inhibition of protein C activity and blocking of tPA binding to endothelial cells. The prevalence of hyperhomocysteinemia in young stroke patients is about 10-16% [25].

Table 3 shows the final diagnoses in our series of 223 patients, between 17 and 46 years of age (111 men and 112 women, median age 36.5), with TIA ($n = 35$; 15.7%) or stroke ($n = 188$; 88.3%) admitted to the Neurological Department of Rome and investigated between September 1991 and July 1999. Patients underwent a diagnostic protocol shown in Table 4.

Table 3. Final diagnosis: distribution for age

Etiological diagnosis	17-29 years	30-46 years	Total
Atherosclerosis	10	39	49
Cardioembolism (PFO)	50 (45)	32 (22)	82
Non-atherosclerotic disease			
Arterial dissection	11	17	28
Vasculitis	12	14	26
Prothrombotic states			
Prot.C/S deficiency	0	2	2
Factor II/V mutation	2	3	5
Migrainous stroke	4	1	5
CADASIL	0	2	2
Undetermined	10	14	24

Table 4. Diagnostic protocol in stroke young patients

Personal and familial history (cerebrovascular risk factors, previous venous and/or arterial events, migraine, oral contraceptives)
General and neurological examination
Laboratory blood tests
Brain CT/MRI
Carotid duplex and transcranial Doppler
Conventional cerebral angiography (23%)
Angio-MRI (25%)
TTE and TEE (78%)
Coagulation and immunological screening (protein C/S, antithrombin III, factor V/II mutation, APC resistance, antiphospholipid antibodies, ANCA, ANA) (85%)
Serological analysis (Chlamydia pneumoniae)

On suspicion of MELAS: serum and CSF lactate and pyruvate and skin and muscle biopsy

In many instances, our patients had multiple potential etiologies. For example, patients with a clear pathogenesis might have had other associated pathologies and conditions (use of oral contraceptives, pregnancy or postpartum state, history of migraine). We did not observe any cerebral ischemic event related to drug abuse or to AIDS, despite specific tests.

References

1. Bogousslavsky J, Pierre P (1992) Ischemic stroke in patients under 45. Neurol Clin 10: 113-124
2. Kristensen B, Malm J, Carlberg B et al (1997) Epidemiology and etiology of ischemic stroke in young adults aged 18 to 44 years in northern Sweden. Stroke 28:1702-1709
3. Caplan LR (1993) Stroke in children and young adults. In: Stroke. A clinical approach. 2nd edn. Butterworth-Heinemann, Boston, MA, pp 469-485
4. Carolei A, Marini C, Ferranti E et al (1993) A prospective study of cerebral ischemia in the young: analysis of pathogenic determinants. Stroke 24:362-367
5. Biller J (1994) Atherosclerotic cerebral infarction in young adults. In: Stroke in children and young adults. Butterworth-Heinemann, Boston, MA, pp 45-56
6. Cardiogenic brain embolism (1989) The second report of the Cerebral Embolism Task Force. Arch Neurol 46:727-743
7. Labovitz AJ, Pearson AC (1993) Cardiac masses and cardiac source of emboli. In: Transesophageal echocardiography: basic principle and clinical applications. Lea & Febiger, Philadelphia, London, pp 106-116
8. Lechat PH, Mas JL, Lascault G et al (1988) Prevalence of patent foramen ovale in young stroke patients. N Engl J Med 318:1148-1152
9. Ranoux D, Cohen A, Cabanes L et al (1993) Patent foramen ovale: is stroke due to paradoxical embolism? Stroke 24:31-34
10. Cabanes L, Mas JL, Cohen A et al (1993) Atrial septal aneurysm and patent foramen ovale as risk factors for cryptogenic stroke in patients less than 55 years of age. A study using transesophageal echocardiography. Stroke 24:1865-1873

11. Lucas C, Moulin T, Deplanque D et al (1998) Stroke patterns of internal carotid artery dissection in 40 patients. Stroke 29:2646-268

12. Bozzao L, Fantozzi LM, Bastianello S et al (1989) Occlusion of the extracranial internal carotid artery in the acute stroke; angiographic findings within six hours. Acta Neurochir (Wien) 100:39-42

13. Cook PJ, Honeybourne D, Lip GYH et al (1998) Chlamydia pneumoniae antibody titers are significantly associated with acute stroke and transient cerebral ischemia. The West Birmingham Stroke Project. Stroke 29:404-410

14. Hart RG, Kanter MC (1990) Hematological disorders and ischemic stroke. A selective review. Stroke 21:1111-1121

15. De Stefano V, Chiusolo P, Paciaroni K et al (1998) Prothrombin G20210A mutant genotype is a risk factor for cerebrovascular ischemic disease in young patients. Blood 91:3562-3565

16. Chaturvedi S, Dzieczkowski J (1998) Multiple hemostatic abnormalities in young adults with activated protein C resistance and cerebral ischemia. J Neurol Sci 159:209-212

17. Levine SR, Brey RL, Sawaya KL et al (1995) Recurrent stroke and thrombo-occlusive events in the antiphospholipid syndrome. Ann Neurol 38:119-124

18. Henderson GV, Kittner SJ, Johns DR (1997) An incidence study of stroke secondary to Melas in the young. Neurology 49:A439

19. Sabbadini G, Francia A, Calandriello L et al (1995) Cerebral autosomal dominant arteriopathy with subcortical infarcts and leukoencephalopathy (Cadasil): clinical, neuroimaging, pathological and genetic study of a large Italian family. Brain 118:207-215

20. Becker WJ (1997) Migraine and oral contraceptives. Can J Neurol Sci 24:16-21

21. Carolei A, Marini C, De Matteis G (1996) History of migraine and risk of cerebral ischaemia in young adults. Lancet 347:1503-1506

22. Headache Classification Committee of the International Headache Society (1998) Classification and diagnostic criteria for headache disorders, cranial neuralgias and facial pain. Cephalgia 8[Suppl 7]:13

23. Grosset DG, Ebrahim S, Bone I et al (1995) Stroke in pregnancy and puerperium: what magnitude of risk? J Neurol Neurosurg Psychiatry 58:129-131

24. Knepper LE, Giuliani MJ (1995) Cerebrovascular disease in women. Cardiology 86:339-348

25. Lindgren A, Brattstrom L, Norrving B et al (1995) Plasma homocysteine in the acute and convalescent phases after stroke. Stroke 6:795-800

26. Fieschi C, Rasura M, Anzini A et al (1996) A diagnostic approach to ischemic stroke in young and middle-aged adults. Eur J Neurol 3:324-330

TRAUMA OPERATIVE PROCEDURES

Update on Trauma Scoring

A.J. Sutcliffe

None of the trauma scores developed in the past 20 years have been entirely satisfactory with regard to their predictive powers. This is a reflection of the fact that scores are usually developed for a specific purpose such as predicting mortality. Subsequently, each score is tested for its ability to predict alternative outcomes. The diverse nature of injury patterns, varying probability of complications and different potential for recovery make it unlikely that a score developed for one purpose will be useful for another purpose. Before we can even begin to develop a trauma score with universal application we must define what we mean by severity and clarify what functions we wish the score to perform.

Anatomical injury severity

Many scores describe in anatomical terms a single injury, or various combinations of injury. The Abbreviated Injury Score (AIS) is an example. The AIS divides the body into six body compartments, and codes the injuries according to severity ranging from 1 (minor) to 6 (fatal). AIS codes are based on clinical experience rather than statistical evidence. At the time of its introduction, the AIS was an important step forward because it was the first score that was widely adopted and used for comparative research. Despite the subjective nature of the scoring system, there is a correlation between the increasing AIS grade of the most severe injury and mortality [1]. But, the AIS was flawed in two respects. First the same score in two different body areas did not necessarily mean that the injuries were comparable with respect to the risk of mortality or morbidity. This point is illustrated in Table 1. Second, the score did not allow for the cumulative effect on the risk of death of two or more injuries. Using a modified form of the AIS, the Injury Severity Score (ISS) was developed as a method for describing patients with multiple injuries and evaluating emergency care [1]. The ISS is the sum of the squares of the highest AIS grade in each of the three most injured body areas. An ISS of 16 or greater is classified as a major injury. The ISS method was much better at predicting mortality than AIS and superseded it as a research tool for comparing different treatment methods. However, even the first description of ISS acknowledged that age is a confounding factor. Mortality increases markedly in proportion to increasing age, particularly in patients with less severe injuries.

Table 1. AIS for two body regions

Score	Head	Chest
5	Brain stem contusion	Severe flail segment
4	Extradural haematoma < 100 ml	Lung laceration with haemothorax
3	Cerebral contusion	Pulmonary contusion
2	Coma < 1 hour	More than 1 rib fracture
1	No loss of consciousness	1 rib fracture

Physiological injury severity

Although AIS and ISS describe severity in terms of anatomical disruption, the score for each injury is often a reflection of the perturbation of physiological homeostasis caused by the injury. For example, a penetrating wound to the heart and severe cerebral contusion score highly and equally because the risk of physiological instability and death is great. A scoring system using physiological rather than anatomical parameters could be useful.

ISS and AIS are often assessed accurately only in retrospect which is not a problem for research or audit. In contrast a physiological score, which can be calculated immediately, is likely to be more useful for triage, helping doctors to communicate the effects of an injury at a given point in time and monitoring the effects of resuscitation and treatment. The Glasgow Coma Scale (GCS) score was one of the first physiological scores and was designed to describe the depth and duration of neurological impairment [2]. Despite its simplicity and universal acceptance, significant inter-observer variation has been demonstrated [3]. This is particularly true when the score is used for intubated patients and this is of concern because the GCS score is included as a component of more sophisticated trauma scoring methods which are used in treatment algorithms and for outcome prediction. In this respect, the work of Ross et al. [4] may be important. For the purposes of triage, the use of the motor component alone has been shown to be as effective as the entire score.

Global physiological derangement was measured first by means of the Trauma Score which described abnormalities of GCS, blood pressure, capillary refill, and respiratory effort and rate. As a triage score it worked reasonably well but its sensitivity and specificity were 80% and 75% respectively. This led to the development of the Revised Trauma Score (RTS).

The unweighted RTS shown in Table 2 is useful for triage but outcome is better predicted when the scores for the different physiological parameters are weighted in favour of GCS and blood pressure. Even better predictions of out-come are achieved when an anatomical score is used in conjunction with a phys-iological score.

Table 2. Revised trauma score

Score	GCS	SBP	RR
4	13 – 15	> 89	10 – 29
3	9 – 12	76 – 89	> 29
2	6 – 8	50 – 75	6 – 9
1	4 – 5	1 – 49	1 – 5
0	3	0	0

To weight score multiply scores for GCS x 0.9368, SBP x 0.7326 and RR x 0.2908. RTS = sum of weighted scores

Combined anatomical and physiological trauma scores

This is the methodology of the Trauma Research Injury Severity Score (TRISS). TRISS utilises the RTS, ISS, age and type of injury (blunt or penetrating) to pre-dict the probability of survival which is displayed on pre-scan charts [5]. The TRISS system includes the M statistic which allows comparison of the original study group with a new group in terms of the distribution and proportions of dif-ferent degrees of injury severity. If the groups are similar, the Z statistic can be used to compare mortality. The pre-scan charts are used to identify unexpected survivors and fatalities Figure 1. This is a crude technique because any fatality below the line indicating a probability of survival of 50% is classed as an unex-pected death. The TRISS and ISS systems may not be as reproducible as previ-ously thought [6]. Other important criticisms of TRISS are the arbitrary division of age, the fact that only the severest injury in a single body area is counted and the difficulty that equal weight is assigned to injuries in the six body regions. Also, no account is taken of the mechanism of injury. For example, TRISS poor-ly predicts mortality after low falls because although the injuries are often mi-nor, most low falls occur in the elderly who have a higher risk. A Severity Char-acterisation of Trauma (ASCOT) was developed to address these issues and is claimed to be a better predictor of mortality than TRISS [7].

Others have claimed that the relatively small gain in predictive accuracy is offset by the increased complexity of ASCOT over TRISS [8]. The story of the development of the TRISS and ASCOT methods illustrates the natural history of many methods of trauma scoring. First a simple score with reasonable predictive accuracy is described. Then others suggest refinements which improve the score's predictive power with regard to the original outcome measure or to im-prove its performance for prediction of alternative outcomes. The refinements

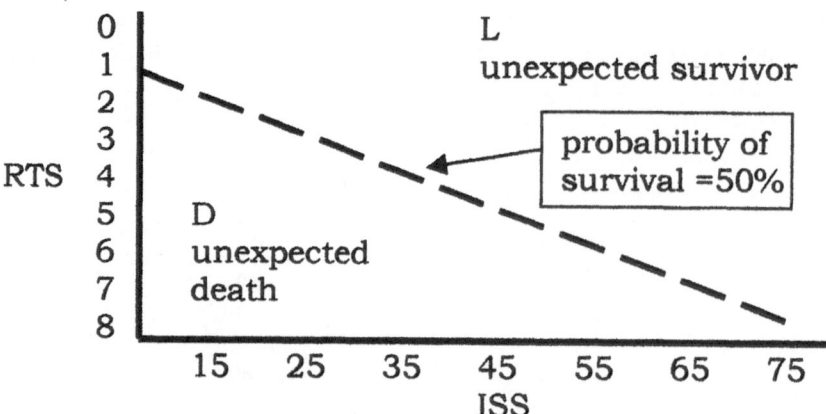

Fig. 1. Diagramatic representation of Prescan chart

usually involve the collection of additional data. The score then becomes difficult to use and labour intensive with regard to data collection and simplifications or alternatives are suggested.

For example, it has been suggested that ISS related to age may predict outcome as well as TRISS and be simpler to use [9]. Another alternative is the New ISS (NISS) which scores the three worst injuries regardless of body region and is believed to be a better predictor of short term mortality [10]. The International Classification of Diseases Severity Score (ICISS) is claimed to be as accurate as TRISS in predicting mortality [11]. An important feature of this method is that it uses ICD codes which are already collected routinely in many hospitals across the world.

Most trauma scores including ISS and TRISS fail to predict accurately hospital length of stay or resource utilisation. It is claimed that ICISS can successfully predict these [11]. It should not be a surprise that scores which accurately predict mortality do not necessarily predict morbidity. Consider a penetrating heart wound and cerebral contusion. They are very different when the healing process and potential for residual disability are considered.

Generic illness severity scores

The scores described so far have been developed specifically for trauma patients. There is evidence to suggest that, although trauma patients can be very expensive to care for, their outcome is usually good compared to patients in some other diagnostic groups. It would be helpful, therefore, if trauma patients could be compared to other patients using a score that was generally applicable.

The Apache II score is a physiological score which is used for intensive care patients. Rhee et al. [12] and McAnena et al. [13] disagree about the effectiveness of APACHE II for predicting outcome after trauma but both groups agree that the addition of an anatomical component to the APACHE II score adds to predictive accuracy.

At present, no score is completely satisfactory for predicting mortality, resource use or length of hospital stay. More importantly, if we wish to improve the quality of care we offer, we need a score which links injury severity to morbidity. This is an even more difficult task. Most people agree that the characteristics of an ideal scoring system would include the features listed in Figure 2.

Clear definitions of injury severity
Small inter observer error in assessment and coding
Simple data collection
High sensitivity and specificity for a range of outcome measures
Applicable for use before admission and in hospital
Applicable to trauma and other illnesses

Fig. 2. Characteristics of the ideal trauma score

It is unlikely that a single scoring system will be simple and yet meet all these requirements. Perhaps therefore, we should agree to develop a limited number of scores with predictive accuracy for a clearly defined set of outcomes such as those suggested in Figure 3.

A means of standardising descriptions of injury or describing injury severity for use as:
– a triage tool
– an audit tool
– a research tool
– a management tool
in order to compare groups of patients to aid clinical decision making, to compare different treatments, to predict mortality or morbidity, to estimate hospital length of stay or to estimate reimbursement costs

---

Fig. 3. Uses for trauma scores

References

1. Baker SP, O'Neill B, Haddon W et al (1974) The injury severity score: a method for describing patients with multiple injuries and evaluating emergency care. J Trauma 14:187-196
2. Teasdale G, Jennett B (1974) Assessment of coma and impaired consciousness. Lancet ii: 81-84
3. Buechler CM, Blostein PA, Koestner A et al (1998) Variations among trauma center's calculation of Glasgow Coma Scale Score: Results of a national survey. J Trauma 45:429-432
4. Ross E, Leipold C, Terregino C et al (1998) Efficacy of the motor component of the Glasgow Coma Scale in trauma triage. J Trauma 45:42-44
5. Boyd CR, Tolson MA, Copes WS (1987) Evaluating trauma care: the TRISS method. J Trauma 27:370-378
6. Zoltie N, de Dombal FT (1993) The hit and miss of ISS and TRISS. Br Med J 307:906-907
7. Champion HR, Copes WS, Sacco WJ et al (1996) Improved predictions from a severity characterization of trauma (ASCOT) over trauma and injury severity score (TRISS): results of an independent evaluation. J Trauma 40:42-49
8. Markle J, Cayten CG, Byrne DW et al (1992) Comparison between TRISS and ASCOT methods in controlling for injury severity. J Trauma 33:326-332
9. Bull JP, Dickson GR (1991) Injury scoring by TRISS and ISS/Age. Injury 21:127-131
10. Brenneman FD, Boulanger BR, McLellan BA (1998) Measuring injury severity: time for a change? J Trauma 44:580-582
11. Rutledge R, Osler T, Emery S et al (1998) The end of the Injury Severity Score (ISS) and the Trauma and Injury Severity Score (TRISS): ICISS, an International Classification of Diseases, ninth revision-based prediction tool outperforms both ISS and TRISS as predictors of trauma patient survival, hospital charges, and hospital length of stay. J Trauma 44:41-49
12. Rhee KJ, Baxt WG, Mackenzie JR et al (1990) Apache II scoring in the injured patient. Crit Care Med 18:827-830
13. McAnena OJ, Moore FA, Moore EE et al (1992) Invalidation of the Apache II scoring system for patients with acute trauma. J Trauma 33:504-507

Trauma Management: From the Field to the Emergency Department

G. Nardi, S. Di Bartolomeo, V. Michelutto

The goal of pre-hospital trauma care is to reduce mortality and morbidity by preventing the development of hypovolaemia, hypoxia, hypercapnia and acidosis, and to ensure, at the same time, the quickest access to a Centre of definitive care and to early surgery when needed.

Trauma is an extremely time-sensitive condition, therefore everything done to and for the patients in the pre-hospital setting must be measured against time. Patients involved in accidents in urban areas usually reach a well equipped hospital in a short time, thus limiting the need for pre-hospital stabilisation. On the contrary patients from rural areas more often need resuscitation and stabilisation on the scene and during transport to the hospital. In an attempt to improve the quality of pre-hospital care, in many health services, physicians, nurses and paramedics are trained to provide advanced life support (ALS) including tracheal intubation, decompression of tension pneumothorax and placement of i.v. lines for fluid resuscitation. Surprisingly there is only a limited number of studies addressing the efficacy of advanced field stabilisation and their results are often controversial. Most American studies [1] were unable to demonstrate any benefit of ALS on the scene, in terms of survival or reduction of hospital stay. In Europe, on the contrary, the large majority of people involved in trauma care strongly support the idea that pre-hospital advanced life support is of paramount importance in reducing mortality and morbidity from trauma. The results of the few available European studies demonstrate a clear benefit of ALS [2, 3]. Several reasons may contribute to explain the discrepancies in the results.

First of all, a high percentage of the authors who investigated the potential advantages of ALS over basic life support (BLS), included in their analysis both blunt and penetrating trauma. As clearly demonstrated by Lerer [4], the key to improve survival in penetrating injuries lies in rapid transportation by the quickest available means including private transportation. Pre-hospital stabilisation for patients with major injuries involving the heart or the large intrathoracic vessels is probably just a waste of time and ALS offers no advantage. On the contrary, many of the blunt trauma patients with multiple trauma due to road traffic accidents (RTA) require prolonged extrication. Prolongation of pre-hospital time without proper resuscitation increases the risk of secondary damage. To reduce study bias and to allow valid conclusions, blunt and penetrating injuries must be analysed individually.

Moreover, many of the investigations were carried on in urban areas where appropriate facilities can be reached in a reasonably short time. The results cannot therefore be easily extrapolated to extra-urban area where the transport time to a Trauma Centre is often prolonged.

However there may be a second and probably more likely explanation for the discrepancies in the conclusions about pre-hospital ALS. Although there is a widespread consensus on the traditional ABCD scheme for diagnosis and early treatment of trauma patients in the pre-hospital setting as well as in the Emergency Room, the same definition "advanced life support" is used as a label for manoeuvres and treatment protocols that are substantially different.

Airway and cervical spine protection

Prevention and treatment of hypoxaemia, hypercapnia, and inhalation is of utter importance in the multiple trauma patient in order to limit secondary injuries. Therefore, securing the airway and ensuring adequate ventilation is one of the most important steps. Endotracheal intubation is the procedure that can afford the best airway control and ventilation, but is an invasive procedure with potentially catastrophic complications. The decision to intubate injured patients at the scene is a difficult one. Intubation in trauma patients may be extremely difficult and an inadequate attempt to intubate may even worsen the injury. Opponents of field intubation claim that it can delay definitive care, increase intracranial pressure and that positive pressure ventilation can worsen shock through diminution of preload [5]. However in a study of over 1000 comatose head injury patients, endotracheal intubation in the field has been shown to significantly improve the outcome of patients with GCS < 9 [6].

Criteria for field intubation in trauma patients are still matter for discussion and they are related both to patient's clinical condition and to the experience of the operator. There is little doubt that general anaesthesia is required for the intubation of a comatose and/or hypoxic patient, who is often combative and has intact pharyngeal reflexes and who is potentially at risk of cranial hypertension. Many more skills than those for intubation of an unconscious, reflex-free patient in cardiac arrest are then expected from the rescue team. Moreover the absolute need to prevent undue movement of the cervical spine adds further difficulties to this procedure when applied to the multitraumatised patient. However field intubation has been proven effective also when performed by paramedics [7]. Effectiveness is still more evident when intubation is done by experienced physicians and is accompanied by other advanced procedures such as aggressive fluid therapy and drainage of tension pneumothorax.

As the aim of endotracheal intubation in the trauma patient is to prevent hypoxia, hypercapnia, and inhalation, indication and timing of field intubation may be summarised as follows: trauma patients must be intubated as the first step in case of apnoea and when the airway can not be made patent with less invasive ways. Intubation should be considered at step B (Breathing) in case of persisting and severe hypoxaemia ($SaO_2 < 85\%$) despite breathing O_2 at high concentration. In case of suspected pneumothorax, the decision whether to intubate before or after chest decompression should be made on the grounds of the degree of respiratory distress. In the patients with patent airways and who are not hypoxic criteria for intubation are based on the level of coma: most authors would agree that patients with GCS lower than 9 benefit from tracheal intubation and artificial ventilation. Moreover Oswalt [8] showed that a delay in tracheal intubation is associated with a mortality rate higher than predicted by the TRISS method also in trauma patients with a GCS lower than 13. In our experience the multiple trauma patients with GCS between 9 and 12 who were intubated on the scene before helicopter transport, had fewer complications than those who were not intubated, although the mortality rate was not significantly different. However a very high level of skills is mandatory in order to intubate on the scene these patients who are often quite reactive.

There are quite a few published data about field intubation in trauma patients and new contributions are extremely welcome. It has been suggested that the left lateral decubitus position affords a more rapid intubation and a better glottic visualisation than the classic kneeling position [9]. Anyway it is difficult to standardise this procedure when the best choice for each case varies greatly with the experience of the operator, the setting (entrapment), the clinical situation (shock, associated facial trauma), and the equipment available. A few points, though, must be kept firm. First of all, prevention of cord lesions due to cervical spine instability is mandatory.

Vilke [10] compared field intubations by nasotracheal route to rapid sequence induction orotracheal intubation and non-induced orotracheal intubation. In this study rapid sequence orotracheal intubation was associated with a higher success rate, fewer complications and a better patient outcome. Orotracheal intubation with manual on-line stabilisation has been proven to be safe in this regard [11] and superior to the nasotracheal route. However, the pre-hospital use of neuromuscular agents can be extremely dangerous in unskilled hands. Moreover an escape plan for failed intubation (e.g. cricothyroidotomy) must be mastered and valid equipment must be always available. For its lower success rate and potential of aggravating base-cranial fractures, nasotracheal intubation should be reserved to the cases in which direct laryngoscopy is impossible (e.g. entrapment).

Breathing

Priority number two after airway control and cervical spine protection is assuring proper ventilation in order to guarantee blood oxygenation and CO_2 removal. Patients who are severely hypoxic and dyspnoeic may benefit from the early onset of artificial ventilation. If the appropriate expertise is available they should be intubated on the scene after rapid sequence induction. Although artificial ventilation may improve oxygenation, positive pressure ventilation may be extremely harmful in case of pneumothorax, unless early recognition and effective treatment of this condition are assured.

Pneumothorax is one of the most frequent and life threatening complications of severe injuries involving the chest. Unrecognised tension pneumothorax is an important cause of preventable death and it is likely to be the most important one in intubated patients under artificial ventilation. Emergency Room AP chest X-ray has a low sensitivity in identifying post-injury pneumothorax and, in case of severe lung contusions or subcutaneous emphysema, a tension pneumothorax may easily be missed. It has been clearly stated that the diagnosis of tension pneumothorax must be made on clinical grounds and the emergency treatment must not be delayed by radiological investigations. The incidence of pneumothorax has not been well defined yet and this may account for a level of awareness lower than that needed. In a recent Italian epidemiological study, over 20% of the major trauma patients developed a unilateral or bilateral pneumothorax [12]. The prevalence of pneumothorax in patients with severe thoracic trauma (AIS $\geq$ 3) was as high as about 50%. In the majority of the cases, pneumothorax was treated by early decompression either on the scene or in the E.R. There are few doubts that emergency decompression of tension pneumothorax is a potentially life-saving procedure and that early detection and treatment of this condition is an important part of pre-hospital ALS strategies. However, once again, there are impressive differences in the percentage of trauma patients who are submitted to thoracic decompression by different ALS teams [13]. Much controversy exists regarding the use of tube thoracostomy in the treatment of a suspected tension pneumothorax in the field. Some authors reported an increased risk of complications after pre-hospital tube insertion with a high rate of malpositioning and up to 30% of organ injury rates [14]. Most of the unfavourable data, however, concern trocar thoracostomy for chest decompression. This technique has a high incidence of complications and must be avoided. Schmidt [15] reported that in a group of 63 trauma patients submitted to pre-hospital tube insertion through blunt dissection, there were no pleural infections and no intraparenchymal tube placements. However in 24% of the patients neither pneumothorax nor haemothorax could be confirmed on the scene and therefore tube thoracostomy turned out to be non-therapeutic. In this study indications for on-scene chest decompression included: decreased breath sounds, chest wall instability, subcutaneous emphysema, penetrating injuries to the chest. The protocol for chest decompression did not include needle decompression or explorative thoracentesis to confirm a suspected pneumothorax before thoracostomy. Tube thoracostomy is the standard treatment inside the hospital. The technique is not difficult to learn, though it does require a high level of skills to be safely performed on the scene. In an extremely interesting study, the group of the EHMS of the London

Royal Hospital, reported that 216 out of 3,113 trauma patients required roadside decompression of at least one pneumothorax [16]. The London group suggests that, in patients under positive pressure ventilation, a simple thoracotomy without insertion of any drainage tube is quicker and simpler and for trauma care carries important advantages.

According to the Italian Resuscitation Council's (IRC) guidelines [17], which have been endorsed by our group, patients presenting with hypoxaemia, hypotension and either subcutaneous emphysema or unilateral severe hypoventilation undergo an explorative thoracentesis on scene. If air under tension is observed, then thoracic decompression is performed. The pre-hospital use of little (2.2 mm $\emptyset$) drains introduced through a large bore needle has been used for several years to provide chest decompression in the field. Although this procedure is considered to be quick and acceptably safe in experienced hands, such a small drainage may not be adequate to treat pneumothorax caused by large pleural lacerations with massive air leak. Recently simple thoracotomy following the techniques suggested by the London group has been successfully introduced in our clinical practice. Although adequate skills are required to perform simple thoracotomy safely, the correct insertion of a chest tube at the roadside may require further experience, bring a non-negligible risk of complications, and add more logistic difficulties. Therefore delaying the insertion of a chest tube until the patient's arrival at the hospital is time saving and reduces complications. This approach is obviously reserved only to patients already intubated and artificially ventilated. Simple thoracotomy has been included in the IRC guidelines and recommended as the quickest and safest way to assure effective decompression of a tension pneumothorax in the field.

Circulation

Fluid administration has long been suggested to avoid hypotension and hypovolaemia, but recently this practice has been questioned. The first concern was raised by Kaweski [18] who, after analysing data from 6,855 patients concluded that mortality rate following trauma is not influenced by pre-hospital fluid administration. A more recent paper from Bickell [19] went further, demonstrating a better outcome in patients who did not receive any pre-hospital infusion. These conflicting results are probably caused by a lack of clear definition of trauma and by a dishomogeneous collection of data. Most of the negative studies concerned trauma patients with penetrating trauma. In penetrating trauma the importance of immediate access to surgery and the haemostatic effect of hypotension are well documented in animal models. The case of the hypotensive multitraumatised patient, who often has associated severe head trauma, is extremely different. The deleterious effect of hypotension in the head trauma patient has been unequivocally demonstrated. Brain injured patients who are hypotensive in the pre-hospital phase have a 15 times higher risk of an unfavourable outcome [20]. The administration of fluids to these patients does not increase intracranial pressure [21]. Updated therapeutic strategies complying with these findings have been established for pre-hospital care of head trauma patients with and without multiple injuries. The need to keep blood pressure high enough to assure brain perfusion despite the loss of autoregulation has been emphasised by the Brain Trauma Foundation guidelines for the management of severe head injury [22]. A systolic blood pressure (SBP) over 120 mmHg or a mean arterial pressure of more than 90 mmHg is considered as the pressure target also in the pre-hospital setting. Similar recommendations have been adopted in Europe [23], although a slightly lower level of SBP (110 mmHg) is accepted as a reasonable target.

The results of studies on penetrating trauma cannot be extrapolated to multiple trauma patients with or without head injury. Many of the lesions responsible for haemorrhage (bone fractures) are self tamponating and thus restoring blood volume and pressure cannot enhance blood losses. In case of haemorrhagic injuries into body cavities (haemoperitoneum, haemothorax) a compromise must be sought between the need to perfuse the organs and the theoretical risk of enhancing haemorrhages. Perfusion of organs is yet more important considering that in the multitraumatised patients access to hospital is often forcibly delayed (e.g. need for extrication) and, once in hospital, access to surgery cannot be as immediate as in penetrating trauma owing to the need for diagnostic procedures. Experimental data demonstrate a higher mortality rate in animals that received no fluid therapy. The best survival rate was achieved with an amount of crystalloids that was twice that of the blood loss [24].

It therefore seems reasonable to differentiate the approach to the hypotensive trauma patient according to the different kind of trauma. Head trauma patients require a higher level of blood pressure than blunt trauma victims who have no injury to the brain, and they will probably benefit from a more aggressive fluid resuscitation. Patients with penetrating injuries to the torso or the abdomen, on the contrary, should receive a limited infusion volume in order to avoid exsanguination. Table 1 shows the guidelines for pre-hospital fluid therapy in the trauma patient, inspired by the principles just described and approved by the Italian Resuscitation Council [18].

Table 1. A suggested differentiated approach to pre-hospital fluid therapy in multiple trauma

	Fluids
Multitraumatised (blunt) with head trauma	The minimum amount with the maximum speed to keep systolic blood pressure > 110 mmHg or mean blood pressure > 90 mmHg
Multitraumatised (blunt) without head trauma	The minimum amount with the maximum speed to keep systolic blood pressure > 90 mmHg
Penetrating trauma	The minimum amount with the maximum speed to keep systolic blood pressure > 70 mmHg

To be effective the infusions must match losses and this often requires large volumes. The maximum speed can be obtained only with flexible bags and pressurisers both of which are to be considered mandatory in the pre-hospital setting. The time-honoured recommendation of two large bore (14 G) i.v. cannulae cannot be overemphasised. Once the infusions are properly started the pursuit of the pressure goals takes place while doing all the other manoeuvres required and during transportation and must not delay access to definite care. If these suggestions are followed blood pressure can be effectively restored without unduly prolonging the pre-hospital time and with beneficial effects on outcome.

Much more controversy exists about the kind of fluids to use. Logistic problems (weight, space), speed of infusion, hypothermia are all factors that are bettered when fluids with the lowest volume for a given circulatory effect are used. Hypertonic solutions also have the theoretical advantage of reducing intracranial pressure and seem to reduce mortality in hypotensive traumatic brain injured patients [25]. No definitive conclusion, though, can be drawn from the present literature. Hypothermia in the multitraumatised patient is a well recognised problem and aggressive fluid resuscitation is an additional risk factor. The body temperature decreases 0.3°C for each litre of infusion at 20°C, much more if the infusions are colder. Therefore, whatever solutions are used, every effort must be made to keep them warm before infusing.

Is ALS effective?

To be effective in terms of reduction of mortality and morbidity the advanced life support manoeuvres, when indicated, have to be performed at the best level. Unfortunately this is often not the case. As an example, in Winchell's study [6] about 50% of trauma patients with GCS < 9 were not intubated by "ALS" teams of paramedics. Patients who were not intubated had a much higher mortality. Nevertheless all the patients were considered as having received advanced life support on the basis that they were treated by an ALS team.

Something similar seems to happen regarding pneumothorax. There are few available data about the frequency of pre-hospital chest decompression performed by an ALS team. Schmidt [13] reported a decompression rate of 0.5% in a series of severely injured patients rescued by an ALS team of paramedics and a rate 20 fold higher for patients with a comparable degree of injuries when rescued by surgeons. A decompression rate ranging around 10% was reported for other ALS teams staffed by skilled physicians [16].

Many studies on pre-hospital fluids reached the conclusion that fluid administration was ineffective in reducing trauma mortality. However in these studies the average amount of fluids administered to hypotensive trauma patients was by far too low to cause any benefit in terms of volaemia. These data, rather than demonstrating the inefficacy of field ALS, reveal an inadequate way of providing advanced care, probably unduly prolonging pre-hospital time.

Within the dispute about the efficacy of field ALS in trauma, there is indeed a problem of definition. Rescue by a so-called "ALS" team does not mean rescue through advanced life support manoeuvres, unless these are performed when indicated and in the right manner. So far very few studies have been performed to understand the impact on mortality and morbidity of "aggressive enough" advanced life support in trauma patients.

In a regional audit [2] on trauma care that enrolled all the victims of involuntary trauma over a population of 1.2 million people, we observed a highly significant reduction in mortality in the group of severe trauma patients rescued by the Emergency Helicopter Medical Service (EHMS) staffed with fully qualified anaesthesiologists in comparison with those rescued by ambulances carrying personnel trained in BLS. In the ALS group all head trauma patients with a GCS < 9 were intubated at roadside; 14% of the trauma victims required pre-hospital chest decompression and patients who were hypotensive on the scene received over 2,000 mls of fluids (colloids and crystalloids) before hospital arrival. In a more recent review of pre-hospital data concerning over 500 comatose trauma patients, the same EHMS team intubated 97% of the patients with a GCS < 9 and 67% of those with a GCS between 9 and 12 on the scene. Pre-hospital mortality for patients with major trauma found alive on the scene was as low as 1.5%.

A precise definition of the meaning of an "ALS strategy" in trauma care is of paramount importance.

In order to identify the best organisation of a pre-hospital trauma emergency service there is a strong need to define which ALS procedures, if any, are useful in the pre-hospital setting and which skills are therefore required. Data collection and quality assurance are also strongly needed.

References

1. Sampalis JS, Lavoie A, Williams JI et al (1993) Impact of on-site care, prehospital time and level of in-hospital care on survival in severely injured patients. J Trauma 34:(2)256-261
2. Nardi G, Massarutti D, Muzzi R et al (1994) Impact of emergency medical helicopter service on mortality for trauma in Nort-East Italy. A regional prospective audit. European J Emerg Med (1)69-77
3. Schuttler J, Schmitz B, Bartsh AC et al (1995) The efficiency of emergency therapy in patients with head-brain, multiple injury. Quality assurance in emergency medicine. Anaesthesist 44(12):850-858
4. Lerer LB, Knottenbelt JD (1994) Preventable mortality following sharp penetrating chest trauma. J Trauma 37(1)6-12
5. Pepe PE (1995) Resuscitation of the patient with major trauma. Current Opin Crit Care 1: 479-486
6. Winchell R, Hoyt DB (1997) Endotracheal intubation in the field improves survival in patients with severe head injury. Arch Surg 132:592-597
7. Frankel H, Rozycki G, Champion H et al (1997) The use of TRISS methodology to validate prehospital intubation by urban EMS providers. Am J Emerg Med 15:630-632

8. Oswalt JL, Hedges JR, Soifer BE (1992) Analysis of trauma intubations. Am J Emerg Med 10:6(511-514)
9. Adnet F, Lapostolle F, Boiron S et al (1997) Optimization of glottic exposure during intubation of a patient lying supine on the ground. Am J Emerg Med 15:1-3
10. Vilke GM, Hoyt DB, Epperson M et al (1994) Intubation techniques in the helicopter. J Emerg Med 12:(2)217-224
11. Criswell JC, Parr MJA (1994) Emergency airway management in patients with cervical spine injuries. Anaesthesia 49:900-903
12. Nardi G, Lattuada L, Scian F and the FVG Major Trauma Study Group (1999) Epidemiological study on high grade trauma 13 Min. Anest 65:6(348-352)
13. Schmidt U, Frame SB, Nerlich ML et al (1992) On-scene helicopter transport of patients with multiple injuries-comparison of a German and an American system. J Trauma 33;4:548-553
14. Baldt MM, Bankier AA, Germann PS et al (1995) Complications after emergency thoracotomy: assessment with CT. Radiology 195:539-543
15. Schmidt U, Stalp M, Gerich T et al (1998) Chest tube decompression of blunt chest injuries by physicians in the field: effectiveness and complications. J Trauma 44:98-101
16. Deakin CD, Davies G, Wilson A (1995) Simple thoracostomy avoids chest drain insertion in prehospital trauma. J of Trauma 39:373-374
17. Italian Resuscitation Council Trauma Committee (1998) Prehospital Trauma Care. IRC ed Compositori Bologna
18. Kaweski SM, Sise MJ, Virgilio RW (1990) The effect of prehospital fluids on survival in trauma patients. Journal of Trauma 30:1215-1218
19. Bickell WH, Wall MJ, Pepe PE (1994) Immediate versus delayed fluid resuscitation for hypotensive patients with penetrating torso injuries. N Engl J Med 331:1105-1109
20. Chestnut RM, Marshall LF, Klauber MR (1992) The role of secondary brain injury in determining outcome from severe head injury. J Trauma 34:216-222
21. Zornow MH, Prough DS (1995) Fluid management in patient with traumatic brain injury. New Horizon 3:488-493
22. Bullock R, Chestnut R, Clifton G (1996) Guidelines for the management of severe head injury. Brain Trauma Foundation, New York
23. Maas AIR (1996) Guidelines for management of severe head injury in adults. In: JL Vincent (ed) 1996 Yearbook of Intensive Care and Emergency Medicine. Springer, pp 707-715
24. Riddez L, Johnson L, Hahn RG (1998) Central and regional hemodynamics during crystalloid fluid therapy after uncontrolled intra-abdominal bleeding. J Trauma 44:433-439
25. Wade CE, Grady JJ, Kramer GC et al (1997) Individual patient cohort analysis of the efficacy of hypertonic saline/dextran in patients with traumatic brain injury and hypotension. J Trauma 42:S61-S65

Intensive Care for Trauma Patients: The First 24 Hours

M.J.A. PARR, J.P. NOLAN

Trauma patients in the Intensive Care Unit require all the complexities of modern day critical care. In an ideal world intensive care management of the seriously injured patient would start in the pre-hospital setting and continue until there was either no longer a requirement or continued treatment was considered to be futile. By definition, multi-trauma patients are critically ill from the time they receive their injuries. In some countries sophisticated pre-hospital intensive care is commenced at the scene by trained physicians but, more commonly, intensive care for trauma patients is commenced in the Emergency Department [1]. Once admitted to the Intensive Care Unit (ICU) several aspects of the continued resuscitation need to be addressed:

- physiological optimisation which requires monitoring and intervention;
- anatomic optimisation which requires continued assessment and planning of interventions including surgery;
- identification of all injuries to avoid missing injuries;
- prevention of late complications, particularly multiple organ failure.

The reasons for admitting trauma patients to an ICU are diverse and include:

- to allow continued airway protection (intubation) and controlled ventilation;
- continued resuscitation in an attempt to achieve appropriate haemodynamic goals. This may require the use of inotropes as well as fluids and blood products;
- the management of severe head injuries;
- the support of organs that are failing or that are likely to fail;
- to permit invasive monitoring that is not available at other hospital sites;
- to correct coagulopathy and major metabolic derangement;
- to permit active rewarming in those patients who are hypothermic;
- to provide a higher level of nursing care to high risk patients e.g. the elderly and those with serious co-morbidity.

Regardless of the indications for admission, the first priority is to repeat a systematic primary survey so that any new problems are detected rapidly. Resuscitation is performed simultaneously with the evaluation of:

- airway with continued cervical spine control if required;
- breathing with support of ventilation;
- circulation and control of haemorrhage;
- disability assessment and prevention of secondary neurological injury;
- exposure while controlling the environment to avoid hypothermia.

Continued intensive care involves identifying commonly missed injuries. Many of these will be minor but a number are potentially life-threatening and include spinal injury, rupture of the thoracic aorta, diaphragmatic rupture, delayed intracerebral haematoma and delayed intra-abdominal pathology.

Initial management in the ICU

Airway

Ensure the tracheal tube is secure and properly located in the trachea, above the carina. Ensure a gastric tube has also been inserted and is correctly positioned. If appropriate, continue cervical spine immobilisation (see below).

Breathing

Check ventilation to both sides of the chest and obtain a chest X-ray as soon as possible. Select an appropriate mode of ventilation and adequate minute ventilation. This will be modified by the presence of severe chest trauma, acute lung injury and severe brain injury. Adjust the inspired oxygen (FiO_2) to maintain the oxygen saturation (SaO_2) > 94%; adjust positive end-expiratory pressure (PEEP) to 5-10 cm H_2O, particularly if a high F_iO_2 (> 0.5) is required. Try to keep peak and mean inspiratory pressures as low as possible and ideally limit the peak inspiratory pressure to < 35 cm H_2O. Check arterial blood gases after each ventilatory adjustment.

Circulation and control of haemorrhage

Confirm adequate intravenous access. Most seriously injured patients will require a central venous catheter (preferably a triple-lumen catheter) both for monitoring and for drug infusions. In selected patients, a pulmonary artery catheter may be useful for estimation of cardiac output and to adjust therapy, however their routine use is probably unnecessary and may even be detrimental [2]. Central venous access may be difficult and, according to one systematic analysis, ultrasound guided vessel location and catheter placement improves success rates and decreases the complications associated with internal jugular and subclavian venous catheter placement [3]. An arterial catheter for monitoring blood pressure and repeat blood-gas analyses will be required in all intubated patients. Infuse warmed fluid until accepted haemodynamic goals (judged on an individual basis) are achieved. In general, these goals are: a mean arterial pressure (MAP) > 80 mmHg, heart rate < 110 beats per minute, central venous pressure (CVP) 10-12 mmHg, and urine output > 50 ml/h. Blood samples should be sent for urea and electrolyte analysis, full blood count, and coagulation studies. In the critically ill patient there is great debate on what haemoglobin concentration should be maintained. It should be sufficient to meet the oxygen delivery requirements of the tissues and often a figure of > 10 g/dl is selected. Lower levels may be tolerated by many patients, however, elderly patients and those with serious co-morbidities (particularly coronary artery disease) may need higher levels [4]. Coagulopathy is common in multi-trauma patients, particularly in association with massive transfusion [5, 6]. If the patient is still bleeding despite appropriate surgery, give platelets to maintain a count > 50 x 10^9/l, fresh frozen plasma (FFP) if the International Normalized Ratio (INR) is > 1.4, and cryoprecipitate if the fibrinogen is < 1 g/l. Keep the patient normothermic, as hypothermia will compound any coagulopathy [7]. There are a number of haemostatic drugs available [8] but none has been evaluated fully in multi-trauma patients. In the face of continued coagulopathy, and if all surgically correctable bleeding has been eliminated it may be reasonable to try these agents and there is anecdotal success attributed to the protease inhibitor, aprotinin (2 million units loading dose, followed by an infusion of 0.5 million units per hour) [9].

Great debate continues on the subject of how much and which fluid should be used in multi-trauma patients [10-14]. The recent discordant meta-analyses reaffirm the complexities of the issues and the difficulties in identifying cause and effect relationships in critically ill patients. Based on current, limited evidence, crystalloid resuscitation may be associated with a lower mortality in trauma patients but methodological limitations preclude any evidence-based recommendations and more study is needed.

Disability

Assess the conscious level of the patient and check the pupillary response to light. Trauma patients requiring intermittent positive pressure ventilation (IPPV) will need sedation and analgesia, ideally to a level at which they are asleep but respond to minor stimuli. Achieving the correct level of sedation and analgesia can be difficult and requires regular assessment and adjustment [15, 16]. Propofol is a particularly useful sedative for trauma patients in the ICU [17]. It is easily titratable, allowing fine control of consciousness, and recovery is rapid even after infusions of many days, which allows accurate evaluation of neurological status. Unlike etomidate, propofol does not impair steroidogenesis [18], and as long as care is taken to maintain cerebral perfusion pressure, it is an effective sedative for patients with serious head-injury [19]. The high cost of propofol prevents many from using it to sedate all patients. Less expensive alternatives include midazolam, and morphine.

Exposure and environment

The whole of the patient needs to be examined but care should be taken to prevent hypothermia (see below). Exposing and examining each region of the body in turn rather than simultaneously reduces unnecessary heat loss.

Evaluation of pre-existing disease (comorbidity)

Often the initial history from severe trauma patients is very limited, inaccurate or non-existent. After admission to the ICU, evidence of pre-existing disease is often revealed by information from third parties or after investigation. An accurate evaluation of comorbidity is very important because many chronic disease processes will have an impact on intensive care management and the outcome after major trauma. Pre-existing liver disease has a prevalence of 0.5% among all trauma patients and has been shown to increase mean duration of hospital stay by up to 36% and mortality by a factor of five [20]. The endocrine system plays a major role in the response to injury, surgery, and sepsis and endocrine dysfunction places the trauma victim at risk of greater morbidity and mortality [21]. Chronic renal disease is associated with fluid retention, electrolyte disturbances, anaemia, platelet dysfunction, malnutrition and, often, underlying disease such as diabetes, hypertension, and coronary artery disease. The mortality and morbidity of trauma increases when the victim has pre-existing renal disease [22]. Pre-existing pulmonary disease predisposes the patient to respiratory complications and further complicates their management [23]. Of all patients over 65 years old, 5.6% will have coronary artery disease [24].

Missed injuries: the secondary and tertiary survey

A detailed secondary survey (head-to-toe examination of the patient) would normally be completed in the Emergency Department but in the emergency situation it is not unusual to postpone this until life-threatening injuries have been dealt with. The risk then arises that the full secondary survey is not performed and injuries are missed. The signs of some injuries may take time to develop or become obvious and may also be missed on a secondary survey. For this reason, it has been suggested recently that a delayed, tertiary survey (within 24 hours) of the trauma patient should be routine practice [25]. In this study of 206 patients, 134 patients (65%) had 309 missed injuries composing 39% of all 798 injuries seen. The tertiary trauma survey detected 56% of early missed injuries and 90% of clinically significant missed injuries within 24 hours. The errors were mainly in clinical assessment and radiology and to a lesser extent were patient-related or technical. The missed injury rate was significantly higher in patients with multiple injuries and in those involved in road crashes. While many missed injuries were minor, clinically significant missed injuries occurred in 30 patients with complications in 11 patients and death in two patients.

Spinal injury

In unconscious trauma patients, there are inconsistencies in the approach to clearing the cervical spine and allowing the removal of immobilisation precautions. There is an over reliance on the lateral cervical spine view alone, which has been shown to be insensitive in this setting [26, 27]. Following significant blunt trauma, the patient's cervical spine cannot be cleared with absolute certainty until an appropriately qualified doctor (typically a senior surgeon) has checked the radiographs and has examined the fully conscious patient. If the whole of the cervical spine, including the C7-T1 junction can not be seen, or if the patient is not alert or has distracting injuries, full precautions should continue [28]. This approach in itself is associated with complications. Hard cervical collars can impair cerebral venous return, causing raised intracranial pressure [29]. Inadequate views on plain X-ray should be supplemented with CT scanning and recommendations for practice management have been published [30, 31]. Some clinicians advocate dynamic flexion and extension views of the cervical spine in unconscious patients [27]; this procedure should be undertaken by experienced clinicians only. While much attention has been paid to improving the diagnosis of cervical spine injuries, fractures of the thoracolumbar (TL) spine have received comparatively little attention. Reports have indicated that back pain and bony tenderness may be absent in some patients with fractures of the thoracolumbar spine which may lead to a delay in diagnosis and an increased risk of neurological damage [32]. Data suggest that patients who are awake, alert, and with no clinical evidence of injury do not require radiological study of the TL spine. Patients with equivocal or positive clinical findings or with altered levels of consciousness should have complete TL spine evaluation [33].

In recognition of the fact that traumatic brain and spinal cord injuries are the leading cause of death and disability for individuals under 50 years of age, the anticipation, prevention, and treatment of sequelae of spinal cord injury are being increasingly stressed [34-39]. In recent years the role of steroids in the early management of spinal cord injury has been evaluated. It is now common practice for cord injury patients to receive methylprednisolone as early as possible, ideally within 3 hours and for this to be maintained for 24 hours. When methylprednisolone is initiated 3 to 8 hours after injury, patients should be maintained on steroid therapy for 48 hours. Interestingly these studies suggest that patients who received the 48-hour regimen and who started treatment at 3 to 8 hours are more likely to improve one full neurological grade at 6 months. They are also likely to have more severe sepsis and pneumonia than patients in the 24-hour methylprednisolone group but similar other complications and mortality. The recommendations have been supported after 1 year follow-up studies [40, 41].

Traumatic rupture of the aorta

The thoracic aorta is at risk in patients sustaining significant deceleration (e.g., fall from a height or high speed road traffic accident). A widened mediastinum may have been overlooked on the original supine chest radiograph. This is a sensitive sign of aortic rupture but is not very specific [42]; 90% of widened mediastinums are due to venous bleeding. If possible an upright chest radiograph should be obtained. This will provide a clearer view of the thoracic aorta. Other signs suggesting rupture of the aorta are:

– wide mediastinum;
– pleural capping;
– left haemothorax;
– deviation of the trachea to the right;
– depression of the left mainstem bronchus;
– loss of the aortic knob;
– deviation of the nasogastric tube to the right;
– fractures of the upper 3 ribs;
– fracture of the thoracic spine.

If an aortic injury is suspected the patient will require an aortogram. A number of centres are now using helical CT and transoesophageal echocardiography to diagnose traumatic aortic ruptures [43-47], but because the sensitivity is more observer-dependent and the manifestations are often subtle, many clinicians still regard the aortogram as the "gold standard". Once a rupture of the thoracic aorta is confirmed, the patient's systolic blood pressure should be maintained at 80-100 mmHg systolic, in an effort to reduce the risk of further dissection or rupture. Beta-blockers (e.g., esmolol) are preferred; vasodilators will increase pulse pressure, which may increase shearing force [47]. The patient should be transferred immediately to the nearest cardiothoracic unit.

Myocardial contusion

The diagnosis of blunt cardiac injury can be suspected following an appropriate mechanism of injury [48, 49]. No single test or combination of tests has been shown to be consistently reliable for detection. Recent evidence based practice guidelines state that an ECG should be performed on admission of all patients who are suspected to have a blunt cardiac injury [31]. If the ECG is normal the risk of having a blunt cardiac injury is insignificant. If the admission ECG is abnormal the patient will require monitoring for at least 24 hours. Thus myocardial contusions resulting from blunt trauma may be detected simply and inexpensively using electrocardiography and careful physical examination. If there is any cardiovascular instability an echocardiogram (transthoracic or transoesophageal) should be obtained. Serum myocardial enzymes and radionuclide studies are non-specific and are not considered predictive of cardiac complications [50]. However, recent studies suggest that circulating cardiac troponin I [51, 52], but not troponin T [53], is of value for the diagnosis of myocardial contusion.

Abdominal injuries

Diaphragmatic rupture occurs in about 5% of patients sustaining severe blunt trauma, frequently to the abdomen rather than to the thorax. It can be difficult to diagnose, particularly when other severe injuries dominate the patient's management. Consequently, diaphragmatic rupture is often not detected until the patient has been admitted to intensive care. Approximately 75% of ruptures occur on the left side. The stomach or colon commonly herniate into the chest and strangulation of these organs is a risk. Diagnosis can sometimes be made on chest X-ray (elevated or loss of hemidiaphragm, gas bubbles above the diaphragm, shift of the mediastinum to the opposite side, nasogastric tube in the chest), particularly with the aid of barium. Once the patient has been stabilised, the diaphragm will require surgical repair. Delayed splenic/hepatic rupture is a rare complication but with the increasing role of conservative management of splenic haematomas it may become more common. Serial examination of haemoglobin and clinical examination of the abdomen supplemented by CT or ultrasound will be required. The introduction of Focused Assessment with Sonography for Trauma (FAST) allows a rapid non-invasive assessment for intra-abdominal free fluid and is likely to have an increasing role in the early identification of intra-abdominal injury [54-56].

Raised intra-abdominal pressure

The abdominal compartment syndrome is a possible result of raised intra-abdominal pressure (IAP) which is a common finding in critically injured trauma patients. A pressure > 20-25 cm H_2O may result in splanchnic ischaemia, renal failure, raised ICP and pulmonary abnormalities if not rapidly treated. The IAP can be reliably estimated from the measurement of bladder pressure via the urinary catheter. The technique is safe and easy and will direct interventions which may result in reduced morbidity and mortality [57, 58]. The presence of raised IAP will increase the need for decompressive surgery and temporary abdominal closures [59, 60].

Rhabdomyolysis

Massive skeletal muscle injury, whether caused by mechanical crush or indirect ischaemia, can result in life-threatening complications. The muscle damage results in high serum concentrations of cardiotoxic or nephrotoxic cations and metabolites (K, PO_4, myoglobin and urate). Hyperkalaemia and hypotension are the most immediate risks of death followed by myoglobinuric renal failure. The renal failure evolves from the combination of renal vasoconstriction, nephrotoxicity, and tubular obstruction by myoglobin plugs and urate. Management includes aggressive intravenous volume replacement followed by mannitol-alkaline diuresis and the use of dialysis when necessary. Diagnosing abdominal compartment syndrome and rhabdomyolysis on a clinical basis is very difficult in the multi-trauma patient. Aggressive, prophylactic fasciotomy may well be indicated and careful monitoring and management of creatine kinase levels will be required [61, 62].

The systemic inflammatory response syndrome

Severe trauma is a potent cause of the systemic inflammatory response syndrome (SIRS [63]), the diagnostic features of which are:
- temperature > 38°C or < 36°C;
- heart rate > 90 beats/min;
- respiratory rate > 20 breaths/min or $PaCO_2$ < 4.3 kPa;
- WBC > 12,000 cells/mm^3, < 4000 cells/mm^3, or > 10% immature (band) forms.

If infection is confirmed, the same diagnostic features define sepsis. A complication of SIRS is the development of "multiple organ dysfunction syndrome" (MODS) which is defined as the "presence of altered organ function in an acutely ill patient such that homeostasis cannot be maintained without intervention" [63]. Crushed and wounded tissues activate complement which in turn triggers a cascade of inflammatory mediators [C3a, C5a, tumour necrosis factor-α (TNF-α), interleukin (IL) 1, IL-6, and IL-8] [64-67]. Large numbers of polymorphonuclear neutrophils (PMNs) are released from bone marrow and depending on the presence of various modulators, the PMNs adhere tightly to endothelium and migrate into the surrounding parenchyma where they are activated to release superoxide anion (O_2^-) [68] and elastase [65]. This inflammatory response plays a key role in the development of acute respiratory distress syndrome (ARDS) and MODS. Although infection may also play a role subsequently, up to 50% of the patients developing organ failure early after trauma, do so in the absence of bacterial infection [66]. Trauma patients developing renal failure as part of MODS will require early renal replacement therapy [typically continuous veno-venous haemodiafiltration (CVVHD)]. As a result of the hypercatabolism associated with severe trauma, these patients have rapidly rising plasma creatinine and urea levels.

Further aims of intensive care are to reduce the incidence of complications, particularly sepsis, multiple organ failure/multiple organ dysfunction syndrome (MODS), acute lung injury (ALI)/acute respiratory distress syndrome (ARDS), acute renal failure, and thromboembolism. To reduce these complications, strategies include early fracture fixation, goal directed therapy, early enteral feeding, immunomodulation, infection control and thromboprophylaxis. While the interventions can be both risky and expensive, the excellent outcome for many of these patients justifies the continued commitment.

References

1. Svenson J, Besinger B, Stapczynski JS (1997) Critical care of medical and surgical patients in the ED: length of stay and initiation of intensive care procedures. Am J Emergency Med 15:654-657
2. Connors AF Jr, Speroff T, Dawson NV et al (1996) The effectiveness of right heart catheterization in the initial care of critically ill patients. JAMA 276:889-897
3. Randolph AG, Cook DJ, Gonzales CA, Pribble CG (1996) Ultrasound guidance for placement of central venous catheters: a meta-analysis of the literature. Crit Care Med 24:2053-2058
4. Hebert PC, Wells G, Blajchman MA et al (1999) A multicenter, randomized, controlled clinical trial of transfusion requirements in critical care. Transfusion Requirements in Critical Care Investigators, Canadian Critical Care Trials Group. N Engl J Med 340:409-417
5. Horsey PJ (1997) Multiple trauma and massive transfusion. Anaesthesia 52:1027-1029
6. Parker RI (1997) Etiology and treatment of acquired coagulopathies in the critically ill adult and child. Crit Care Clin 13:591-609
7. Patt A, McCroskey BL, Moore EE (1988) Hypothermia-induced coagulopathies in trauma. Surg Clin North Am 68:775-785
8. Mannucci PM (1998) Hemostatic drugs. N Engl J Med 339:245-253
9. Valentine S, Williamson P, Sutton D (1993) Reduction of acute haemorrhage with aprotinin. Anaesthesia 48:405-406
10. Hambly PR, Dutton RP (1996) Excess mortality associated with the use of rapid infusion system at level 1 trauma center. Resuscitation 31:127-133
11. Schierhout G, Roberts I (1998) Fluid resuscitation with colloid or crystalloid solutions in critically ill patients: a systematic review of randomised trials. BMJ 316:961-964
12. Human albumin administration in critically ill patients: systematic review of randomised controlled trials by the Cochrane Injuries Group Albumin Reviewers (1998) BMJ 317:235-240
13. Choi PT, Yip G, Quinonez LG, Cook DJ (1999) Crystalloid vs. colloid in fluid resuscitation: a systematic review. Crit Care Med 27:200-210
14. Nolan J (1999). Fluid replacement. In: Yates D (ed) Trauma: the science of success. Br Med Bull 55 (in press)
15. Carroll KC, Atkins PJ, Herold GR et al (1999) Pain assessment and management in critically ill postoperative and trauma patients: a multisite study. Am J Crit Care 8:105-117
16. Park GR (1997) Sedation, analgesia and muscle relaxation and the critically ill patient. Can J Anaesthesia 44:R40-R51
17. Beller JP, Pottecher T, Lugnier A et al (1988) Prolonged sedation with propofol in ICU patients: recovery and blood concentration changes during periodic interruptions in infusion. Br J Anaesth 61:583-588
18. Aitkenhead AR, Pepperman ML, Willatts SM et al (1989) Comparison of propofol and midazolam for sedation in critically ill patients. Lancet 2:704-709

19. Farling PA, Johnston JR, Coppel DL (1989) Propofol infusion for sedation of patients with head injury in intensive care. Anaesthesia 44:222-226
20. Gomez GA, Jacobson LE, Asensio JA, Nauta RJ (1994) Pre-existing liver disease in the trauma patient. Crit Care Clin 10:555-566
21. Boulanger BR, Gann DS (1994) Management of the trauma victim with pre-existing endocrine disease. Crit Care Clin 10:537-554
22. Cachecho R, Millham FH, Wedel SK (1994) Management of the trauma patient with pre-existing renal disease. Crit Care Clin 10:523-536
23. O'Brien GM, Criner GJ (1994) Chronic pulmonary disease in the trauma patient. Crit Care Clin 10:507-522
24. Wilson RF (1994) Trauma in patients with pre-existing cardiac disease. Crit Care Clin 10:461-506
25. Janjua KJ, Sugrue M, Deane SA (1998) Prospective evaluation of early missed injuries and the role of tertiary trauma survey. J Trauma 44:1000-1006
26. Gupta KJ, Clancy M (1997) Discontinuation of cervical spine immobilisation in unconscious patients with trauma in intensive care units - Telephone survey of practice in south and west region. BMJ 314:1652-1655
27. Lockey AS, Handley R, Willett K (1998). "Clearance" of cervical spine injury in the obtunded patient. Injury 29:493-497
28. Woodring JH, Lee C (1993) Limitations of cervical radiography in the evaluation of acute cervical trauma. J Trauma 34:32-39
29. Raphael JH, Chotai R (1994) Effects of cervical collar on cerebrospinal fluid pressure. Anaesthesia 49:437-439
30. Mirvis SE, Shanmuganathan K (1995) Imaging of acute cervical spine trauma. J Intens Care Med 10:15-33
31. Pasquale M, Fabian TC (1998) Practice management guidelines for trauma from the Eastern Association for the Surgery of Trauma. J Trauma 44:941-956
32. Meek S (1998) Lesson of the week: fractures of the thoracolumbar spine in major trauma patients. BMJ 317:1442-1443
33. Durham RM, Luchtefeld WB, Wibbenmeyer L et al (1995) Evaluation of the thoracic and lumbar spine after blunt trauma. Am J Surg 170:681-684
34. Chiu WT, Liu A, Chen SY (1995) Recent developments in the management of spinal cord injuries. Curr Opin Crit Care 1:494-502
35. Gimenez Y, Ribotta M, Privat A (1998) Biological interventions for spinal cord injury. Curr Opin Neurol 11:647-654
36. el Masry WS, Short DJ (1997) Current concepts: spinal injuries and rehabilitation. Curr Opin Neurol 10:484-492
37. Faden AI (1997) Therapeutic approaches to spinal cord injury. Advances in Neurology 72:377-386
38. McBride DQ, Rodts GE (1994) Intensive care of patients with spinal trauma. Neurosurg Clin North America 5:755-766
39. Marion DW (1998) Head and spinal cord injury. Neurologic Clinics 16:485-502
40. Bracken MB, Shepard MJ, Holford TR et al (1997) Administration of methylprednisolone for 24 or 48 hours or tirilazad mesylate for 48 hours in the treatment of acute spinal cord injury. Results of the third national acute spinal cord injury randomized controlled trial. National acute spinal cord injury study. JAMA 277:1597-1604
41. Bracken MB, Shepard MJ, Holford TR et al (1998) Methylprednisolone or tirilazad mesylate administration after acute spinal cord injury: 1-year follow up. Results of the third national acute spinal cord injury randomized controlled trial. J Neurosurg 89:699-706
42. Maggisano R, Cina C (1990) Traumatic rupture of the thoracic aorta. In: McMurty RY, McLellan BA (eds) Management of blunt trauma. Williams & Wilkins, Baltimore, pp 206-226
43. Smith MD, Cassidy JM, Souther S et al (1995) Transesophageal echocardiography in the diagnosis of traumatic rupture of the aorta. N Eng J Med 332:356-362

44. Goarin JP, Catoire P, Jacquens Y et al (1997) Use of transesophageal echocardiography for diagnosis of traumatic aortic injury. Chest 112:71-80
45. Durham RM, Luchtefeld WB, Wibbenmeyer L et al (1994) Computed tomography as a screening exam in patients with suspected blunt aortic injury. Ann Surg 220:699-704
46. Fabian TC, Richardson D, Croce MA et al (1997) Prospective study of blunt aortic injury: multicenter trial of the American Association for the Surgery of Trauma. J Trauma 42:374-383
47. Fabian TC, Davis KA, Gavant ML et al (1998) Prospective study of blunt aortic injury. Helical CT is diagnostic and antihypertensive therapy reduces rupture. Ann Surg 227:666-677
48. Pretre R, Chicott M (1997) Blunt trauma to the heart and great vessels. N Eng J Med 336: 626-632
49. Roxburgh JC (1996) Myocardial contusion. Injury 27:603-605
50. Christensen MA, Sutton KR (1993) Myocardial contusion: new concepts in diagnosis and management. Am J Crit Care 2:28-34
51. Edouard AR, Benoist JF, Cosson C et al (1998) Circulating cardiac troponin I in trauma patients without cardiac contusion. Intensive Care Med 24:569-573
52. Adams JE 3rd, Davila-Roman VG, Bessey PQ et al (1996) Improved detection of cardiac contusion with cardiac troponin I. Am Heart J 131:308-312
53. Ferjani M, Droc G, Dreux S et al (1997) Circulating cardiac troponin T in myocardial contusion. Chest 111:427-433
54. Smith RS (1997) The focused abdominal ultrasound examination for trauma. Curr Opin Crit Care 3:455-459
55. Schuster-Bruce M, Nolan J (1999) Priorities in the management of blunt abdominal trauma. Curr Opin Crit Care 4 (in press)
56. Scalea TM, Rodriquez A (1999) Focused assessment with sonography for trauma (FAST): results from an international consensus conference. J Trauma 46:466-472
57. Ivatury RR (1997) Abdominal compartment syndrome. Curr Opin Crit Care 3:443-447
58. Nathens AB, Boulanger BR (1998) The abdominal compartment syndrome. Curr Opin Crit Care 4:116-120
59. Sugrue M, Jones F, Janjua KJ et al (1998) Temporary abdominal closure: a prospective evaluation of its effects on renal and respiratory physiology. J Trauma 45:914-921
60. Harman PK, Kron IL, McLachlan HD et al (1982) Elevated intra-abdominal pressure and renal function. Ann Surg 196:594-597
61. Brumback RA, Feeback DL, Leech RW (1995) Rhabdomyolysis following electrical injury. Seminars in Neurology 15:329-334
62. Abassi ZA, Hoffman A, Better OS (1998) Acute renal failure complicating muscle crush injury. Seminars in Nephrology 18:558-565
63. American College of Chest Physicians/Society of Critical Care Medicine Consensus Conference (1992) Definitions for sepsis and organ failure and guidelines for the use of innovative therapies in sepsis. Crit Care Med 20:864-874
64. Roumen RMH, Hendriks T, Ven van der-Jongekrijg J et al (1993) Cytokine patterns in patients after major vascular surgery, hemorrhagic shock and severe blunt trauma. Relation with subsequent adult respiratory distress syndrome and multiple organ failure. Ann Surg 218:769-776
65. Roumen RMH, Redl H, Schlag G et al (1995) Inflammatory mediators in relation to the development of multiple organ failure in patients after severe blunt trauma. Crit Care Med 23: 474-480
66. Waydhas C, Nast-Kolb D, Jochum M et al (1992) Inflammatory mediators, infection, sepsis, and multiple organ failure after severe trauma. Arch Surg 127:460-467
67. Donnelly TJ, Meade P, Jagels M et al (1994) Cytokine, complement, and endotoxin profiles associated with the development of the adult respiratory distress syndrome after severe injury. Crit Care Med 22:768-776
68. Botha AJ, Moore FA, Moore EE et al (1995) Early neutrophil sequestration after injury: a pathogenic mechanism for multiple organ failure. J Trauma 39:411-417

Intensive Treatment of the Patient with Hepatic Trauma

B. KREMŽAR, A. ŠPEC-MARN

Injury to the liver is suspected in all patients with penetrating or blunt trauma that involves the lower chest and upper abdomen. Numerous analyses have shown that isolated liver injury with the exception of severe injury is relatively unimportant as a cause of death or serious complications. Results have demonstrated that the pattern of associated organ injuries is a major determinant of complications and of the ultimate outcome of patients with hepatic injuries. Severe blunt brain trauma is the most important associated injury seen in conjugation with blunt hepatic trauma [1].

In general, death from liver injury can be divided into two groups. The mortalities that occur within the first 24-48 hours are largely due to uncontrolled bleeding as a result of the initial injury, but uncorrectable coagulopathy as a result of inadequate resuscitation, hypothermia, acidosis and dilutional effects may complicate surgical hemorrhage. The single most important factor influencing late death after liver trauma is the development of intra-abdominal sepsis.

Intensive therapy of patients with hepatic trauma should be started as soon as possible to prevent the development of several complications [2].

The pathophysiology of hepatic dysfunction

Under normal circumstances, the liver has a very limited level of auto-regulation of blood flow and the centrilobular area is at a watershed of blood flow and oxygen availability. In situations of low oxygen delivery, oxygen availability to many tissues is reduced but in particular to the cells towards the center of the liver lobules.

Hepatic blood flow is approximately 100 ml/min per 100 g, and represents about 25% of cardiac output. The liver is supplied by two large vessels: the hepatic artery and the portal vein. The hepatic artery carries only 20% of the total blood flow passing to the liver but it provides up to 45-50% of hepatic oxygen supply. The portal vein provides 75% of the total hepatic blood flow and only 50-55% of the hepatic oxygen supply. Portal venous blood is partially deoxygenated in the preportal organs and tissues (stomach, intestines, spleen and pancreas) and it is rich in nutrients (provides 80% of nutrient requirements) and other substances absorbed by the gastrointestinal tract [3].

The liver vasculature plays a vital role as a blood reservoir and it is mainly mediated by the sympathetic nervous system. During hemorrhage the liver may deliver out up to 500 ml of blood to the systemic circulation. It is known that relatively mild hypovolemia, with a loss of only 10% of circulating volume results in a 40% reduction in splanchnic blood, subsequently causing tissue hypoxia [3]. Direct hepatic injury, shock, hepatic venous stasis and/or hypoxemia will constitute additional insults to the liver parenchyma. All these factors are responsible for triggering and initiating pathologic mechanisms which lead to hepatic ischemia. The low-flow ischemic insult to the liver results in a depletion of cellular energy stores, altered cellular homeostasis, and ultimately, failure of cellular energy function. Even when reperfusion is initiated, liver failure occurs.

Reperfusion of tissue after a period of ischemia is known to show signs of accentuated vascular and endothelial injury. Activated neutrophils and oxygen radicals formed by xanthine oxidase have been suggested to play a major pathogenetic role in a variety of inflammatory reactions associated with ischemia-reperfusion injury by deterioration of the microvascular blood flow. It has been proved that besides ischemic trauma to hepatic tissue further cellular damage occurs during the phase of reperfusion which might explain the deterioration of liver function in spite of successful resuscitation. Colletti et al. observed that local expression of hepatic epithelial neutrophil activating protein produced in response to TNF-α is an important mediator of the local neutrophil-dependent hepatic injury associated with hepatic ischemia-reperfusion injury [4].

Recent observations showed an improvement in hepatic macro- and microhemodynamics, as well as in survival rates after warm ischemia of the liver following treatment with N-acetylcysteine, a glutathione precursor. Glutathione is an important cellular defense against oxidative stress. N-acetylcysteine given after ischemia is effective in replenishing depleted glutathione stores, improving glutathione homeostasis, ameliorating bile output (ATP regeneration), and increasing survival [5, 6].

Consequences of hepatic dysfunction

It is believed that alterations in liver function may adversely affect the overall response of hospitalized patients to critical illness and trauma. Some authors have even suggested that the liver is the pivotal organ which determines the adequacy of the stress response. Following hemorrhagic shock, bacterial translocation to the mesenteric lymphatics and portal vein may occur. Liver with impaired function cannot resist the invasion of translocated bacteria and endotoxins, which then subsequently enter the systemic circulation. In addition to being a potential source of infection, this bacterial translocation appears to serve as a trigger for the release of cytokines and other cellular mediators that may, in turn, activate or further perpetuate the inflammatory and hypermetabolic response to injury. Thus, besides gut dysfunction, impaired liver function may play a major role in the initiation and propagation of a systemic inflammatory response and multiple organ failure [7].

Apart from the direct effect of endotoxins on hepatocytes, they may also activate Kuppfer cells to release mediators with specific effects on hepatocyte metabolism synthesis. Tumor necrosis factor (TNF) and interleukins inhibit albumin synthesis and increase synthesis of acute-phase proteins. They also decrease the concentration of zinc in blood, which is then transported into the liver cells where it is utilized for liver regeneration. When liver function is impaired, drug metabolism is also changed.

Severe liver injury is almost always associated with severe blood loss with consequent inadequate oxygen delivery (DO_2) and oxygen consumption ($\dot{V}O_2$) which leads to tissue hypoxia. Mixed venous O_2 saturation (SvO_2) is the best indicator, easily available, of the balance between oxygen supply and oxygen demand [8]. In spite of this conclusion, it is known for years that a normal SvO_2 should not be considered as a sole criteria to insure optimal DO_2 in critically ill patients, because a flow-limited regional oxygen consumption may potentially exist despite the presence of a normal SvO_2 [9]. Dahn et al. performed a study on the influence of hepatic venous oxygen saturation ($ShvO_2$) on the synthetic response of the liver to metabolic stress. They found that various hepatic processes are affected differentially by stress conditions and flow alterations that may exist during critical illness. It was concluded that regional venous oximetry may play an important role in detection of hepatic functional impairment [10].

Intensive therapy

After surgery, a patient's treatment is continued in the intensive care unit (ICU), where efforts are made to protect and to support liver function. This can be achieved by prevention or adequate treatment of most important early and late complications and by continuous monitoring of liver function [11].

Mechanical ventilation

The remaining part of liver parenchyma after injury is very susceptible to hypoxia. This is why we keep the patient on a ventilator for at least 24 hours. For sedation we use midazolam as the analgetic-fentanyl. The parameters of controlled ventilation should be carefully selected in order to avoid an unnecessary intrathoracic pressure increase which may impede venous return, thereby decreasing cardiac output. Reduced CO as well as arterial hypotension should be avoided. For the same reason we should be careful with PEEP especially if the patient is dehydrated. Other important factors which may have an influence on the reduction of total liver blood flow are hypocapnia and vasoactive agents. Hypocapnia might be iatrogenic if the patient is mechanically hyperventilated.

Vasoactive agents

The effect of vasoactive agents on hepatic blood flow is determined by the innervation and adrenoreceptor population of the hepatic vasculature. Hepatic arteries have α-adrenergic constrictor, β-2 dilator, and DP-dilator receptors. The portal vein has only α-adrenergic constrictor receptors. Dobutamine can selectively increase gastric mucosa blood flow (+ 77%) with only a 10% increase in CI, suggesting a vasodilating effect of dobutamine on gastric circulation. The combination norepinephrine-dobutamine is superior (increase in pHi and hepato-splanchnic blood flow, decrease in lactate) to epinephrine, while addition of dopamine (low dose) to norepinephrine makes it possible to increase splanchnic blood flow [12].

Regulation of body temperature

After the operation, patients are quite often hypothermic. Besides heat loss during the massive transfusion of cold blood and fluids, we should also take into account enormous heat loss during long surgical procedures with open abdominal cavity, as a cause of hypothermia and suppressed hepatic thermogenesis. This is sometimes the reason for prolonged postoperative hypothermia which exists in spite of routine preventive and therapeutic measurements.

Hypothermia is known to prolong the prothrombin time ratio and the partial thromboplastin time ratio. Hypothermia induces a qualitative platelet dysfunction. Hypothermia may cause severe arrhythmia, compromising cardiac function and leading to acidosis.

Patients often shiver in an attempt to produce heat. Shivering can increase oxygen consumption to as much as five times normal level [13]. Hypokalemia is often observed in association with postoperative hypothermia necessitating caution in administration of $NaHCO_3$, insulin, calcium (they move K^+ into cells) or digitalis. Lethal dysrhythmias may occur in this setting.

Hypothermia can be prevented by taking aggressive measures toward heat conservation. The greatest heat loss takes place in the first hour of anesthesia probably as a result of exposure, prepping and peripheral vasodilatation during induction. A drop in body temperature as much as 1.3°C during the first hour of anesthesia has been noted in elective surgical patients. It is important to institute preventive measures early enough to achieve success. The most important measures are:

– operating room temperature above 21°C

– humidification and warming of inspired gases

– use of blood and fluids warmers

– use of heating blanket

In ICU, warming is continued with administration of warm fluids and blood products. Large volumes of coagulation factors should be reserved until after the hypothermia has been corrected.

Fluid and electrolyte management

The assessment of fluid loss during the operation is quite difficult even with the measurements of CVP and PWP with Swan-Ganz catheter. This is why we should pay special attention during the early postoperative period to balance the fluids and electrolytes. First two days after the surgery or trauma, the patient should be in positive fluid balance, because of great sequestration of fluids into the third space. Between the third and fifth days an inverse reaction is expected, therefore we should be very careful not to overload the patient. We must reduce the load of fluids.

Routine control of electrolytes and acid-base status is necessary even several times per day. As has already been mentioned, hypokalemia and metabolic acidosis are mostly present immediately after the admission of the patient into ICU. With the correction of acidosis we should be very careful, especially if the patient is hypothermic and hypokalemic. In addition, the subsequent occurrence of metabolic alkalosis is possible as the consequence of citrate turnover into bicarbonate after massive transfusion.

Alkalosis is very dangerous because the unload of oxygen to tissues is diminished as a result of the shift in oxyhemoglobin dissociation curve to the left. Alkalosis is also difficult to correct. This is why metabolic acidosis should be corrected carefully.

Nutritional support

Nutritional support for patients with liver resection or hepatic trauma is of the utmost importance since the liver requires adequate nutrition for regeneration. It is important to start with enteral nutrition as soon as possible because of its beneficial effect on hepatic function. In fact, enteral nutrition protects abdominal organs from ischemic injury by increasing mesenteric blood flow, diminishes the invasiveness of gut bacteria, improves gut mass, decreases bacterial translocation, improves survival, decreases hypermetabolism, protects the liver from injury during shock, improves protein synthesis and increases the rate of wound healing [14]. Taken into account that nutrition is considered part of the prevention and therapy of liver insufficiency after liver trauma, one should carefully consider the use of specialized nutritional substrates because substrate intolerance may result from the central metabolic role of the liver. The goal of nutritional support for the patient after liver trauma should be to provide for the increased catabolic needs with substances that cause minimal complications.

The patients should be carefully and fully assessed before beginning any nutritional intervention [15]. Otherwise the patient requires:

- 35-40 kcal/kg day (non protein)
- 25-40% should be provided as fat
- no more than 5 mg/kg min glucose
- maintain blood glucose level at less than 200 mg/dl (11.7 mM)
- supplement insulin if necessary
- if hypertriglyceridemia develops, administer lipids once a week to avoid essential fatty acid deficiency
- maintain positive nitrogen balance
- in severe hepatic failure, use solutions with high branched-chain and low aromatic amino acid contents

The liver is chief regulator of carbohydrate metabolism through:

- glycogenesis
- glycogenolysis
- gluconeogenesis

Insulin and glucagon are of major importance in this regulatory process because the liver degrades both these hormones.

We administer up to 150 g glucose as a 5% or 10% solution in continuous infusion in 24 hours, for the first two days because of these reasons:

- the liver parenchyma which is not injured should not be overloaded;
- paradoxical hypoglycemia can occur because of increased secretion of insulin and decreased degradation by insufficient liver function. That should be especially expected after resection of greater than 70% of liver parenchyma. Besides the insulin and glucagon involved in hypoglycemia the proposed etiology of hypoglycemia involves both glycogen depletion and decreased gluconeogenesis.

The most clinically significant metabolic problems associated with hepatic failure involve protein metabolism. Protein synthesis is depressed because of the reduction of hepatic parenchyma. The liver participates in the:

- deamination of amino acids
- formation of urea for removal of ammonia
- formation of plasma proteins
- transamination

Amino acids normally metabolized by the liver (methionine, glutamine) and aromatic amino acids (tryptophan, phenylalanine and tyrosine), accumulate in hepatic insufficiency while branched-chain amino acid (BCAA) levels are decreased (leucine, isoleucine, valine).

Beside standard amino acid solutions, we use solutions which contain higher percent of arginine which accelerates the conversion of ammonia into urea. In that way we can prevent the occurrence of hyperammonemia which often accompanies large liver resections. In severe hepatic failure is advisable to use high-BCAA, low-aromatic amino acid solutions.

To prevent hypoalbuminemia as the consequence of decreased synthesis, loss due to hemorrhage and hemodilution, the patient should be given solutions of 20% albumin to keep the level in blood over 30 g/l.

The liver participates in the metabolism of lipids. Oxidation of long-chain fatty acids to ketones takes place in the liver. The primary hepatic alteration in fat metabolism is the accumulation of triglycerides, known as fatty liver.

The liver is a principal vitamin storage site, which might be limited in hepatic insufficiency. A number of vitamins, especially A, D, E, K, B complex, thiamin and folic acid may be deficient. In fact the liver is a great gland with an external secretion of bile which is most important for lipid metabolism and for absorption of fat insoluble vitamins (A, D, E, K).

Iron and zinc deficiencies may be present and serum copper levels may be decreased. It is well documented that Zn moves to the liver cells where it is utilized for liver regeneration.

Drug and hormone metabolism is also reduced. This may have practical importance as drugs metabolized by hepatic microsomal enzymes are commonly used in the ICU: barbiturates, benzodiazepins, narcotic analgesics, theophylline, etc.

The liver plays an important role in inactivation of the following hormones:
- estrogens
- corticosteroids
- thyroxin
- vasopressin

Coagulation disorders

Special attention has to be paid to coagulation disorders either because of massive transfusion or because of depressed synthesis of coagulation factors. The liver has several functions within the coagulation system:
1. it is responsible for the synthesis of most plasmatic coagulation and fibrinolysis factors:
   - factors II, VII, IX, X (prothrombin complex) and V
   - plasminogen
2. it is the production site for numerous inhibitors of the coagulation and fibrinolytic system:
   - Antithrombin III (ATIII)

- α_s-antiplasmin
- α_2-macroglobulin
- α_1-antitrypsin

3. the reticuloendothelial system (RES) of the liver is primarily involved in the elimination of activated and inactivated coagulation and fibrinolysis factors:
   - 50-80% of RES is in the form of Kupffer's cells

Disorders of hemostasis are dependent of the level of hepatic insufficiency, underlying diseases, percent of liver resections, amount of blood transfused and several other accompanying factors.

In correspondence with the half-life, factor VII falls first, followed by II, X, IX. The fibrinogen level does not fall until there is progressive destruction of the hepatic tissue; this is always a sign of severe liver dysfunction.

Treatment of coagulation disorders is directed at prevention of hemorrhagic diathesis resulting from impaired synthesis of the coagulation factors, consumption coagulopathy and micro- and macrothrombotic events. For substitution of coagulation factors it is essential to give fresh frozen plasma. Vitamin K increases the activities of the prothrombin complex factors. This response is a useful test for hepatic function, and therefore can provide information about hepatocellular damage (Koller test). If prothrombin time shortens after the application of vitamin K, liver function is considered to be normal; if not liver failure is suspected. Prothrombin complex should only be given if hemostasis potential has been completely exhausted.

The most advanced methods of prevention and treatment of severe coagulation disturbances are based on the coagulations and fibrinolysis inhibitors. This is especially important if heparin has to be used. Among these, ATIII is believed to have a particularly high potential and is one of the strongest known natural anticoagulants which is synthesized by liver hepatocytes and might be decreased in liver insufficiency.

Assessment of liver tests

Icterus is not an infrequent occurrence in the first week after operation, which we mostly explain as a consequence of intrahepatic cholestasis because of rapid liver regeneration [13]. But there are several other reasons for postoperative jaundice which is a complex diagnostic and therapeutic clinical problem. For that reason, it is advantageous to relate icterus to the three basic mechanisms:

1. prehepatic defect - an increased pigment load;
2. intrahepatic defect - impaired bilirubin conjugation and/or excretion due to some abnormality of hepatocellular function;
3. posthepatic defect - an inability to excrete conjugated bilirubin.

The predisposing factors for jaundice are:

- hypoxia, hypotension

- raised intrathoracic pressure with decreased liver blood flow
- direct endotoxins
- hemolysis of transfused blood
- resorption from hematomas
  It is important to pay some attention to liver function tests as well:
- indirect bilirubin: hemolytic, hepatocellular
- direct bilirubin: cholestatic, extrahepatic
- SGOT and LDH reflect structural and functional integrity of the hepatocyte
- alkaline phosphatase reflects integrity of biliar ductal endothelium
- albumin is an indicator of hepatic synthesis capacity
- prothrombin

Late complications

Advance treatment of the patient in ICU is directed to the prevention of late complications. The most important is prevention of intra-abdominal sepsis (the second commonest cause of hepatic-related death), which depends on debridment of devitalized tissue, on a careful search for biliary leaks and on efficient drainage [13]. Several risk factors are important: age, shock, mechanism of injury, additional injuries to other organs and inadequate antibiotic therapy. The most important risk factor for development of inhoald abscess or sepsis is massive transfusion, especially hemorrhage in abdominal cavity.

There is experimental evidence for the adjuvant effect of hemoglobin in the development of valuabled sepsis. Hemoglobin may reduce normal tolerance to bacterial contamination by the inhibition of bacterial absorption from the peritoneal cavity, inhibition of PNL chemotaxis and intracellular killing, or by a direct enhancement of bacterial growth, so that blood transfusion may result in impaired immune function. Prolonged hemorrhage leads to hypothermia, poor tissue perfusion and ineffective distribution of antibiotics. It is interesting to note that most of the pathogens are enteric organisms (translocation of bacteria). If the packs are the source of infection one might expect more growth organisms. However the prevalence of grown-enteric organisms suggests another source. Hypotension and shock have been shown to alter the colonic mucosa so that these organisms can enter into portal system. Shock also causes a breakdown in hepatic RES, thus the hepatic Kupffer's cells are unable to clear the microorganisms.

Antibiotics that we usually give to patients with liver resection are those which penetrate and concentrate well in liver bile ducts and are less toxic. Some cephalosporins seem to fulfill these criteria (cefoperazone, cefotaxime, cefuroxime).

Other complications that we could be aware of and that we could expect are: hemorrhage, stress ulcer, renal insufficiency, bile fistulas, and hemobilia.

Conclusions

It appears likely that the liver contributes to the genesis of multiple organ dysfunction by virtue of its ability to interact with other organ systems. The management of the pathophysiologic process of hepatic dysfunction in liver trauma patients consists of prevention through vigorous resuscitative efforts, careful attention to respiratory and other organs, and early nutritional support, preferably through the use of enteral nutrition.

References

1. Rivkind A, Siegel JH, Dunhum CM (1989) Patterns of organ injury in blunt hepatic trauma and their significance for management and outcome. J Trauma 29:1398-1415
2. Scott CM, Grasbergerer RC, Heeran TF et al (1988) Intraabdominal sepsis after hepatic trauma. Am J Surg 155:284-288
3. Ramsay G, Runcie C (1989) Hepatic dysfunction in shock. In: Vincent JL (ed) Update in intensive care and emergency medicine. Springer, Berlin Heidelberg New York, pp 386-375
4. Colletti LM, Kunkel SL, Walz A et al (1996) The role of cytokine networks in the local liver injury following hepatic ischemia/reperfusion in the rat. Hepatology 23:506-514
5. Koeppel TA, Lehmann TG, Thies JC et al (1996) Impact of N-acetylcysteine on the hepatic microcirculation after orthotopic liver transplantation. Transplantation 61:1397-1407
6. Fukuzawa K, Emre S, Senyuz O et al (1995) N-acetylcysteine ameliorates reperfusion injury after warm hepatic ischemia. Transplantation 59:6-9
7. Schiano TD, Ehrenpreis ED (1998) Gut and hepatobiliary dysfunction. In: Hall JB, Schmidt GA, Wood LDH (eds) Principles of critical care. Mc Graw-Hill, New York, pp 1223-1236
8. Gattinoni L, Brazzi L, Pelosi P (1996) Does cardiovascular optimization reduce mortality. In: Vincent JL (ed) Yearbook of intensive care and emergency medicine. Springer, Berlin Heidelberg New York, pp 308-318
9. Dahn MS, Lange MP, Jacobs LA (1988) Central mixed and splanchnic venous oxygen saturation monitoring. Intensive Care Med 14:373-378
10. Dahn MS, Lange MP, Benn S (1999) The influence of hepatic venous oxygen saturation on the liver's synthetic response to metabolic stress. Proc Soc Exp Biol 221:39-45
11. Kaku N (1987) Short-term and long-term changes with blunt liver injury. J Trauma 27: 607-614
12. Martini C, Viviand X, Potie F (1997) Use and misuse of catecholamines: combination in septic shock patients. In: Vincent JL (ed) Yearbook of intensive care and emergency medicine. Springer, Berlin Heidelberg New York, pp 289-304
13. Hawker F (1993) Liver trauma. In: Park GR (ed) Critical care management. WB Saunders, London, pp 356-371
14. Zaloga GP, Roberts PR (1997) Early enteral feeding improves outcome. In: Vincent JL (ed) Yearbook of intensive care and emergency medicine. Springer, Berlin Heidelberg New York, pp 701-714
15. Jolliet P, Pichard C, Biolo G et al (1999) Enteral nutrition in intensive care patients: a practical approach. Clin Nutr 18(1):47-56

Mistakes in the Management of Trauma Patients

M. FISHER

There have been many studies in recent times on errors occurring in the management of hospitalised patients. In the Quality in Australian Health Care Study [1, 2] 16.6% of 14,655 admissions to hospital had an adverse event leading to disability of prolonged stay: 31% were categorised as injuries, poisoning, or toxic drug effects, 34.6% of adverse events were related to technical performance, 15.8% failure to act on available information, 11.8% failure to arrange investigation, procedure or consultation, and 10.9% lack of care and attention or failure to attend.

Why should trauma patients be associated with a higher incidence of errors in management?

Most studies on trauma patients show an increased mortality and morbidity when injuries are missed [3-6].

The management of trauma patients is more circumscribed and defined that most groups of patients. There are well defined protocols, excellent courses (such as the ATLS courses), and the basic diagnosis is usually obvious. Why then do studies find a high incidence of errors, even in units with extensive experience with dedicated trauma teams?

Additional medical process of history, differential diagnosis, investigations, diagnosis and definitive treatment is not appropriate in many cases of trauma. Penetrating trauma with shock, for example, is usually an indication for urgent surgery, which may preclude a careful examination. However, interrupting the diagnostic work-up because of a need for urgent surgery did not appear to be a major source of error in penetrating trauma [4].

Multiple trauma in many hospitals is managed by people from different disciplines. When management becomes the priority other aspects of the injury may be overlooked. In particular, the presence of acute head injury may lead to immediate surgery or Computerised Axial Tomography (CT Scan).

In many hospitals the tradition of emergency rooms run by junior staff continues.

Changes have occurred in trauma management which have predicated changes to systems. Such changes include the early fixation of fractures which may require long operating theatre sessions leaving the care of the patient largely to anaesthetists and admitting hypothermic patients to the intensive care units. CT scanning has meant unstable and partially resuscitated patients need transport from the resuscitation room to X-ray, often accompanied by junior staff and inferior monitoring and resources.

Deficiencies in knowledge can occur. Even in the United States there is a high incidence of misinterpretation of gunshot wounds by surgeons [7]. McLaughlan, Jones and Guly found a 32%, 48%, and 80% correct interpretation of X-rays from trauma patients in junior, experienced junior, and senior doctors, respectively [8].

Missed injuries in trauma: findings from some recent studies

Hirshberg et al. described 123 missed injuries in 117 patients requiring re-operation over a 10 year period in a hospital with a large trauma service and 85% of these patients had penetrating trauma. Delayed haemorrhage was the most common presentation (64 injuries) and the colon, thoracic vessels, chest wall vessels, and diaphragm were the most common sites. Delayed diagnosis directly contributed to 20 deaths and three patients died of their original injuries. 18 missed injuries were discovered on repeat physical examination. 46 injuries were missed on judgmental and technical difficulties during the diagnostic work-up, and 43 were missed at operation. Deviation from established protocols accounted for the greater proportion of those missed during work-up. Injuries missed because of a decision to abandon diagnostic work-up in favour of urgent intervention were least common.

Junjua et al. found 309 missed injuries in 134 out of 206 patients with blunt trauma studied, prospectively [9]. A tertiary trauma survey of 24 hours detected 56% of missed injuries and 905 of clinically significant missed injuries. Over half the errors were in clinical assessment, 83 in radiology and only 4 technical. The majority of missed injuries were soft tissue and only 12 patients had missed visceral injuries. Two patients died of missed C1-C2 fractures. Three unstable cervical spine fractures were missed by specialized radiologists. 35 of 83 missed radiological injuries were present on initial films and missed by treating physicians.

In another tertiary trauma survey, before ambulation or on regaining consciousness, 41 missed injuries in 399 patients (90% blunt trauma) including 28 fractures and 11 thoracic and abdominal injuries were detected [3].

Rizoli et al. found 59 of 432 patients with blunt trauma had missed injuries. 35% were detected on repeat examination and 28% when consciousness was regained. They concluded repeated physical assessment was the most effective way of diagnosis and patients who were obtunded, intubated, or had severe anatomical injuries were at the highest risk of missed injuries [10]. Conversely, Robertson et al. did not find a higher incidence of missed injuries when trauma patients had depressed mental status [11]. Blunt trauma produces more missed injuries than penetrating trauma [3, 6, 11].

Muckhart and Thompson found 18 patients with missed injuries. Failure to perform investigations accounted for seven and a further seven were missed at laparotomy. The mortality and morbidity was increased after missed injuries and the presenting diagnoses were multi organ failure, ARDS, persistent peritonitis, persistent pleural effusion and absent femoral pulse [6].

Davis et al. studied 22,577 patients in 6 trauma centers [12]. There were 76 preventable deaths and 505 occurred after errors in management in the Intensive Care unit as opposed to during resuscitation (36%) and operative errors (14%).

The ICU errors described were not errors specific to trauma patients, but were rather ICU complications occurring in trauma patients such as iatrogenic pneumothorax, sepsis and deep vein thrombosis.

Transport factors

Air transport and evacuation was associated with missed injury in one study, in particular eye injuries (50% missed), cervical spine injuries (33% missed), crush injuries (33% missed), fractures (25% missed) and a significant number of chest and abdominal injuries [13]. Robertson et al. showed that inter-hospital transport increases the incidence of missed injuries [11].

Diagnostic difficulties

Penetrating injury to both chest and abdomen increases the risk of both unnecessary surgery and missed illness. The authors of the study emphasised the unreliability of decisions based on abdominal examination and chest tube drainage [14].

Blow et al. showed that diagnostic peritoneal lavage (DPL) gave a more rapid diagnosis than CT scans in 1,182 patients with blunt trauma [15]. There were no missed injuries. The DPL patients spent considerably less time in the ER in spite of not being transported to CT. Their study included patients with haemodynamic instability and head injury. However, it should be remembered that if a CT of the head is indicated, modern scanners require little extra time to scan abdomen, pelvis or chest. Further, Metzger et al. found that patients with small bowel injury who did not have signs of peritonitis on admission had the diagnosis missed by DPL, ultrasound and X-ray, but the injuries were detected within 24 hours in 7/11 patients with CT and ultrasound [16]. Conversely, Bloom et al. found that lack of evidence and negative CT scans lead to a missed diagnosis in 445 of patients and emphasised that a 'seat belt sign' should be a reason of suspect [17].

Phillips et al. found a 25% false negative rate with DPL in perforating injuries of the small bowel after blunt trauma [18] and other authors note that CT scan has an error rate of 1-3% [19].

Errors of concern in practice

Chance fractures are usually high speed seat belt injuries causing distraction fractures of the upper lumbar spine. 50% of these patients have intra-abdominal injuries [20]. These patients in practice seem particularly vulnerable to deterioration during transport, and DPL or laparotomy should be considered prior to transport. The converse may apply in these patients. Patients who present with intra-abdominal catastrophes related to MVA in particular may have their spinal injury overlooked.

Head injury without other injuries is rarely associated with hypotension or shock and the presence of either should lead to DPL in the former case and urgent laparotomy or angiography in the latter. Chesnut et al. [21] found 21 of 248 head injured patients with early hypotension had no discernable extracranial cause for their hypotension. 15 patients had a diffuse injury on CT scan and 16 had received mannitol or frusemide early.

The following are important impressions of the author and are not supported by data.

The recommended DVT prophylaxis for patients with spinal injuries is a sequential compression device and low molecular weight heparin. Since introducing this therapy we have seen a number of patients with spinal injury and after elective spinal surgery develop extradural haematomata, some with disastrous consequences. This situation is similar to the patients who have been described. Epidural anaesthesia and low molecular weight heparin should be used with caution in this group of patients until further safety data appears.

25 years ago a surgeon suggested to me that any patient who needs two litres or more of blood or colloid in the first 24 hours postoperatively needs a re-exploration. I have seen two negative operations based on this criteria in the subsequent 25 years.

Recommendations to minimise missed injuries in the ICU

Admission of a trauma patient to intensive care should lead to a thorough physical examination both on admission, when awake, and prior to ambulation, sitting out of bed or discharge to the word. Transferred patients should be assumed to have missed injuries until cleared by physical examination, DPL if indicated, and imaging.

No one diagnostic test (ultrasound, DPL, CT scan) is infallible in detecting serious intestinal injury.

In blunt trauma the neck should be treated as unstable until cleared by plain x-rays and flexion extension films if the patient cannot cooperate with physical examination. CT Scan and plain films do not detect unstable ligamentous injuries [22].

The development of any signs of deterioration in the intensive care unit, in particular organ failure or loss of blood volume, should lead to a further search for missed injuries, particularly internal injuries.

The need for more than 2 litres of blood or colloid in the first 24 hours post-operatively should lead to a search for haemorrhage and angiography or re-operation should be considered.

Patients with significant head injuries who are to undergo lengthy orthopaedic procedures should have ICP monitoring [23, 24]. The decisions regarding early fracture fixation in head injured patients should be carefully considered in individuals rather than following a blanket protocol [25].

Patients should be actively warmed intra-operatively and post-operatively.

X-rays taken on admission should be reviewed by a radiologist as soon as possible.

Patients with seat belt injuries should be treated with a high index of suspicion for intestinal injury, which may be missed on initial assessment and may not be associated with haemodynamic instability.

References

1. Wilson RM, Runciman WB, Gibberd RW et al (1995) The Quality in Australian Health Care Study. Med J Aust 163:458-471
2. Wilson RM, Harrison BT, Gibberd RW, Hamilton JD (1999) An analysis of the causes of adverse events from the Quality in Australian Health Care Study. Med J Aust 170:411-415
3. Enderson BL, Reath DB, Meadors J et al (1990) The tertiary trauma survey: a prospective study of missed injury. J Trauma 30:666-669
4. Hirshberg A, Wall MJ, Allen Mk, Mattox KL (1994) Causes and patterns of missed injuries in trauma. Am J Surg 168:299-303
5. Sung CK, Kim KH (1996) Missed injuries in abdominal trauma. J Trauma 41:276-278
6. Muckart DJJ, Thomson Sr (1991) Undetected injuries; a preventable cause of increased morbidity and mortality. Am J Surg 162:460
7. Collins KA, Lantz PE (1996) Interpretation of fatal, multiple, and existing gunshot wounds by trauma specialists. J Forens Sci 39:94-99
8. McLauchlan CA, Jones K, Guly HR (1998) Interpretation of trauma radiographs by junior doctors in accident and emergency departments: a cause for concern? J Accid Emerg Med 14:295-298
9. Janjua KJ, Sugrue M, Deane Sa (1998) Prospective evaluation of early missed injuries and the role of tertiary trauma survey. J Trauma 44:1000-1007
10. Rizoli SB, Boulanger BR, McLellan BA, Sharkey PW (1994) Injuries missed during initial assessment of blunt trauma patients. Accident Analysis and Prevention 26:681-686

11. Robertson R, Mattox R, Collins T et al (1996) Missed injuries in a rural trauma centre. Am J Surg 172:564-568
12. Davis JW, Hoyt DB, McArdle MS et al (1992) An analysis of errors causing morbidity and mortality in a trauma system: A guide for quality improvement. J Trauma 32:660-665
13. Linn S, Knoller N, Giligan CG, Dreifus U (1997) The sky is a limit: errors in prehospital diagnosis by flight physicians. Am J Emerg Med 15:316-320
14. Hirshberg A, Wall MJ, Allen Mk, Mattox KL (1995) Double jeopardy: Thoracoabdominal injuries requiring surgical intervention in both chest and abdomen. J Trauma 39:225-231
15. Blow O, Bassam D, Butler K et al (1998) Speed and efficiency in the resuscitation of blunt trauma patients with multiple injuries: the advantage of diagnostic peritoneal lavage over abdominal computerised tomography. J Trauma 44:287-290
16. Metzger J, von Flue M, Babst R, Harder F (1995) Small bowel injuries in blunt abdominal trauma - a diagnostic problem. Swiss Surgery 5:222-225
17. Bloom AI, Rivkind A, Zamir G et al (1996) Blunt injury of the small intestine and mesentery - the trauma surgeons Achilles heel? Eur J Emerg Med 3:85-91
18. Phillips TF, Brotman S, Cleveland S, Cowley RA (1983) Perforating injuries of the small bowel from blunt trauma. Ann Emerg Med 12:75-79
19. PachterHL, Feliciano DV (1996) Complex hepatic injuries. Surg Clin North Am 76:763-782
20. Gumley G, Taylor TKF, Ryan MD (1982) Distraction fractures of the lumbar spine. J Bone Joint Surg 64B:520-525
21. Chesnut RM, Gautille T, Blunt BA et al (1998) Neurogenic hypotension in patients with severe head injuries. Jnl of Trauma - Injury Infection & Critical Care 44(6):958-963; discussion 963-964 Jun
22. Pasquale M, Fabian TC and the East Ad Hoc Committee on Practice Management Guideline Development (1998) Practice management guidelines for trauma from the Eastern Association for the surgery of trauma. J Trauma 44:941-957
23. Scalea TM, Scott JD, Brumback RJ et al (1999) Early fracture fixation may be 'just fine' after head injury: No difference in neurological outcomes. J Trauma 46:839-846
24. Kalb DC, Ney AL, Rodriguez JL et al (1998) Assessment of the relationship between timing of fixation of fracture and secondary brain injury in patients with multiple trauma. Surgery 124:739-744
25. Velmahos GC, Arroyo H, Ramicone E et al (1998) Timing of fracture fixation in blunt trauma patients with severe head injuries. Am J Surg 176:324-329

FOCUS ON NEUROTRAUMA

Integrated Intensive Care Management of Severe Head Injury

N. STOCCHETTI, L. LONGHI, S. MAGNONI

Patients with severe head injury require timely and aggressive treatment. They are potentially exposed to multiple life-threatening lesions, which cannot be properly treated by a single specialist; they can be better tackled by a team. Only the availability of the right expertise at the right time could offer, in fact, the best surgical and medical therapy required.

Aim of this chapter is to describe:

– the threats and main lesions to be treated;
– how to identify and treat them;
– how to integrate the information and the necessary expertise.

Severe head injury, cerebral and systemic damage

Severe head injury is associated with systemic disturbances that can, in turn, exacerbate cerebral damage itself. A great proportion of head injuries suffers from associated injuries to the limbs, thorax and abdomen; even in case of "pure" head trauma, however, the systemic physiology is disturbed, since the regulatory function of the brain is altered. Extra-cranial injuries have a direct impact on outcome by itself and through their consequences, such as arterial hypotension and shock or respiratory failure. A better understanding of the relationship between brain and systemic events after injury is necessary in order to plan appropriate interventions.

Brain vulnerability

After head injury the brain becomes more vulnerable to further damage, such as a secondary ischemic insult. The mechanisms of such enhanced vulnerability are not totally clear, but involve both the microvasculature and the cerebral tissue. The capability of increasing cerebral blood flow in response to hypotension, for instance, is greatly reduced after trauma. Neurons themselves appear more vulnerable, and a number of potential mediators contributing to this vulnerability has been identified [1].

Primary and secondary brain damage

The structural damage initially determined by a direct or indirect injury to the cerebral tissue is called primary brain damage. In case of trauma, this injury is determined by an energy transmission to the brain tissue itself, with consequent compressions and deformations, while in other situations it may be the result of a critically inadequate supply of oxygen and essential substrates. More frequently, the initial damage involves neurons but it may also affect the glia and cerebral vascular structures [2]. It may produce a deformation of superficial structures, as in the case of contusions and lacerations, or have deeper consequences and cause axonal and vascular shearings.

Many experimental researches have been devoted to the comprehension of the pathophysiological events started by insults and responsible for the secondary damage. It is now possible to recognize that, irrespective of the different course or sequences, all kinds of injuries have a limited number of biochemical destructive chain reactions in common. These reactions may progressively affect the cerebral tissue through vicious circles and feed-forward processes.

The initial damage tends to worsen and to determine a final damage that will be more serious than that caused directly by the initial impact. The sequence of events leading to final damage is called secondary damage.

Insults superimposed to the damaged brain

Occasionally, further unfavourable events, called insults, are superimposed to the initial damage. Such insults are generally events that produce a deterioration of the relationship between the supply of substrates to the tissue and the metabolic needs of the tissue itself. Typically, insults cause ischemia, either because they determine a deterioration of the oxygen transport (as in case of anemia, hypo-oxygenation or arterial hypotension), or because they cause a decline in the energy requirements of the tissue, such as in epileptic crises or during hyperthermia. The main causes of intracranial systemic insults are shown in Table 1.

Secondary insults have been repeatedly identified in the various phases of the treatment of head-injured patients. Generally such insults have been measured at the hospital admission, where a greater incidence of arterial hypotension over hypoxemia has been found. However, when the insults have been measured on the scene of the trauma, through helicopter emergency crews, hypoxemia was more frequent than arterial hypotension.

Within the intensive care units insults are quite frequent also: whenever they are accurately documented, for example through computerized systems, more than half the patients suffer repeated insults during their hospital stay.

Insults can worsen morbidity and mortality. Data from the Traumatic Coma Data Bank suggest that mortality due to head injury alone significantly increases in case of concurrent hypotension or hypoxemia. The association of head injury with other insults, such as intracranial hypertension and reduced cerebral perfusion pressure, has also been linked to worse outcome. The role of insults in the worsening of cerebral damage is well documented in the laboratory, but is very difficult to prove in the clinical setting. In fact, it is very difficult to determine whether the insults are simply associated with the damage, whether they are a consequence of a particularly serious cerebral damage or whether they cause the damage. As a general rule, however, insults must be deemed deleterious and must be identified early and treated aggressively.

Table 1. Intra- or extracranial insults

Intracranial insults:
Intracranial hypertension
Mass lesions
Oedema
Hydrocephalus
Infections
Seizures
Alterations of regional and global flows
Damage caused by free radicals and excitotoxic substances
Extracranial insults:
Arterial hypotension
Hypoxia
Anemia
Hyperthermia
Hyper/hypocapnia
Electrolyte anomalies (mainly hyponatremia)
Hypo/hyperglycemia
Alterations of the acid-base balance

Treatment of severe head injury

Optimal treatment of head injury requires a system [3, 4]. This system should provide fast and qualified rescue, capable of restoring oxygenation and perfusion directly at the accident scene. A reasonable system should refer the right patient to the right hospital and, once in the hospital, it should concentrate resources to expedite diagnosis and treatment. The first approach to the severely head-injured patient must be a combined medical and surgical effort. The proportion of surgical cases varies depending upon the referral system, the epidemiology of injury and local policies. On average, in many centres 50% of cases are felt to require emergency surgery.

Severe head injury is a surgical emergency

Supportive intervention is necessary to preserve cerebral perfusion and oxygenation after trauma, but effective therapy is most often surgical. There is no substitute for prompt and complete surgical intervention. In case of severe abdominal bleeding, or after pericardial tamponade, as in case of acute epidural hematoma, there is no place for deferred decisions. The attending team must identify the most urgent lesions and plan a reasonable sequence of interventions. Delayed diagnosis or treatment of a surgical intracranial mass may cause permanent tissue damage and increases morbidity and mortality.

Intracranial and extracranial surgery

The first cause of secondary cerebral damage is the enlargement of intracranial masses. The removal of these masses is mandatory, but the necessary prerequisite is the adequacy of perfusion and a preserved coagulation.

It is meaningless, and very often hopeless, to begin the evacuation of a hematoma when there is another source of systemic bleeding (such a spleen rupture) which has not been treated.

Successful neurosurgery becomes possible after stabilization, which sometimes requires the surgical repair of extracranial bleeding organs. They have, therefore, the priority when multiple surgical interventions are necessary.

Limb fractures are an additional challenge. Early treatment can reduce late complications [5-8] but this concept has been recently questioned [9].

Intensive care of severe head injury

Goals

The main goal of intensive care in head injury is to prevent, limit or eliminate further secondary cerebral damage. Primary cerebral damage can only be prevented or limited at the moment of impact, and is not suitable for treatment later on. Secondary cerebral damage, on the contrary, is a dynamic process that develops, and often starts, in the hours/days following the initial injury. Therefore it could be prevented or treated. This goal can be achieved by combining careful observation and monitoring with a prompt and targeted correction of the disturbances.

Monitoring

Despite the advancements in technology, the clinical control of the patient remains mandatory. An evaluation of the neurologic reactivity must be repeated at least every hour with a consistent methodology and must be registered in such a way that any changes can be easily recorded. A first evaluation is possible using the Glasgow Coma Scale together with the observation of the pupillary diameter and reactivity to light.

Repeated cerebral CT scans are necessary in comatose patients. A first scan must be executed at the hospital admission, after stabilizing ventilation and circulation. Early CT scans are essential and can show the existence of masses that require urgent surgical treatment. If a CT scan is executed too early it might not show incipient lesions that have not yet reached a considerable size.

Intracranial pressure

Intracranial pressure (ICP) is a physiologic parameter that has considerable importance in the maintenance of a normal cerebral function. Under normal conditions it remains fairly stable, since mechanisms of adjustment exist and variations of short duration are well tolerated. An increased ICP may cause distortion of the cerebral structures and/or decrease of cerebral blood flow, both resulting in regional or global cerebral ischemia.

Increased ICP can be an emergency "per se", but it is always a consequence, and is more properly treated when the causes of increased intracranial volume have been identified. Cerebral perfusion pressure (CPP) is estimated as the difference between mean arterial pressure and ICP (CPP = MAP-ICP). A raised ICP, sufficient to compromise CPP, can cause permanent brain damage and death [10, 11] and therefore ICP must be measured and treated rapidly.

It has been reported that according to the severity of coma and to the effacement of basal cisterns visible on the CT scan, it is possible to identify patients with more than a 50-60% probability of developing an ICP persistently greater than 20 mmHg [12, 13].

A recent paper [14] reports the frequent occurrence of increased ICP also in cases who did not meet the CT scan criteria of increased intracranial content. According to these findings, increased ICP may be suspected in all comatose head-injured patients, and therefore indications for monitoring may be further extended.

ICP may be useful also in deciding if and when an indication for surgery exists. By monitoring ICP the evolution of cerebral contusions can be followed, and if they cause a refractory high ICP, the surgical approach can be reconsidered. ICP control is also crucial after surgical evacuation of masses; a rise in ICP allows the detection of secondary or delayed lesions before a severe clinical deterioration occurs [15].

The usefulness of ICP monitoring has been questioned even in trauma; in fact a prospective randomized clinical trial demonstrating that by aggressively monitoring and treating head-injured patients their outcome will significantly improve is still unavailable [16, 17].

Unfortunately the arguments in favor of or against ICP monitoring are based on historical comparisons, while an appropriate study, randomizing patients to different levels of monitoring and care, cannot be contemplated.

Different kinds of ICP monitoring devices have been described, but the systems can be summarized according to the point at which the pressure is detected. Epidural, subdural, ventricular and intraparenchymal devices are currently available. Each device carries some specific advantages, disadvantages and risks. The gold standard is still represented by the ventricular catheter, which allows the acquisition of a better waveform, the drainage of cerebral-spinal fluid (CSF), and the determination of Pressure Volume Index (PVI) and related measurements.

In our experience subdural catheters filled with saline and connected to an external piezoelectric transducer are inexpensive and suitable for routine clinical use [18, 19].

The risk of dampening the pressure wave must be considered; a low-pressure flushing device may be attached to the catheter providing 1-2 ml/hour of saline to the system. This, however, is seldom necessary.

Intraparenchymal devices are easily placed in emergency situations and are widely used; unfortunately they are costly and cannot be reset to zero.

The main complications in ICP monitoring are related to the insertion of the catheter (brain damage and hemorrhage due to the penetration of the brain parenchyma) or to the contamination of the ICP system by bacteria (meningitis or ventricular infections) [20-22]. Almost all major complications can be avoided. Intracranial hemorrhage from brain penetration results from multiple punctures in the presence of coagulopathies. Coagulative deficits are not uncommon during the first phase of a multiple trauma but they are usually of mild degree. If a major coagulopathy is suspected any invasive procedure should be deferred until the coagulopathy has been corrected. Infections are the other major concern in ICP monitoring. The rate of infection can be reduced under 5% by a careful surgical technique and a meticulous care in the ICU [23]. In our experience the rate of infection, prospectively studied in a large series [22], was below 3%.

Jugular bulb saturation

Arterio-jugular oxygen difference is a useful estimate of the relationship between cerebral blood flow and cerebral oxygen consumption.

Although this method has limitations and must therefore be cautiously used, it is undoubtedly useful:

– to identify dangerous situations of desaturation;
– to identify the correct level of $PaCO_2$ set during artificial ventilation. An excessive reduction of CO_2 may induce dangerous cerebral blood flow reductions. It is not unusual, especially during the first hours of treatment, to discover jugular desaturations associated with inappropriate ventilatory setting (excessive hyperventilation).

Jugular saturation should be monitored continuously, but the debate on the reliability of the signals produced by the fiberoptic catheters is still open. Desaturation should be checked through planned samples and CO-oximeter readings every time the respiratory parameters change, in order to optimize the level of CO_2. Such check must also be repeated:

– routinely, every 12 hours
– whenever the clinical situation changes, and
– whenever ICP is greater than 25 mmHg or CPP is below 70 mmHg

Medical therapy

As for all patients in the ICU, therapy is aimed at maintaining the homeostasis of the various organs. Those aspects are not discussed in this chapter; we shall focus here on the treatment of intracranial hypertension. A stable ICP above a certain threshold lasting at least 5 minutes must be considered a serious emergency and treated with determination. The identification of the threshold must at least consider the following two factors:

– age: until 6 years of age normal ICP is not greater than 5 mmHg;
– time elapsed from the trauma: while during the first days 20 mmHg is considered the threshold for treatment in adult patients, subsequently values of ICP < = 25 mmHg with CPP > 70 mmHg are deemed acceptable.

The first step is to distinguish between hyper-acute and threatening ICP rises which require the immediate execution of a CT scan to capture the potential indications for surgery, and ICP rises where it is possible to proceed with relative ease to:

– rule out any causes of intracranial hypertension that can be resolved more easily
– then explore the intracranial causes of the current hypertension.

The aims of the treatment are not only to restore a stable ICP below the threshold, but also to restore an adequate cerebral perfusion pressure. In adult patients CPP values must be at least 70 mmHg. For older patients suffering from arterial hypertension such value is probably too low.

The treatment is essentially based on the following procedures:

1. sedation
2. cerebrospinal fluid (CSF) drainage
3. mannitol
4. hyperventilation

Sedation: It guarantees an adequate deafferentation of the patient, an appropriate adjustment to artificial ventilation, and may help reduce cerebral oxygen consumption.

Liquor drainage: Whenever ventricular catheters are available, CSF can be subtracted. CSF withdrawal, which must be gradual and maintain the collection tank at an adequate height in order to avoid sudden pressure gradients, helps reduce the intracranial volume.

Mannitol: Mannitol infusions, in doses of 0.3-0.5 g/kg, may effectively reduce intracranial hypertension. The mechanisms through which the drug acts are not entirely clear, and include effects on the vessels (initial increase of cerebral blood flow, followed by an increase in cerebral vascular resistance) and on the cerebral tissue. The use of mannitol is not free of complications:

- mannitol should not be given in case of dehydration, hypovolemia, or hyponatremia;
- mannitol should not be given for long periods because it can cross the damaged blood brain barrier. After crossing the barrier the drug accumulates in the cerebral tissue and retains water in the tissue itself.

Hyperventilation: Although criticized for the possible deleterious effects of an excessive cerebral vasoconstriction induced by hypocapnia, hyperventilation is effective in controlling intracranial pressure.

The reduction of partial tension of CO_2 determines an increase of the cerebral interstitial pH followed by vasoconstriction, and a reduction of the cerebral blood flow and of the total cerebral blood content. This decrease of intracranial volume determines a reduction of intracranial pressure that might restore an adequate cerebral perfusion pressure. There is a paradox in this treatment, because it uses a reduction of flow in order to obtain an increase in perfusion, and in that paradox lies the potential danger of the treatment. When using hyperventilation very low levels of CO_2 should be avoided and the extent of hypocapnia should be guided by retrograde jugular saturation.

Whenever the usual treatments should prove ineffective, more extreme therapies, such as barbiturates and surgical decompression, might become necessary. Indications for those extreme treatments are based on two considerations:

1. there must be the opportunity to stop the ongoing pathological process, and
2. there must be recoverable nervous tissue.

Generally speaking, these conditions are met in case of young patients suffering from acute deterioration, with preserved brain oxygen consumption. They are less likely to be found in older patients, with metabolic cerebral activity clearly depressed and with evidence of established brain stem damage. The decision to use extreme treatments should be taken early, because in case of severe intracranial hypertension, any delay causes progressive damages and worse results.

Barbiturates

The extreme medical treatment consists in the use of barbiturates. They must be employed with particular attention to the hemodynamic instability. Before infusing Pentotal it is extremely important to verify that central venous pressure is adequate and that arterial pressure is at the limit. A catecholamine infusion, which could be necessary to support arterial pressure, must be planned. In non-emergency conditions a complete hemodynamics monitoring with cardiac catheterization is necessary to control the hemodynamic parameters during the barbiturate infusion.

A barbiturates bolus is infused (250 mg in 2 minutes followed by other infusions up to 1-2 gr) and then an infusion of 4-8 gr/die is added. The aim of this treatment is not to induce a barbiturate coma but to bring ICP below the threshold value. It is essential to protect the patient from decubitus lesions due to peripheral hypoperfusion.

Decompression

If the extreme medical treatment cannot bring ICP under control, surgical decompression must be considered. The same questions arising when extreme medical treatment must be decided, arise even more seriously when a functional surgical decompression must be executed if the presence of surgically removable masses has been already ruled out.

Conclusion: rules for integrated care

Severe brain injury induces a cascade of events capable of amplifying the initial damage. Insults superimposed to the direct effect of trauma may worsen outcome. Intracranial hypertension is a common event after brain injury and is the result of increased intracranial volume. Appropriate monitoring may guide therapeutic interventions toward specific targets.

The overall management is based on the strict co-operation of many professionals, who should combine their expertise in a profitable way. There are, therefore, many level of integration of care:

– during the rescue phase
– during the early hospital admission
– during the ICU stay

   In all of them, the combination of skills provides the best chances of success.

   Integration, however, does not happen by chance. It has to be planned and pursued, and is the result of commitment and unified direction rather than the natural outcome of unregulated, spontaneous willingness.

References

1. DeWitt DS, Jenkins LW, Prough DS (1995) Enhanced vulnerability to secondary ischemic insults after experimental traumatic brain injury. New Horizons 3:376-377
2. Graham DI, Adams JH, Doyle D et al (1993) Quantification of primary and secondary lesions in severe head injury. Acta Neurochir S57:41-48
3. Pitts LH (1988) The neurosurgeon and neurotrauma care system design. Clin Neurosurg 34; 30:618-629
4. American Congress of Emergency Physicians (1993) Guidelines for trauma care systems. Ann Emerg Med 22:1079-1100
5. Goris RJA, Gimbrere JSF, Niekerk JLM et al (1982) Early osteosynthesis and prophylactic mechanical ventilation in the multitrauma patient. J Trauma 22;11:895-903
6. Johnson KD, Cadami A, Seibert GB (1985) Incidence of adult respiratory distress syndrome in patients with multiple musculoskeletal injuries: effect of early operative stabilization of fractures. J Trauma 25;5:375-384
7. Ten Duis HJ, Nijsten MWN, Klasen HJ et al (1988) Fat embolism in patients with an isolated fracture of the femoral shift. J Trauma 28;3:383-390
8. Charash WE, Fabian TC, Croce MA (1994) Delayed surgical fixation of femur fractures is a risk factor for pulmonary failure independent of thoracic trauma. J Trauma 37:667-672
9. Poole GL, Miller JD, Agnew SG (1992) Lower extremity fracture fixation in head-injured patients. J Trauma 32;5:654-659
10. Narayan RK, Greenberg RP, Miller JD et al (1981) Improved confidence of outcome prediction in severe head injury. J Neurosurg 54:751-762
11. Marmarou A, Anderson RL, Ward JD et al (1991) Impact of ICP instability and hypotension on outcome in patients with severe head trauma. J Neurosurg 75:59-66
12. Miller JD (1987) ICP monitoring - Current status and future directions. Acta Neurochir 85: 80-86
13. Narayan RK, Kishore PRS, Becker DP et al (1982) Intracranial pressure: to monitor or not to monitor? A review of our experience with severe head injury. J Neurosurg 56:650-659
14. O'Sullivan MG, Statham PF, Jones PA et al (1994) Role of intracranial pressure monitoring in severely head-injured patients without signs of intracranial hypertension on initial computerized tomography. J Neurosurg 80:46-50
15. Bullock R, Hanneman CO, Murray L et al (1990) Recurrent hematomas following craniotomy for intracranial mass. J Neurosurg 72:9-14
16. Colohan ART, Alves WM, Gross CR et al (1989) Head injury mortality in two centers with different emergency medical services and intensive care. J Neurosurg 71:202-207
17. Stuart GG, Merry GS, Smith JA et al (1983) Severe head injury managed without intracranial pressure monitoring. J Neurosurg 59:601-605
18. Yano M, Kobayashi S, Otsuka T (1988) Useful ICP monitoring with subarachnoid catheter method in severe head injuries. J Trauma 28:476-480
19. Sugiura K, Hayama N, Tachisawa T et al (1985) Intracranial pressure monitoring by a subdurally placed silicone catheter: technical note. Neurosurgery 16;2:241-244
20. Clark WC, Muhlbauer MS, Lowrey R et al (1989) Complications of intracranial pressure monitoring in trauma patients. Neurosurgery 25:20-24
21. Mayhall CG, Archer NH, Lamb VA et al (1984) Ventriculostomy-related infections: A prospective epidemiologic study. New Engl J Med 310: 553-559
22. Rossi S, Buzzi F, Paparella A et al (1998) Complications and safety associated with ICP monitoring: a study of 542 patients. Acta Neurochir 71[Suppl]:91-93
23. Pickard JD, Czosnyka M (1993) Management of raised intracranial pressure. J Neurol Neurosurg Psychiatry 56:845-858

METABOLISM, ARTIFICIAL NUTRITION, CRRT

Organ Transplantation and Metabolism

G. Sganga, M. Castagneto

The metabolic response to surgical trauma has been characterized by the production of a variety of mediators, such as interleukins, which interact within a complex neuroendocrine alteration in the hormonal balance that regulates body metabolism.

These mechanisms shift the metabolic balance from a state of homeostasis to one of oxidative catabolism and muscle proteolysis. At the same time, the liver is activated to increase production of acute phase proteins that are essential in the primary humoral aspects of host defense and damage control, at the expense of other hepatic proteins.

In transplant patients, this immunomediated inflammatory response is affected by the presence of the graft, the clinical rejection episodes, and the immunosuppressive therapy [1].

Moreover, in transplant patients, it is very important to consider not only the pathophysiological changes following the surgical trauma, but also the preoperative clinical condition and particularly the preoperative organ dysfunction: on both these two conditions depend the biohumoral response, the ability of the graft to restore an adequate function and the rate of postoperative complications.

Candidates for organ transplantation are patients suffering from a terminal disease usually unresponsive to medical therapy. These patients present specific problems related to the organ involved (e.g. hepatic failure, heart failure, end-stage renal disease, respiratory insufficiency, complicated diabetes) with general metabolic alterations that suppress local as well as systemic immune and neuroendocrine response and the patient's stress response profile with increased risk of sepsis.

In these patients transplantation represents a severe trauma to an organism on the verge of metabolic compensation whose only chance of survival depends on the immediate function of the transplanted organ together with proper intensive care management.

Pretransplant assessment

Among the preoperative problems we must consider the pathophysiological status of the patient and particularly the metabolic derangements due to the specific organ dysfunction and to the underlying diseases.

All patients waiting for organ transplantation are suffering at least from one end stage organ failure and usually present some clinical evidence of malnutrition.

They have, together with specific clinical and biohumoral signs of organ failure (e.g. end stage hepatic failure, end stage renal disease, heart failure, pulmonary insufficiency, complicated diabetes), a severe alteration of the whole metabolism which affects the inflammatory and immunological response (antibody production, mediator and cytokine response) and then the susceptibility of the organism to the surgical stress and eventually an overall increase in systemic infections.

All these patients, beyond the primary organ failure, can have a lot of underlying diseases (e.g. diabetes, hypertension, cardiac, pulmonary and metabolic diseases), which can increase the surgical risk and the amount of postoperative complications.

Cadaver transplant is usually an unplanned event and thus patients on the waiting list must be kept under periodical clinical control.

Postoperative complications

Among the postoperative problems, we must include all the clinical and pathophysiolocal events related directly to the transplanted organ and to the ability to achieve an immediate graft function (degree of organ failure, type of transplanted organ, organ preservation, cold ischemia time, etc.), together with the organism's response to the surgical stress (general and specific surgical trauma) and the effects related to the immunosuppressive therapy.

The ability of the new organ to restore an adequate postoperative function depends both on the physiological functional reserve of the individual type of organ (resistance to ischemia time and organ preservation) and on the clinical conditions of the donor and of the recipient.

An immediate function after organ transplantation is strictly related to a good postoperative period, which means a good prognosis: the complete recovery of the patient depends on continuous organ function.

During and after surgery great care is taken to ensure adequate peripheral oxygenation, nutritional support and the correct water-electrolyte balance required to restore graft function.

Usually, patients who need an organ transplantation are suffering very complicated metabolic derangement due to the primary organ failure and/or to the artificial organ support: the real possibility of survival in most circumstances is related to the immediate organ function and of course to the intensive therapeutic support.

From the metabolic point of view, the metabolic activation after surgical trauma entails a greater activity of the cell oxidation systems, with an increase in oxygen consumption ($\dot{V}O_2$) and metabolic rate (MR) accompanied by an increase in cardiac output (CO), in an attempt to guarantee maximum oxygen flow when demand is at its peak.

The proteolytic effect aims at supplying aminoacids for protein synthesis at a time when the latter is stimulated and the exogenous calorie-protein supply is insufficient or even absent. The consequence is considerable nitrogen and 3-methylhistidine loss (hypercatabolism), correlated with the severity of trauma and worsened by the onset of infections, which often entails a negative nitrogen balance in spite of optimal nutritional supply.

This new pathophysiologic situation characterized by hypermetabolism and hypercatabolism induces considerable changes in substrate utilization.

While there are abundant and accessible endogenous reserves, the organism seems to be affected by severe malnutrition and the protein reserves are disintegrated to meet requirements which could normally be met by resorting to more specifically energetic substrates.

In recent years, the role of oxygen free radicals has been emphasized, as bioproducts of the revascularization of the new organ and as products of the ischemia-reperfusion damage, although in the clinical setting there are no definitive data on the relationship between this biohumoral damage and the organ functional damage.

At the same time there is no specific evidence that the clinical use of antioxidants drugs after organ transplantation improves the postoperative organ function.

It is very easy to recognize the fundamental role of the immediate graft function: that is evident in heart and lung transplantation where it represents the basis of survival. In the case of transplantation of splanchnic organs, primary graft non-function generally results in multiorgan damage and failure.

In kidney and pancreas graft, primary non-function can be readily compensated by artificial organ support (hemodialysis, medical therapy and insulin administration).

In liver transplantation the primary hepatic graft non-function commonly precipitates a multiple organ failure syndrome (MOFS) reversible only with prompt retransplantation.

In fact for hearts, lungs and livers, patient survival and early adequate function are considered to be synonymous; for kidneys, inadequate function is defined as the need for dialysis in the first postoperative week.

The cold ischemia time and the time required by the new organ to achieve good functionality represent two very critical points in terms of survival of the graft and of the patient.

The ischemia-reperfusion syndrome can be reduced by improving organ preservation and by reducing the cold ischemia time.

The surgical procedure for organ transplantation represents a general surgical trauma and includes specific problems due to the ischemia-reperfusion syndrome, the acute immunological reaction and any particular problems related to the type of the organ transplanted: all these factors, of course, have a different impact on the pathophysiological status of the patient.

Among the non-specific risk factors we can include the surgical stress response, (hypermetabolism, hypercatabolism, acute phase protein synthesis, posttraumatic immunosuppression, the need for increasing oxygen delivery and oxygen transport, the need to support the hyperdynamic state and the cardiac output) [2].

All these changes require an appropriate functional organ reserve and, from the therapeutic point of view, adequate support of the metabolic, hemodynamic and cardiorespiratory function.

Among the specific risk factors of particular relevance are the events related to the transplanted organ (e.g. hemorrhage in liver transplantation; ventricular insufficiency in heart transplantation, etc.) and to the whole pathophysiological derangement due to the severity of the surgical trauma and the degree of the immunosuppressive therapy.

Late deterioration of graft function brings the patient back to the pretransplant condition with aggravation due to the immunosuppressive state.

In summary, the clinical problems of organ transplantation are related to four major factors:

a) the recipient's status, namely the selection and pretransplant assessment;
b) perioperative events;
c) immediate late, continuing graft function;
d) immunosuppression.

These elements contribute, together or separately, to the success or failure of the transplant.

Nutritional assessment

Within all these elements the nutritional status of the patient together with the intrinsic nutritional status of the transplanted organ seem to play an important role in preventing and/or minimizing systemic complications as well as complications related to organ malfunction and/or organ rejection.

The parameters used to assess malnutrition in the preoperative period in patients who are waiting for organ transplantation do not differ from those used in patients waiting for general surgery.

Clinical, anthropometric, biohumoral and immunological parameters assess the nutritional status.

Anyway, it is very important to determine the degree of malnutrition, which must be correlated to the severity of the disease, and to the degree of organ dysfunction.

On the other hand, it is very useful to adjust the nutritional therapy in view of the metabolic derangement of the individual patient and the type of organ alterations.

Any given organ dysfunction or failure needs different nutritional formulas, looking at the better pharmacological effects of the individual nutrients in order to obtain an adequate positive nitrogen balance, avoiding severe side effects.

The causes of malnutrition can be different in patients awaiting organ transplantation, on the basis of the organ failure.

In end stage hepatic failure, the most common metabolic alteration is a defect of protein synthesis and the most common causes of malnutrition are due to anorexia, asthenia, intestinal malabsorption, recurrent infections, and a primary defect in the utilization of normal substrates, particularly aminoacids.

In end stage renal disease there is a prevalent hypermetabolism and hypercatabolism; the causes of malnutrition are related to the anorexia, uremia, hemodialysis, and to the underlying disease.

In pulmonary insufficiency, the main metabolic derangement is due to alterations of oxygen delivery and oxygen transport and malnutrition is due to anorexia, recurrent infections, hypoxia, or associated pancreatic insufficiency.

Whatever the causes, certainly malnutrition is closely related to an increase of postoperative complications, especially septic complications, which are much more frequent and severe because of the concomitant immunological reaction and the immunosuppressive therapy.

In liver transplantation Shaw and co-workers [3] identified a predictive equation for death in the first six months after transplantation. The scoring method is based on the high degree of correlation between survival probability and various preoperative and operative patient characteristics. Among the significant parameters are the presence of encephalopathy, ascites, the degree of malnutrition, the operative blood loss and amount of blood transfusions, and the presence of coagulopathy.

The metabolic response to the surgical trauma is closely related to the type of organ transplanted, but in all patients also to preoperative nutritional status.

All the patients present a surgical stress response after transplantation, with an increase of the resting energy expenditure (REE) and of 24-hour urinary urea nitrogen (UUN).

Only after liver transplantation, Shanbhogue et al. [4] showed that the patients in the early period after surgery are hypercatabolic (increased tissue breakdown) but not hypermetabolic compared with their stable state before transplantation.

Metabolic patterns in the donors

More recently, particular emphasis has been focused on the nutritional status of the cadaver donor: particularly it has been shown that the nutritional status of the donor may affect the outcome of the liver transplantation. However, many donors staying in the intensive care unit for a long period are in a reduced nutritional state.

In an experimental model in pigs, Sadamori et al. [5] demonstrated better liver function and bile production in liver transplanted pigs using organs from donors fed orally (group II) or treated by i.v. 20% glucose (group III) than from a control group of fasted pigs on i.v. normal saline (group I). In the same groups of animals the glycogen content in the liver at harvesting, which was completely consumed in group I, was well preserved after reperfusion in groups II and III.

The mean survival time was 37.2 days in group III, 9.8 days in group II and only 5.8 days in group I.

Conclusions

The success of organ transplantation is related to proper patient selection and timing of transplantation, proper prophylaxis and correct surgical technique.

Good graft function represents the fulcrum between the patient's recovering and progressive deterioration of his/her illness aggravated by the immunosuppressive state.

In relation to this delicate balance between the risks and benefits of immunosuppression, an aggressive approach to the recipient's preparation for transplantation in the perioperative intensive care and in the lifetime (graft-patient) follow-up is mandatory.

In this view, preoperative correction of malnutrition and postoperative identification of metabolic disorders due to surgical stress and the immunobiological response to the new organ are critical factors on which the survival of both graft and organism may depend.

After organ transplantation, artificial nutrition plays a critical role and has to be addressed to the metabolic derangements of the whole organism, bearing in mind the primary organ dysfunction or failure.

Today artificial nutrition, either enteral or parenteral, can effect a modulation of the immune system: there is evidence that artificial nutrition can have effects on:

- cell-cell communication;
- cytokine production;
- prostaglandin milieu;
- cell-mediated immune response;
- hypermetabolic and hypercatabolic syndrome.

The use of new substrates is strongly encouraged in organ transplantation.

New lipids have a wide range of immunomodulatory potencies (modulation of eicosanoid synthesis, changes in all membrane properties, changes at receptor bindings, etc.), pharmacological modification of prostaglandin milieu (blockage of PG synthesis, etc.), and faster hydrolysis with lower effects on the immune system.

New aminoacids (glutamine, arginine) can improve the cumulative nitrogen balance and can promote rapid proliferation of cells of the gut and of the immune system.

New factors (growth factors, etc.) are still under investigation and, in the case of organ transplantation, the cumulative effect on metabolism and on the immune response is still not clear.

The intention is to prevent, recognize and treat immediately any adverse immunological or infectious event.

References

1. Castagneto M, Sganga G, Serino F (1996) Risposta biomorale, compenso funzionale e complicanze nel trapianto d'organo. Atti Soc Ital Chir 4:281-284
2. Sganga G, Gangeri G, De Gaetano A, Castagneto M (1992) Metabolic aspects in complicated surgery. In: Gullo A (ed) Recent Advances in Anaesthesia Pain Intensive Care and Emergency, A.P.I.C.E., Trieste, pp 383-391
3. Shaw BW Jr, Wood RP, Gordon RD et al (1985) Influence of selected patient variables and operative blood loss on six-month survival following liver transplantation. Semin Liv Dis 5(4): 385-393
4. Shanbhogue RL, Bistrian BR, Jenkins RL et al (1987) Increased protein catabolism without hypermetabolism after human orthotopic liver transplantation. Surgery 101(2):146-149
5. Sadamori H, Tanaka N, Yagi T et al (1995) The effects of nutritional repletion on donors for liver transplantation in pigs. Transplantation 27;60(4):317-321

Clinical Aspects of Nutrition in Acute Renal Failure

H.P. KIERDORF

The mortality of acute renal failure has not changed in the last 20 years [1-4] despite progress in intensive care and extracorporeal treatment. This is mainly due to an increasing incidence of multiple organ failure (MOF) including acute renal failure (ARF) [2-4]. Major changes in the treatment of ARF in the intensive care unit (ICU) in the last 20 years were the development of continuous renal replacement therapy (CRRT) and the improvements in the nutritional management. CRRT offers the opportunity thanks to the unlimited fluid exchange to adapt nutritional support to the individual needs of these critically ill patients [4]. There is no doubt that the principles of nutrition in ARF in the ICU fundamentally differ from those used in the treatment of patients with end-stage renal failure (ESRF) [5]. The concept of a diet with reduced protein intake and the exclusive use of essential amino acids (EAA) can not be transferred to the nutritional support of ARF patients [6]. The problems of such a transfer will be discussed.

ARF patients are substantially different from patients with ESRF; also, they need amino acid (AA) in their nutrition as originally shown by Abel et al., who recorded improved survival in ARF patients with additional AA input compared to the administration of glucose alone [8]. Since then the question of whether a better survival rate is due to protein intake by AA or to an improvement in nutritional input has been controversial [9-11]. Another aspect is that ARF has today become a hypercatabolic disease, which is usually part of a MOF, a syndrome in which there is little doubt that nutritional treatment is one of the cornerstones of modern intensive care [5].

The aim of this review will be to analyse the changes in nutritional support of ARF patients according to changes in their clinical status and the increasing severity of the accompanying disease. It will analyse the metabolic impact of uremia on metabolism and it will discuss the type and composition of nutrients of critically ill hypercatabolic ARF patients.

Metabolic changes associated with ARF or extracorporeal treatment

Several metabolic troubles have been associated with ARF. However, it is often difficult to distinguish ARF-related alterations from those due to the underlying disease following sepsis, injury or other severe illness.

Protein metabolism

One major metabolic abnormality in ARF is accelerated protein catabolism, leading to a negative nitrogen balance, thus endangering these critically ill patients independently of the underlying disease [12]. Enhanced protein degradation and release of amino acids from skeletal muscle [13, 14], combined with a slightly increased hepatic protein synthesis result in a strong negative nitrogen balance [14]. Skeletal muscle proteolysis is a "physiological" reaction in this hypercatabolic condition, leading to a redistribution of amino acids to the liver for gluconeogenesis [15], synthesis of acute phase proteins [16], reparation of epithelium in the bowel [17] and glutamine release to lymphocytes and granulocytes [18]. As a consequence of alterations in amino acid metabolism in ARF, i.e. reduced tyrosine clearance and increased cystine and histidine clearance, the plasma concentration of amino acids and their individual utilisation is altered [19]. Proteolysis, especially in skeletal muscle is attributed to endocrine changes (insulin resistance and glucagon, catecholamines, growth factors) [15, 20], the release of mediators of MOF, such as tumour necrosis factor and other interleukins [21-24] and circulating proteolytic enzymes [25-27]. In addition the form of extracorporeal treatment in these patients also influences metabolic pathways. During conventional hemodialysis up to 1-3 g amino acids are lost every hour [28, 29], leading to a protein loss of up to 10 g in every treatment, which increases during consecutive amino acid infusion [30]. Acetate-hemodialysis has been shown to increase muscle proteolysis [31] and oxygen consumption [32], but it seems questionable whether this is true for modern dialysis therapy, especially for bicarbonate-hemodialysis.

CRRT also leads to a significant daily loss of amino acids and protein. The AA concentration in the hemofiltrate reaches 0.2-0.3 g/L, resulting in a daily loss of up to 10-15 g AA per day. [34, 35]. Since AA have a sieving coefficient close to 1.0, the loss of AA in the hemofiltrate is determined by their plasma concentration.

Carbohydrate metabolism

Glucose intolerance has been widely reported in ARF [10, 36]. This is probably due to a post receptor defect rather than to impaired insulin sensitivity since the insulin concentration needed for glucose uptake is normal. This might mirror the same situation encountered in severe sepsis or injury [37]. On the other hand muscular glycogen synthesis is impaired [38].

Hepatic gluconeogenesis, as mentioned above, is accelerated with enhanced hepatic extraction of gluconeogenetic amino acids [15, 38] and cannot be suppressed by increased glucose input [39]. Glucose is a small molecule with a molecular weight of 180 and is therefore eliminated in every CRRT with a daily loss of 50-100 g according to the amount of haemofiltrate and glucose plasma concentration. This daily energy loss of 200-500 kcal must be taken into account [30, 33, 35, 40]. It appears, however, that CRRT does not lead to a loss of insulin [40]. The metabolic changes in carbohydrate metabolism are even more complicated, as in animal experiments a reduction in both the production and hepatic removal of insulin, following bilateral nephrectomy in dogs, has been demonstrated [41]. In the same study a reduced insulin metabolism, leading to increased plasma insulin levels due to a decreased insulin degradation and excretion was described.

Lipid metabolism

Hypertriglyceridemia is the main symptom in ARF according to disturbed metabolism of lipids and fatty acids by impaired lipolysis [5, 42]. Cholesterol, especially high density lipoprotein cholesterol, is decreased [5, 43, 44]. Compared to ESRF patients, carnitine seems to play no role in lipid abnormalities or disturbed fatty acid metabolism in ARF patients. Due to an increased release from the skeletal muscle, carnitine levels are in the upper normal range or are increased in critically ill patients with ARF [45]. The elimination of parenterally administered lipid solutions in critically ill patients with ARF is reduced by more than 50%, both for long chain and medium chain triglycerides [46]. Due to the high molecular weight lipids are not eliminated during CRRT or hemodialysis

Metabolic changes associated with MOF

For patients with MOF a slightly increased metabolic rate leading to an increase of energy consumption up to 50-70% after major burns and severe head injuries had been described [49, 50]. Unfortunately most of these data are not so accurate as they seem, since, one problem in these critically ill patients is that accurate measurement of energy expenditure is not easy [51]. Despite this difficulty, it is important to note that even in critically ill patients with severe sepsis a recorded energy expenditure in excess of 2700 kcal/d is uncommon [52].

The complete pathogenesis of hypermetabolism is unclear [53], but the changes in carbohydrate, lipid and protein metabolism does not seem to differ significantly in the critically ill with or without ARF. Insulin resistance in septic [54] and thermally injured patients [55] is the hallmark of carbohydrate metabolism, reflecting abnormalities in both liver and muscle glucose and glycogen metabolism (see above). Unlike healthy subjects in whom fat oxidation can be suppressed by large amounts of carbohydrates, hypermetabolic patients behave abnormally in that such suppression cannot be achieved, even when plasma insulin is controlled [52, 54]. As is the case in ARF patients, lipid metabolism is characterized by an impairment of lipolysis [42], leading to hypertriglyceridemia [44]. The changes in protein metabolism are the same as those described in ARF patients [56]. In conclusion, the pathogenesis and derangements leading to metabolic changes as a result of sepsis, injury, MOF and ARF are similar.

Practical applications

Energy, amino acid and micronutrient requirements

As mentioned above, energy expenditure is generally normal in patients with uncomplicated ARF [57], while sepsis or MOF may increase expentidure in ARF patients by 20-40% [57-59]. Substrate requirements in critically ill patients with ARF are mainly determined by the accompanying vital function disturbances as mentioned above. Even in severe sepsis energy expenditure does not exceed 2500 kcal/d and complications with an excessive input of calories may occur. Especially with high intravenous carbohydrate intake [5, 60] the total calories administered should not exceed 30-40 kcal/kg/day. Earlier recommendations of up to 50 kcal/kg/day [61] increase the risk of dangerous side effects in ARF patients. In CRRT or haemodialysis glucose elimination during treatment should be taken into account, while fat is not eliminated during any extracorporeal therapy. There is no doubt that AA input is beneficial for critically ill patients. In sepsis daily nitrogen excretion varies between 16 and 40 g/d [62-64], according to the severity of the disease. The same level nitrogen excretion is described for MOF patients with or without ARF [11, 64-66]. Protein malnutrition has been identified as an independent predictor for outcome in MOF patients [9, 66, 67]. The aim of AA substitution in this situation is to reduce the negative nitrogen balance, which is difficult due to the severity of the disease [68, 69]. Nitrogen excretion studies have shown that ARF patients lose 1.2-1.5 g protein/kg/day, but only a few studies have attempted to define the optimal amino acid intake in critically ill ARF patients. Most of these studies date from the early eighties [11, 61, 70] with a very low nitrogen administration level compared to modern studies [71]. One of the reasons was the extracorporeal treatment available, limiting the protein intake to 21 or 42 g per day in one study [11] as the authors subsequently referred with a critical approach [72]. This is not the case if modern CRRT is used. In a prospective study we demonstrated a significant reduction in protein catabolism with adapted amino acid intake in a group of 30 patients with MOF, including ARF. All patients were treated by CRRT. The patients received 30 kcal/kg/day of energy (carbohydrate: lipid = 2:1), 10 patients 0.7 g amino acid/kg/day, 10 patients 1.5 g amino acid/kg/day and in 10 patients amino acid administration was adapted to daily nitrogen loss averaged at 1.74 g/kg/day. We could not reach a positive nitrogen balance, but could show a significantly improved nitrogen balance in the two groups with higher nitrogen input [73, 74]. In this study an amino acid loss of 5-7 g/day was demonstrated. We therefore concluded that the critically ill with ARF during CRRT need a minimal amino acid input of about 1.5 g/kg body weight.

Little is known about the requirements of micronutrients in critically ill ARF patients. In experimental ARF vitamin E and selenium deficiency decrease the recovery rate of the kidneys [75]. The same is true for a decreased oxygen radical scavenger system [76]. A zinc deficiency is common in MOF patients [77]. Story et al. recently published small or undetectable micronutrients loss in CRRT, while compared to healthy volunteers all MOF patients with or without ARF had significantly lower median blood concentrations of vitamin C, vitamin E, copper, selenium and zinc [78].

Since water soluble micronutrients are lost during every extracorporeal treatment, nutrition must include a supplement of all water soluble vitamines [5]. In CRRT a daily removal of folic acid of about 700 nmol and of 80 nmol of pyridoxal-5-phoshate has been described [79]. Excessive doses of vitamin C should be avoided, as more than 250 mg/d may aggravate ARF, leading to secondary oxalosis [80]. Fat soluble vitamins E and D should be administered, while vitamin A and K levels increase during ARF [5, 81].

No established guidelines for trace elements have been described for the nutrition of ARF patients in the ICU, so we substitute a mixture of zinc, selenium, magnesium, manganese, cobalt and copper twice a week. Overdosage must be avoided, as ARF may interfere with the normal metabolism of trace elements and AS intoxication has been described [5].

Which nutritional substrates to substitute amino acids, carbohydrates and fat?

One of the essential questions in obtaining the ideal nutrition mixture for ARF-patients is whether to apply EAA only, or AA solutions containing EAA and non essential amino acids (NEAA) as recently used in the ICU. The use of EAA solutions is based on a concept developed for the treatment of patients with chronic renal failure [82]. Such a treatment does not take into account either the specific metabolic problems of critically ill patients with ARF, nor the fact that the application of EAA alone is suitable only if done orally, which is often impossible in the critically ill [83]. Subsequently general amino acid solutions containing EAA and NEAA with no special composition were used especially in the ICU for critically ill patients [5]. Three main reasons have been suggested for the use of such a mixture: first, in critically ill patients many NEAA are not readily synthesized but are needed because of their physiologic functions [84]. Secondly, specific NEAA (histidine and arginine) might conditionally become essential in ARF [85]. Thirdly many NEAA are extracted by the liver from plasma, as these amino acids are metabolized in gluconeogenesis (see above). It is unknown whether any solutions especially developed for ARF patients with a higher amount of gluconeogenetic AA and branched-chain AA might play any role in nutritional treatment [86]. In conclusion, the best amino acid solution for critically ill ARF patients has not been defined yet; however, the exclusive administration of EAA is today obsolete and the use of any AA solution for ICU patients may be useful in these patients. Alternative carbohydrates, such as xylitol, sorbitol or fructose offer no advantages over glucose and may have hazardous side effects. Lactacidosis, induction or prolongation of ARF and an increasing consumption of ATP, leading to a dramatic reduction of phosphate [87-89] have been described. Therefore, glucose seems to be the main energy substrate in critically ill patients with ARF. As mentioned above, due to insulin resistance in some cases, a continuous intake of insulin is necessary to maintain a plasma glucose concentration of about 10 mmol/l, but an intake of more than 3-5 g glucose/kg/day should be avoided. Over this maximum limit lipogenesis, hepatomegaly by fatty infiltration, cholostasis and increased carbon dioxide production can occur [60, 90]. In nearly all cases it is not possible and not even desirable to cover the whole energy requirement by glucose alone. Administration of fat or glucose is not recommended today but, rather, the application of a combination of fat and glucose whenever possible [91-93] although no clinical studies exist about which energy mixture is the best in nutritional management of ARF patients in the ICU. Combining glucose and lipids agrees with the trend in general intensive care to shift to a fuel preference of lipids [91-93]. Lipid solutions have the advantage to cover energy demand in high concentration at a low osmolality with a diminished carbon dioxide production, which may be advantageous in mechanically ventilated patients [94]. It is at present unclear whether ARF patients will benefit from the use of medium chain triglycerides as compared to fat solutions with long chain triglycerides [95]. As mentioned above, the elimination of both is equally delayed in ARF patients [46]. We start with 0.5 g lipids/kg/day, increasing the dosage to a maximum of 1.5 g/kg/day under regular control of the plasma triglyceride and glucose concentration, in order to choose the best individual ratio of lipids to carbohydrate for each patient.

How to administer nutrition?

There is no doubt that in the critically ill, enteral nutrition has important advantages over parenteral feeding and it is generally agreed that enteral feeding should be used for all patients who can tolerate it [5, 96, 97]. The major advantages of this form of feeding have often been demonstrated. Protection of the gastrointestinal mucosa [97] and reduced bacterial translocation [98] have been described. Enterally administered nutrition even in small amounts will maintain normal intestinal function [99]. Oral feeding is nearly impossible in the critically ill, therefore enteral nutrition is often administered using a soft feeding tube usvally placed with tip in the stomach. Especially in unconscious patients, the insertion of the tube under endoscopic control beyond the pyloric sphincter seems to have some advantages. Fix compositions of enteral nutrients are often of little use in ARF patients because of their high potassium and/or sodium concentration. It is necessary to mix different components to adapt enteral feeding with special reference to the protein demand of these patients. The advantages of enteral feeding in experimental ARF have been shown recently by Mouser et al. [100].

In patients with disturbed gastrointestinal motility, parenteral nutrition is necessary. Despite the general problems of this such nutrition, technique is well established [101]. Any subsequent complications seem to be attributable to the technique rather than to ARF or MOF themselves [72, 85]. One minor advantage of the parenteral application of nutrients is a better fluid balancing of these patients, as in many critically ill resorption of enterally administered nutrition is unclear and balancing errors may occur.

Specific problems of extracorporeal treatment on nutrition

When conventional dialysis treatment is used, especially in anuric patients, despite daily haemodialysis, hyperhydration frequently occurs during intermittent treatment due to parenteral feeding as fluid overload is one of the most common problems encountered during extracorporeal treatment in critically ill patients with ARF. This often leads to an insufficient nutrition in these patients, since in cases of fluid overload nutrition is often neglected and malnutrition becomes a problem [102]. Due to the high fluid turnover rate, no limitations on fluids are necessary in CRRT techniques [74]. All forms of nutrition can be adapted without restriction to the needs of hypercatabolic patients, even in cases of anuria. Recent studies show that MOF patients benefit greatly from CRRT, thanks to the unlimited supply of energy and amino acids and to the steady control of azotemia [69, 70, 103-105]. CRRT eliminates the effect of malnutrition on the mortality rate of these patients.

Conclusion

Our conclusions for ARF patients with MOF on parenteral nutrition are reported on Table 1. They are based on the following:

- nutritional therapy in critically ill patients with ARF does not depend on the impairment of renal function but on the severity of the underlying MOF. The nutrition of these patients must be adapted to the rules of nutritional treatment of other critically ill patients;
- there is no doubt that enteral nutrition should be used whenever possible, since undefined resorption may result in balancing errors;
- ARF per se does not have consequences on energy expenditure;

Table 1. Example of a total parenteral nutrition in a critically ill patient with ARF treated by continuous hemofiltration. ICU means intensive care unit. Composition of BCAA (branched-chain amino acids) - enriched solution is detailed in [86]

	Energy amount Kcal/kg bw/day	Volume ml/day
Energy		
Glucose 40 (50)%	20-25 (30)	700-1000
Fat 20 (10)%	8-12	200-400
Amino Acids		
ICU solution (10%) or	4-8	700-1200
BCAA solution	4-8	700-1200

Additional ingredients: Water-soluble vitamines daily, Vitamin D + E and micronutrients twice a week

– nutrition in ARF patients differs from that in ESRF patients. There is absolutely no role for the sole application of EAA in ARF. Tailored AA administration up to 1.5-1.7 g/kg/day is necessary to reduce negative nitrogen balance in hypercatabolic patients;

– no data exist about the composition of AA solutions, however any ICU solution can be used;

– an energy dose of 25-35 kcal/kg/day should be administered as a glucose (3-5 g/kg/day) and lipid solution (up to 1.5 g/kg/day) according to the clinical condition of the patients;

– CRRT offers the opportunity to nourish each patient according to individual needs, so there is no reason to reduce nutrition because of extracorporeal treatment. In every extracorporeal treatments the amino acid and glucose loss must be taken into account.

References

1. Butkus DE (1983) Persistent high mortality in acute renal failure. Arch Intern Med 2:209-212
2. Sieberth HG, Kierdorf H (1989) Is continuous haemofiltration superior to intermittent dialysis and haemofiltration treatment? Adv Exp Med Biol 260:181-192
3. Cameron JS (1990) Acute renal failure thirty years on. Q J Med 74:1-2
4. Kierdorf H (1995) The nutritional management of acute renal failure in the intensive care unit. New Horizon 3:700-718
5. Druml W (1993) Nutritional support in acute renal failure. Clin Nutr 12:196-207
6. Berlyne GM, Bazzard FJ, Booth EM et al (1967) The dietary treatment of acute renal failure. Q J Med 141:59-65
7. Kleinknecht D, Junkers R, Chanard J et al (1972) Uremic and non-uremic complications in acute renal failure. Evaluation of early and frequent dialysis on prognosis. Kidney Int 1: 190-194
8. Abel RM, Beck CH, Abbott WM et al (1973) Improved survival from acute renal failure after treatment with intravenous essential L-amino acids and glucose. N Engl J Med 288:695-698

9. Mault JR, Bartlett RH, Deckert RE et al (1983) Starvation: A major contributing factor to mortality in acute renal failure. Trans Am Soc Artif Intern Organs 29:390-394
10. Feinstein EI, Blumenkrantz J, Healy M et al (1981) Clinical and metabolic responses to parenteral nutrition in acute renal failure. Medicine 60:124-137
11. Feinstein EI, Kopple JD, Silberman H et al (1983) Total parenteral nutrition with high or low nitrogen intakes in patients with acute renal failure. Kidney Int 24:S319-S323
12. Wolfe RR, Jahoor F, Hartl WH (1989) Protein and amino acid metabolism after injury. Diabetes Metab Rev 5:149-164
13. Flugel-Link RM, Salusky IB et al (1983) Protein and amino acid metabolism in the posterior hemicorpus of acutely uremic rats. Am J Physiol 244:615-623
14. Lacy WW (1969) Effect of acute uremia on amino acid uptake and urea production by perfused rat liver. Am J Physiol 216:1300-1305
15. Hasselgren PO, Pedersen P, Sax HC et al (1988) Current concepts of protein turnover and amino acid transport in liver and skeletal muscle during sepsis. Arch Surg 123:992-999
16. Roth E, Funovics J, Schulz F, Karner J (1980) Biochemische Methoden zur Bestimmung des klinischen Eiweißkatabolismus. Infusionsther Klin Ern 6:306-309
17. Souba WW, Smith RJ, Wilmore DW (1985) Glutamine metabolism by the intestinal tract. J Par Ent Nutr 9:608-617
18. Schauder P (1990) Glutamine metabolism in human lymphocytes. Clin Nutr 9:36-37
19. Druml W, Burger U, Kleinberger G et al (1986) Elimination of aminoacids in acute renal failure. Nephron 42:62-67
20. Frayn KN, Little RA, Maycock PF, Stoner HB (1985) The relationship of plasma catecholamines to acute metabolic and hormonal responses to injury in man. Circ Shock 16:229-240
21. Baracos V, Rodemann HP, Dinarello CA, Goldberg AL (1983) Stimulation of muscle protein degradation and prostaglandin E_2 release by leukocyte pyrogen (interleukin-1). N Engl J Med 308:553-558
22. Clowes GHA, George BC, Villee CA, Saravis CA (1983) Muscle proteolysis induced by a circulating peptide in patients with sepsis or trauma. N Engl J Med 308:545-552
23. Nathan CF (1987) Secretory products of macrophages. J Clin Invest 79:319-326
24. Zamir O, Hasselgren PO, Kunkel SL et al (1992) Evidence that tumor necrosis factor participates in the regulation of muscle proteolysis during sepsis. Arch Surg 127:170-174
25. Hörl WH, Heidland A (1980) Enhanced proteolytic activity: cause of protein catabolism in acute renal failure. Am J Clin Nutr 33:1423-1427
26. Hörl WH, Stepinski J, Gantert C et al (1981) Evidence for the participation of proteases on protein catabolism during hypercatabolic renal failure. Klin Wochenschr 59:751-757
27. Heidland A, Schaefer RM, Heidbreder E, Hörl WH (1988) Catabolic factors in renal failure: Therapeutic approaches. Nephrol Dial Transplant 3:8-16
28. Young GA, Parsons FM (1966) Amino nitrogen loss during haemodialysis, its dietary significance and replacement. Clin Sci 31:299-307
29. Kopple JD, Swendseid ME, Shinaber JH, Umezawa CY (1973) The free and bound amino acids removed by hemodialysis. Trans Am Soc Artif Intern Organs 14:309-311
30. Wolfson M, Jones MR, Kopple JD (1982) Amino acid losses during hemodialysis with infusion of aminoacids and glucose. Kidney Int 21:500-506
31. Alverstrand A, Gutierrez A, Wahren J et al (1987) Protein catabolism in sham hemodialysis: the effect of different membranes. Blood Purif 5:269-275
32. Mault JR, Bartlett RU, Dechert RE et al (1982) Oxygen consumption during hemodialysis for acute renal failure. Trans Am Soc Artif Intern Organs 28:514-516
33. Blumenkrantz MJ, Gahl GM, Kopple JD et al (1981) Protein losses during peritoneal dialysis. Kidney Int 19:593-602
34. Davenport A, Will EJ, Davidson AM (1993) Improved cardiovascular stability during continuous modes of renal replacement therapy in critically ill patients with acute hepatic and renal failure. Crit Care Med 21:328-338

35. Davies SP, Reaveley DA, Brown EA, Kox WJ (1991) Amino acid clearences and daily losses in patients with acute renal failure treated by continuous arteriovenous hemodialysis. Crit Care Med 19:1510
36. De Fronzora, Tobin JD, Rowe JW, Andres R (1978) Glucose intolerance in uremia. Quantification of pancreatic beta cell sensitivity to glucose and tissue sensitivity to insulin. J Clin Invest 62:425-434
37. Fröhlich J, Schölmerich J, Hoppe-Seyler G et al (1974) The effect of acute uremia on gluconeogenesis in isolated perfused rat livers. Europ J Clin Invest 4:453-458
38. May RC, Clark AS, Goheer MA, Mitch WE (1985) Specific defects in insulin-mediated muscle metabolism in acute uremia. Kidney Int 28:490-497
39. Cianciaruso B, Bellizzi V, Napoli R et al (1991) Hepatic uptake and release of glucose, lactate and amino acids in acutely uremic dogs. Metabolism 40:261-290
40. Bellomo R, Colman PG, Caudwell J et al (1992) Acute continuous hemofiltration with dialysis: effect on insulin concentrations and glycemic control in critically ill patients. Crit Care Med 20:1672-1676
41. Cianciaruso B, Sacca L, Terracciano V et al (1987) Insulin metabolism in acute renal failure. Kidney Int 32:S109-S112
42. Druml W, Zechner R, Magometschnigg D et al (1985) Post-heparin lipolytic activity in acute renal failure. Clin Nephrol 23:289-293
43. Naschitz JE, Varak C, Yeshurun D (1983) Reversible diminished insulin requirement in acut failure. Postgrad Med J 59:269-271
44. Druml W, Laggner A, Widhalm K et al (1983) Lipid metabolism in acute renal failure. Kidney Int 24:S139-S142
45. Wanner C, Riegel W, Schaefer RM et al (1989) Carnitine and camitine esters in acute renal failure. Nephrol Dial Transplant 4:951-956
46. Druml W, Fischer M, Sertl S et al (1992) Fat elimination in acute renal failure: Long chain versus medium chain triglycerides. Am J Clin Nutr 55:468-472
47. Cuthbertson DP (1942) Post-shock metabolic response. Lancet I 433-437
48. Wilmore DW, Kinney JM (1981) Panel report on nutritional support of patients with trauma or infection. Am J Clin Nutr 34:1213-1222
49. Davies JWL (1982) Physiological responses to burning injury. Academic Press, New York
50. Clifton GI, Robertson CS, Choi SC (1986) Assessment of nutritional requirements of head-injured patients. J Neurosurg 64:895-901
51. Barison RD (1990) The measurement of energy expenditure: instrumentation, practical considerations, and clinical application. Respir Care 35:640-659
52. Stoner HB, Little RA, Frayn KN et al (1983) The effect of sepsis on the oxidation of carbohydrate and fat. Br J Surg 70:32-35
53. Liddell MJ, Daniel AM, MacLean LD et al (1979) The role of stress hormones in the catabolic metabolism of shock. Surg Gynecol Obstet 149:822-830
54. White RH, Frayn KN, Little RA et al (1987) Hormonal and metabolic responses to glucose infusion in sepsis studied by the hyperglycaemic glucose clamp technique. J Parent Ent Nutr 11:345-353
55. Little RA, Henderson A, Frayn KN et al (1987) The disposal of intravenous glucose studied using glucose and insulin clamp techniques in sepsis and trauma in man. Acta Anaesth Belg 38:275-279
56. Long CL, Jeevanandam M, Kim BM et al (1977) Whole-body protein synthesis and catabolism in septic man. Am J Clin Nutr 30:1340-1344
57. Schneeweiß B, Graninger W, Stockenhuber F et al (1990) Energy metabolism in acute and chronic renal failure. Am J Clin Nutr 52:596-601
58. Bouffard Y, Viale JP, Annat G et al (1987) Energy expenditure in the acute renal failure patient mechanically ventilated. Intens Care Med 13:401-406
59. Soop M, Forsberg E, Thörne A et al (1989) Energy expenditure in postoperative multiple organ failure with acute renal failure. Clin Nephrol 31:139-143

60. Sax HC, Talamini MA, Brackett K et al (1986) Hepatic steatosis in total parenteral nutrition: failure of fatty infiltration to correlate with abnormal serum hepatic enzyme levels. Surgery 100:697-703
61. Spreiter SC, Meyers BD, Swenson RS (1980) Protein energy requirements in subjects with acute renal failure receiving intermittent hemodialysis. Am J Clin Nutr 33:1433-1438
62. Roth E, Funovics J, Sporn P et al (1981) Parenterale Ernährung beim septischen Patienten. Intensivmed 18:97-101
63. Radrizzani D, Iapichino G, Cambisano M et al (1988) Peripheral, visceral and body nitrogen balance of catabolic patients, without and with parenteral nutrition. Intensive Care Med 14:212-216
64. Behrendt W, Kierdorf H (1992) Stoffwechsel und Ernährung bei Sepsis. Intensiv und Notfall 17:96-101
65. Knochel JP (1985) Complications of total parenteral nutrition. Kidney Int 27:489-495
66. Bartlett RH, Mault JR, Deckert RE et al (1986) Continuous arteriovenous hemofiltration: Improved survival in surgical acute renal failure? Surgery 100:400-408
67. Bartlett RH (1985) Energy metabolism in acute renal failure. In: Sieberth HG, Mann H (eds) Continuous arteriovenous hemofiltration (CAVH). Karger, Basel, pp 194-203
68. Rennie MJ (1985) Muscle protein turnover and the wasting due to injury and disease. Br Med Bull 41:257-264
69. Bessey PQ (1990) Nutritional support in critical illness. In: Deitch AE. Multiple organ failure. Thieme, Stuttgart, New York, pp 126-149
70. Lopez-Martinez J, Caparros T et al (1980) Nutrition parenteral en enfermos septicos con fracaso renal agudo en fase poliurica. Rev Clin Esp 157:171-178
71. Bellomo R, Martin H, Parkin G et al (1991) Continuous arteriovenous haemodiafiltration in the critically ill. Influence on major nutrient balances. Intensive Care Med 17:399-402
72. Feinstein EI (1985) Parenteral nutrition in acute renal failure. Am J Nephrol 5:145-149
73. Kierdorf H, Kindler J, Sieberth HG (1986) Nitrogen balance in patients with acute renal failure treated by continuous arteriovenous haemofiltration. Nephrol Dial Transplant 1:72
74. Kierdorf H (1991) Continuous versus intermittent treatment: Clinical results in acute renal failure. Contrib Nephrol 93:1-12
75. Nath KA, Paller MS (1990) Dietary deficiency of antioxidants exacerbates ischemic injury in the rat kidney. Kidney Int 38:1109-1117
76. Joannidis M, Bonn G, Pfaller W (1989) Lipid peroxidation - An initial event in experimental acute renal failure. Renal Physiol Biochem 12:47-55
77. Golden MHN, Golden BE, Harland PSEG et al (1978) Zinc and immuno competence in protein-energy malnutrition. Lancet 1:1226-1229
78. Story DA, Ronco C, Bellomo R (1999) Trace element and vitamin concentration and losses in critically ill patients treated with continuous venovenous hemofiltration. Crit Care Med 27:220-223
79. Fortin MC, Amyot SL, Geadah D, Leblanc M (1999) Serum concentrations and clearances of folic acid and pyridoxal-5-phosphate during venovenous continuous renal replacement therapy. Intensive Care Med 25:594-598
80. Friedman AL, Chesney RW, Gilbert EF et al (1983) Secondary oxalosis as a complication of parenteral alimentation in acute renal failure. Am J Nephrol 3:248-252
81. Druml W, Schwarzenhofer M, Apsner R, Hörl WH (1998) Fat-soluble vitamines in patients with acute renal failure. Miner Electrolyte Metab 24:220-226
82. Bergstrom J, Furst P, Noree LU (1975) Treatment of chronic uremic patients with protein-poor diet and oral supply of essential amino acids. I. Nitrogen balance studies. Clin Nephrol 3:187-194
83. Fürst P, Ahlberg M, Alvestrand A, Bergström J (1978) Principles of essential amino acid therapy in uremia. Am J Clin Nutr 31:1744-1755
84. Druml W (1989) Nutritional importance of non-essential amino acids. J Clin Nutr Gastroenterol 4:71-75

85. Druml W, Bürger U, Kleinberger G et al (1986) Elimination of amino acids in acute renal failure. Nephron 42:62-67
86. Kierdorf H, Stehle P, Behrendt W et al (1991) Influence of a new amino acid (AA) solution with increased amount of essential and branched-chain AA on protein catabolism in acute renal (ARF) and multiple organ failure (MOF). Clin Nutr 10[Suppl 2]:57-58
87. Craig GM, Crane CW (1971) Lactic acidosis complicating liver failure after intravenous fructose. Brit Med J 211-216
88. Förster H, Meyer E, Ziege M (1970) Erhöhung von Serumharnsäure und Serumbilirubin nach hochdosierten Infusionen von Sorbit, Xylit und Fructose. Klin Wochenschr 48:878-879
89. Evans GW, Phillips G, Mukherjee TM et al (1973) Identification of crystals deposited in brain and kidney after xylitol administration by biochemical, and electron diffraction methods. J Clin Path 26:32-36
90. Burke JF, Wolfe RR, Mullany CJ et al (1979) Glucose requirements following burn injury. Ann Surg 190:274-279
91. Romanosky AJ, Bagby GJ, Bockman EL et al (1980) Free fatty acid utilization by skeletal muscle after endotoxin administration. Am J Physiol 239:E391-E395
92. Spitzer JJ, Bagby GJ, Meszaros K, Lang CH (1988) Alteration in lipid and carbohydrate metabolism in sepsis. J Parenter Enteral Nutr 12:553-558
93. Schneeweiß B, Graninger W, Ferenci P et al (1992) Short term energy balance in patients with infections: Carbohydrate-based versus fat-based diets. Metabolism 41:125-130
94. Christman JW, McCain RW (1993) A sensible approach to the nutritional support of mechanically ventilated critically ill patients. Intensive Care Med 19:129-136
95. Sobrado J, Moldawer LL, Pomposelli JJ et al (1985) Lipids emulsions and reticuloendothelial system function in healthy and burned guinea pigs. Am J Clin Nutr 9:559-565
96. McArdle AH, Palmason C, Mozency I, Brown RA (1981) A rationale for enteral feeding as the preferable route for hyperalimentation. Surgery 90:616-623
97. Kudsk KA, Crose MA, Fabian TC et al (1991) Enteral versus parenteral feeding. Effects on septic morbidity after blunt and penetrating abdominal trauma. Ann Surg 215:503-513
98. Zaloga GP (1991) Bedside method for placing small bowel feeding tubes in critically ill patients. A prospective study. Chest 100:1643-1646
99. Deitch EA, Winterton J, Berg R (1987) The gut as a portal of entry for bacteremia. Role of protein malnutrition. Ann Surg 207:681-692
100. Mouser JK, Hak EB, Kuhl DA et al (1997) Recovery from ischemic acute renal failure is improved with enteral compared with parenteral nutrition. Crit Care Med 25:1748-1754
101. Lee HA, Sharpstone P, Ames AC (1967) Parenteral nutrition in renal failure. Postgrad Med J 43:81-91
102. Paganini EP, O'Hara P, Nakamoto S (1984) Slow continuous ultrafiltration in hemodialysis resistant oliguric acute renal failure patients. Trans Am Soc Artif Intern Organs 30:173-178
103. Weisse L, Danielson BG, Wikstroem B et al (1989) Continuous arteriovenous haemofiltration in the treatment of 100 critically ill patients with acute renal failure: report on clinical outcome and nutritional aspects. Clin Nephrol 31:184-189
104. Geronemus R, Schneider N (1984) Continuous arteriovenous haemodialysis: A new modality for treatment of acute renal failure. Trans Am Soc Artif Intern Organs 30:610-613
105. Ronco C (1993) Continuous renal replacement therapies for the treatment of acute renal failure in intensive care patients. Clin Nephrol 40:187-198

The Tricks and Traps of Enteral Nutrition

G.J. DOBB

Many aspects of the approach to nutrition of critically ill patients have changed over the last decade even though the clinical problems are unchanged. Surgery, sepsis, trauma, burns and other causes of critical illness increase metabolic rate but sick patients are unable to eat because of impaired consciousness, sedation or recent surgery, or because their appetite is decreased. A large negative nitrogen balance can accumulate quickly with loss of muscle, delayed wound healing and reduced resistance to infection. It is now clear that the negative nitrogen balance cannot be reversed completely even with active nutritional support, but this should not prevent nutritional issues being considered in every patient needing intensive care.

The aims of nutritional support defined by the American Society for Parenteral and Enteral Nutrition [1] include:
- detection and correction of pre-existing malnutrition
- prevention of progressive protein energy malnutrition
- optimising patient's metabolic state
- reducing morbidity and time to convalescence

Trap: underestimation of pre-existing malnutrition

Critical illness often occurs after a period of illness with weight loss made greater by poor appetite, unattractive hospital food or fasting for procedures or surgery. Initial clinical assessment with a dieting history and clinical examination is important to define nutritional status and the need to minimise further deterioration. Surveys show up to one third of hospital inpatients have unrecognised malnutrition [2]. Indices commonly equated to poor nutritional status include a body mass index (body mass kg/height m^2) of less than 19 kg/m^2, weight loss of more than 10% of body weight over 3 months, or mid arm muscle circumference index below the 5th percentile (mid arm circumference cm – 3.14 x triceps skin fold thickness).

Tricks: Subjective clinical assessment appears to be no worse than more complex measures or techniques as an indicator of nutritional status [3, 4]. Hypoalbuminaemia and lymphopaenia are too non-specific to be useful in critically ill patients [3, 4].

Trap: delaying the start of enteral feeding

Early enteral feeding benefits patients after trauma and burns [5, 6]. It may be beneficial in other groups of critically ill patients but this remains controversial [7], particularly for patients with shock or gut mucosal ischaemia. It is known that enteral nutrition plays an important role in maintaining normal gut function, mucosal integrity and the normal gut bacterial flora [8], though human gut mucosa appears more resistant to atrophy than that of animals used in experimental studies - after no enteral feeding for two weeks mucosal mass can be unaffected [9]. Nevertheless, current consensus favours early enteral feeding and there is anecdotal evidence that establishing feeds early helps maintain gastric emptying.

Tricks: Consider starting enteral nutrition after initial resuscitation of the patient i.e. within 3-4 hours of intensive care unit admission. Commonly, the volume of enteral nutrition is increased in steps to the estimated requirement but this process is usually unnecessary and not of proven value unless prolonged starvation precedes the start of enteral nutrition. Nevertheless, it can be difficult to establish enteral feeding in some patients (Table 1) even if a naso- or orogastric tube is in place, the gut is not obstructed, not ischaemic and has not been resected. Bowel sounds correlate poorly with successful enteral nutrition, especially in mechanically ventilated patients [10]. Absent bowel sounds should not delay a trial of enteral nutrition. Recent upper gastrointestinal surgery [11] or pancreatitis [12] are not contraindications to enteral nutrition provided the nutrition is given through a jejunal feeding tube.

Table 1. Conditions associated with large gastric aspirates or difficulty in establishing enteral nutrition

Retroperitoneal haematoma
Intraperitoneal sepsis, blood or inflammation (e.g. pancreatitis)
Renal or biliary colic
Brain injury
Septicaemia or other cause of persistent shock (e.g. cardiogenic)
Electrolyte abnormalities: hypokalaemia, hypomagnesaemia, hypo- or hypercalcaemia
Metabolic abnormalities - diabetic ketoacidosis, myxoedema, acute porphyria, hepatic encephalopathy, anaemia, hypoxaemia
Drugs: narcotics, sedatives, anticholinergics
Immobilisation (e.g. paraplegia)

Chronic gastric emptying problems e.g. duodenal scarring, diabetic gastro-paresis, previous gastroparesis, previous truncal vagotomy, can become evident when nasogastric feeding and regular gastric aspiration are used during an episode of critical illness. Difficulty with nasogastric feeding is particularly common after traumatic brain injury [13] and does not appear to be just related to the opiates many of these patients receive.

Trap: giving up on enteral nutrition too easily

If patients are difficult to feed by the enteral route it is seductively easy to turn to parenteral nutrition. However, parenteral nutrition should only be considered if enteral nutrition is impossible. Enteral nutrition is cheaper and parenteral nutrition is associated with a greater risk of infective complications [14]. Parenteral fat emulsions possibly interfere with bacterial clearance [15]. Well nourished patients easily manage without nutritional support for up to five days if enteral nutrition is not possible [1]. While parenteral nutrition provides a viable alternative to starvation [16] the only contraindications to enteral nutrition are bowel obstruction, high output jejunal or ileal fistula, very extensive bowel resection and severe gut ischaemia.

Tricks: Enteral nutrition is usually started through a nasogastric tube. If patients are heavily sedated and ventilated, initial feeding through an oro-gastric tube reduces bleeding during insertion, and sinusitis. Nasal intubation is relatively contraindicated in patients with a base of skull fracture because of the risk of intracranial placement.

If nasogastric aspirates are persistently greater than 200-300 ml several tricks are available. Gastric aspirates are usually least with the patient lying right side down with the pylorus dependent. If gastric aspirates remain large, cisapride 10 mg nasogastrically 6 hourly will usually reduce the volume [17]. Alternatives are metoclopramide which has been shown to reduce aspirate volume once patients are established on feeds [18], domperidone 10-20 mg orally or 30-60 mg rectally every 4-8 hours, or erythromycin. Domperidone's efficacy has not been demonstrated in an adequate clinical trial and the high frequency of nausea associated with erythromycin often makes it unsuitable. If these measures are unsuccessful, transpyloric placement of a feeding tube should be considered. Many suitable tubes are commercially available in sizes 8-12 FG in varying designs. All have a wire stylet or guidewire to facilitate insertion and many are provided with a weighted tip despite there being little evidence that this assists transpyloric placement, but weighted tubes are easier to pass from oesophagus to stomach [19]. A soft 110 cm or more 8 FG hygromer-coated self lubricating tube with a metal stylet and a weighted non-bulbous tip is suitable for most adult patients.

Spontaneous passage of fine bore feeding tubes from stomach to duodenum is reported to occur in 15-50% of patients, though the proportion appears to be at the lower end of this range or less in patients needing intensive care, especially if they have large gastric aspirates. Prokinetic drugs including cisapride 10 mg 6 hourly, metoclopramide 10-20 mg intravenously 6 hourly or erythromycin 100-200 mg intravenously have been used to promote transpyloric placement but if they have been ineffective in reducing gastric aspirate volumes the chances of success seem low. It is quicker and more certain to guide the enteral feeding tube through the pylorus using endoscopy or fluoroscopy to a position with the tip in the jejunum or distal duodenum. Routine transpyloric placement of feeding tubes is unnecessary and, in comparison with intragastric feeding, the effect on the frequency of complications has been inconsistent [20]. Gastric feeding tubes are misplaced in 0.3-4% of blind insertions [21]. The tip position should always be confirmed by X-ray before feeding begins though this policy has been challenged in paediatric practice [22] with the inability to aspirate more than 10 ml of an aliquot of insufflated air being strongly associated with transpyloric positioning.

In some centres [23] it is common to fashion a feeding jejunostomy at the time of laparotomy for major upper gastrointestinal surgery or in critically ill patients. This overcomes problems associated with intragastric feeding but complications, including leaks, peritonitis and wound infection, are common compared to nasojejunal intubation [24].

Trap: expensive feeds are better feeds

A wide variety of enteral feeding products are available in both liquid and powder forms. The liquid feeds tend to be more expensive but are convenient, sterile and avoid the trouble and cost of preparation. When assessing the suitability of a feed the factors to consider are:

- energy to nitrogen ratio
- energy ratio of carbohydrate to fat
- energy density (kJ or Cal/ml)
- fibre content
- electrolyte content
- form of amino acids
- distribution of amino acid content
- other supplements

Enteral feed formulations designed for specific patient groups [4] e.g. trauma patients, are more expensive, but evidence of patient benefit from a very high nitrogen-to-energy ratio and other specific modifications needs careful evaluation.

Elemental feeds with protein as peptides or amino acids have no advantage over standard feeds for critically ill patients [25]. Although they have been recommended for use after prolonged fasting and in patients with short bowel syndrome, radiation enteritis, pancreatitis and pancreatic insufficiency, elemental feeds do not protect intestinal growth factors from auto-digestion [26] whereas standard protein sources do provide protection.

The addition of glutamine to enteral feeds has a strong theoretical basis. Glutamine is the most abundant amino acid in plasma but its plasma concentration decreases during critical illness. It has a major role as the main nitrogen transporter of nitrogen from sites of synthesis (muscle and liver) to sites of utilisation (gut, lymphocytes and lung), is a precursor of nucleotides and glutathione, and is a major metabolic fuel of the enterocytes of the gut mucosa, lymphocytes and macrophages [27]. Most commercial enteral feeds contain minimal or no glutamine because it is unstable in solution. Although experimental studies suggest it should be beneficial [28, 29] and some [30, 31] but not all [32] preliminary clinical studies are promising, the benefit of glutamine supplementation in patients needing intensive care has still to be confirmed.

"Immune-enhancing" enteral feeds supplemented with arginine, nucleotides and omega-3 fatty acids have been heavily promoted. Arginine is a non-essential amino acid in adults but also stimulates prolactin, growth hormone, glucagon and insulin release and is a precursor of nitric oxide. In both experimental and clinical studies arginine improves indirect measures of immune function [33, 34] but an effect on outcome in critically ill patients has not been shown [35]. In guinea pigs with peritonitis giving large amounts of arginine – 6% of total energy – decreased survival. Nucleotides are part of a normal diet and can be synthesised from glutamine. In experimental studies restriction of dietary nucleotides can reduce resistance to infection [36]. Normally the bacteria dying in the gut lumen provide more nucleotides than contained in "nucleotide supplemented feeds". Nucleotide supplements have not been shown to improve patient outcome. Dietary supplements of omega-3 fatty acids reduce monocyte production of interleukin 1α, interleukin 1β and tumour necrosis factor in human volunteers [37]. The effect of omega-3 fatty acids supplements in animal models of sepsis has been variable. Patients given fish oil as their fat source after abdominal surgery had a non-significant trend to reduced infection in a preliminary study but the effect of omega-3 fatty acids in isolation is not well studied.

The best studied feed combining arginine, nucleotide and omega-3 fatty acid enhancement is "Impact" (Sandoz Nutrition, Minneapolis, MH, USA). Other products available include "Immune-Aid" (McGaw Inc, Irvine, CA, USA) also supplemented with glutamine and branched chain amino acids and "Replete" (Clintec Nutrition, Deerfield, IL, USA) with glutamine and omega-3 fatty acids. The effect of these feeds on patient outcome remains controversial. Many studies are in surgical rather than critically ill patients. Well designed clinical trials are still needed to confirm any role for these products in intensive care. However, the current weight of evidence is in their favour [38] and the cost-benefit ratio overall seems plausible.

Most newer enteral feeds contain a source of fibre. The bacterial breakdown products of fibre: acetate, proprionate and butyrate are important substrates for the cells of the colonic mucosa. Although no adverse effects have been reported from including fibre in enteral feeds, published clinical trials do not provide firm evidence for its routine inclusion [39].

Tricks: In practice, a feed that is lactose-free, near isotonic, providing two thirds of non-protein energy as carbohydrate and with a caloric to nitrogen ratio of 100-150:1gN$_2$ (420-630MJ:1gN$_2$) suits most patients. The electrolyte content of feeds can be important in critically ill patients and varies widely between different feeds. Sodium restriction may be needed in patients with heart failure or oedema and restriction of potassium and magnesium intake in patients with renal failure. When fluid restriction is a priority, feeds are available with an energy density of 1.5 or 2.0 Cal/ml (6.3-8.4 kJ/ml).

The requirements of critically ill patients for vitamin and trace elements are poorly defined but it is likely there are important interactions with the pathophysiology of critical illness. Most commercial feeds contain the standard recommended daily allowance for vitamins in a volume containing approximately 2000 Cal (8.4 MJ). Critically ill patients probably need more than the recommended daily allowance for at least some vitamins [40] and losses of the water soluble vitamins (e.g. folic acid, vitamin C) will be increased by continuous haemodiafiltration. Supplements additional to the content of enteral feeds should therefore be given to patients in intensive care.

In patients who are glucose intolerant or patients being weaned from mechanical ventilation who have carbon dioxide retention, a reduced carbohydrate load can facilitate glycaemic control and minimise the respiratory quotient. Up to two thirds of non-protein energy may be provided as fat.

Trap: enteral feeding appears simple and benign

Although the complication rate associated with enteral nutrition is low, this does not mean that complications are absent (Table 2).

Tricks: Complications can be reduced by close patient observation and monitoring. The position of the feeding tube tip should be confirmed radiologically before feeds are started.

Whenever possible, patients should be nursed head up to minimise regurgitation. Nursing head up reduces the frequency of nosocomial pneumonia during enteral nutrition [41], probably by reducing microaspiration.

Pseudo-obstruction can be a troublesome problem during enteral feeding but usually responds to neostigmine 2.5 mg intravenously [41].

Many of the other complications can be reduced by close attention to the feed content and administration.

Table 2. Some of the complications reported in association with enteral nutrition

Related to feeding tube insertion
    Trauma and bleeding
    Perforation: retropharyngeal space, oesophagus, stomach
    Pneumomediastinum, pneumothorax
Related to the presence of a feeding tube
    Patient discomfort
    Erosion of nares
    Sinusitis
    Aerophagy
    Tube displacement or obstruction
    Wound infection, leaks, peritonitis (gastrostomy, jejunostomy)
Related to feed misplacement
    Pneumonitis
    Pleural effusion or empyema
Related to feeding
    Nausea, regurgitation, vomiting
    Abdominal distention
    Pulmonary aspiration of feed
    Intestinal pseudo-obstruction
Interaction with medications (reduced absorption)
Related to feed content
    Hyperglycaemia
    Hypercarbia
    Azotaemia
    Electrolyte abnormality (especially low potassium, magnesium phosphate and zinc)
    Deficiency disorders after long term use

Conclusion

Nutritional support should be a routine consideration during intensive care. The many products and devices now available make it easy to provide but there are still traps for the unwary. A few tricks and close attention to detail can increase the chances of successful enteral nutrition and reduce the risk of complications.

References

1. American Society for Parenteral and Enteral Nutrition Board of Directors (1993) Guidelines for the use of parenteral and enteral nutrition in adult and pediatric patients. FPEN 14:1SA-52SA
2. Nightingale JMD, Walsh N, Bullock ME et al (1996) Three simple methods of detecting malnutrition on medical wards. J Roy Soc Med 89:144-148
3. Manning EMC, Shenkin A (1995) Nutritional assessment in the critically ill. Crit Care Clin 11:603-634
4. Chan S, McCowen KC, Blackburn GL (1999) Nutrition management in the ICU. Chest 115: 145S-148S

5. Chiarelli A, Enzi G, Casadei A et al (1990) Very early nutrition supplementation in burned patients. Am J Clin Nutr 51:1035-1039
6. Moore E, Jones T (1986) Benefits of immediate jejunostomy feeding after major abdominal trauma: a prospective randomised study. J Trauma 26:874-880
7. Revelly JP, Berger M, Chiolero R (1999) The haemodynamic response to enteral nutrition. In: Vincent JL (ed) Yearbook of intensive care and emergency medicine. Springer, Berlin, pp 105-114
8. Dobb GJ (1992) Enteral nutrition for the critically ill. In: Vincent JL (ed) Yearbook of intensive care and emergency medicine. Springer, Berlin, pp 609-619
9. Guedon C, Schmitz J, Lerebours E et al (1986) Decreased brush border hydrolase activities without gross morphologic changes in human intestinal mucosa after prolonged total parenteral nutrition of adults. Gastroenterology 90:373-378
10. Shelly MP, Church JJ (1987) Bowel sounds during intermittent positive pressure ventilation. Anaesthesia 42:207-209
11. Carr CS, Ling KDE, Boulos P et al (1996) Randomised trial of safety and efficacy of immediate postoperative enteral feeding in patients undergoing gastrointestinal resection. BMJ 312: 869-871
12. McClare SA, Greene LM, Snider HL et al (1997) Comparison of the safety of early enteral vs parenteral nutrition in mild acute pancreatitis. JPEN 21:14-20
13. Norton JA, Olt LG, McClain C et al (1988) Intolerance to enteral feeding in the brain injured patient. J Neurosurg 68:62-66
14. Moore F, Feliciano D, Andrussy R et al (1992) Early enteral feeding, compared with parenteral, reduces septic complications: the results of a meta-analysis. Ann Surg 216:172-183
15. Pomposelli JJ, Bistrian BR (1994) Is total parenteral nutrition immunosuppressive? New Horizons 2:224-229
16. Sandstrom R, Drott C, Hyltander A et al (1993) The effect of postoperative intravenous feeding (TPN) on outcome following major surgery evaluated in a randomised study. Ann Surg 217:185-195
17. Spapen HD, Duinslaeger L, Diltoer M et al (1995) Gastric emptying in critically ill patients is accelerated by adding cisapride to a standard enteral feeding protocol: results of a prospective, randomised, controlled trial. Crit Care Med 23:481-485
18. Jooste CA, Mustoe J, Colle G (1999) Metoclopramide improves gastric motility in critically ill patients. Intensive Care Med 25:464-468
19. Paz HL, Weinar M, Sherman MS (1996) Motility agents for the placement of weighted and unweighted feeding tubes in critically ill patients. Intensive Care Med 22:301-304
20. Spain DA, DeWeese C, Reynolds MA et al (1995) Transpyloric passage of feeding tubes in patients with head injuries does not decrease complications. J Trauma 39:1100-1102
21. Dobb GJ (1990) Enteral nutrition. Clin Anaesthesiol 4:531-557
22. Harrison AM, Clay B, Grant MJ et al (1997) Nonradiographic assessment of enteral feeding tube position. Crit Care Med 25:2055-2059
23. Mizrahi S (1988) Use of grooved needle in catheter jejunostomy technique. JPEN 12:419
24. Adams MB, Seabrook GR, Quebbeman EA et al (1986) Jejunostomy. A rarely indicated procedure. Ann Surg 121:236-238
25. Mowatt-Larssen CA, Brown RO, Wojtysiak SL et al (1992) Comparison of tolerance and nutritional outcome between a peptide and a standard enteral formula in critically ill hypoalbuminaemic patients. JPEN 16:20-24
26. Playford RJ, Woodman RC, Clark P et al (1993) Effect of luminal growth factor preservation on intestinal growth. Lancet 341:866-867
27. Hall JC, Keel K, McCauley R (1996) Glutamine. Br J Surg 83:305-312
28. Zapata-Sirvent RL, Hansbrough JF, Ohara MM et al (1994) Bacterial translocation in burned mice after administration of various diets including fiber- and glutamine-enriched enteral formulas. Crit Care Med 22:690-696
29. Gianotti V, Alexander JW, Gennari R et al (1995) Oral glutamine decreases bacterial translocation and improves survival in experimental gut-origin sepsis. JPEN 19:69-74

30. Jones C, Palmer TE, Griffiths RD (1999) Randomised clinical outcome study of critically ill patients given glutamine-supplemented enteral nutrition. Nutrition 15:108-115
31. Hammarqvist F (1999) Randomised trial of glutamine-enriched enteral nutrition on infectious morbidity in patients with multiple trauma. JPEN 23:43-44
32. Jensen GL, Miller RH, Talabiska DG et al (1997) A double-blind, randomised study of glutamine-enriched compared with standard peptide-based feeding in critically ill patients. Am J Clin Nutr 64:615-621
33. Barbul A (1986) Arginine: biochemistry, physiology and therapeutic implications. JPEN 10: 227-238
34. Daly JM, Reynolds JV, Thorn A et al (1988) Immune and metabolic effects of arginine in the surgical patient. Ann Surg 208:512-523
35. Brown AO, Hunt H, Mowatt-Larssen CA et al (1994) Comparison of specialised and standard enteral formulas in trauma patients. Pharmacotherapy 14:314-320
36. Daly JM (1995) Specific nutrients and the immune response: from research to clinical practices. J Crit Care Nutr 2:24-29
37. Alexander JW (1998) Immunonutrition: the role of omega-3 fatty acids. Nutrition 14:627-633
38. Zaloga GP (1998) Immune-enhancing enteral diets: where's the beef? Crit Care Med 26: 1143-1146
39. Scheppach W, Burghardt W, Bartram P et al (1990) Addition of dietary fiber to liquid formula diets: the pros and cons. JPEN 14:204-209
40. Demling RH, DeBiasse MA (1995) Micronutrients in critical illness. Crit Care Clin 11:61-673
41. Ponec RJ, Saunders MD, Kimmey MB (1999) Neostigmine for the treatment of acute colonic pseudo-obstruction. N Engl J Med 341:137-141

Update on CRRT Therapy

P. Rogiers

Since continuous hemofiltration was first described by Peter Kramer as a new form of renal replacement therapy, it has undergone a lot of changes, making it a widely accepted treatment for acute renal failure in critically ill patients. Concomitantly, new insights into the pathogenesis of severe sepsis and septic shock have led to a recent form of immunomodulating therapy for septic shock. In the past decade hemofiltration has gained more importance as a possible treatment of severe sepsis and septic shock. Indeed, various experimental studies have been performed in acute endotoxic or septic shock in different animal models in vivo, focusing on the hemodynamic response. At the same time in vitro studies have studied the removal of different cytokines, both by convection and adsorption.

Clinical studies have been performed in patients with sepsis and septic shock to study clinical outcome and removal of cytokines. This paper will mainly focus on the application of CRRT in sepsis and septic shock.

In vivo experimental studies in sepsis

Animal research on hemofiltration has yielded various results. Some authors found only minor or even no effects, while others demonstrated impressive hemodynamic improvement. During endotoxic shock in pigs, Stein et al. [1] showed that low-volume CAVH (20 ml/kg/h) did not significantly influence hemodynamics. During septic shock in dogs, Freeman et al. [2] demonstrated that moderate-volume CAVH (60 ml/kg/h) failed to improve hemodynamics or survival rate. In a dog model with live E. coli sepsis, Gomez et al. [3] showed that low-volume (27 ml/kg/h) CAVH increased cardiac contractility, but the hemodynamic variables were not significantly compromised during their study. In canine with E. coli sepsis, the same group of investigators [4] recently reported that the combination of low-volume CAVH (16 ml/kg/h) and phenylephrine could restore stroke volume, suggesting that low-volume CAVH alone may not be sufficient to improve hemodynamics in these conditions. However in endotoxic rats, Heidemann et al. [5] were able to improve short term survival with CAVH (22-48 ml/kg/h) and this was associated with the removal of thromboxane B2. In pigs with Staphylococcus aureus sepsis, Lee et al. [6] showed that CAVH (133 ml/kg/h) did not alter arterial blood pressure, but survival significantly increased with hemofiltration.

Considering that the removal of the so-called 'middle-molecules' is a convective process, Grootendorst et al. decided to apply much higher volumes of ultrafiltration. They studied the effect of high-volume CVVH (162 ml/kg/h or 6 L/h) in pigs with endotoxic shock [7, 8], and found that CVVH was associated with greater arterial blood pressure and cardiac output, as well as right ventricular ejection fraction. In another model of gut ischemia and reperfusion in pigs, the same authors reported that CVVH, started before clamping of the superior mesenteric artery, significantly increased arterial blood pressure, improved cardiac function, reduced macroscopic gut damage, and improved 24-hour survival [9].

We studied the effects of CVVH with two different ultrafiltrate rates (107 and 214 ml/kg/h or 3 and 6L/h respectively) in a canine model of acute endotoxic shock and were able to demonstrate positive hemodynamic effects in the high-volume group [10]. In a study using again low-volume hemofiltration (33 ml/kg/h), Murphey et al. were not able to demonstrate any cardiopulmonary improvement in a porcine model of acute endotoxin shock [11].

Role of the membrane

Hemofilters were originally designed for treatment of chronic renal failure. Until recently, cuprophane, a cellulose-based material, has been the most commonly used membrane material. Triacetate and hemophane are examples of modified cellulose structure, which results in enhanced biocompatibility. Most of these cellulosic membranes are low-flux, i.e. permeable to smaller, lower-molecular weight molecules. Synthetic polymers used for hemofilters are polycarbonate, polysulphone, polyacrylonitrile (PAN and AN69) and polymethylmethacrylate (PMMA). Most of these synthetic membranes are high-flux, i.e. permeable to larger, higher-molecular-weight molecules. Synthetic membranes are generally more biocompatible than cellulose membranes. Because of their biocompatibility and their high permeability, synthetic membranes are widely used for hemofiltration, allowing convective removal of small molecules such as urea and creatinine and also ions. These membranes have a sieving coefficient of 0.55 for myoglobin, whose molecular weight is 17000 daltons, i.e. very close to that of TNF-alpha (16500 daltons). By using these membranes the TNF-alpha monomer and various cytokines that are responsible for myocardial dysfunction, can theoretically be removed by convection. The biological form of TNF however is a trimer that has a molecular weight which is too big to pass hemofiltration membranes.

Removal of mediators of sepsis

A number of mediators like eicosanoids, cytokines (tumor necrosis factor or TNF, interleukins 1, 6, 8) endothelin and platelet-activating factor (PAF) are involved in the development of septic shock. Is there experimental or clinical evidence that hemofiltration can remove these mediators?

Experimental studies

Because of their biocompatibility and their high permeability, synthetic membranes are widely used for hemofiltration, allowing convective removal of small molecules such as urea, creatinine and also ions. Lonneman et al. [12] showed significant removal of TNF and IL-1, using AN69 and polysulphone membranes in an in vitro dialysis system. These data were confirmed by others [13-16]. In vitro, hemofiltration [R1] of a 1% albumin solution containing TNF and IL-1, through a variety of filters, resulted in higher sieving coefficients of the two cytokines than expected. This was due to a 32% binding effect by the membranes [14]. Because of its high molecular weight, endotoxin cannot be readily removed from circulation, but endotoxin fragments can be eliminated. An interesting technique is the specific adsorption of endotoxin with polymyxin using different systems of hemofiltration [17, 18]. In vivo, Sato et al. [19] showed that hemoperfusion using a polymyxin B fiber column can decrease circulating endotoxin and TNF levels in live E. coli shock in dogs.

Obviously, the potential benefits related to hemofiltration are not restricted to the elimination of cytokines. Complement factors (molecular weight 10,000 to 12,000), beta-endorphine (molecular weight 4000), bradykinin (molecular weight 1060), or arachidonic acid metabolites (molecular weight 600) can also be removed from the circulation. In particular, arachidonic acid metabolites including prostacyclin, thromboxane, and leukotrienes have been shown to be removed by hemofiltration in animals and in patients [20, 21], and this has been suggested to be related to some hemodynamic improvement.

Clinical studies

Elliott et al. [22] could detect considerable amounts of TNF and IL-1 in the ultrafiltrate of patients treated with CAVHD or CVVHD. Despite removal of considerable amounts of TNF with CVVH in patients with multiple organ failure, Kierdorf et al. [23] found no reduction in plasma TNF levels. Millar et al. [24] found a reduction in serum TNF, but not in IL-6 or IL-8 plasma levels in children with multiple organ failure treated with hemofiltration. Andreasson et al. [25] and Journois [16] found that hemofiltration can reduce complement levels after cardiopulmonary bypass. In patients with sepsis and acute renal failure,

Bellomo et al. [26] could detect considerable amounts of IL-6 and IL-8 in the ultrafiltrate. In patients with acute renal failure and sepsis, van Bommel et al. [27] found that TNF can be removed from circulation mainly by adsorption and that IL-1 and IL-6 are removed by convection. In septic patients treated with CVVH, Hoffmann et al. [28, 29] could not demonstrate significant removal of TNF, IL-1, IL-6, or IL-8, but complement levels could significantly be lowered. Incubation of lymphocytes with ultrafiltrate from these septic patients stimulated TNF release and suppressed IL-2 and IL-6 release. Tonnessen et al. [30] found significant removal of TNF and IL-6 in septic patients treated with CAVH. Despite considerable amounts of TNF and IL-6 in the ultrafiltrate of septic patients, Sander et al. [31] did not find decrease in plasma cytokine levels. CVVH with PAN filters decreased factor D levels resulting in reduced complement activation in critically ill patients with acute renal failure [32]. However, in a recent study performed by Kellum et al. [33], CVVH resulted in a decrease in plasma TNF levels while levels of IL-6, IL-8, soluble L-selectin and endotoxin remained unchanged.

So, despite removal of mediators with hemofiltration, plasma levels seldomly decrease. These substances tend to have an endogenous clearance that largely exceeds the clearance by extracorporeal techniques. Therefore, some authors believe that hemofiltration in sepsis in futile [34, 35].

Clinical studies in critically ill patients with sepsis

Very few of these were obtained prospectively and historical controls were used in most cases. Different hemofilters and volumes were used making comparison between these studies very difficult. Another drawback is the limited number of patients thereby making statistical analysis difficult to interpret. Moreover, since most of the studies were performed in patients with already established acute renal failure, the positive effects could be the result of a better metabolic and fluid balance control.

Timing may be very important. In one study in patients with post-traumatic acute renal failure early and late application of CRRT were compared. survival improved when CRRT was applied early [36].

New forms of CRRT

Recently continuous renal replacement therapy is being used more often in other indications beside acute renal failure. Because conventional hemofiltration failed to show clear beneficial effects in sepsis, other forms are being developed and employed.

High-volume hemofiltration has been studied most extensively, especially in experimental conditions in animals, and to a lesser extent in patients. Recently Bellomo [37] compared high-volume hemofiltration to conventional hemofiltration in human septic shock, and found a significant need of vasopressor requirement in the high-volume group.

It has also recently been shown that hemofiltration using high-pore membranes can be beneficial in sepsis. By enlarging filter pore size the cut-off point of the membrane increases from 40 kdalton to about 80 kdalton, resulting in convective removal of larger molecules responsible for sepsis syndrome. Two experimental studied have shown hemodynamic improvement [38] and an increase in survival rate [39]. However, these experimental data still need to be confirmed clinically.

Hemoperfusion with adsorptive devices

An interesting technique is the specific adsorption of endotoxin with polymyxin (PMX-F) using different systems of hemoperfusion [17, 18]. The endotoxin-neutralizing capacity of PMX-F has been tested ex vivo by incubating PMX-F with E coli endotoxin, and subsequently injecting the solution intravenously in mice or rabbits. All ex vivo experiments showed marked improved survival in animals treated with the mixed PMX-F/endotoxin solution compared with pure endotoxin [40, 41]. In vivo, Sato et al. [19] showed that hemoperfusion using a polymyxin B fiber column can decrease circulating endotoxin and TNF levels in live E. coli shock in dogs. In patients no prospective randomized clinical trials have been performed to date. Several uncontrolled trials were published, showing decrease of endotoxin levels and reversal of the hyperdynamic syndrome [42, 43]. No conclusions can be drawn from the mortality data since these studies were not randomized, or controlled. A second problem is that hemoperfusion was initiated rather late in the phase of sepsis, wheras earlier application could possibly be more beneficial and maybe prevent organ failure and death.

Another method in the treatment of sepsis by means of extracorporeal devices could be coupled filtration and adsorption. The innovation with this technique is that plasma is first separated by means of a conventional plasmafiltration system and this plasma then runs over an adsorptive column. Finally the 'purified' plasma is given back to the patient. The potential advantage is that activation of neutrophils and cytokine release is minimal or even absent, since all the cells are first separated from the plasma before reaching the adsorptive column. This has been tested in vitro by Tetta et al. [44] showing efficient removal of cytokines from the plasma. In vivo animal experiments with this technique are currently performed.

One of the latest developments and results of modern bio-engineering is the bio-artificial kidney. Recent reports with this bioartificial renal tubule assist device showed improved metabolic and endocrinological functions [45].

Conclusions

Although CRRT has undergone a remarkable evolution since its first description more than 20 years ago, we should not forget that patient care and cure is the main goal. Hemofiltration still remains an invasive technique, that can be dangerous for the patient. Therfore it should only be applied by experienced centers with enough skilled nursing and medical staff members. Despite the enthusiasm of many research centers multicenter, randomized clinical trials investigating the role of different forms of CRRT in various indications were not feasible. These planned trials should focus on clinical outcome measures and not on levels of mediators. Unless we succeed in setting up these clinical trials in the next decade, there will always remain 'believers' and 'non-believers'.

References

1. Stein B, Pfenninger E, Grunert A et al (1990) Influence of continuous hemofiltration on hemodynamics and central blood volume in experimental endotoxic shock. Intensive Care Med 16:494-499
2. Freeman BD, Yatsiv I, Natanson C et al (1995) Continuous arteriovenous hemofiltration does not improve survival in a canine model of septic shock. J Am Coll Surg 180:286-292
3. Gomez A, Wang R, Unruh H et al (1990) Hemofiltration reverses left ventricular dysfunction during sepsis in dogs. Anesthesiology 73:671-685
4. Mink SN, Jha P, Wang R et al (1995) Effects of continuous arteriovenous hemofiltration with systemic vasopressor therapy on depressed left ventricular contractility and tissue oxygen delivery in canine Escherichia coli sepsis. Anesthesiology 83:178-190
5. Heidemann SM, Ofenstein JP, Sarnaik AP (1994) Efficacy of continuous arteriovenous hemofiltration in endotoxic shock. Circ Shock 44:183-187
6. Lee PA, Matson JR, Pryor RW et al (1993) Continuous arteriovenous hemofiltration therapy for Staphylococcus aureus induced septicemia in immature swine. Crit Care Med 21:914-924
7. Grootendorst AF, van Bommel EFH, van der Hoven B et al (1992) High-volume hemofiltration improves hemodynamics of endotoxin-induced shock in the pig. J Crit Care 7:67-75
8. Grootendorst AF, van Bommel EFH, van der Hoven B et al (1992) High volume hemofiltration improves right ventricular function of endotoxin induced shock in the pig. Intensive Care Med 18:235-240
9. Grootendorst AF, van Bommel EF, van Leengoed LA et al (1994) High volume hemofiltration improves hemodynamics and survival of pigs exposed to gut ischemia and reperfusion. Shock 2:72-78
10. Rogiers P, Zhang H, Smail N et al (1999) CVVH improves cardiac performance by mechanisms other than TNF attenuation during endotoxic shock. Crit Care Medicine (in press)
11. Murphey ED, Fessler JF, Bottoms GD et al (1997) Effects of continuous venovenous hemofiltration on cardiopulmonary function in a porcine model of endotoxin-induced shock. J Vet Res 58:408-413
12. Lonneman G, Schindler R, Dinarello CA et al (1993) Removal of cytokines by hemodialysis membrane in vitro. In: Faist E, Meakins J, Schildberg FW (eds) Host defense dysfunction in trauma, shock and sepsis. Springer, Berlin Heidelberg New York 613-623
13. Barrera P, Janssen EM, Demacker PN et al (1992) Removal of interleukin-1 beta and TNF from human plasma by in vitro dialysis with polyacrylonitrile membranes. Lymphokine Cytokine Res 11:99-104
14. Goldfarb S, Golper TA (1994) Pro-inflammatory cytokines and hemofiltration membranes. J Am Soc Nephrol 5:228-232

15. Nagaki M, Hughes RD, Lau JYN et al (1991) Removal of endotoxin and cytokines by adsorbents and the effects of plasma protein binding. Int J Artif Organs 14:43-50
16. Journois D (1995) Complement fragments and cytokines: production and removal as consequences of hemofiltration. In: Sieberth HG, Stummvoll HK, Kierdorf H (eds) Continuous extracorporeal treatment in multiple organ dysfunction syndrome. Contrib Nephrol Basel Karger 116:80-85
17. Cheadle WG, Hanasawa K, Gallinaro RN et al (1991) Endotoxin filtration and immune stimulation improve survival from gram-negative sepsis. Surgery 110:785-792
18. Jaber BL, Barrett TW, Cendoroglo Neto M et al (1998) Endotoxin removal by polymyxin-B immobilized derivative fibers during in vitro hemoperfusion of 10% human plasma. ASAIO J Jan-Feb;44(1):54-61
19. Sato T, Orlowski JP, Zborowski M (1993) Experimental study of extracorporeal perfusion for septic shock. ASAIO J 39:M790-M793
20. Gotloib L, Barzilay E, Shustak A et al (1986) Hemofiltration in septic ARDS. The artificial kidney as an artificial endocrine lung. Resuscitation 13:123-132
21. Bellomo R (1995) Continuous hemofiltration as blood purification in sepsis. New Horizons 3:732-737
22. Elliott D, Wiles C, Reynolds H et al (1994) Removal of cytokines in septic patients using continuous venovenous hemodiafiltration (letter). Crit Care Med 22:718-719
23. Kierdorf H, Melzer H, Weissen D et al (1992) Elimination of tumor necrosis factor by continuous venovenous hemofiltration (abstract). Ren Fail 14:98
24. Millar AB, Armstrong L, van der Linden (1993) Cytokine production and hemofiltration in children undergoing cardiopulmonary bypass. Ann Thorac Surg 56:1499-1502
25. Andreasson S, Güthberg S, Berggren H et al (1993) Hemofiltration modifies complement activation after extracorporeal circulation in infants. Ann Thorac Surg 56:1515-1517
26. Bellomo R, Tipping P, Boyce N (1995) Interleukin-6 and interleukin-8 extraction during continuous venovenous hemodiafiltration in septic acute renal failure. Renal Failure 17:457-466
27. van Bommel EFH, Hesse CJ, Jutte NHPM et al (1995) Cytokine kinetics (TNF-alpha, IL-1b, IL-6) during continuous hemofiltration: a laboratory and clinical study. In: Sieberth HG, Stummvoll HK, Kierdort H (eds) Continuous extracorporeal treatment in multiple organ dysfunction syndrome. Contrib Nephrol Basel Karger 116:62-75
28. Hoffmann J, Hartl W, Deppisch et al (1995) Hemofiltration in human sepsis: evidence for elimination of immunomodulary substances. Kidney International 48:1563-1570
29. Hoffmann J, Hartl W, Deppisch R et al (1996) Effect of hemofiltration on hemodynamics and systemic concentrations of anaphylatoxins and cytokines in human sepsis. Intensive Care Med 22:1360-1367
30. Tonnesen E, Hansen M, Hühndorf K et al (1993) Cytokines in plasma and ultrafiltrate during continuous arteriovenous hemofiltration. Anaesth Intens Care 21:752-758
31. Sander A, Armbruster W, Sander B et al (1995) The influence of continuous hemofiltration on cytokine elimination and cardiovascular stability in the early phase of sepsis. Contrib Nephrol 116:99-103
32. Gasche Y, Pascual M, Suter PM et al (1996) Complement depletion during haemofiltration with polyacrilonitrile membranes. Nephrol Dial Transplant 11:117-119
33. Kellum JA, Johnson JP, Kramer D et al (1998) Diffusive vs convective therapy: effects on mediators of inflammation in patients with severe systemic inflammatory response syndrome. Crit Care Med 26:1995-2000
34. Schetz M, Ferdinande P, Van den Berghe G et al (1995) Removal of pro-inflammatory cytokines with renal replacement therapy: sense or nonsense? Intensive Care Med 21:169-176
35. Rodby RA (1998) Hemofiltration for SIRS: Bloodletting, twentieth century style? Crit Care Med 26:1940-1942
36. Gettings LG, Reynolds HN, Scalea T (1999) Outcome in post-traumatic acute renal failure when CRRT is applied early versus late. Intensive Care Med 25:805-813
37. Bellomo R, Balwin I, Cole, Ronco C (1998) Preliminary experience with high-volume hemofiltration in human septic shock. Kidney Int [Suppl]May;66:S182-S185

38. Kline JA, Gordon BE, Williams et al (1999) Large-pore hemodialysis in acute endotoxin shock. Crit Care Med 27(3):588-596
39. Lee PA, Weger GW, Pryor RW et al (1998) Effects of filter pore size on efficacy of continuous arteriovenous hemofiltration therapy for Staphylococcus aureus-induced septicemia in immature swine. Crit Care Med 26:730-737
40. Hanasawa K, Tani T, Kodama M (1989) New approach to endotoxic and septic shock by means of polymyxin B immobilized fiber. Surg Gynecol Obstet 168:323-331
41. Kodama M, Hanasawa K, Tani T (1990) New therapeutic method against septic shock-Removal of endotoxin using extracorporeal circulation. Adv Exp Med Biol 256:653-664
42. Kodama M, Aoki H, Tani T, Hanasawa K (1993) Hemoperfusion using a polymyxin B immobilized fiber column for the removal of endotoxin. In: Levin J, Alving CR, Munford RS, Stutz PL (eds) Bacterial endotoxin: recognition and effector mechanisms. Amsterdam, The Netherlands, Elsevier Science Publishers, pp 389-398
43. Aoki H, Kodama M, Tani T, Hanasawa K (1994) Treatment of sepsis by extracorporeal elimination of endotoxin using polymyxin B-immobilized fiber. Am J Surg 167:412-417
44. Tetta C, Cavaillon JM, Schulze M et al (1998) Removal of cytokines and activated complement components in an experimental model of continuous plasma filtration coupled with sorbent adsorption. Nephrol Dial Transplant 13:1458-1464
45. Humes HD, Mac Kay SM, Funke AJ, Buffington DA (1999) Tissue engineering of a bioartificial renal tubule assist device: in vitro transport and metabolic characteristics. Kidney Int 55:2502-2514

Haemofiltration in Neonates

G. Zobel, S. Rödl, B. Urlesberger

Acute renal failure is defined as the cessation of renal function with or without changes in urinary output. The incidence of acute renal failure in neonatal intensive care units is highly variable, ranging from 1 to 8% [1]. When conventional therapy fails to control fluid and metabolic balances, renal replacement therapy has to be instituted [2]. Of the available methods intermittent hemodialysis and peritoneal dialysis are not always feasible in critically ill patients for technical as well as clinical reasons [3]. Continuous hemofiltration, either driven in the arterio-venous or veno-venous mode, is an alternative continuous renal replacement therapy (CRRT) to control fluid and metabolic balances in critically ill patients [4, 5]. In 1977 Kramer et al. first described continuous arterio-venous hemofiltration (CAVH) as a method for extracorporeal renal support in oliguric adults with diuretic resistant fluid overload [6]. In 1985 the first reports on CAVH in neonates were published by Lieberman et al. and Ronco et al. [7, 8]. In 1989 we reported that CAVH is feasible in critically ill preterm infants to control fluid overload and metabolic derangement [9]. A variety of techniques, such as suction support, predilution, or intermittent or continuous hemodialysis, and pump driven or veno-venous hemofiltration have been described to increase the efficiency of CAVH [10-14].

Vascular access: Adequate vascular access is extremely important for CAVH in neonates. The catheters have to be short with a relative large inner diameter to minimize the resistance to blood flow. The umbilical vessels can be used for blood access in neonates during the first week of life. However, the resistance of standard umbilical catheters is rather high [15]. Short 20-22 G cannulas inserted into the radial or brachial arteries usually provide adequate blood flow in newborns. Radial and brachial arteries are punctured directly whereas femoral artery catheters are placed percutaneously using the Seldinger technique. The internal jugular vein should be used for blood return because its cannulation is safe and easy in neonates. The venous catheter should be short with a large inner diameter to optimize blood flow through the circuit. We now use 4 Fr catheters (Medcomp, Medical Components Inc., Harleysville, USA) placed with standard Seldinger technique for blood return in neonates.

For pump-driven hemofiltration we prefer the use of two 4-5 Fr single lumen catheters (Medcomp, Medical Components Inc., Harleysville, USA) in neonates. The tip of the catheter has to be placed into the mid of the right atrium to provide adequate drainage of venous blood.

Extracorporeal circuit: Different hemofilter systems (Amicon Minifilter®, Amicon Minifilter Plus®, Amicon Corp., Lexington, MA; Miniflow 10® Hospal Lyon, France; Gambro FH 22®, Gambro Corporation, Hechingen, FRG) are available for CRRT in neonates. Hemofilter characteristics are given in Table 1. The membrane surface area ranges from 0.015 m² to 0.2 m² and the priming volume from 3.7 to 15 ml. The hemofilter system is rinsed with 1L 0.9% saline solution containing 5000 IU of heparin. The system is primed with heparinized blood (3 IU/ml) immediately before starting the procedure.

Table 1. Characteristics and operational data of hemofilters for neonates ($n = 33$)

	Minifilter (old/new)	Miniflow 10	Minifilter plus	FH-22
Material	**Polysulfone**	**Polyacrilonitrile**	**Polysulfone**	**Polyamide**
Length of fibers (cm)	8/12.7	21	12.7	11.5
Diameter of fibers (μm)	1100/1100	240	570	220
Surface area (m²)	0.015/0.021	0.042	0.08	0.2
Filling volume (ml)	6/7.6	3.7	15	13
Number of fibers	60/60	264	450	2400
Qb (ml/min)	7.6 ± 2.2	15.5 ± 2.2 *	25.1 ± 2.8 **	13.3 ± 2.5 +
Qf (ml/min/m²)	1.8 ± 0.2	7.6 ± 1.6 **	7.3 ± 0.8 **	9.1 ± 2.3 **
HF-exchange (h)	26.1 ± 6.3 ++	51.5 ± 11 *	80.8 ± 24.1 *	29.2 ± 9.5 ++
Duration of CRRT (h)	63.1 ± 11	246 ± 107 *	127 ± 44 *	100 ± 20 *, §
No of neonates	11	7	5	10
S/NS	8/3	5/2	1/4	8/2

* $p < 0.05$ vs Minifilter, ** $p < 0.01$ vs Minifilter, + $p < 0.05$, ++ $p < 0.01$ vs Minifilter plus, § $p < 0.05$ vs Miniflow 10
Qb, blood flow; Qf, ultrafiltration rate; HF, hemofilter; h, hours; CRRT, continuous renal replacement therapy; S, survivors; NS, nonsurvivors

Anticoagulation: Anticoagulation is usually achieved with unfractioned heparin. Patients with a normal coagulation status initially receive a heparin bolus of 50-100 IU/kg followed by a continuous infusion of 10-20 IU/kg/h into the arterial line of the extracorporeal device. Heparinization is controlled by partial thromboplastin time (PTT) measurements in the systemic circulation 3-4 times a day. PTT is maintained at 20-30 sec over baseline. AT III is kept at 80%, fibrinogen > 100 mg/dl, and platelets > 50.000 mm³.

Fluid balancing and replacement fluid: The ultrafiltrate is partially or totally replaced according to the clinical situation. The bicarbonate based ultrafiltrate substitution is warmed by a fluid warmer system (Hotline®, Level 1 Technologies Inc., Rockland, MA, USA) before infusion and consists of sodium 145 mmol/L, calcium 1.84 mmol/L, magnesium 0.53 mmol/L, chloride 115 mmol/L, lactate 3.16 mmol/L, and bicarbonate 35 mmol/L (Hemosol BO, Hospal Lyon, France). Potassium is added as required up to 4.5 mmol/L. Fluid in- and output can be either controlled by the nurses on an hourly basis or continuously by a microprocessor controlled fluid balance system (Amicon Equaline® system, Amicon Corp., Lexington, MA, USA) using the weight change program. The ultrafiltrate, the replaced ultrafiltrate substitution fluid, and the fluid balance are continuously displayed on the control panel.

Continuous arterio-venous hemofiltration: During CAVH blood is driven through the highly permeable hemofilter by the patient´s arteriovenous pressure gradient, producing an ultrafiltrate that is partially or totally replaced with an appropriate replacement solution.

Continuous veno-venous hemofiltration: For pump-driven hemofiltration a roller pump (Gambro AK 10® blood monitor, Gambro Corporation, Hechingen, FRG) with pressure alarms, an air trap, an air bubble detector, and small blood lines (Gambro A-5.124-B3®, V-5.109-X®, Gambro Comp., Hechingen, FRG) are used. The roller pump enables blood flow rates from 12-50 ml/min. Pressure tracings are performed immediately before the roller pump and after the hemofilter.

Continuous hemodiafiltration: During CHDF the CAVH or CVVH cicuit is modified by the addition of slow countercurrent dialysate flow into the ultrafiltrate-dialysate compartment of the hemofilter. CHDF can be driven in the spontaneous or pump-driven mode. The bicarbonate-based dialysate is administered in a countercurrent way to blood flow. The produced ultrafiltrate is partially or totally replaced by a volumetric pump.

Patients

From June 1985 to June 1999 33 critically ill neonates (22 males/11 females) with a mean age of 9.8 ± 1.4 days and a mean body weight 3.1 ± 0.1 kg underwent continuous arterio-venous ($n = 17$) or veno-venous ($n = 16$) renal support at the pediatric or neonatal ICUs of the Children's Hospital, University of Graz. All patients were on mechanical ventilation and 88% needed vasopressor support. Indications for continuous extracorporeal renal support were: acute renal failure, low cardiac output, multiple organ system failure, diuretic resistant hypervolemia, and metabolic crisis in inborn errors of metabolism.

Results

CAVH: Seventeen neonates were treated with CAVH. Operational data are given in Table 2. The pre-CAVH serum creatinine and urea levels were 2.4 ± 0.3 and 88 ± 7.6 mg/dl, the post-CAVH levels were 2.2 ± 0.3 and 93 ± 10 mg/dl, respectively. CAVH was well tolerated by all patients. Frequent clotting of the hemofilter was observed in 3 neonates with rather low blood flow. Local bleeding at the catheter entrance site was observed in 4 patients and severe bleeding in 1 patient. Femoral artery cannulation resulted in transient ischemia of the leg in 2 neonates.

Table 2. Operational data during continuous renal replacement therapy in critically ill neonates ($n = 33$)

	CAVH ($n = 17$)	CVVH ($n = 16$)
Qb (ml/min)	7.0 ± 0.5	20.8 ± 1.7 *
Qf (ml/min/m²)	3.3 ± 0.4	9.4 ± 2.0 *
Duration (h)	123 ± 39	108 ± 25
HF-exchange (h)	26.8 ± 6.0	55.1 ± 12.2 *
Survival rate (%)	65	68

* $p < 0.01$ vs CAVH
CAVH, continuous arteriovenous hemofiltration; CVVH, continuous venovenous hemofiltration; Qb, blood flow; Qf, ultrafiltration rate; h, hours; HF, hemofilter

CVVH: Sixteen neonates were treated with pump-driven hemofiltration (Table 2). The pre-CVVH serum creatinine and urea levels were 1.5 ± 0.1 and 72 ± 10 mg/dl, the post-CVVH levels were 1.3 ± 0.2 and 77 ± 4.0 mg/dl, respectively. Complications included partial thrombosis of the vena cava superior or inferior in 3 patients, and cardiocirculatory compromize in one neonate with severe metabolic crisis.

CHDF: The mean ultrafiltration rates during CHF were 1.06 ± 0.2 ml/min. Adding a dialysate solution at a rate of 5 ml/min in a countercurrent fashion to blood flow the ultrafiltration rate decreased by 20% and whereas urea and creatinine clearances increased by 300%.

Clinical advances in CRRT

Today, CRRT is the method of choice to maintain adequate metabolic control in the critically ill anuric adult as well as pediatric patients. CAVH is a simple method of renal replacement therapy by which fluid and solutes can be removed from the body by convective transport. Without using a pump, the blood is driven through the hemofilter device only by the arterio-venous pressure gradient. The major determinants for ultrafiltrate production are the surface area and the permeability of the hemofilter membrane and the transmembrane pressure across the hemofilter membrane. The transmembrane pressure depends on the blood flow through the hemofilter device, the colloidosmotic pressure and the negative pressure on the ultrafiltrate side of the hemofilter created by the distance between the hemofilter and the ultrafiltrate collection bag. The blood flow during CAVH depends on the arterio-venous pressure gradient, length and diameter of blood lines and catheters, and blood viscosity. It allows good control of fluid overload and metabolic imbalances and provides hemodynamic stability. In addition, it allows adequate nutrition and unlimited medication. The risks are bleeding and thrombosis. A disadvantage is its rather low urea clearance insufficient to control azotemia in hypercatabolic states. In 1995 Ronco published his experience with CRRT (CAVH) in neonates and small infants using 4 different Minifilter versions [16]. CRRT lasted from 1-32 days, blood flow ranged from 13-48 ml/min producing ultrafiltration rates from 0.6-2.9 ml/min. The overall survival rate of the 26 patients was 46%. Technical or clinical complications were very rare. The author concluded that CAVH is a simple, safe, and effective extracorporeal renal replacement technique for neonates and small infants in conditions in which hemodialysis or peritoneal dialysis are contraindicated. CAVH was well tolerated by our critically ill neonates. Problems included low blood flow rates through the hemofilter device associated with low ultrafiltration rates and frequent hemofilter clotting and local bleeding at the catheter entrance site.

To improve urea clearance in critically ill patients with multiple organ system failure, CAVHDF and CVVH have been introduced recently. During CHDF the dialysate solution passes on the ultrafiltrate side of the filter countercurrent to blood flow. Contact between blood and dialysate accross the membrane allows diffusion of solutes into the ultrafiltrate compartment by a diffusion gradient. In addition, since blood pressure in the device creates a transmembrane pressure gradient, an element of ultrafiltration is automatically added. The ultrafiltration rates of CAVHDF permit administration of hyperalimentation solutions as well as fluid removal in hypervolemic patients. CAVHDF has the advantages of CAVH in terms of simplicity and sufficient removal of excess plasma water and has the capability of increased solute removal.

Recently Gouyon et al. reported urea clearance rates during CAVH and CAVHD in 7 anesthetized adult rabbits which were given urea infusions [17]. For this experiment a 800 cm^2 polysulfone hemofilter was used. Operational parameters were comparable during CAVH and CAVHD. Urea clearance increased by 285% during CAVHD. In contrast to our findings they observed an increase in ultrafiltration rates during CAVHD by 47%. In our experience with polysulfone and polyacrilinitrile filters in small infants urea clearance improved substantially during CHDF.

CVVH is another extracorporeal renal support system which allows higher ultrafiltration rates and urea/creatinine clearances [5, 18]. Inserting a pump into the extracorporeal system blood flow and ultrafiltration rates are no longer dependent on the patient's blood pressure.

Falk et al. reported the successful use of CVVH and CVVHD in the acute management of metabolic crises associated with inborn errors of metabolism

[19]. Two of the 4 treated patients were neonates with acute accumulation of branched chain amino acids (BCAA) due to maple syrup urine disease (MSUD). CVVH and CVVHD allowed a significant reduction in BCAA. Thompson et al. showed that CVVH rapidly decreased circulating levels of various toxic metabolites in two neonates with MSUD and fatty acid oxidation defect, respectively [20]. Both neonates rapidly improved clinically. The authors concluded that CVVH should have broad application in the acute management of metabolic decompensation in a broad range of inborn errors of intermediary metabolism.

In our experience blood flow and ultrafiltration rates were significantly higher during pump-driven hemofiltration than during spontaneous hemofiltration. In addition, the hemofilter running time was significantly longer in the pump-driven mode [18]. However, CVVH is technically more difficult, especially in small infants when a double-lumen catheter is used. This problem can be overcome by using 2 single-lumen catheters and placing the suction catheter in the upper part of the right atrium to optimize drainage of blood into the extracorporeal device.

In conclusion, continuous hemofiltration either driven in the arterio-venous or veno-venous mode is an effective method of renal support in critically ill neonates. Both methods allow good control of fluid, electrolyte and acid-base balances. CAVH requires arterial cannulation and the procedure is blood pressure dependent resulting in lower ultrafiltration rates and shorter hemofilter running time. The pump driven mode allows constant blood flow and ultrafiltration rates with excellent control of azotemia even in hypercatabolic states. The use of a pump makes the procedure more complex, but it can be performed in every pediatric/neonatal ICU without dialysis trained staff. The use of CAVHDF substantially increases urea clearances while maintaining the simplicity and safety of the CAVH system. CVVHDF permits the highest urea clearance rates and is indicated in emergency conditions such as severe metabolic crisis due to inborn errors of metabolism.

References

1. Brion LP, Satlin LM, Edelmann CM (1994) Renal disease. In: Avery GB, Fletcher MA, Mac-Donald MG (eds) Neonatology pathophysiology and management of the newborn. Lippincott, Philadelphia, pp 815-833
2. Schetz M, Lauwers PM, Ferdinande P (1989) Extracorporeal treatment of acute renal failure in the intensive care unit: a critical view. Intensive Care Med 15:349-357
3. Maxwell LG, Fivush BA, McLean RH (1987) Renal failure. In: Rogers MC (ed) Textbook of pediatric intensive care. Williams and Wilkins, Baltimore, pp 1001-1055
4. Lauer A, Saccaggi A, Ronco C et al (1983) Continuous arteriovenous hemofiltration in the critically ill patient. Ann Intern Med 99:455-460
5. Storck M, Hartl WH, Zimmerer E et al (1991) Comparison of pump-driven and spontaneous continuous hemofiltration in postoperative acute renal failure. Lancet 337:452-455

6. Kramer P, Wigger W, Rieger J et al (1977) Arteriovenous hemofiltration: A new and simple method for the treatment of overhydrated patients resistant to diuretics. Klin Wochenschr 55:1121-1122
7. Lieberman KV, Nardi L, Bosch JP (1995) Treatment of acute renal failure in an infant using continuous arteriovenous hemofiltration. J Pediatr 106:646-649
8. Ronco C, Brendolan A, Bragantini L et al (1986) Treatment of acute renal failure in newborns by continuous arteriovenous hemofiltration. Kidney Int 29:908-915
9. Zobel G, Ring E, Müller WD (1989) Continuous arteriovenous hemofiltration in preterm infants. Crit Care Med 17:534-536
10. Geronemus R, Schneider N (1984) Continuous arteriovenous hemodialysis: a new modality of treatment for acute renal failure. Trans ASAIO 30:610-613
11. Kaplan AA (1985) Pre vs postdilution for continuous arteriovenous hemofiltration. Trans ASAIO 31:28-31
12. Zobel G, Kuttnig M, Ring E (1990) Continuous arteriovenous hemodialysis in critically ill infants. Child Nephrol Urol 10:196-198
13. Zobel G, Ring E, Trop M et al (1988) Suction supported continuous arteriovenous hemofiltration in children. Blood Purif 6:37-42
14. Ellis EN, Pearson D, Robinson L et al (1993) Pump-assisted hemofiltration in infants with acute renal failure. Pediatr Nephrol 7:434-437
15. Jenkins RD, Harrison HL, Jackson EC et al (1991) Continuous renal replacement in infants and toddlers. Contrib Nephrol 93:245-249
16. Ronco C (1995) Acute renal failure in the neonate: Treatment by continuous renal replacement therapy. In: Bellomo R, Ronco C (eds) Update in intensive care and emergency medicine. Acute renal failure. Springer, Berlin, pp 246-264
17. Gouyon JB, Petion AM, Huet F et al (1994) Urea removal by hemofiltration and hemodiafiltration. Biol Neonate 65:36-40
18. Zobel G, Ring E, Kuttnig M et al (1991) Continuous arteriovenous hemofiltration versus continuous venovenous hemofiltration in critically ill pediatric patients. Contr Nephrol 93: 257-260
19. Falk MC, Knight JF, Roy LP et al (1994) Continuous venovenous hemofiltration in the acute treatment of inborn errors of metabolism. Pediatr Nephrol 8:330-333
20. Thompson GN, Butt WW, Shann FA et al (1991) Continuous venovenous hemofiltration in the management of acute decompensation in inborn errors of metabolism. J Pediatr 118:879-884

DRUGS IN ICU
USE, ABUSE AND MISUSE

Use, Abuse and Misuse of Drugs in the ICU: Muscle Relaxants

G. CONTI, R. MARELLA, M.C. MARINI

Guidelines to the use of muscle relaxants in ICU

Twenty years ago, muscle relaxants were frequently used in the ICU in almost all critically ill patients (91%), but ten years later a large survey reported frequent use of nondepolarizing muscle relaxants in only 16%, and recently, only 1% of adults and 5% of neonatal and other paediatric patients were therapeutically paralysed, because of new sedative techniques [1].

The following are suggested as essential for starting of the use of muscle relaxants in the ICU:

– neuromuscular monitoring equipment should be available and used at appropriate intervals;
– patients must be sedated (sedatives, narcotics), to avoid awakening psychoses;
– patients should be receiving appropriate mechanical respiratory support, because of drug-induced paralysis;
– the unit's nursing staff should be appropriately trained and understand the implications of the use of muscle relaxants [2].

The main indication is adaptation to the mechanical respiratory support of patients.

Another indication is to increase chest wall compliance in the presence of high airway pressure (as in ARDS patients) [3], even though the results seem to be lower than expectations and similar to those already obtained with deep sedation [4].

Other indications are:

– improving the interaction between patient and ventilator, reducing the respiratory muscle work and muscle oxygen consumption;
– preventing uncoordinated respiratory movements, reducing peak airways pressures and the risk of barotrauma;
– allowing "permissive hypercapnia" to improve gas exchange;
– avoiding and preventing shiver (in burns, hypothermia, and post-surgery patients);

– avoiding uncoordinated and dangerous movements during specialized procedures such as X-ray, transport, extracorporeal oxygenation;
– in patients with critically raised intracranial pressure to prevent coughing on
  tracheal suction or other movements not controlled by the simple use of hyp-
  notic agents [5];
– allowing anaesthesiological and surgical procedures;
– to facilitate treatment in medical conditions such as tetanus, status epilepticus, status asthmaticus, strychnine poisoning.

Some of these indications may be considered relative because sedation can
often be enough.

Before using muscle relaxants in critically ill patients it is necessary to observe some precautions, which must be respected to avoid complications such
as:

– checking the ventilator circuit and avoiding the disconnection;
– avoiding the exclusive use of muscle relaxants but always combining it with
  neurovegetative sedation and optimal analgesia [6];
– monitoring neuromuscular function, avoiding oedematous zones [7] to
  choose the kind of muscle relaxant, the mode of administration, and the kind
  of electrical excitation in the appropriate way [8] (Table 1).

Table 1. Crucial points in the choice of muscle relaxants in ICU

Onset speed
Cardiovascular effects
Hepatic and renal metabolism
Histamine release
Cumulative effect
Rapid antagonism
Knowledge of action
Possibility of administration by bolus or by continuous infusion
Capacity of evocation or inhibition of hepatic enzymatic system
Production of active metabolites
Interaction with other drugs
Cost

During the administration of muscle relaxants we must consider the additive
effect of many drugs that are used in the ICU, such as some antibiotics [9]
(Table 2) and other drugs or clinical conditions that influence the activity of
muscle relaxants [10].

Table 2. Antibiotic effects on neuromuscular blockade

Antibiotic	Increase of neuromuscular blockade	
	Depolarizing	Nondepolarizing
Neomycin	yes	Yes
Streptomycin	Yes	Yes
Gentamicin	Yes	Not studied
Kanamycin	Yes	Yes
Polymyxin A	Yes	Not studied
Polymyxin B	Yes	Yes
Tetracycline	Yes	Not studied
Lincomycin	Yes	Not studied
Clindamycin	Yes	Not studied

Muscle diseases caused by or associated with the use of muscle relaxants

Many authors have reported muscle diseases in critically ill patients and have attributed this to nondepolarizing neuromuscular blocking agents. In critically ill patients evidence has shown [11], after percutaneous muscle biopsy, a massive reduction in the concentration of glutamine (72%), free aminoacids and percentage of phosphorylated creatine (22%) in presence of 19% of muscular water. Trauma patients with either septic condition or surgical complications have a greater risk of developing muscle disease. Rhabdomyolysis has been described and correlated to the use of steroid muscle relaxants. Furthermore cases of polineuropathy, cachectic myopathy, panfascicular necrosis of muscle fibres, quadriplegic myopathy with necrosis of myofibrils, and atrophy by degeneration have been recorded [12]. These cases often implicate alterations in nervous conduction with reduced capacity of potential and abnormal spontaneous activity. The severity of these neuromyopathies has led various ICUs to adopt valid guidelines for administering the correct dosage of muscle relaxant. Mercatello [13] evaluated motor deficits in patients with encephalopathy, myopathy and peripheral neuropathy, remarking on the use of pancuronium, vecuronium and atracurium as possible pathologic causes. According to Tobias [14] electromyographic alterations can persist for many years after treatment. Despite multiple aetiologies and risk conditions muscle relaxants are often, still today, frequently used, even at high dosages, often with disregard for the function of important organs and emunctories. However, he monitoring of neuromuscular function allows the use of minimal daily dosage with optimum results, especially for i.v. administrations of short duration. More specifically, real muscle disease can be caused by protracted administration of muscle relaxants. Some diseases are characterized by atrophy of both type I and type II fibres (or twitch fibres with slow conduction or red fibres), more sensitive to NMBS and fibres having a faster conduction (II) more sensitive to depolarizing muscle relaxants [15]. Furthermore, a destructive myopathy characterized by slight inflammation of motor nerves whilst sensory perception remains relatively preserved has been described; this pathology is different from the critical illness polyneuropathy because it is found almost exclusively in muscle. Importantly, muscular disease can be divided in two groups [16]: those related to alteration in clearance and metabolism and those related to neuromuscular disease. Associated disease (burns and sepsis) can lead to different up-regulations of receptors, not only after i.v. administration of nondepolarizing muscle relaxants but also after administration of depolarizing muscle relaxants, which often can induce hyperkalaemia. To prevent protracted paralysis of pharmacokinetic origins it is essential to monitor the neuromuscular function even if small doses are still able to cause receptorial proliferation. Among the causes of delayed weaning from ventilator Lemaire [17] reports fatigue and wasting of respiratory muscles, critically ill polyneuritis and/or myopathy, and prolonged i.v. administration of a high dosage of steroid and/or non-depolarizing muscle relaxants. It has been shown that a difficult weaning can be caused by prolonged used of muscle relaxants, whether or not in association with other drugs. Bolton [18] suggests that for a correct diagnosis of myopathy, which often is associated with septic condition, disuse atrophy, trauma and alterations of capillary permeability, we should consider muscle biopsy, elecrophysiological examinations and dosages of creatinephosphokinase. Anatomic alterations are often characterized by degeneration of the peripheral nervous fibres, by muscle atrophy caused by denervation and central necrosis of muscle, as observed in septic myopathy, or by denervation atrophy with diffuse necrosis.

The effects of muscle relaxants on the CNS in the ICU

Many authors have been interested on the potential toxic effect that these drugs could have on the CNS, once they pass through the blood brain barrier.

A very important subject of many studies has been a metabolite of atracurium, called laudanosine, which has some strychnine-like effects [19] and which represents, for his quantity (43% of atracurium) and effects, the most important metabolite.

Laudanosine, compared to its precursor, has a longer half-life with a short clearance; in critically ill patients the half-life increases five-fold, and clearance decreases. For this reason the use of cisatracurium is suggested.

Although the use of long infusion with high blood concentrations of these drugs in critically ill patients has never induced seizures, this possibility must be considered, especially given the very high liquoral concentration, which reaches seven time the normal liquoral value [20].

Many authors did not find high liquoral values [21] and in experimental studies they stated that the action of laudanosine was different from strychnine. Non-depolarizing muscle relaxants should not pass through the blood brain barrier of the normal subject because they are quaternary substances having a strong positive charge.

In addition, some studies on sensory neurons have experimentally demonstrated that among the extracellular effects of pancuronium there is a reduction in Na^+ flow both in the opened and closed channels [22].

Has paralysis some effect on chest wall in mechanically ventilated, sedated patients?

To evaluate the separate effect of sedation and paralysis on chest wall and respiratory system mechanics of mechanically ventilated [4], critically ill patients, 13 critically ill patients were enrolled in this study. All were affected by diseases involving both lungs and chest wall mechanics (ARDS in 4 patients, chest trauma in 4 patients, cardiogenic pulmonary oedema with fluid overload in 5 patients).

Respiratory system and chest wall mechanics were evaluated during constant flow controlled mechanical ventilation in basal conditions (i.e. with the patient under apnoeic sedation) after paralysis with pancuronium bromide (Table 3). We simultaneously recorded airflow, tracheal pressure, oesophageal pressure and tidal volume; with the end-inspiratory and end-expiratory airway occlusion technique we could evaluate respiratory system and chest wall elastance and resistances. Lung mechanics were evaluated by subtracting chest wall from respiratory system data. All data obtained with the patient sedated with thiopental or propofol and after muscle paralysis were compared using the Student t test for paired data. The administration of pancuronium bromide to sedated patients induced a complete muscle paralysis without producing significant modification of either the viscoelastic or the resistive parameters of the chest wall and respiratory system.

Table 3. Modifications of the respiratory system, chest wall and lung mechanics before and after paralysis in 13 mechanically ventilated, sedated patients. (Ers, El, Ecw elastance of the respiratory system; lungs and chest wall respectively, Rcw resistance of the chest wall, RRS max total resistance of the respiratory system; RRS min minimal resistance of the respiratory system)

	Apnoeic sedation	Sedation + paralysis
Ers (cm H_2O/l)	24.9 ± 11	24.7 ± 10.9
Ecw (cm H_2O/l)	10.6 ± 3.1	10.7 ± 2.9
El (cm H_2O/l)	14.2 ± 9.5	14.3 ± 9.1
Rcw (cm H_2O/l s)	1.9 ± 0.5	2 ± 0.9
RRS max (cm H_2O/l s)	12.5 ± 4.3	11.9 ± 3
RRS min (cm H_2O/l s)	6.6 ± 2.9	6.6 ± 2.8
ΔRRS (cm H_2O/l s)	5.7 ± 1.9	5.2 ± 1.7

This study demonstrates the lack of additive effects of muscle paralysis in mechanically ventilated, sedated patients. Also in view of the possible side effects of muscle paralysis, our results question the usefulness of generalized administration of neuromuscular blocking drugs in mechanically ill patients.

References

1. Durbin CG (1991) Neuromuscular blocking agents and sedative drugs. Crit Care Clin 7 (3): 489-506
2. Elliot JM, Bion JF (1995) The use of neuromuscular blocking drugs in the intensive care practice. Acta Anaesth Scand 39[Suppl 106]:70-82
3. Sharpe MD (1992) The use of muscle relaxants in Intensive Care Unit. Can J Anaesth 39(9): 949-962
4. Conti G, Vilardi V, Rocco M et al (1995) Paralysis has no effect on chest wall and respiratory system mechanics of mechanically ventilated, sedated patients. Intens Care Med 21:808-812
5. Werba A, Gilly H, Weindlmayr-Goettel M et al (1992) Porcine model for studying the passage of non-depolarizing neuromuscular blockers through the blood brain barrier. Br J Anaesth 69:382-386
6. Berger J, Waldrom RE (1995) Analgesia, sedation and paralysis in the intensive care unit. Am Fam Physician 51(1):166-172
7. Casale LM, Siegel R (1993) Neuromuscular blockade in the ICU. Chest 104(5):1639-1640
8. Sharpe MD (1992) The use of muscle relaxants in the Intensive Care Unit. Can J Anaesth 39(9):949-962
9. Isenstein DA, Venner DS, Duggan J (1992) Neuromuscular blockade in the Intensive Care Unit. Chest 102:1258-1266
10. Shapiro BA, Warren J, Egol AB et al (1995) Practice parameters for sustained neuromuscular blockade in the adult critically ill patient: an executive summary. Crit Care Med 23(9):1601-1605
11. Gamrin L, Essen P, Forsberg AM et al (1996) A descriptive study of skeletal muscle metabolism in critically ill patients: free amino acids, energy-rich phosphates, protein, nucleic acids, fat, water and electrolytes. Crit Care Med 24(4):575
12. Bolton CF (1993) Neuromuscular complications of sepsis. Intens Care Med 19:S58-S63
13. Mercatello A, Coronel B, Mosckovtchenko JF (1995) La neuropathie de réanimation: un defi pour le futur. Ann Fr Anesth Réanim 14:209-212
14. Tobias J, Lynch A, McDuffee A et al (1995) Pancuronium infusion for neuromuscular block in children in the pediatric Intensive Care Unit. Anaesth Analg 81:13-16
15. Silverman DG, Mirakhur RK (1994) Non-depolarizing relaxants of the 1990s. In: Silverman DG (ed) Neuromuscular block in perioperative and intensive care. JB Lippincott Company, Philadelphia, pp 200-216
16. Watling SM, Dasta JF (1994) Prolonged paralysis in Intensive Care Unit patients after the use of neuromuscular blocking agents: a review of the literature. Crit Care Med 22(5):884-893
17. Lamaire F (1993) Difficult weaning. Intens Care Med 19:S69-S73
18. Bolton CF (1994) Muscle weakness and difficulty in weaning from the ventilator in the critical care unit. Chest 106(1):1-2
19. Al-Muhandis WM, Lauretti GR, Pleuvry BJ (1991) Modification by drugs use in anaesthesia of CNS stimulation induced in mice by laudanosine and strychnine. Br J Anaesth 67:608-613
20. Eddleston JM, Harper NJN, Pollard BJ et al (1989) Concentrations of atracurium and laudanosine in cerebrospinal fluid and plasma during intracranial surgery. Br J Anaesth 63:525-530
21. Gwinnutt CL, Edleston JM, Edwards D et al (1990) Concentration of atracurium and laudanosine in cerebrospinal fluid plasma in three intensive care patients. Br J Anaesth 65: 829-832
22. Maestrone E, Magnelli V, Nobile (1994) Extracellular pancuronium affects sodium current in chick embryo sensory neurones. Br J Pharmachol 11:283-287

Use of Corticosteroids in the Severely Ill Patient

M. ANTONELLI, M. PASSARIELLO

Besides primary and secondary adrenal insufficiency, many medical conditions benefit from the use of corticosteroids because of their anti-inflammatory and immunosuppressive activity. Several mechanisms are involved in the suppression of inflammation by the glucocorticoids, and many remain to be elucidated. Glucocorticoids inhibit the recruitment of leukocytes and monocyte-macrophages into affected areas and the synthesis of a great variety of chemotactic substances and other factors that mediate increased capillary permeability, vasodilatation, and contraction of various nonvascular smooth muscles. All natural and synthetic glucocorticoids act by binding a specific cytoplasmic glucocorticoid receptor. The complex glucocorticoid receptor has the ability to enter the nucleus of the cell and bind specific sites of DNA and control transcription of glucocorticoid-regulated genes. At present the list of substances whose synthesis or release is inhibited by glucocorticoids includes arachidonic acid and its metabolites (prostaglandins and leukotrienes), platelet activating factor (PAF), the nitric-oxide pathway, tumor necrosis factor (TNF) and many interleukins. Glucocorticoids can thus control the synthesis or release of substances involved in onset and evolution of inflammation [1-7].

A list of diseases and conditions that can benefit from corticosteroids is given in Table 1.

Table 1. Conditions in which corticosteroids are of proven efficacy

Primary and secondary adrenal insufficiency
Immunologic diseases (rheumatoid arthritis, etc.)
Renal diseases (nephrotic syndrome)
Allergic diseases
Bronchial asthma
Ocular inflammations
Skin diseases (dermatitis, etc.)
Diseases of gastrointestinal tract (celiac sprue, Crohn's disease, chronic ulcerative cholitis)
Cerebral edema
Malignancies (bone marrow, solid organs)
Hematological diseases (thrombocythemia, hemolytic anemia, etc.)
Diseases of the liver (cirrhosis)
Transplantation

Table 2. Published studies on the use of corticosteroids in patients with severe infections

Author	No. of pts	Patients	Control group	Random	Prospective	Drug evaluated	Dose	Duration	Outcome
Schumer 1976 [10]	172	Septic shock	Yes	Yes	Yes	Methylprednisolone / Dexamethasone	30 mg/kg / 3 mg/kg	Repeated if necessary after 4 h	Reduced mortality
Sprung 1984 [11]	59	Septic shock	Yes	Yes	Yes	Methylprednisolone / Dexamethasone	30 mg/kg / 6 mg/kg	Repeated if necessary after 4 h	Shock reversal / No reduction of overall mortality
Bone 1987 [13]	381	Severe sepsis, shock	Yes	Yes	Yes	Methylprednisolone	30 mg/kg	24 h	No benefit
Veterans Administration 1987 [12]	223	Sepsis	Yes	Yes	Yes	Methylprednisolone	30 mg/kg followed by 5 mg/kg	9 h	No benefit
Luce 1988 [14]	75	Septic shock	Yes	Yes	Yes	Methylprednisolone	30 mg/kg x 4	24 h	No benefit
Hoffman 1984 [19]	38	Typhoid fever	Yes	Yes	Yes	Dexamethasone	3 mg/kg	NA	Reduced mortality (10% vs 55.6%)
Ajao 1984 [20]		Typhoid fever perforation	Yes	Yes	Yes	Methylprednisolone / Dexamethasone	NA	NA	Reduced mortality
Gagnon 1990 [21]	23	Pneumocystis carinii pneumonia in AIDS	Yes	Yes	Yes	Methylprednisolone	40 mg x 4	7 days	Reduced mortality
Lucas and Ledgerwood 1981 [51]	114	Hypovolemic shock	Yes	Yes	Yes	Methylprednisolone	1 gr in OR + 3.578 mg/day (average)	3 days	No benefit
Sladen 1976 [50]	10	Shock lung syndrome	No	No	No	Methylprednisolone	30 mg/kg x 4	48 h	Reduced mortality
Weigelt 1985 [53]	81	Pulmonary failure	Yes	Yes	Yes	Methylprednisolone	30 mg/kg x 4	48 h	No benefit
Odio 1991 [18]	101	Bacterial meningitis	Yes	Yes	Yes	Dexamethasone	0.15 mg/kg x 4	4 days	Reduced mortality / Reduced neurologic sequelae
Bernard 1987 [54]	99	ARDS	Yes	Yes	Yes	Methylprednisolone	30 mg/kg x 4	24 h	No benefit
Meduri 1991 [60]	8	Late ARDS	No	No	No	Methylprednisolone	Bolus 2 mg/kg 2-3 mg/kg x 4	Until extubation	Reduction LIS
Meduri 1994 [61]	25	Late ARDS	No	No	No	Methylprednisolone	Bolus 200 mg 2-3 mg/kg x day	Until extubation	Reduction LIS / Improvement PaO_2/FiO_2
Meduri 1995 [62]	9	Late ARDS	No	No	No	Methylprednisolone	Bolus 200 mg 2-3 mg/kg x day	Until extubation (average 6 weeks)	Reduction in plasma and BAL inflammatory cytokines (TNF-α, IL-6)
Bollaert 1998 [36]	41	Septic shock	Yes	Yes	Yes	Hydrocortisone	100 mg x 3	≥ 5 days	Increased shock reversal / 28-day mortality reduction of 31%
Meduri 1998 [63]	24	Late ARDS	Yes	Yes	Yes	Methylprednisolone	2 mg/kg	32 days	Improvement LIS / Improvement MODS score / Reduced mortality

The use of corticosteroids during infectious diseases, especially sepsis, and during acute respiratory distress syndrome (ARDS) is still controversial. In these situations corticosteroids have been used for their anti-inflammatory activity but criticized because of their immunosuppressive action. The recent concept of occult relative adrenal insufficiency occurring in the critically ill patient may explain a positive impact of corticosteroid therapy on mortality and outcome.

Corticosteroids in sepsis and septic shock

Severe infection, sepsis and septic shock are responsible for high morbidity and mortality among critically ill patients. Despite aggressive fluid resuscitation, broad-spectrum antibiotic therapy and new life-support devices, mortality attributable to septic shock did not improve over the last decades and remains a major concern.

The anti-inflammatory properties of corticosteroids have encouraged researchers to evaluate their therapeutic activity in severe infections, while being aware of their important side effects and their immunosuppressive action. Whether corticosteroids exert a beneficial or detrimental effect on outcome is still uncertain. The first study that suggested the use of corticosteroids in patients with severe systemic infection was published in 1951 [8] but the first prospective, randomized trial was published in 1963 [9] (Table 2). Schumer [10] in 1976 demonstrated with a prospective, randomized, double-blind study that the use of corticosteroids (methylprednisolone and dexamethasone) significantly lowered the mortality rate in a population of septic patients.

In the 1980s new large clinical trials evaluated the effect of steroids on mortality [11-13].

Sprung et al. [11] reported that glucocorticoids did not significantly improve the overall hospital mortality rate in patients with septic shock, despite a significant enhancement of short-term survival and shock reversal. A multicenter trial [12] showed that there was no difference in mortality between the steroid-treated patients and the placebo group; the resolution of secondary infection was, however, significantly higher in patients receiving placebo than in those receiving active drug. Similarly Bone et al. [13] and Luce et al. [14] did not find different mortality rates between the steroid-treated patients and patients who received placebo, confirming that in patients receiving steroids, significantly more deaths were related to secondary infection. In the subgroup of septic patients with renal failure, corticosteroids worsened shock and mortality rate increased after treatment. All these studies concluded that the use of high-dose corticosteroids provides no benefit in the treatment of severe sepsis or septic shock and should therefore not be used. In 1992 the guidelines of the Infectious Diseases Society of America [15] stated that the routine use of glucocorticoids was not recommended for the treatment of sepsis and septic shock; however, their use was accepted for specific infectious diseases for which its efficacy was proven, like bacterial meningitis in children [16-18], typhoid fever [19, 20], or *Pneumocystis carinii* pneumonia in patients with acquired immunodeficiency syndrome [21, 22]. In 1995 two meta-analyses [23, 24] of past clinical trials confirmed these principles.

More recently, the concept of adrenocortical deficiency in critically ill patients renewed interest in the use of corticosteroids in sepsis. Several investigators [25-28] showed that a low cortisol response to a short corticotropin stimulation test was associated with high mortality in septic shock patients with relative adrenocortical insufficiency. The reduced serum cortisol response to corticotropin in some critically ill patients seems related either to a super-maximal stimulation of the hypothalamic-pituitary-adrenal axis, or to interference with the normal corticosteroid-synthesis [25]. Despite elevated serum cortisol levels, these patients have a blunted response to corticotropin and show a low cortisol reserve. The notion of total adrenal insufficiency (occurring in 2-3% of critically ill patients [29-31]) has been gradually replaced by the concept of occult or relative adrenal insufficiency, which might contribute to a fatal outcome, especially in the presence of multi-organ failure. Although the significance and the prognostic value of the corticotropin test have been challenged [32, 33], two studies [34, 35] showed that the infusion of replacement doses of hydrocortisone in septic patients under catecholamines was associated with rapid hemodynamic improvement and weaning from inotropic and vasoactive support.

Bollaert et al. [36] reported that the administration of low dose hydrocortisone (300 mg/day for more than 5 days) in 42 septic shock patients under catecholamines was associated with an improved and faster shock reversal and reduction of 28-day mortality. The proportion of patients with recovery from shock was similar in responders and non-responders to the corticotropin test, and both groups benefited from hydrocortisone. Reversal of relative adrenocortical insufficiency due to cortisol supplementation cannot fully explain the improvement of hemodynamics and the beneficial effect on survival. Corticosteroids may reverse the desensitization and down-regulation of the adrenergic receptor [37, 38] and restore the vascular tone. Prolonged exposure to β-adrenergic agonists induces a loss of their hemodynamic effectiveness [39, 40]. This desensitization is apparently a result of both down-regulation of receptors (i.e. a decrease in their number) and uncoupling of the receptor from adenylate cyclase [41, 42]. Glucocorticoid-mediated transcriptional regulation of β-adrenergic receptors has been reported [43]. This desensitization occurs 72 h after catecholamine infusion; only after this period do glucocorticoids seem effective in restoring normal sensitivity of the adrenergic receptor and normalizing the vascular tone [44].

Corticosteroids in ARDS

Acute respiratory distress syndrome (ARDS) is a clinical and pathophysiologic entity characterized by acute and diffuse endothelial and epithelial damage of the lung with increased vascular permeability. The mortality rate associated with ARDS is 60-70%, without improvement over the last 20 years despite new developments in supportive therapy [45]. The anti-inflammatory properties of corticosteroids have been thought to be effective in this syndrome. Investigations on the use of corticosteroids in the prevention and treatment of ARDS led to controversial results.

High-dose corticosteroid treatment was recommended for ARDS in the 1970s because of its effect on the hemoglobin dissociation curve [46], on cardiac output [47], and for reducing pulmonary venous spasm [48]. Bowers [49] reported that high-dose corticosteroids were able to reduced pulmonary permeability in animal experimental models. Sladen [50] found a PaO_2 increase after corticosteroids in patients with "shock lung", while Lucas and Ledgerwood [51] found that in patients at risk for post-transfusion ARDS treated with corticosteroids there was an increase of central venous pressure and a decrease of PaO_2. Sibbald [52] in 1981 concluded that high-dose methylprednisolone may reduce alveolo-capillary permeability in early ARDS due to sepsis; conversely Weigelt et al. [53] found no decrease in the development of ARDS in high-risk surgical patients after steroid treatment.

Bernard [54] in 1987 reported that high-dose methylprednisolone (four doses of 30 mg/kg every 6 h) did not affect outcome in patients with established ARDS.

In the late 1980s a new impulse to research came from the definition of the so-called cytokine network that plays an important role in the onset, evolution and regulation of inflammation in the lung as in any other anatomical site. Cytokines are soluble proteins secreted by specific challenged cells and possess autocrine and paracrine activities.

Pulmonary cytokines are produced either by local cells, like macrophages, endothelial cells, pneumocytes, and fibroblasts, or by other cells such as neutrophils, lymphocytes, and platelets migrating into the lung from other sites. Inflammatory cytokines are known to mediate the injury to the endothelial and epithelial cells of the lung and amplify fibroblast proliferation, deposition of collagen and promotion of fibrosis [55].

In a study of 30 mechanically ventilated patients at risk for ARDS, high concentrations of cytokines, namely tumor necrosis factor (TNF), were found in the bronchoalveolar lavage fluid, supporting the concept of local production of this cytokine in ARDS [56].

Recurrent lung injury due to a persistent elevation of plasma inflammatory cytokines (IL-1β and IL-6) levels is predictive of poor outcome [57]. Similar finding were reported in 14 patients with hematological malignancies and severe sepsis, most of whom died of ARDS and septic shock, despite severe leukopenia, supporting the idea that several perturbed cells other than leukocytes sustain cytokine production [58]. Pulmonary fibroproliferation is a frequent finding in late ARDS and is associated with persistent inflammation.

Although the release of cytokines is essential for immunologic regulation, acute and exaggerated production or persistent release can have devastating effects. Eighty-five percent of patients with ARDS survive the initial insult [59]; the major causes of late death, frequently unrecognized, are pulmonary fibrosis and sepsis secondary to nosocomial pneumonia. Cytokine-mediated pulmonary inflammation and fibrosis are often associated with fever and leukocytosis, making the clinical distinction from secondary sepsis even more difficult. The hypothesis that fibrosis of the late ARDS may be steroid-responsive was tested by Meduri [60,61]: methylprednisolone (2-3 mg/kg every 6 h until extubation), administered to ARDS patients for an average time of 36 days, was associated with a significant improvement of PaO_2/FiO_2 ratio, chest X-ray densities, and Lung Injury Score (LIS). The same investigator [62, 63] found that prolonged corticosteroid treatment in late ARDS patients lowered plasma and BAL inflammatory cytokines levels with simultaneous clinical improvement and reduced mortality. Recent findings suggest that although a short corticosteroid therapy may not be beneficial in the early phase of ARDS, prolonged administration of steroids may blunt the cytokine-mediated fibrotic process and thus improve outcome.

Conclusion

The use of corticosteroids in sepsis and acute respiratory distress syndrome has been variably approved and criticized. The latest investigations suggest that in patients with advanced catecholamine-treated septic shock corticosteroid therapy may provide shock reversal and reduce the mortality rate. Similarly lung fibrosis and the recurrent cytokine-mediated inflammation responsible for the poor outcome of patients with late ARDS may be prevented or reduced by the long-term administration of steroids. No differences in efficacy, however, have been observed between the various glucocorticoids tested.

References

1. Packard BD, Weiler JM (1983) Steroids inhibit activation of the alternative amplification pathway of complement. Infect Immunol 40:1011-1019
2. Moncada S, Higgs A (1993) The L-arginine-nitric oxide pathwway. N Eng J Med 329:2002-2012
3. Hammerschmidt DE, White JG, Graddock PR et al (1979) Corticosteroids inhibit complement-induced granulocyte aggregation: A possible mechanism for their efficacy in shock states. J Clin Invest 63:798-893
4. Skubits KM, Craddock LR, Hammerschmidt DE et al (1981) Corticosteroids block binding of chemotactic peptide to its receptor on granulocytes and cause disaggregation of granulocyte aggregates in vitro. J Clin Invest 68:13-20
5. Dhainaut JF, Mira JP (1993) The role of platelet activating factors in sepsis. In: Gartner JD, Calandra T, Carlet J (Eds) Mediators of sepsis: From pathophysiology to therapeutic approaches. Maurice Rapid Colloquia. Baum, Paris, Flammarion
6. Beutler B, Krochin N, Milsark I et al (1986) Control of cachectin (tumor necrosis factor) synthesis: Mechanisms of endotoxin resistance. Science 232:977-980
7. Parant M, Le Contel C, Parant F et al (1991) Influence of endogenous glucocorticoid on endotoxin-induced production of circulating TNF-alpha. Lymphokine Cytokine Res 10:265-271
8. Hahn EC, House HB, Rammelkamp CH et al (1951) Effect of cortisone on acute streptococcal infections and post-streptococcal complications. J Clin Invest 30:274-281
9. Bennet IL, Finland M, Hamburger M et al (1963) The effectiveness of hydrocortisone in the management of severe infections. JAMA 183:462-465
10. Schumer W (1976) Steroids in the treatment of clinical septic shock (1963). Ann Surg 184:333-339
11. Sprung CL, Caralis PV, Marcial EH et al (1984) The effect of high dose corticosteroids in patients with septic shock. N Eng J Med 311:1137-1143
12. The Veterans Administration Systemic Sepsis Cooperative Study Group (1987) Effect of high-dose glucocorticoid therapy on mortality in patients with clinical signs of sepsis. N Eng J Med 317:659-665
13. Bone RC, Fisher CJ, Clemmer TP et al (1987) A controlled clinical trial of high-dose methylprednisolone in the treatment of severe sepsis and septic shock. N Eng J Med 317:653-658
14. Luce JM, Montgomery AB, Marks JD et al (1988) Ineffectiveness of high-dose methylprednisolone therapy in preventing parenchymal lung injury and improving mortality in patients with septic shock. Am Rev Resp Dis 138:62-68
15. McGowan JE, Chesney PJ, Crossley KB et al (1992) Guidelines for the use of systemic glucocorticoids in the management of selected infections. J Infect Dis 165:1-13
16. Havens PL, Wendelberg KJ, Hoffmann GM (1989) Corticosteroids as adjunctive therapy in bacterial meningitis. Am J Dis Child 143:1051-1055
17. Lebel MH, Freij BJ, Syrogiannopulos GA et al (1988) Dexamethasone therapy for bacterial meningitis. N Eng J Med 319:964-971
18. Odio CM, Fainzegicht I, Paris M et al (1991) The beneficial effect of early dexamethasone administration in infants and children with bacterial meningitis. N Eng J Med 324:1525-1531
19. Hoffman SL, Punjabi NH, Kumala S et al (1984) Reduction of mortality in the chloramphenicol-treated severe typhoid fever by high-dose dexamethasone. N Eng J Med 310:82-88
20. Ajao OG, Ajao A, Johnson T (1984) Methylprednisolone sodium succinate in the treatment of typhoid perforation. Trans R Soc Trop Med Hyg 78:573-576
21. Gagnon S, Boota AM, Fischl MA et al (1990) Corticosteroids as adjunctive therapy for severe *Pneumocystis carinii* pneumonia in the acquired immunodeficiency syndrome. A double-blind, placebo-controlled trial. N Eng J Med 323:1444-1450
22. The National Institute of Health - University of California Expert Panel for Corticosteroids as Adjunctive Therapy for Pneumocystis Pneumonia (1990) Consensus statement on the use of corticosteroids as adjunctive therapy for Pneumocystis pneumonia in the acquired immunodeficiency syndrome. N Eng J Med 323:1500-1504

23. Lefering R, Neugebauer EAM (1995) Steroid controversy in sepsis and septic shock: A meta-analysis. Crit Care Med 23:1294-1303
24. Cronin L, Cook DJ, Carlet J et al (1995) Corticosteroid treatment for sepsis: A critical appraisal and meta-analysis of the literature. Crit Care Med 23:1430-1439
25. Lamberts SWJ, Bruining HA, De Jong FH (1997) Corticosteroid therapy in severe illness. N Eng J Med 337:1285-1292
26. Rothwell PM, Udwadia ZF, Lawler PG (1991) Cortisol response to corticotropin and survival in septic shock. Lancet 337:582-583
27. Moran JL, Chapman MJ, O'Fathartaigh MS et al (1995) Hypocortisolemia and adrenocortical responsiveness at onset of septic shock. Intensive Care Med 20:489-495
28. Soni A, Pepper GM, Wyrwinski PM et al (1995) Adrenal insufficiency occurring during septic shock: Incidence, outcome and relationship to peripheral cytokine levels. Am J Med 98: 266-271
29. Drucker D, Shandling M (1985) Varial adrenocortical function in acute medical illness. Crit Care Med 13:477-479
30. Jurney TH, Cockrell JL Jr, Lindberg JS et al (1987) Spectrum of serum cortisol response to ACTH in ICU patients: correlation with degree of illness and mortality. Chest 92:292-295
31. Sainsbury JR, Stoddart JC, Watson MJ (1981) Plasma cortisol levels: a comparison between sick patients and volunteers given intravenous cortisol. Anaesthesia 36:16-21
32. Bouachour G, Tirot P, Gouello JP et al (1995) Adrenocortical function during septic shock. Intensive Care Med 21:57-62
33. Bouachour G, Roy PM, Guiraud MP (1995) The repetitive short corticotropin stimulation test in patients with septic shock. Ann Intern Med 123:962
34. Briegel J, Forst H, Hellinger H et al (1991) Contribution of cortisol deficiency during septic shock. Lancet 338:507-508
35. Schneider AJ, Voerman HJ (1991) Abrupt hemodynamic improvement in late septic shock with physiologic doses of glucocorticoids. Intensive Care Med 17:436-437
36. Bollaert PE, Charpentier C, Levy B et al (1998) Reversal of late septic shock with supraphysiologic doses of hydrocortisone. Crit Care Med 26:645-650
37. Barnes PJ (1995) Beta-adrenergic receptors and their regulation. Am J Resp Crit Care Med 152:838-860
38. Walker BR, Williams BC (1992) Corticosteroids and vascular tone: Mapping the messenger maze. Clin Sci 82:597-605
39. Colucci WS, Wright RF, Braunwald E (1985) New positive inotropic agents in the treatment of congestive heart failure. N Eng J Med 314:290-296
40. Spitzer JA, Rodriguez de Turco EB, Deauciuc IV et al (1989) Receptor changes in endotoxemia. In: Passmore JC (ed) Perspectives in shock research. Liss, New York, pp 95-106
41. Sibley DR, Lefkovitz RJ (1985) Molecular mechanisms of receptor desensitization using the beta-adrenergic receptor-coupled adenylate cyclase system as a model. Nature 317:124-129
42. Colucci WS, Alexander RW, Williams GH, Braunwald E (1981) Decreased lymphocyte beta-adrenergic-receptor density in patients with heart failure and tolerance to the beta-adrenergic agonist pirbuterol. N Eng J Med 305:185-190
43. Collins S, Caron MG, Lefkowits RJ (1988) Beta-adrenergic receptors in hamster smooth muscle cells are transcriptionally regulated by glucocorticoids. J Biol Chem 263:9067-9070
44. Saito T, Takanashi M, Gallagher E et al (1995). Corticosteroid effect on early beta-adrenergic down-regulation during circulatory shock: hemodynamic study and beta-adrenergic receptor essay. Intensive Care Med 21:204-210
45. Asbaugh DG, Bigelow DB, Petty TL, Levine BE (1967) Acute respiratory distress in adults. Lancet 2:319-323
46. McConn R, Del Guercio LRM (1971) Respiratory function of blood in the acutely ill patient and the effect of steroids. Ann Surg 174:436-450
47. Lozman J, Dutton RE, English M, Powers SR (1975) Cardiopulmonary adjustments following single high dose administration of methylprednisolone in traumatized man. Ann Surg 181:317

48. Kusaijma K, Wax SD, Web WR (1974) Effects of methylprednisolone on pulmonary microcirculation. Surg Gynecol & Obstet 139:1
49. Bowers R, Brigham KL (1978) Methylprednisolone prevents endotoxin induced high lung vascular permeability in the awake sheep. Clin Res 444
50. Sladen A (1976) Methylprednisolone: pharmacologic dose in shock lung syndrome. J Thorac Cardiovasc Surg 71:800-806
51. Lucas CE, Ledgerwood AM (1981) Pulmonary response of massive steroids in seriously injured patients. Ann Surg 194:256-261
52. Sibbald WJ, Anderson RR, Reid B et al (1981) Alveolo-capillary permeability in human septic ARDS: effect of high dose corticosteroid therapy. Chest 79:133-142
53. Weigelt JA, Norcross JF, Borman KR, Snyder WH (1985) Early steroid therapy for respiratory failure. Arch Surg 120:536-540
54. Bernard GR, Luce JM, Sprung CL et al (1987) High-dose corticosteroids in patients with the adult respiratory distress syndrome. N Eng J Med 317:1565-1570
55. Elias JA, Freundlich B, Kern JA, Rosenbloom J (1990) Cytokine networks in the regulation of inflammation and fibrosis in the lung. Chest 97:1439-1445
56. Raponi GM, Antonelli M, Gaeta A et al (1992) Tumor necrosis factor in serum and bronchoalveolar lavage of patients at risk for ARDS. J Crit Care 7:183-188
57. Meduri GU, Headley S, Kohler G et al (1995) Persistent elevation of inflammatory cytokines predicts a poor outcome in ARDS. Plasma IL-1beta and IL-6 levels are consistent and efficient predictors of outcome over time. Chest 107:1062-1073
58. Antonelli M, Raponi GM, Martino P et al (1995) High IL-6 serum levels are associated with septic shock and mortality in septic patients with severe leukopenia due to hematological malignancies. Scand J Infect Dis 27:381-384
59. Montgomery AB, Stager MA, Carrico CJ, Hudson LD (1985) Causes of mortality in patients with the adult respiratory distress syndrome. Am Rev Respir Dis 132:485-489
60. Meduri GU, Belenchia JM, Estes RJ et al (1991) Fibroproliferative phase of ARDS. Clinical findings and effects of corticosteroids. Chest 100:943-952
61. Meduri GU, Chinn AJ, Leeper KV et al (1994) Corticosteroid rescue treatment of progressive fibroproliferation in late ARDS. Patterns of response and predictors of outcome. Chest 105: 1516-1527
62. Meduri GU, Headley S, Tolley E et al (1995) Plasma and BAL cytokine response to corticosteroid rescue treatment in late ARDS. Chest 108:1315-1325
63. Meduri GU, Headley, Golden E, Carson SJ (1998) Effect of prolonged methylprednisolone therapy in unresolving acute respiratory distress syndrome. A randomized clinical trial. JAMA; 280:159-165

ADVANCES IN CPR

On Field Resuscitation

M.A. Baubin

Besides the treatment of the severely injured patient or seriously ill infant, cardiopulmonary resuscitation (CPR) is one of the most challenging and emotional situations for an out-of-hospital emergency medicine team. In the so-called industrial world, the most common cause of adult sudden cardiac arrest (CA) is ischaemic heart disease. Despite the individual history and treatment of each patient, people with primary CA represent the most homogeneous group in emergency medicine. Thus, they are the best group on which to judge the quality of emergency medical service (EMS). For uniform data management in cardiac arrest patients the "Utstein Style" was developed and is now accepted worldwide [1].

Basic life support (BLS) and defibrillation are the only interventions which have been shown unequivocally to improve long-term survival [2]. The time factor is most important for a positive outcome during resuscitation, intervals of 30 seconds each can be crucial.

Epidemiology

About one CPR situation per 1000 inhabitants occurs each year. Return of spontaneous circulation (ROSC) at the scene, hospital admission but especially hospital discharge are outcome criteria. Hospital discharge rates vary between 2% and 20%. The optimum are patients discharged without neurological deficit in a cerebral performance category of 1-2.

In adults the most common primary arrhythmia at the onset of cardiac arrest is ventricular fibrillation (VF). The overwhelming majority of survivors come from this group. VF is an eminently treatable rhythm, but the chances of successful defibrillation decline substantially 7-10% with the passage of each minute. Amplitude and waveform of VF deteriorate rapidly reflecting the depletion of myocardial high energy phosphate. The rate of decline in success depends in part upon the provision and adequacy of basic life support (BLS). As a result, the priority is to minimise any delay between the onset of cardiac arrest and the administration of defibrillation shocks.

CPR guidelines and practice

Especially when time is of the essence, uniform treatment guidelines are of great importance. In CA situations they must be mandatory. Thus, each CA team member knows exactly what to do and what has to be done next. After 10 minutes of uniform advanced cardiac life support (ACLS) according to the guidelines the team leader, if he is a physician can consider alternative methods.

Recent CPR algorithms were published by the European Resuscitation Council (ERC) in 1998 [2]. They are based on the statements of the International Liaison Committee on Resuscitation (ILCOR), which was founded to encourage global cooperation between national and international CPR organisations.

Modified for the on field resuscitation, the "chain of survival" preferably includes bystander CPR, sometimes initiated by the EMS dispatcher (so-called "dispatcher CPR"), early defibrillation and bag-valve-mask ventilation with 100% oxygen by the first tier, intravenous access, catecholamine administration, intubation, stabilisation and transport to the emergency department by the second tier.

Various emergency systems are used: emergency medical technician (EMT) staffed first tiers followed by paramedic- or physician-staffed second tiers, or nurse-staffed systems. In some systems EMTs or paramedics with or without certification to defibrillate, insert the laryngeal mask (LM), intubate or administer certain drugs. In CPR situations the authorisation to make a declaration of death has an important influence on out-of-hospital management. If a paramedic is not allowed to declare a person dead, the patient must be transported to the hospital under CPR conditions. This has a drastic influence on statistical outcome results.

BLS and AED

BLS is important because it restores and maintains cerebral and coronary blood flow with transportation of oxygen and energy. Optimal BLS performance can ensure up to 30% of normal blood flow. Bag-valve-mask ventilation with 100% oxygen is standard for the first tier or BLS team arriving at the scene. Tidal volumes of 400 ml to 600 ml are sufficient for adequate chest movement, but the new guidelines recommend a chest compression rate of 100/min.

New techniques for external chest compression (ECC) have been developed and are still under trial, most notably ECC with active compression decompression (ACD), and CPR performed either by the BLS team or the ACLS team. Unfortunately, at present there are no clinical data showing unequivocal improvement in outcomes.

Other methods like vest CPR, the thump or abdominal counterpulsation also failed to show improvement.

In many countries early defibrillation with first-responder or semi-automated defibrillators (AED) are becoming more and more common. There is still discussion on whether the biphasic truncated waveform is more efficient than the monophasic waveform. First of all, the ACLS team must order an AED immediately.

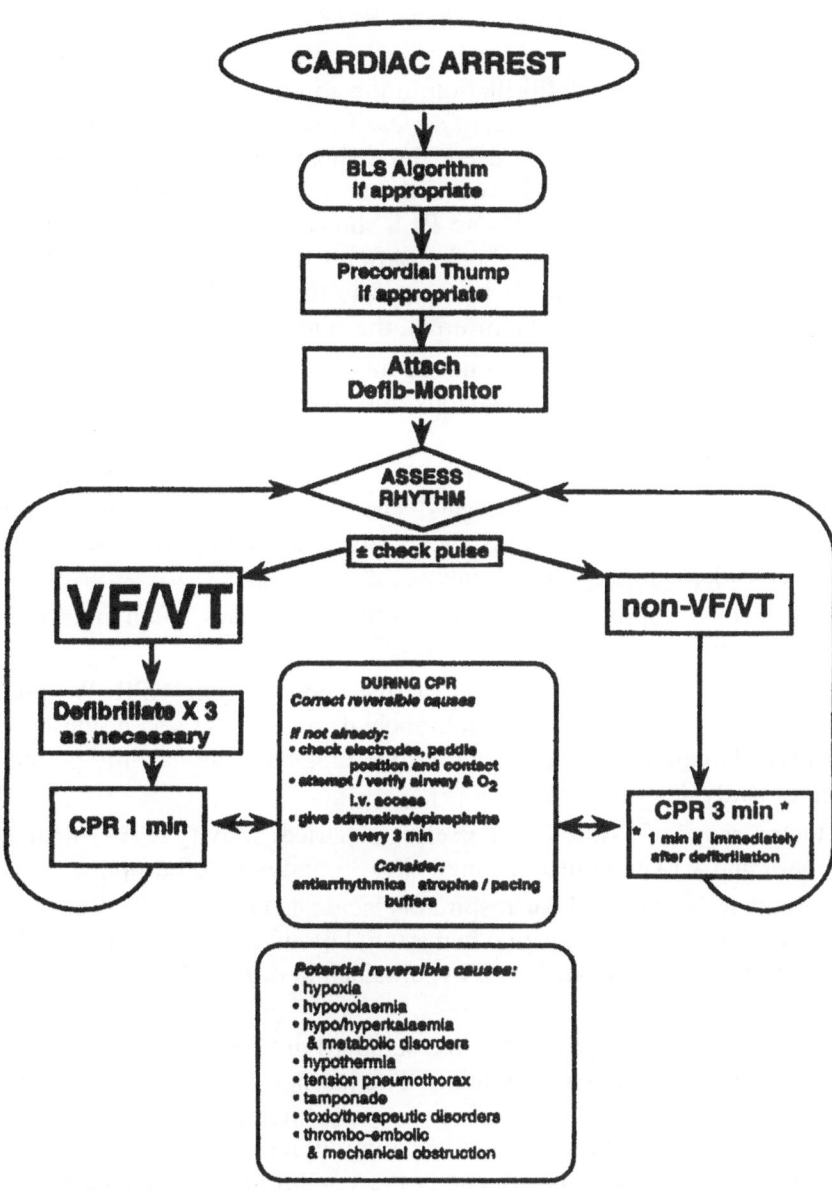

Fig. 1. The ERC ACLS Algorithm

ACLS

As soon as the ACLS team arrives at the scene the team leader checks the patient again and confirms the diagnosis of the BLS team. The next step is to obtain an adequate ECG signal. This can be done by receiving the signal by defi pads or cutaneous electrodes. According to the new guidelines, one should discriminate only between VF or pulseless ventricular tachycardia (VF/VT) and non VF/VT. When the ECG signal shows VF/VT, the precordial thump can be the first step of ACLS.

VF/VT is treated with defibrillation in the adult at 200, 200, 360 J and then at 360, 360, 360 J for all subsequent series. To reduce the transthoracic impedance, defibrillation pads can be used: three shocks of each series must be applied in about 45-60 seconds. Between the first and the second and the second and the third shock of each series no BLS should be performed in order not to prolong the time between the shocks. After each particular shock the team leader judges the ECG signal. If it is equal to the signal before the shock, the next shock is applied; but if it is different, the central pulse needs to be checked.

The time between a series must not be more than 60 seconds. These intervals are used for insertion of an intravenous line (best: jugularis externa), drug administration and/or intubation.

Some treatments like defibrillation or catecholamine administration should be performed at certain time intervals. The rescuer who performs ventilation counts each ventilation: eight BLS cycles (five chest compressions/one ventilation) are considered to take one minute.

Simultaneously applied automatic ventilating strokes often interfere with chest compression.

Adrenalin/epinephrine is the drug of first choice during CPR. We prefer to administer it intravenously; the endobronchial route is the second-best alternative. Although, neither absorption within the lungs nor the half-life period have been sufficiently determined to date [3].

In the presence of asystole or pulseless electrical activity (PEA) with bradycardia one can try to administer a single 2 to 3 mg dosage of atropine.

Bicarbonate is indicated for respiratory acidosis and after 15 min of unsuccessful CPR. It can also be given when arterial blood gases show a pH < 7.1 or a BE < – 10 or in CA associated with hyperkalaemia or following tricyclic antidepressant overdose.

Endobronchial intubation is the gold standard in CPR to obtain a reliable airway and prevent subsequent aspiration. The laryngeal mask airway (LMA) offers an alternative to tracheal intubation, and although it does not absolutely guarantee against aspiration, the incidence in reported series is low. A third feasible option for airway management is the combitube, but it requires special training and is not in routine use in hospitals.

If PEA is present one must consider the four "H"s (hypoxia, hypovolaemia, hypo/hyperkalaemia, hypothermia) and the four "T"s (tension pneumothorax, tamponade, toxic/therapeutic disorders, thrombo-embolic and mechanical obstruction).

Some centres try thrombolysis if CPR is performed without primary success. To date no data have been published.

Special situations

Despite these common rules for the treatment of primary CA, some extraordinary situations require a modified approach. For cardiac arrest due to trauma, mass accidents, septic shock, poisoning, drug overdose, anaphylaxis, hypovolaemia, hypothermia, near-drowning or -burying by avalanches, special recommendations exist. This is also true for CPR in children and newborns.

Considering all these details of CPR, quality assurance demands that BLS as well as ACLS be trained regularly by the team under the supervision of highly experienced instructors. Both societies, AHA and ERC, offer ACLS provider and instructor courses.

Environment

On field resuscitation requires great team expertise: all guidelines should be known inside out and the manual skills must be performed precisely.

Although theoretical training forms the basis, practising CPR in emergency situations is always different.

Beside ensuring optimal CPR efforts and fast diagnosis, the team leader has to get an overview of the environment very quickly. He has to recognise any dangerous situation for the patient or the emergency team. It is important that enough space be established for the team and the equipment. The equipment itself has to be placed so that the team leader can observe the monitor at all times. Sometimes it is necessary to move the patient from the actual scene to another place or into the ambulance for treatment or transport purposes. In about 60% of cases there are relatives or bystanders at the scene, who witnessed the collapse; they are important for additional information. Once CPR has been started, these persons should be asked for their names and any steps undertaken by them. Later it will probably be necessary to inform them about the outcome of the patient. If a relative started CPR prior to the professionals the physician should include him or her in the decision to withdraw or break-off the procedures. Sometimes, especially in the drug scene, bystanders do not recognise the critical nature of the situation and only impede effective help.

Decision making and ethics

CPR managers have to know the factors influencing outcome as mentioned above and take them into consideration when deciding to discontinue CPR efforts. Monitoring of etCO$_2$ or of potassium can be helpful for the decision-making process. The most important factors for continuing or withdrawing CPR efforts are: biological age, the patient's history and last will. Moreover, the period between CA and onset of CPR, the duration and quality of CPR efforts, the primary rhythm and also the experience of the physician strongly influence CPR results. Nursing homes often have a record of the patient's history, but this is often not true for the unknown patient on the field or at home.

Future aspects

A lot of topics in CPR research are under discussion and have been debated even at recent ERC meetings.

A "50/2" chest compression/ventilation rate is discussed when CPR is started by bystanders [5]. To avoid fears surrounding artificial ventilation, it is under discussion whether lay persons should be taught only chest compression without ventilation. It is argued that in cardiac arrest patients there is enough oxygen in the lungs and the blood for at least the first three to five minutes of CA. The rescue team will start artificial ventilation.

Early defibrillation on field but also in the hospital should become general practice. In addition, more research is necessary to clarify bio-technical effects such as waveforms and energy content.

The laryngeal mask is considered a better airway approach than the face mask; and with moderate degree of training on insertion, the LM could become a possibility for paramedical personnel.

In animal CPR research vasopressin was found to be an alternative or a even better vasopressor as adrenalin/epinephrine [4]. Recently, a multicentre study was started under the patronage of the ERC to test vasopressin versus adrenalin in a randomised, double blind, out-of-hospital trial.

Open-chest cardiac massage after mini-thoracotomy was recently reported in an on field CPR situation [5]. Furthermore, a small device was developed for direct cardiac massage after making a small incision in the thorax wall [6].

Conclusions

In conclusion, on field resuscitation is a discipline requiring comprehensive experience, a stable personality in each team member and optimal working conditions for the entire team. Evidence-based CPR performance is specified in international guidelines. CPR research will open new concepts for ameliorating CPR results.

References

1. Task Force of the European Resuscitation Council, American Heart Association, Heart and Stroke Foundation of Canada, Australian Resuscitation Council (1991) Recommended guidelines for uniform reporting of data from out-of-hospital cardiac arrest: the 'Utstein Style'. Resuscitation 22:1-26
2. Bossaert L (1998) European Resuscitation Council Guidelines for Resuscitation. Elsevier, Amsterdam
3. Schüttler J (1991) Pharmakotherapie des Kammerflimmerns. Anaesthesist 40:172-179
4. Lindner KH, Prengel AW, Pfenninger EG et al (1995) Vasopressin improves vital organ blood flow during closed-chest cardiopulmonary resuscitation in pigs. Circulation 91:215-221
5. Craig R, Clarke K, Coats TJ (1999) On scene thoracotomy: a case report. Resuscitation 40: 45-47
6. Buckman RF Jr, Badellino MM, Mauro LH et al (1995) Direct cardiac massage without major thoracotomy: feasibility and systemic blood flow. Resuscitation 29:237-248

The Chain of Survival: Focus on Early Defibrillation

F. KETTE

It is widely known that survival from cardiac arrest is critically time-related. The correctness of the cardio-pulmonary resuscitation maneuvers alone is not sufficient to preserve the full neurological function if too many minutes elapse from the moment of the collapse.

About one decade ago Cummins et al. introduced one of the most important concepts in the setting of the emergency cardiac care, the "Chain-of-Survival" [1]. This concept pointed out that more people can survive sudden cardiac death not only when a single action is performed, but rather when a particular sequence of interventions is performed. When a heart attack occurs, the recognition of the symptoms and signs is of paramount importance. This should allow prompt activation of the emergency medical service. Several conditions, however, have to be taken into account before the activation of the emergency system, for example, may spend an eyewitness several minutes trying to locate a telephone and may not know the correct emergency number [2]. Indeed, beside the general awareness of lay people in recognizing the symptoms of a heart attack, several studies have demonstrated that an eyewitness may phone friends, relatives, neighbors, or their own physician before calling the emergency number. This yields a considerable delay which, in turn, accounts for much lower likelihood of survival. Mayron et al. observed that the activation of a three digits emergency phone number after having used the local numbers, increased the percentage of the calls made in less than one minute from 63% to 82% [3]. Accordingly, awareness of the signs and symptoms of a heart attack and the knowledge of the correct number to activate constitute the first steps for a proper emergency intervention.

An additional delay is due to the call-processing time, which is the time required by the dispatcher to send the proper vehicle and personnel. Accordingly, from the activation to the arrival of the personnel on the scene (ambulance response time) several minutes may then elapse. Commonly, an attempt to reduce this time interval is to improve the number of the ambulances [4]. However, after a certain level, an increase in the number of the vehicles failed to significantly reduce the response time. Hallstrom et al. demonstrated that an 80% increase in the number of the ambulances reduced the average response time by 1 minute only. It was then suggested that such 1-minute reduction could be achieved by increasing the education of the lay people and therefore augmenting their awareness about sudden cardiac death.

CPR alone, namely ventilation and precordial compression, only rarely restore spontaneous cardiac function, but never if the ventricles are fibrillating. The importance of the prompt administration of the Basic Life Support allows the maintenance of a minimal amount of flow to the vital organs, heart and brain. It may be therefore said that CPR maneuvers gain precious minutes by preserving the rapid deterioration of these organs [5, 6].

In fact the great majority of the people (50 to 85%) experience cardiac arrest collapse because of ventricular arrhythmia away from a hospital setting [7, 8]. Ventricular tachicardia may be triggered and this can rapidly evolve in ventricular fibrillation (VF). Other times ventricular fibrillation may develop following a torsade-de-point or it may originate immediately as VF [7]. When out of hospital ambulatory patients were under monitor control, more than 60% of the 157 patients who had cardiac arrest developed ventricular tachycardia first. This lasted from few seconds to several minutes before evolving into ventricular fibrillation. The torsade de point was observed in about 8% of the instances, whereas VF developed instantaneously in another 13% of the cases [7]. Although this group of patients belonged to a selected population of heart disease patients, it is likely that these conditions usually represent what occurs in the sudden cardiac deaths.

Only a quick defibrillation can restore a viable rhythm. The evidence of the importance of the early defibrillation was also supported by experiences in cardiac rehabilitation programs. When the patients were monitored and had the chance to be immediately defibrillated, the resuscitation rates ranged from 85 to 100% with full neurological recovery [7, 9, 10]. Unfortunately, most of the patients who experience cardiac arrest outside the hospital are unmonitored. The patient may remain pulseless for several minutes and the rhythm can be identified only after arrival of the ambulance personnel. The lack of oxygen may rapidly lead to a progressive loss of the energy substrates: a coarse ventricular fibrillation evolves into a progressive fine VF and subsequently into asystole. This explains the lower percentage of the ventricular fibrillation found on the scene [11].

The inverse relationship between delay to first defibrillation and survival is now well recognized. In the out-of-hospital setting Weaver et al. demonstrated that, in the absence of CPR, from the collapse to the first countershock there is a 5% decrease in survival rate for every minute elapsed [8]. Comparable results were more recently demonstrated by Kette et al. in a prospective observational study on out-of-hospital cardiac arrests in Friuli-Venezia Giulia (Italy). Defibrillation performed within 4 minutes was associated with the highest return of spontaneous circulation (ROSC) (92%) and the highest hospital discharge (54%). However, as the minutes passed there was a progressive decline in both, ROSC and hospital discharge. After 14 minutes from the collapse 32% of the patients were still successfully defibrillated, but none was discharge alive from hospital [11]. Similar results were observed when cardiac arrest occurred in the hospital wards. Those patients who developed VF were more likely to be resuscitated when defibrillation was performed within the first minutes.

These data strongly support the need to improve the diffusion of the defibrillators, but their use by non-physicians is still questioned and regulated by strict laws in many countries. In the USA when earlier programs on defibrillation stated that only paramedics could defibrillate [12, 13], the time between collapse and their arrival on the scene averaged more than 12 minutes. Consequently, the results were quite poor and only a very modest survival rates was documented [14]. To reduce such critical time interval, programs spreading the use of defibrillators among other categories were started. The availability of the defibrillators to the emergency medical technicians (EMTs) demonstrated that they were able to use the device correctly as the paramedics [15, 16].

One step forward which enhanced the utilization of the defibrillators by non-physicians was the introduction of the automated and semi-automated external defibrillators (AEDs). These devices are highly accurate and eliminate the need for adequate training in the rhythm recognition. By simply attaching the adhesive paddles on the patient's thorax, the AED analyzes his rhythm and applies the electric shock. It is then responsibility of the operator to ensure the safety of the scene and to impede that the patient be touched during the electrical shock. This kind of device, called shock-advisory, has almost totally replaced the fully automated defibrillators. Some of the companies producing AEDs have also removed the screen from the device as it is not required by the user to look at the waveform. The operator is guided by the vocal apparatus whether or not to defibrillate.

Different degrees of success have been reported after the use of the AEDs by the EMTs. Before the wide institution of the AEDs, survival rates averaged 3% in several communities. Afterwards, in the same communities, the survival ranged from 10% to 20% and rose up to 26% in one community [16-18].

Although the training in the use of the AED requires little time, the defibrillation has to be combined with the other interventions recommended by the links of the chain of survival. In refractory ventricular fibrillation, CPR must be interposed with the electrical shocks in order to provide some oxygen. Walter et al., in a study aimed to evaluate the correctness of the interventions by the EMTs, observed that only one third of about 100 rescuers conducted the maneuvers properly. One error occurred in 36% of the cases, two errors in 22% and three errors in the remaining 8%. The most important mistakes were related to the missing order to stand clear (23%) and to the omitted interposed CPR (35%) [19].

According to all these evidences, the universal algorithm was set to administer the electrical shock, if appropriate, as quickly as possible. Attention was also paid to the details which render the defibrillation more successful, such as the best paddle position, the presence of a pacemaker, transcutaneous therapies and, more importantly, safety during electrical shocks. One paddle must be positioned at the level of the fifth left intercostal space on the anteriore axillary line whereas the second one has to be placed just below the right clavicula. With this position, the current flow crosses the whole myocardial mass. If a pacemaker is located under the skin the paddle must be placed at a distance of 12-15 cm. All cutaneous nitrates must be removed. With regards to safety during the electrical shocks, everyone must stand clear at the moment of defibrillation, and the team leader will assure the safety by saying loudly "I am clear, you are clear, everybody is clear".

Either by using manual or semi-automated defibrillators, the first shock will deliver an energy of 200 J. This energy has been selected as the lowest one capable of converting the rhythm without producing excessive myocardial lesions. If unsuccessful, the second shock must be administered without any delay at the same 200 J energy. The rationale of such choice is related to the decrease of the impedance occurring particularly after the first shock. With a reduced impedance, yet maintaining the 200 joules, the amount of current flowing through the heart is higher. This mechanism augments the likelihood to convert the malignant rhythm. Only after the second shock, if unsuccessful, must the energy for the defibrillation be increased to 360 J, and the third shock is given without interrupting the sequence. The AEDs are automatically set to deliver the first two energies at 200 J and the third one at 360. There are, however, circumstances in which the semi-automated device has to be reset. This is the case when VF is converted following the second shock, and VF reoccurs after a short interval of pulsatile rhythm. In this case the subsequent energy has to be the one which restores a viable rhythm. If the AED is still on, the operator has to manually modify the energy in order to remain at 200 J.

To reduce the size and costs of the defibrillators in order to increase their diffusion, a relatively new technique of shock delivery was adopted. This was based on a different waveform of the current administration. The waveform determines the amount of energy received by the patient and the time over which the energy is delivered. The "new" waveform is denominated biphasic because of the two phases and the two polarity waveforms, in contrast to the monophasic waveform normally utilized in all other defibrillators. This method, however, has been widely adopted for almost two decades in the implantable defibrillators. This methodology was used even earlier in the former Soviet Union where Gurvich observed that the biphasic damped sine waveform required a significant lower amount of energy than monophasic defibrillation. However, despite the major efficacy demonstrated by this kind of defibrillation, it was the cost and the size which hampered its practical applicability. Only in the last decade have new engineering technologies rendered the construction of these new defibrillators feasible for their use as external devices.

Basically, the reasons of the slower energy used is related to the automatic calculation of the transthoracic impedance. Since impedance determines the time over which the shock is delivered (usually it does in a range within 5 to 40 m/sec), the length may be shorter (less than 5 m/sec) or longer (more than 40 m/sec). The effects can be respectively an inefficieny to defibrillate or an increased risk or recurrence of VF. Accordingly, by instantaneously measuring the transthoracic impedance, lower energy would be delivered within the appropriate time.

The results of the biphasic defibrillation are now reported in both, experimental and clinical studies [20-22]. There is evidence that lower biphasic energies (180-190 J) are as effective as the traditional monophasic 200 J energies. In addition, the lower damage to the myocardial fibers is well documented [23].

At the present time there are several on-going studies to investigate this particular technological aspect. Also under investigation is the possibility to defibrillate at once or to proceed with some short phase of precordial compression to provide a partial myocardial oxygenation [24]. It cannot be excluded that some modification of the algorithm will occur in the future. Until then, early defibrillation remains a milestone in ventricular fibrillation with well established efficacy if applied as soon as possible.

References

1. Cummins RO, Ornato JP, Thies WH, Pepe PE (1991) Improving survival from sudden cardiac arrest: the "Chain of Survival" concept. Circulation 83:1832-1847
2. Stults KR (1987) Phone first. J Emerg Med Services 12:28
3. Mayron R, Long RS, Ruiz E (1984) The 911 emergency telephone number: impact on emergency medical system access in a metropolitan area. Am J Emerg Med 2:491-493
4. Graf WS, Polin SS, Pagel BL (1973) A community program for emergency cardiac care: a three-year coronary ambulance-paramedic evaluation. JAMA 226:156-160
5. Cummins RO, Eisenberg MS (1985) Prehospital cardiopulmonary resuscitation: is it effective? JAMA 253:2408-2412
6. Bossaert L, Van Hoeeyweghen R (1989) Cerebral resuscitation study group: bystander cardiopulmonary resuscitation (CPR) in out-of-hospital cardiac arrest. Resuscitation [Suppl]17: S55-S69
7. Bayes de Luna A, Coumel P, Leclercq JF (1989) Ambulatory sudden cardiac death: mechanisms of production of fatal arrhythmia on the basis of data from 157 cases. Am Heart J 117:151-159
8. Weaver WD, Cobb LA, Hallstrom AP et al (1986) Factors influencing survival after out-of-hospital cardiac arrest. J Am Coll Cardiol 7:752-757
9. Hossack KF, Hartwig R (1982) Cardiac arrest associated with supervised cardiac rehabilitation. J Cardiac Rehab 2:402-408
10. Van Camp SP, Peterson RA (1986) Cardiovascular complications of outpatient cardiac rehabilitation programs. JAMA 256:1160-1163
11. Kette F, Sbrojavacca R, Rellini GL et al (1998) Epidemiology and survival rate of out-of-hospital cardiac arrest in north-east Italy: the FACS Study. Resuscitation 36:153-159
12. Roth R, Stewart RD, Rogers K, Cannon GM (1984) Out-of-hospital cardiac arrest: factors associated with survival. Ann Emerg Med 13:237-243
13. Wright D, James C, Marsden AK, Mackintosh AF (1989) Defibrillation by ambulance staff who have extended training. BMJ 299:96-97
14. Eisenberg MS, Horwood BT, Cummins RO et al (1990) Cardiac arrest and resuscitation: a tale of 29 cities. Ann Emerg Med 19:179-186

15. Eisenberg MS, Hallstrom AP, Copass MK et al (1984) Treatment of ventricular fibrillation: emergency medical technicians defibrillation and paramedic services. JAMA 251:1723-1726
16. Stults KR, Brown DD, Schug VL, Bean JA (1984) Prehospital defibrillation performed by emergency medical technicians in rural communities. N Engl J Med 310:219-223
17. Eisenberg MS, Copass MK, Hallstrom AP (1980) Treatment of out-of-hospital cardiac arrest with rapid defibrillation by emergency medical technicians. N Engl J Med 302:1379-1383
18. Bachman JW, McDonald GS, O'Brien PC (1986) A study of out-of-hospital cardiac arrests in northeastern Minnesota. JAMA 256:477-483
19. Walters G, D'Auria D, Glucksman E (1992) Automated external defibrillation: implications for training qualified ambulance staff. Ann Emerg Med 21:692-697
20. Bardy GH, Gliner BE, Kudenchuk PJ et al (1995) Truncated biphasic pulses for transthoracic defibrillation. Circulation 91:1768-1774
21. Greene HL, Di Marco JP, Kudenchuk PJ et al (1195) Comparison of monophasic and biphasic defibrillating pulse waveform for transthoracic cardioversion. Am J Coll Cardiol 75:1135-1139
22. Bardy GH, Marchlinski FE, Sharma AD et al (1996) Multicenter comparison of truncated biphasic shocks and standard damped sine wave monophasic shocks for transthoracic ventricular defibrillation. Circulation 94:2507-2514
23. Jones JL, Jones RE, Balasky G (1987) Microlesion formation in myocardial cells by high intensity electric field stimulation. Am J Physiol 253:H480-H486
24. Sato Y, Weil MH, Sun S et al (1997) Adverse effects of interrupting precordial compression during cardiopulmonary resuscitation. Crit Care Med 25:733-736

EVIDENCE-BASED MEDICINE AND POLICY IN THE ICU

Evidence-Based Medicine in the ICU

J.-L. VINCENT

Current financial constraints across the medical sector, accompanied by increasing litigation by patients and/or relatives, has resulted in increasing pressure on physicians of all specialties to account for their actions and supply supported reasoning for their actions. In this context, evidence-based medicine (EBM) has been promoted as a tool to provide physicians with the necessary means to evaluate the current basis for any proposed intervention. Essentially, EBM must be seen as an approach to literature appraisal and application, and requires the ability to accurately assess the weight carried by the various levels of evidence and to integrate all the evidence available in an overall assessment of the intervention in question. EBM is thus an approach to clinical practice based on knowledge of the evidence, and the strength of that evidence, on which practice is based [1]. Increasingly EBM has become the buzz word for 'good' medical practice.

The randomized controlled trial

EBM stresses the need for physicians to base their actions on sound clinical evidence, preferably derived from that 'gold-standard' - the randomized, controlled (double-blind) trial (RCT). EBM classically divides the literature according to the strength of the evidence with RCTs providing grade I and II evidence (Table 1). However, in intensive care medicine, RCTs are notoriously difficult to perform, and EBM must rely more heavily on other study designs and clinical experience. In an ideal world, all new and established interventions would indeed be tested by large, double-blinded RCTs. Randomization controls for unknown and unmeasured variables between groups, and random assignment to treatments, especially when blinded, removes the potential of bias [2]. However, in many fields, especially intensive care, RCTs are frequently not practical or appropriate, and many established therapeutic interventions have never been tested by RCT. Indeed, when a group of intensive care examination candidates were asked to list accepted therapeutic interventions which have been shown to reduce mortality in intensive care unit patients, less than half were able to supply an answer, demonstrating the lack of RCT-based evidence in this field [3]. In

Table 1. Levels of evidence based on literature appraisal of a proposed treatment [13, 14]

Level I: Randomized trials with low false positive and low false negative errors, i.e., a randomized trial showing a statistically significant benefit of treatment, or a trial showing no effect but which was large enough to exclude any possible beneficial effect (i.e., small 95% confidence intervals)

Level II: Randomized trials with high false positive and/or high false negative errors, i.e., a trial with a non statistically significant trend in favor of treatment, or a trial showing no effect but with the distinct possibility of a beneficial effect (i.e., with very large 95% confidence intervals). Pooling of the data of two small level II trials by meta-analysis may result in overall level I evidence

Level III: Non-randomized concurrent cohort comparisons between contemporaneous patients who did and did-not receive the treatment

Level IV: Non-randomized historical cohort comparisons between current patients who received treatment and former patients (from the same institution or from the literature) who did not

Level V: Case series without controls

this study, candidates could find only eight therapeutic interventions which had been shown by RCT to reduce mortality (Table 2), and for most of these interventions although one RCT may have shown improved outcome others demonstrated no effect or a harmful effect [3], highlighting the limitations to basing treatment recommendations on the results of a single RCT. A similar study was recently conducted in registrants at a large international symposium on intensive care and emergency medicine. Here, there was evident confusion about which accepted therapeutic interventions had in fact been tested in a RCT, with respondents listing interventions, such as fluid challenge and percutaneous tracheostomy, which have never been subject to a RCT (unpublished data). The fact that an intervention is not supported by RCT-based evidence does not necessarily mean it is of no value.

There are many reasons why an RCT may not be practical or appropriate [4]. In the critically ill population, one of the main problems is the heterogeneous nature of the intensive care population. Intensive care unit patients are a group of people of varying ages, underlying pathologies, complications, treatments, etc., and yet frequently they are grouped together under the label 'critically ill' for purposes of clinical trial inclusion. It is perhaps not surprising that RCTs of anti-sepsis treatments in such a mixed bunch of patients have failed to show benefit. Indeed, subgroup analysis in several of these large RCTs has shown benefit [5, 6] suggesting that in the septic population, smaller RCTs in more carefully selected populations may provide more valuable information.

Another problem in intensive care medicine is the often complex and confusing terminology. Definitions of common disease processes are often inadequate and incomplete. For example, many trials of septic patients have employed the SIRS [7] criteria, but these are so sensitive that almost all intensive care unit patients meet them [8]. Patients with myocardial infarction can be selected accord-

Table 2. Therapeutic interventions listed by candidates of the Belgian Board Examination in Intensive Care Medicine as having been shown in RCTs to reduce mortality [3]

Therapeutic intervention	Relevant RCTs
Open lung approach in ARDS	[15]
Early nutritional support	[16-19]
Supranormal oxygen delivery	[20-27]
N-acetylcysteine in acetaminophen intoxication	[28]
N-acetylcysteine in ARDS	[29-32]
Non-invasive respiratory support	[33-38]
Hypothermia in severe head trauma	[39, 40]
Corticosteroids in spinal trauma	[41, 42]

ing to EKG changes and raised levels of cardiac enzymes, but the classification of septic patients is less clear-cut.

Ethical considerations may also preclude testing an intervention by RCT. For example, no ethical board would accept a trial randomizing critical care patients to ICU or general ward care, or one which assessed the benefits of mechanical ventilation against no intervention in patients with respiratory failure. Cardiopulmonary resuscitation could not be refused in the patient with cardiorespiratory arrest merely for the benefits of a RCT, and what doctor would stand and watch a patient bleed to death for the sake of evaluating the benefits of a blood transfusion. In such cases, and many others, evidence must come from other sources including observational studies. RCTs and non-randomized studies can provide complementary evidence and clinicians must be aware of the strengths and weaknesses of each method [9].

Practicing EBM in the ICU

So, does the general shortage of RCT-based evidence in the ICU mean that the intensivist is exempt from practicing EBM, or that he/she should not use those interventions which have not been proved to be effective by RCT - of course not. While acknowledging that the RCT provides the highest level of evidence, EBM recognizes that this is not to the exclusion of all other studies and experience. Indeed, this would be a misinterpretation of the principles of EBM. Many aspects of clinical practice cannot and will never be tested by RCT, and in these situations, clinical experience and observation provide essential evidence.

EBM has been described as the sum of five key aspects [10]:

1. that clinical and health care decisions should be based on the best patient and laboratory-based evidence

2. that it is the problem in question rather than individual habits, customs or protocols, that determines the nature of the evidence to be researched

3. that identifying the best evidence needs full integration of epidemiological and biostatistical methods with personal experience

4. that the results of the critical appraisal of evidence are of value only if applied directly to influence patient management

5. that our application and assessment of the evidence for each problem are repeatedly reviewed as new evidence becomes available

In essence, the practice of EBM can be divided into two fundamental aspects, literature appraisal and clinical experience, which when combined together will give the full analysis of the intervention in question for any individual patient [11]. Critical literature appraisal includes conducting an efficient search of the literature, selecting relevant studies and applying rules of evidence to determine their validity, and thereby determining the level of evidence for or against the proposed intervention. These skills must be learned, yet are not often included in medical school programs. With the continuing exploding volume of literature, and the rapid development and introduction of new therapies, it is vital that techniques of literature appraisal are taught to enable the physician to keep up to date with the latest advances. However, literature appraisal must be complemented by clinical experience based on a traditional medical training with a sound knowledge of the pathophysiology of disease. The results of clinical trials can only be applied to a specific patient in the light of the pathophysiology of their disease process. In addition, some knowledge of the individual patient including their past history, emotional and psychological needs, and treatment preferences, is a necessary part of the application of EBM [11]. Literature appraisal can inform but clinical experience determines how the evidence should be integrated into a patient's care [12].

Conclusion

EBM is a tool to assist the clinician in assessing the literature, to complement not replace clinical experience and training. Literature appraisal is the cornerstone of EBM, but when applied without appropriate clinical knowledge and expertise is of little relevance to the physician and of no help to the patient.

References

1. Cook DJ, Sibbald WJ, Vincent JL, Cerra FB (1996) Evidence based critical care medicine: What is it and what can it do for us? Crit Care Med 24:334-337
2. Kunz R, Oxman AD (1998) The unpredictability paradox: review of empirical comparisons of randomised and non-randomised clinical trials. Br Med J 317:1185-1190
3. Vincent JL (1999) Which therapeutic interventions in critical care medicine have been shown to reduce mortality in prospective, randomized, clinical trials? A survey of candidates for the Belgian Board Examination in Intensive Care Medicine. Crit Care Med (in press)
4. Black N (1996) Why we need observational studies to evaluate the effectiveness of health care. Br Med J 312:1215-1218
5. Reinhart K, Wiegand-Lohnert C, Grimminger F et al (1996) Assessment of the safety and efficacy of the monoclonal anti-tumor necrosis factor antibody-fragment, MAK 195F, in patients with sepsis and septic shock: a multicenter, randomized, placebo-controlled, dose-ranging study [see comments] [published erratum appears in Crit Care Med 1996 Sep;24(9):1608]. Crit Care Med 24:733-742
6. Baudo F, Caimi TM, de Cataldo F, et al (1998) Antithrombin III (ATIII) replacement therapy in patients with sepsis and/or postsurgical complications: a controlled double-blind, randomized, multicenter study [see comments]. Intensive Care Med 24:336-342
7. Anonymous (1992) American College of Chest Physicians/Society of Critical Care Medicine Consensus Conference: definitions for sepsis and organ failure and guidelines for the use of innovative therapies in sepsis. Crit Care Med 20:864-874
8. Bossink AW, Groeneveld J, Hack CE, Thijs LG (1998) Prediction of mortality in febrile medical patients: How useful are systemic inflammatory response syndrome and sepsis criteria? Chest 113:1533-1541
9. McKee M, Britton A, Black N et al (1999) Methods in health services research. Interpreting the evidence: choosing between randomised and non-randomised studies. BMJ 319:312-315
10. Sackett DL, Rosenberg WM (1995) The need for evidence-based medicine. J R Soc Med 88:620-624
11. Anonymous (1992) Evidence-based medicine. A new approach to teaching the practice of medicine. Evidence-Based Medicine Working Group. JAMA 268:2420-2425
12. Sackett DL, Rosenberg WM, Gray JA et al (1996) Evidence based medicine: what it is and what it isn't [editorial]. BMJ 312:71-72
13. Cook DJ, Guyatt GH, Laupacis A, Sackett DL (1992) Rules of evidence and clinical recommendations on the use of antithrombotic agents. Chest 102:305S-311S
14. Cook DJ (1995) Clinical trials in the treatment of sepsis: An evidence-based approach. In: Sibbald WJ, Vincent JL (eds) Clinical trials for the treatment of sepsis. Springer, Heidelberg, pp XIX-XXXI
15. Amato MB, Barbas CS, Medeiros DM et al (1998) Effect of a protective-ventilation strategy on mortality in the acute respiratory distress syndrome. N Engl J Med 338:347-354
16. Moore EE, Jones TN (1986) Benefits of immediate jejunostomy feeding after major abdominal trauma - A prospective, randomized study. J Trauma 26:874-881
17. Moore FA, Moore EE, Jones TN et al (1989) TEN versus TPN following major abdominal trauma - Reduced septic morbidity. J Trauma 29:916-922
18. Moore EE, Moore FA (1991) Immediate enteral nutrition following multisystem trauma: a decade perspective. J Am Coll Nutr 10:633-648
19. Kudsk KA, Croce MA, Fabian TC et al (1992) Enteral versus parenteral feeding. Effects on septic morbidity after blunt and penetrating abdominal trauma. Ann Surg 215:503-511
20. Shoemaker WC, Appel PL, Kram HB et al (1988) Prospective trial of supranormal values of survivors as therapeutic goals in high-risk surgical patients. Chest 94:1176-1186
21. Shoemaker WC, Appel PL, Kram HB (1992) Role of oxygen debt in the development of organ failure sepsis, and death in high-risk surgical patients. Chest 102:208-215
22. Fleming A, Bishop M, Shoemaker W et al (1992) Prospective trial of supranormal values as goals of resuscitation in severe trauma. Arch Surg 127:1175-1179

23. Boyd O, Grounds RM, Bennett ED (1993) A randomized clinical trial of the effect of deliberate perioperative increase of oxygen delivery on mortality in high-risk surgical patients. JAMA 270:2699-2707

24. Yu M, Levy MM, Smith P et al (1993) Effect of maximizing oxygen delivery on morbidity and mortality rates in critically ill patients: a prospective, randomized, controlled study. Crit Care Med 21:830-838

25. Hayes MA, Timmins AC, Yau EH et al (1994) Elevation of systemic oxygen delivery in the treatment of critically ill patients. N Engl J Med 330:1717-1722

26. Gattinoni L, Brazzi L, Pelosi P et al (1995) A trial of goal-oriented hemodynamic therapy in critically ill patients. SvO$_2$ Collaborative Group. N Engl J Med 333:1025-1032

27. Bishop MH, Shoemaker WC, Appel PL et al (1995) Prospective, randomized trial of survivor values of cardiac index, oxygen delivery, and oxygen consumption as resuscitation endpoints in severe trauma. J Trauma 38:780-787

28. Keays R, Harrison PM, Wendon JA et al (1991) Intravenous acetylcysteine in paracetamol induced fulminant hepatic failure: a prospective controlled trial. BMJ 303:1026-1029

29. Jepsen S, Herlevsen P, Knudsen P et al (1992) Antioxidant treatment with N-acetylcysteine during adult respiratory distress syndrome: a prospective, randomized, placebo-controlled study. Crit Care Med 20:918-923

30. Suter PM, Domenighetti G, Schaller MD et al (1994) N-acetylcysteine enhances recovery from acute lung injury in man. A randomized, double-blind, placebo-controlled clinical study. Chest 105:190-194

31. Domenighetti G, Suter PM, Schaller MD et al (1997) Treatment with N-acetylcysteine during acute respiratory distress syndrome: a randomized, double-blind, placebo-controlled clinical study. J Crit Care 12:177-182

32. Bernard GR, Wheeler AP, Arons MM et al (1997) A trial of antioxidants N-acetylcysteine and procysteine in ARDS. The Antioxidant in ARDS Study Group. Chest 112:164-172

33. Bott J, Carroll MP, Conway JH et al (1993) Randomised controlled trial of nasal ventilation in acute ventilatory failure due to chronic obstructive airways disease [see comments]. Lancet 341:1555-1557

34. Brochard L, Mancebo J, Wysocki M et al (1995) Noninvasive ventilation for acute exacerbations of chronic obstructive pulmonary disease. N Engl J Med 333:817-822

35. Kramer N, Meyer TJ, Meharg J et al (1995) Randomized, prospective trial of noninvasive positive pressure ventilation in acute respiratory failure. Am J Respir Crit Care Med 151:1799-1806

36. Wysocki M, Tric L, Wolff MA et al (1995) Noninvasive pressure support ventilation in patients with acute respiratory failure. A randomized comparison with conventional therapy. Chest 107:761-768

37. Wedzicha JA (1996) Non-invasive ventilation for exacerbations of respiratory failure in chronic obstructive pulmonary disease. Thorax 51[Suppl 2]:S35-S39

38. Wood KA, Lewis L, Von Harz B, Kollef MH (1998) The use of noninvasive positive pressure ventilation in the emergency department: results of a randomized clinical trial. Chest 113:1339-1346

39. Clifton GL, Allen S, Barrodale P et al (1993) A phase II study of moderate hypothermia in severe brain injury. J Neurotrauma 10:263-271

40. Marion DW, Penrod LE, Kelsey SF et al (1997) Treatment of traumatic brain injury with moderate hypothermia. N Engl J Med 336:540-546

41. Bracken MB, Shepard MJ, Collins WF et al (1990) A randomized, controlled trial of methylprednisolone or naloxone in the treatment of acute spinal-cord injury. Results of the Second National Acute Spinal Cord Injury Study. N Engl J Med 322:1405-1411

42. Bracken MB, Shepard MJ, Holford TR et al (1997) Administration of methylprednisolone for 24 or 48 hours or tirilazad mesylate for 48 hours in the treatment of acute spinal cord injury. Results of the Third National Acute Spinal Cord Injury Randomized Controlled Trial. National Acute Spinal Cord Injury Study. JAMA 277:1597-1604

The Performance of an ICU

G.J. Dobb

Intensive Care Units (ICUs) are extremely complex organisations with multiple internal and external functions. The focus in the assessment of ICU performance has, appropriately, been on external performance as indicated by patient outcome. However, many aspects of a unit's function contribute to the overall external perception of its performance. Some of these, listed in Table 1, can be considered as measures of "internal" performance or non-clinical performance but there is evidence that they play a major part in determining the "external" or clinical performance of the unit. Comparisons between ICUs show the organisation of intensive care affects patient outcome [1-3] and that within a single unit changes in organisation affect the unit's performance [4, 5].

The concept of "performance" is also complex but includes elements of:
- effectiveness - the effect of care on mortality and health;
- efficiency - the effect per unit of cost;
- satisfaction - acceptability to patients, their relatives, and staff, including the ability to meet external demand.

Internal performance

A unit's external "reputation" is greatly affected by aspects of its internal performance. In part this is because information on clinical performance is often regarded as confidential, but also internal performance is usually evident to the healthcare workers within the unit who change jobs and roles to create referral patterns that ultimately affect workload and case mix.

The criteria listed in Table 1 are internally rather than "customer" orientated, even though the education, research and administrative work of an ICU produces useful external results. Most organisations accept that their staff are their most important asset. This is especially true in intensive care which needs skilled nurses and other staff working closely together in a team environment to optimise care delivery. Staff who demonstrate a clear understanding and competence with the equipment they are using foster patients' and their relatives' confidence and trust [6].

Table 1. "Internal" performance criteria

Staff related:
– staff satisfaction
– staff turnover
– staff appraisal (if benchmarked against external criteria)
Teaching/education:
– participation rates in teaching sessions
– success of staff in external examinations
– student satisfaction/performance assessment
Research:
– publications
– postgraduate students/research fellow numbers
– participation in multicentre clinical trials
– presentations at scientific meetings
– award of competition grants
– participation in medical journals, grant review boards, etc.
Administration:
– participation in hospital/system administration
– timeliness and completeness of compliance with reporting standards
– compliance with admission and discharge criteria
Quality improvement:
– outcome of performance audits
– critical incident reporting
– equipment servicing and fault recognition
– peer review processes
– compliance with unit guidelines

Clinical audit has been defined as, "A systematic critical analysis of the quality of medical care, including procedures used in diagnosis and treatment, use of resources and the resulting outcome for the patient" [7]. It can address any aspect of patient care including the nursing and paramedical services with a process of information collecting and evaluation being used to identify deficiencies against defined criteria [8]. Correction of deficiencies can then be assessed by repetition of the audit to determine if performance has improved.

Critical incident reporting provides a means of identifying recurrent problems in intensive care and improving patient safety [9]. For example, a review of 3600 reported incidents suggests that inadequate nurse staffing precipitates more incidents and compromises performance [10].

External performance

The primary focus of external performance by ICUs has been on patient mortality, usually expressed as a standardised mortality ratio (SMR) derived from comparison with published datasets and "corrected" for differences in illness severity and (sometimes) case mix. This information is being published in publicly available "league tables" of hospital and ICU performance [11] and the SMR has been recommended as the basis for identifying high performance ICUs [12]. The validity of this approach has been challenged and, at least in neonatal intensive care [13], mortality and risk adjusted mortality do not appear to be reliable indicators of hospital performance or best practice.

Standardised mortality as a performance indicator

It is obvious that ICU mortality varies with the severity of illness of patients admitted, and also to some extent with case mix. The systems used include APACHE II [14], APACHE III [15], SAPS II [16] and MPM II [17], of which APACHE II is the most widely used and most commonly cited general purpose prediction model for adults. PRISM [18] and PIM [19] are similar systems designed for use in children. Other systems have been developed for patients with traumatic injuries – ISS [20] and TRISS [21] – as a group in which the general purpose prediction models perform poorly, and also for many other groups of critically ill patients within specific disease categories e.g. cardiothoracic surgery, pancreatitis, liver failure in which APACHE II, for example, performs reasonably well in some studies.

Nevertheless, the general purpose prediction models are relatively crude measures and, in particular, the SMR is influenced by many factors (Table 2). Recommendations have been put forward to minimise the effects of lead time bias, deal with multiple admissions and to standardise the time point for assessment of mortality at 90 days after the first major ICU admission [12], but mortality remains a very crude measure of performance, or even the overall effectiveness of intensive care delivery. If used as a "performance indicator" the SMR should be stated with its confidence limits and interpreted with care and insight.

Table 2. Factors influencing standardised mortality ratios for intensive care

Variation in data definition between units
Variation in data collection
The mortality prediction model used
Variations in case mix
Bias from delayed ICU admissions ("lead time" bias)
Source of patient admission
Care after ICU discharge if hospital mortality is used
ICU discharge policy if ICU mortality is used
The distribution of illness severity scores

Other measures of the effectiveness of intensive care

Intensive care or hospital mortality can indicate the short term effectiveness of intensive care, but additional information is provided by longer term follow up i.e. 6 months or one year, and assessment of quality of life at these times. Although there is increased interest in later outcomes from intensive care, little information exists on the interaction between late outcome and quality of life and the shorter term mortality for a unit. Overall, quality of life assessments are reported infrequently in the ICU literature and are of limited methodological quality [22]. Comparisons between units have not been made, perhaps because of the difficulty in separating the effects of the underlying disease from those of the performance of intensive care. The instruments available include the Health Status Questionnaire of the self administered Medical Outcomes Study Short Form Survey (SF-36), the Nottingham Health Profile, and the Perceived Quality Of Life scale. The acceptability, validity and reliability of the SF-36 in adult patients after discharge from an ICU were all found to be satisfactory though it is time consuming to administer [23], and a questionnaire designed specifically for critically ill patients [24] also has acceptable validity and reproducibility in this patient population. Quality of life six months after intensive care varies with the underlying diagnosis, rather than age or the severity of illness [25]. Patients admitted with an acute illness generally have decreased quality of life but patients admitted with pre-existing ill health, particularly those in whom this was surgically corrected, report significant improvement [26]. Overall, however, patients who have been admitted to intensive care have a lesser quality of life at six months than the general population [26, 27], though even after surviving acute respiratory distress syndrome [28] or combined multiple organ failure and renal failure [29] the quality of life is perceived as good or acceptable. Impairments in the mental health domains of the SF-36 may be related to traumatic experiences during intensive care [28], suggesting an area in which ICU performance needs to be assessed in greater detail.

End points other than mortality may provide more sensitive measures of intensive care effectiveness. These might include the development of additional organ failures, complications of procedures, nosocomial infection rates and duration of ICU stay and ICU readmission rates. All of these will also be influenced by case mix and illness severity, but could be used as performance indicators. Little published information is available on the correlation between these measures and other measures of ICU performance. In Australia the frequency of pneumothorax after central vein catheterisation, accidental extubation and ICU readmission have been adopted as national "clinical indicators". In a surgical setting morbidity does appear to be related to other assessments of the process of healthcare delivery [30] including the technical competence of staff, relationship to other services, co-ordination of work and monitoring of the quality of care.

Readmission rates to ICU are easy to measure. The Society of Critical Care Medicine's Quality Indicators Committee ranked readmission to ICU within 48 hours as the best indicator of ICU quality [31] but the evidence supporting this is slight. Patients readmitted to the ICU have worse outcomes [32, 33] but it has not been shown that keeping these patients in the ICU for longer would have altered their outcome [31]. As with other performance indicators for intensive care, the readmission rate is affected by case mix [33], but is also affected by factors that are poorly corrected for by ICU scoring systems such as alcohol dependence [34] and by the availability of high dependency care [35]. It is therefore not surprising that ICU readmission rates correlate poorly with other ICU performance indicators [32].

Efficiency of intensive care

Recent emphasis on ICU costs has resulted in economic evaluations being part of the assessment of most innovative treatments in intensive care [36]. However, precise tracking of costs for intensive care is complex and studies have used such different methods for allocation of capital overhead and indirect costs that comparisons are virtually impossible [37]. An alternative method of measuring resource use [38] derives a Resource Use Performance Index (RUPI) calculated from a regression equation for hospital length of stay with a greater weighting for ICU days than those on the hospital ward, but this approach and the associated plotting of RUPI against clinical performance has not been assessed outside the United States and practice patterns differ in other settings.

The Therapeutic Intervention Scoring System (TISS) was also developed in the United States but has been both simplified and assessed in other settings [39]. A preliminary study reports a correlation between daily TISS score and ICU costs for days after the first [40] – the first day costs were approximately 50% greater than subsequent days – but the same group has suggested the association not sufficiently robust to assess individual patients in the ICU, particularly for high cost patient days [41].

More detailed information collected by computerised clinical information systems should provide more precise estimates of individual patient costs to assist in describing the efficiency of intensive care. Commercial hospital organisations are already using this information to benchmark ICU performance efficiency between different facilities. In the public sector the greatest emphasis has been on compliance with budget targets as a measure of ICU and clinical manager performance.

Satisfaction with intensive care

"Consumer" satisfaction is an important performance indicator for most organisations. Many ICU patients are unable to express their satisfaction with the services provided and later assessment by questionnaire can be misleading because so many have incomplete or no memory of their stay. Pain [42, 43], noise [43-45], loss of privacy, the ICU environment, complications of treatment, communication [43] and emotional support received from staff may all contribute to patient satisfaction but benchmarks against which to judge whether performance is acceptable are completely absent. The Intensive Care Unit Environmental Stressor Scale [43] needs further validation but provides a potentially useful approach.

Other ICU "consumers" include the patients' relatives, referring physicians and surgeons and the staff, many of whom will rotate from other areas of the hospital. Working in an ICU is stressful for the staff and this may reduce job satisfaction [46]. Interestingly, while factors related to organisational structure and process improved staff satisfaction, a study in 25 critical care units [47] found no significant association with severity adjusted patient mortality, though this may reflect the limitations of severity adjustment models for between unit comparisons. In another study [48] that compared the effects of change from an open to a closed ICU organisation both staff satisfaction and clinical outcomes were improved.

Improving ICU performance

General guidelines in improving ICU performance have been published by the European Society of Intensive Care Medicine [49]. Performance may be improved through changes in the organisational structure or the process of intensive care. The process of intensive care includes the timeliness of service delivery, access to intensive care, the appropriateness of interventions and treatments, the frequency of adverse events and the response to adverse events. Process performance is assessed by comparison of actual performance against "best practice" or clinical practice guidelines. After identifying problems, solutions must be developed and introduced into ICU practice for patients to benefit. In the jargon of quality improvement this is the "Plan-Do-Study-Act" cycle [50]. There is some evidence that this approach can improve ICU performance, for example, by reducing the frequency of nosocomial lower respiratory infections in mechanically ventilated patients [51]. Overall, however, its impact on the performance of healthcare professionals and patient outcome in many different settings has been disappointing [52]. Audit, the assessment of its findings and the implementation of findings are time and resource intensive but without the "Study" and "Act" components performance improvement will be suboptimal.

Conclusion

"ICU performance" is difficult to define. Like good wine, it is easier to recognise than quantitate. The whole is greater than the sum of the parts for it requires all those working in an ICU to work well as a team and integrate with all other hospital services to provide optimum service delivery in all aspects. Excellent ICU performance includes rapid admission of the right patients, efficient and caring treatment to best practice standards and expeditious discharge to ongoing care. Quality staff, good interpersonal relationships and close communication are prerequisites which will be enhanced by active commitment to continually improving ICU performance.

References

1. Kanus WA, Wagner DP, Zimmerman JE et al (1993) Variations in mortality and length of stay in intensive care units. Ann Int Med 111:753-761
2. Miranda DR, Ryan DW, Schaufeli WB et al (eds) (1998) Organisation and management of intensive care: a prospective study in 12 European countries. Springer, Berlin
3. Pronovost PJ, Jenckes MW, Dorman T et al (1999) Organisational characteristics of intensive care units related to outcomes of abdominal surgery. JAMA 281:1310-1317
4. Hanson CW, Deutschman CS, Anderson HL et al (1999) Effects of an organised critical care service on outcomes and resource utilisation: a cohort study. Crit Care Med 27:270-274
5. Kern H, Kox WJ (in press) Impact of standard procedures and clinical standards on cost- effectiveness and intensive care unit performance in adult patients after cardiac surgery. Intensive Care Med
6. Stroud R (1997) Kreuzer Award 1997. The effects of technology on relatives in critical care environments. Nurs Crit Care 2:272-275
7. Department of Health, UK (1989) Working for patients (White Paper). London HMSO
8. Shaw CD (1990) Criterion based audit. BMJ 300:649-651
9. Beckmann U, Baldwin I, Hart GK et al (1996) The Australian incident monitoring study in intensive care: HIMS-ICU. An analysis of the first year of reporting. Anaesth Intens Care 24:320-329
10. Beckman U, Baldwin I, Durie M et al (1998) Problems associated with nursing staff shortage: an analysis of the first 3600 incident reports submitted to the Australian incident monitoring study (AIMS-ICU). Anaesth Intens Care 26:396-400
11. Linde-Zwirble WT, Angus DC (1998) Can scoring systems assess ICU performance? J Intensive Care Med 13:155-157
12. Teres D, Higgins T, Steingrub J et al (1998) Defining a high performance ICU system for the 21st century: a position paper. J Intensive Care Med 13:195-205
13. Parry GJ, Gould CR, McCabe CJ et al (1998) Annual league tables of mortality in neonatal intensive care units: longitudinal study. BMJ 316:1931-1935
14. Knaus WA, Draper EA, Wagner DP et al (1985) APACHE II: a severity of disease classification system. Crit Care Med 13:818-828
15. Knaus WA, Wagner DP, Draper EA et al (1991) The APACHE III prognostic system: risk prediction of hospital mortality for critically ill hospitalised adults. Chest 100:1619-1636
16. Le Gall JR, Lemeshow S, Saulnier F (1993) A new simplified acute physiology score (SAPS II) based on a European/North American multicenter study. JAMA 270:2957-2963
17. Lemeshow S, Teres D, Klar J et al (1993) Mortality prediction models (MPM II) based on an international cohort of intensive care unit patients. JAMA 270:2478-2486

18. Pollack MM, Ruttimann UE, Getson PR (1988) Pediatric risk of mortality (PRISM) score. Crit Care Med 16:1110-1116
19. Shann F, Pearson G, Slater A et al (1997) Paediatric index of mortality (PIM): a mortality prediction model for children in intensive care. Intensive Care Med 23:201-207
20. Baker SP, O'Neil B, Haddon W (1974) The injury severity score: a method for describing patients with multiple injuries and evaluating emergency care. J Trauma 14:187-196
21. Boyd CR, Tolson MA, Copes WS (1987) Evaluating trauma care: the TRISS methods. J Trauma 27:370-378
22. Heyland DK, Guyatt G, Cork DJ et al (1998) Frequency and methodologic quality of quality-of-life assessments in the critical care literature. Crit Care Med 26:591-598
23. Chrispin PS, Scotton H, Rogers J et al (1997) Short Form 36 in the intensive care unit: assessment of acceptability, reliability and validity of the questionnaire. Anaesthesia 52:15-23
24. Fernandez RR, Cruz JJ, Mata GV (1996) Validation of a quality of life questionnaire for critically ill patients. Intensive Care Med 22:1034-1042
25. Hurel D, Loirat P, Saulnier F et al (1997) Quality of life 6 months after intensive care: results of a prospective multicenter study using a generic health status scale and a satisfaction scale. Intensive Care Med 23:331-337
26. Ridley SA, Chrispin PS, Scotton H et al (1997) Changes in quality of life after intensive care: comparison with normal data. Anaesthesia 53:195-202
27. Brooks R, Kerridge R, Hillman K et al (1997) Quality of life outcomes after intensive care. Comparison with a community group. Intensive Care Med 23:581-586
28. Schelling G, Stoll C, Haller M et al (1998) Health related quality of life and post traumatic stress disorder in survivors of the acute respiratory distress syndrome. Crit Care Med 26: 651-659
29. Gopal I, Bhonagiri S, Ronco C et al (1997) Out of hospital outcome and quality of life in survivors of combined acute multiple organ and renal failure treated with continuous veno venous hemofiltration/hemodiafiltration. Intensive Care Med 23:766-772
30. Daly J, Forbes MG, Young GJ et al (1997) Validating risk adjusted surgical outcomes: site visit assessment of process and structure. National VA Surgical Risk Study. J Am Coll Surg 185:341-351
31. Angus DC (1998) Grappling with intensive care unit quality - does the readmission rate tell us anything? Crit Care Med 26:1779-1780
32. Cooper GS, Sirio CA, Rotondi AJ et al (1999) Are readmissions to the intensive care unit a useful measure of hospital performance? Medical Care 37:399-408
33. Chen LM, Martin CM, Keenan SP et al (1998) Patients readmitted to the intensive care unit during the same hospitalisation: clinical features and outcomes. Crit Care Med 26:1834-1841
34. Maxson PM, Schultz KL, Berge KH et al (1999) Probable alcohol abuse or dependence: a risk factor for intensive care readmission in patients undergoing elective vascular and thoracic surgical procedures. Mayo Clin Proc 74:448-453
35. Fox AJ, Owen-Smith O, Spiers P (1999) The immediate impact of opening an adult high dependency unit on intensive care occupancy. Anaesthesia 54:280-283
36. Rubenfeld GD (1998) Cost effectiveness considerations in critical care. New Horizons 6: 33-40
37. Elliott D (1997) Costing intensive care services: a review of study methods, results and limitations. Aust Crit Care 10:55-63
38. Rapoport J, Teres D, Lemeshow S et al (1994) A method for assessing the clinical performance and cost effectiveness of intensive care units: a multicenter inception cohort study. Crit Care Med 22:1385-1391
39. Miranda DR, Rijk A, Schau Feli W (1996) Simplified therapeutic intervention scoring system: the TISS – 28 items – results from a multicenter study. Crit Care Med 24:64
40. Edbrooke DL, Stevens VG, Hibbert CL et al (1996) A new method of accurately identifying costs of individual patients in intensive care: the initial results. Intensive Care Med 23:645-650

41. Mills GH, Hibbert CL, Edbrooke DL (1998) Can TISS be used to accurately reflect the daily costs of care for individual patients in the intensive care unit? Intensive Care Med 24[Suppl 1]:S59

42. Carroll KC, Atkins PJ, Herold GR et al (1999) Pain assessment and management in critically ill postoperative and trauma patients: a multisite study. Am J Crit Care 8:105-107

43. Novaes MA, Aronovich A, Ferraz MB et al (1997) Stressors in ICU: patients' evaluation. Intensive Care Med 22:1282-1285

44. Tsiou C, Eftymiatos D, Theodossopoulou E et al (1998) Noise sources and levels in the Evgenidion Hospital intensive care unit. Intensive Care Med 24:845-847

45. Moore MM, Nguyen D, Nolan SP et al (1998) Interventions to reduce decibel levels in patient care units. Am Surgeon 64:894-899

46. Goodfellow A, Varnam R, Rees D et al (1997) Staff stress in the intensive care unit: a comparison of doctors and nurses. Anaesthesia 52:1037-1041

47. Mitchell PH, Shannon SE, Cain KC et al (1996) Critical care outcomes: linking structures, processes and organisational and clinical outcomes. Am J Crit Care 5:353-363

48. Carson SS, Stocking C, Podsadecki T et al (1996) Effects of organisational change in the medical intensive care unit of a teaching hospital: a comparison of "open" and "closed" formats. JAMA 276:322-328

49. Thijs LG, Members of the Task Force European Society of Intensive Care Medicine (1997) Continuous quality improvement in the ICUs' general guidelines. Intensive Care Med 23: 125-127

50. Berwick DM (1998) Developing and testing changes in delivery of care. Ann Intern Med 128: 651-656

51. Joiner GA, Salisburg D, Bollin GE (1996) Utilising quality assurance as a tool for reducing the risk of nosocomial ventilator associated pneumonia. Am J Med Qual 11:100-103

52. Thomson MA, Oxman AD, Davis DA et al (1998) Audit and feedback to improve professional practice and healthcare outcomes (Parts I and II). In: Bero L, Grilli R, Grimshaw J, Oxman A (eds) Collaboration on effective professional practice module of the Cochrane database of systematic reviews. Cochrane Library (database on disk and CD-ROM) Issue 1. The Cochrane Collaboration. Update Software, Oxford

Care of Dying Patients in ICU

M. FISHER

After the Second World War there was a tremendous expansion of therapeutic options, especially in relation to the support of ventilation and circulation. This technology changed the medical profession to the point where death was considered a failure and the traditional medical skills in dealing with death and dying were lost.

Subsequently changes in society's expectations and a relative disenchantment with technology have fostered a desire to make the intensive care environment more humane, particularly by avoiding inappropriate life support which prolongs dying in the absence of a reasonable expectation of a return to a level of function acceptable to the patient.

The fundamental goals have been summarized by G.R. Dunstan who stated [1]: "The success of intensive care is not... to be measured only by the statistics of survival, as though each death were a medical failure. It is to be measured by the quality of lives preserved or restored, the quality of the dying and by the quality of relationships involved in each death".

Principles
Alternative treatment versus withdrawal of care

Perhaps the worst statement a doctor can make to a patient or relative is that nothing more can be done. Reaching a point where cure is impossible should lead to a different form of care in which the goals are alleviation of suffering, provision of a quiet and dignified environment, and encouragement of patient and family to communicate, touch and deal with "unfinished business". In these circumstances the focus of treatment shifts. Caring for the family unit as a whole assumes a high priority.

Attention is paid to the removal of unnecessary equipment which may impair the patient's appearance, to the provision of unrestricted visiting, to the elimination of unnecessary procedures or investigations (particularly those which may cause discomfort), and to determination and fulfillment of the needs of the group collectively and individually. Unnecessary drugs are withdrawn and analgesia optimized.

The ICU as an environment for palliative care

Good management of death and dying produces feelings of a job well done rather than failure, and produces the benefits of realistic expectations, better interpersonal relationships, and consequently improved teamwork. The rewards to the clinician provided by a well managed death may be as great as those provided by a cure.

Patients admitted to an intensive care unit and their relatives seek a "job description" or a behaviour pattern with which they are comfortable. This behaviour pattern is established from observation of the activity that occurs in the unit. The manner in which staff interact with each other and with the patient is crucial. An atmosphere of quiet competence and efficiency engenders confidence in relatives whereas interpersonal hostility, noise and drama provoke anxiety and hostility.

It is helpful to humanize the intensive care area. Noise reduction, windows with a view, pictures and privacy all assist to provide contrast to the technology. Provision of personal items such as picture, books or toys ameliorate the technological hostility of the environment. Giving patients clothing where possible, rather than hospital gowns or nursing them naked is a major step in restoring dignity.

If the relationship between the staff and the family unit has been of sufficient quality since admission. We believe it is of benefit to both parties to keep the patient in the unit, although the ICU is a limited resource and it may become necessary to transfer the patient. If that is necessary contact with the family and patient should be maintained.

Communication

There should be honest communication with the patient (when possible) and family from the day of admission. There is a benefit in minimising the number of communicators since minor differences in explanations are often magnified in the minds of relatives, providing an impression of discord and disagreement. Attention should be given the needs of relatives. We believe it is very important for clinicians to provide leadership and direction in the introduction of discussions regarding choices or alternative forms of care. Since physicians have a considerable ability to influence the attitudes and decisions of patients and families in this regard [2], they have a responsibility to exercise this power with care.

Practical application of ethical principles

The decision to withdraw treatment does not occur at a single moment but evolves as determined by events. Involvement of clinicians and family is a progressive undertaking in the course of the patient's illness.

Medical consensus

The first item to be established is medical consensus that active, supportive treatment is no longer warranted. This requires accurate diagnosis and a consideration of the data relating to outcome and quality of life. In the absence of such consensus, active treatment is often continued, but with some limitations. A further time period of active treatment and subsequent review are organised.

Medical and nursing consensus

The nursing staff who will be the continuing providers of bedside care to patient and family should be involved early. Efforts should be made to contact any nurse who has shown particular interest in the patient and family, or expended considerable energy in the patient's care. Sternburg [3] emphasises the importance of nursing participation in the decision making process, noting the frustration experienced by nurses required to participate in care they may feel is inappropriate. The importance of group involvement is two fold: individual bias may be balanced, and support for the major participants enlisted.

Establishment of person to be involved in discussions

If the patient is competent, rational, and reasonably cognisant of the disease process, therapeutic options and prognosis should be discussed with the patient. Fear, pain, stress and psychological disturbances must considered and minimised. Critically ill patients are rarely competent and so surrogates, usually family members, are involved in discussions. Rapin [4] notes the difficulties that may arise when families become involved in the decision making process, emphasising unrealistic demands and suggests the family should not make decisions as to the treatment in borderline cases, but that the views of the family unit should figure in the physician's calculations in choosing an optimal therapeutic course. What data exists suggests that surrogates often have little insight into the patient's wishes.

Establishment of resource person

The person holding discussions with either the patient or family must be someone significantly involved in the active care of the patient. Trust and credibility is earned by being involved in bedside care and communicating early. To avoid apparent conflict of opinions a single resource person is preferable.

Consensus with patient or relatives

We seek agreement on a medical management plan, and never permission to change and withdraw treatment. This is the approach the majority of people want. Discussion with overseas colleagues suggest that in most societies outside the USA it is rare for relatives to wish to bear the burden of decision making, but wish to participate in the process. Making decisions which lead to the inevitable death of a loved one, constitutes apparently, an unwelcome burden. The relatives and/or patient are given ime to consider this proposal and seek other advice. If agreement is not reached a discussion at a later date is arranged, supportive therapy continues, and the inappropriateness of further intervention should be established. If agreement is reached the decision is fully documented in the records, and an effort made to fill the needs of patients and relatives in terms of emotional, social and spiritual aspects. The hospital corridor is a poor place to communicate. Relatives are encouraged to ask questions and express feelings and reassured that they are not required to behave in a manner which is uncomfortable for them.

A management plan is activated

Artificial forms of life support are maintained until the patient and relatives have had time together. It is important that the resource person regularly visit the patient and relatives at the bedside. Pastoral and social workers should be available, if desired. When the physician is comfortable that the patient, relatives and staff have had sufficient time to accept the irreversability of death, and the patient is painfree, supportive therapy may be withdrawn preferably in a gentle manner. In most cases removal of inotropic agents or reduction of inspired oxygen concentration will lead to death over a period of time. Formal disconnection of patients from ventilators is more likely to be followed by rapid demise. Patients who are to be disconnected from artificial ventilation should be sedated rather than permitted to experience discomfort and acute breathlessness. We discourage patients who wish to be disconnected from artificial ventilation while awake and unsedated, as this causes more distress to the patient, relatives and staff.

After death

The resource person should see the relatives after death and the family should be given the opportunity to contact the physician if problems related to the bereavement occur or unanswered questions become a problem.

Two common enquiries both before and after a death are whether small children should see the relative before and after death, and whether relatives should view the body after death. There is considerable opinion about the benefits of viewing the body after death which is not supported by data [5], and our attitude is to encourage the participants to decide for themselves, and to support this decision.

Dealing with death causes stress and suffering in those delivering care as well as in those who are receiving or observing the care. The key to managing staff problems is prevention by adequate support during and after the event by means of support ranging from a session at the local pub or with a skilled counsellor.

Conclusion

We believe that the concept of death as a medical failure is outdated and that there is a need for doctors to be more involved and aware of the process and the issues. These issues require urgent public debate. It may be that if funds for healthcare are to be reallocated to other Government departments the medical profession has a responsibility to ensure the money is spent on social necessities. As Berger [6] wrote "I do not know what a human life is worth. I only know that the question will not be answered by word, but in the active creation of a more humane environment".

Whenf a humane environment is created in the intensive care unit the problems regarding withdrawal of treatment may be dealt with by health care providers, patients and families in a sensible and beneficial manner without recourse to committees or courts. The major principle in establishing such an environment is the creation of trust between consumer and clinician. Early frank, open and realistic discussion between consumer and someone close to the patient. The preparedness of health care providers to discuss and undertake alternative treatment is essential in the prevention of an undignified "high technology death" and in the waste of resources.

References

1. Dunstan GR (1985) Hard questions in intensive care. Anaesthesia 40:479-482
2. Pelligrino ED (1992) Doctors must not kill. J Clin Ethics 3:95-102
3. Sternberg M (1988) The responsible powerless. Nurses and decisions about resuscitation. J Cardiovasc Nursing 3:47-56
4. Rapin M (1987) The ethics of intensive care. Int Care Med 13:300-303
5. Editorial (1988) Seeing the body after death. Brit Med J 297:999
6. Berger J (1964) A Fortunate Man. Allen Lane, London

Cost-Effectiveness in the ICU

D. REIS MIRANDA, M. JEGERS

A Medline search for cost-effectiveness in the ICU documents the importance attributed to the issue.

Some studies address the use of the facilities:

Senaratne et al. [1], for example, determined the feasibility and the cost-effectiveness of direct discharge from the coronary care unit (CCU) to their home, of 497 consecutive patients after acute myocardial infarction. The post-discharge course was evaluated six weeks later. In comparison to historical controls, the authors concluded that the new discharge strategy resulted in a cost saving of Cdn. $4,044.01 per patient. The design of this study was however rather inappropriate, and the comparison made with the historical group of patients cannot be accepted.

After a computerised computer search using the key words *intermediate care unit*, *respiratory care unit* and *step-down unit*, Keenan et al. [2] only found three studies that fulfilled their selection criteria. They concluded that: "To date, the evidence in the literature is insufficient to determine under which circumstances, if any, these units are a cost-effective alternative technology to the traditional institution with only ICU and general ward beds".

Other studies address therapeutic interventions:

With a prospective and randomised design, Raoof et al. [3] studied the effect of kinetic and mechanical percussion therapy (requiring the use of more expensive beds) in a group of mechanically ventilated patients with lung atelectasis, in comparison to another group of patients receiving manual repositioning and manual percussion. The resolution of the lung atelectasis was more effective and quicker in the first group, with clear impact on the clinical condition of the patients; several of the patients in the second group required bronchoscopy for recurring lung atelectasis. Although the authors knew the cost involved with the use of the special bed in the first group of patients, and calculated the cost of each bronchoscopy, they did not elaborate further on the cost-effectiveness of the studied intervention.

Barba et al. [4] studied, in 48 ICU patients randomly divided into two groups, the cost-effectiveness of percutaneous tracheotomy under bronchoscopic guidance versus standard tracheotomy. Without clinical and outcome differences between the two groups, the average saving related to the studied intervention amounted to US $3,335 per patient. These savings corresponded to costs otherwise incurred by the standard tracheotomy procedure (e.g., operating theatre, anaesthesia, etc.).

Finally, other studies address the use of new pieces of equipment:

Kollef et al. [5] studied the use of a hygroscopic condenser humidifier (HCH) versus heated water humidification (HWH), randomly applied to 147 patients requiring mechanical ventilation. At patient level, the experiment lasted for a maximum of seven days. A carefully selected set of clinical variables did not show significant differences between the two groups. The cost per patient of the HCH (US $16), however, was less than half of the cost of the HWH ($38).

Ceelen et al. [6] divided 29 patients after abdominal aortic aneurysm requiring surgical repair into a group receiving open surgical repair, and a group in which closed repair was performed by the endovascular introduction of a gelatin coated graft. The patients receiving the endovascular graft had: shorter operating time; no need for blood transfusion; shorter ICU stay; lower associated morbidity (e.g. pulmonary dysfunction, ileus, limb oedema). The calculated costs involved with both procedures, however, were not different: in the endovascular repair group, the money saved with the lower hospitalisation cost was consumed by the expensive gelatin coated graft.

All these (and comparable) studies only partially reflect the true underlying mechanisms explaining cost differences. A more comprehensive approach should consider the ICU as a social system in which several simultaneous processes take place. This point will be developed in the next section.

The system approach to health care

Health care is often appropriately approached as a social system. A system is usually a collection of interrelated work processes, activities and tasks, such that the collection and the interrelationships together avoid disorder [7]. From an economic point of view, a system is characterised by two major elements: the resources it consumes (its inputs); and the services or goods it produces (its outputs). In large organisations, such as health care organisations, the system can be divided into sub-systems. The reason for this is that sub-systems can be so different regarding the various elements in their structures that each sub-system should be considered a system "in its own right".

The ICU, for example, is one of the sub-systems of the hospital care system. Of course it is important for the successful functioning of the hospital system that the major organisational and work processes, activities and tasks in the ICU are interrelated in a purposeful manner with those of the other hospital sub-systems, such as anaesthesia, internal medicine, surgery, etc.

The various elements of the sub-system in the ICU are known and should be analysed into detail. Here we are usually not talking of sub-sub-systems, but of processes of care.

Processes are the throughput of systems, transforming the inputs into the outputs of the system. Looking in more detail, the interrelation of processes is usually such that the output of one process is the input of another process. A classical example could be the output/input liaison observed between operating theatre ↔ ICU ↔ ward ↔ home; another example could be: mechanical ventilation ↔ weaning ↔ rehabilitation. The important difference between these two examples is that the first relates to the input/output of a whole (sub)system, whereas the second concerns the output/input liaison of a particular set of interrelated processes within a given (sub)system.

Process of care is therefore the organisation of selected operations leading to a desired outcome of care. In the ICU, the processes of care are mainly related to the functioning of vital human organs and systems, the primary mission of each unit. The overall process of care in the ICU, assuring survival and health improvement, can therefore be divided into various sub-processes of care: e.g. respiratory, cardiovascular, renal, metabolic care, etc. Each of these sub-processes is, on its own, the purposeful organisation of selected operations expected to lead to a previously planned outcome. Respiratory support, for example, is composed by the operations of mechanical ventilation, sedation, physiotherapy, postural drainage, etc. Each of these operations can be further decomposed into tasks, such as choice of drug, preparation and insertion of infusion set, administration of drug, monitoring of effect, and titration of dosage in the case of sedation. As a matter of fact, some operations to consider can be very complex and are better approached as a sub-process of care (e.g. particular modes of mechanical ventilation requiring specific operations and tasks). Just as for processes, each operation, and each task, should have a defined mission and a measurable outcome.

The application of cost-effectiveness analysis (CEA) to health care, approached from a system perspective, is very useful indeed, as it allows the objective evaluation of the different elements of the system. What is important to remember here is that the CEA of a system, or any of its elements, relates to the process of transforming the input of the element under analysis into its respective output. If the output considered is equally influenced by any other process of transformation, this has necessarily to be included in the analysis. In the case of Ceelen et al. [6], the intervention performed in the operating theatre influenced the outcome in the ICU. The integration of both processes of care was not appropriately done, and the benefits of the intervention might have been grossly underestimated (the targeted outcomes of the intervention were not prospectively defined).

The cost

Simply put, cost-effectiveness analysis in the ICU is the evaluation of the cost of alternative courses of care aiming at the same effect. In order to compare the costs of the alternatives under analysis, it is necessary to carefully, and as exhaustively as possible, determine the cost of each of them. To be correctly performed, this operation of costing involves a detailed knowledge of the processes of care and the resources used.

The operation of costing will not be discussed in this chapter. It has to be said, however, that this operation, though laborious and time consuming, is certainly accessible to intensive care professionals. The important recommendation is that the design, and the development of the study, is performed with the collaboration of someone of the staff of the financial department of the hospital. The costing procedures are to be done regularly, but not continuously. In other words, once cost has been calculated, recalculation (other than simple annual checks) is required whenever the process of care changes, or whenever purchase prices change.

If the system approach to the ICU was applied, as indicated above, detailed identification of the various elements of each process of care will allow their cost to be calculated. It will be also noted that some of the identified elements are specific to a given process. Others, however, are common to several processes. The cost of each process is therefore the sum of the cost of the elements of care of which it is composed.

This methodology, however, is not often employed. The cost figures are quite often derived from administrative information such as hospital billing. It has been shown on several occasions, however, that this practice can provide very inaccurate results [8] as it is based on charges, however determined, and not on the value of the inputs consumed.

The Foundation for Research on Intensive Care in Europe (FRICE), has started a project in ICU's of 14 European countries (website at www.frice.nl). This project (EURICUS-III) aims at harmonising the budgeting and costing procedures in the ICUs of the countries of the European Union by the use of standard definitions and guidelines developed by the Department of Micro-economics for the Profit and Not for Profit Sectors of the Free University of Brussels (VUB), Belgium. The guidelines are incorporated in a very friendly software. The use of this software is readily integrated with a system approach to costing in the ICU.

The procedure of costing may have the objective of attributing "selling prices" (or costs to be refunded by external payers) to the various activities of the ICU. In this case, all costs should be considered [9]. More often, however, the costing procedures aim at supporting the comparison of alternative courses of care (e.g., CEA). In this case, only the costs directly related to the alternatives under comparison are relevant [9] and therefore the costs common to all alternatives considered can be ignored. Besides being more appropriate, this makes the procedure easy and accessible to the ICU staff, as it does not require them to get into rather more complex (and clearly specialist) reasoning and computation. Three of the studies indicated above [3-5] are classical examples of simple CEA aiming at the improvement of tasks and activities of processes of care in the ICU.

Effectiveness

Effectiveness concerns the evaluation of the outcomes of the interventions under analysis. To a certain extent, effectiveness is synonymous with performance (or carrying out a defined task).

In the medical literature a number of variables are inappropriately used as a measure of ICU effectiveness. One classical example concerns the use of standard mortality ratios (SMRs) for the evaluation of the effectiveness or performance of ICUs. Based upon methodology arguments, it is today clear that the regression of SMRs cannot be considered the gold standard of performance of ICUs [10].

In the last decade, health economists have become increasingly interested in intensive care. This is a very important and welcome development. Mutual understanding and collaboration between the relevant disciplines will improve the appropriate progress of health systems. Based on sound microeconomic theoretical grounds, the economists argue that the effectiveness of all medical interventions has to be evaluated in terms of the overall benefits to the society, whereas the measures available and applied cover some (smaller or larger) part of these benefits. Mortality 6 or 18 months after discharge, for example, has become a common end-measurement variable, but is probably one of the weakest benchmarks for evaluating the quality (effectiveness) of processes of care. Other benchmarks mentioned are for example life years gained, or the more comprehensive quality-adjusted life year (QALY) variable (which provokes a lot of fundamental discussion among professional economic researchers [11, 12]). These end-points are today the only standard accepted by many authors and journals, regardless of the subject addressed. In itself, the view is not wrong. It simply cannot be applied universally. Let us take the example of the GUSTO study [13] comparing two thrombolytic agents in the treatment of acute myocardial infarction. The study addresses the clear cycle of one cause, one sickness, one organ, leading to a high rate of physical and mental handicap, and to a high mortality rate; medication of the cause (by whichever element of the hospital care system) will have a direct and measurable effect upon outcome. In this case, late outcomes are appropriate. In the case of Selective Decontamination of the Digestive Tract (SDD), however, the choice of late outcomes for the evaluation of the effectiveness of the method is not appropriate: SDD eliminates and/or prevents the growth of aerobic gram-negative bacteria in the digestive tract; these bacteria are known to be only one of the causes of several infections; infection, on the

other hand, is one of the major causes of organ system failure, which often causes death in the ICU. The importance of the processes of care of the ICU system
in the care of infection ↔ organ failure ↔ death is undisputed. The analysis of
the (cost-)effectiveness of SDD should be performed at process of care level. Its
analysis at hospital care system level is irrelevant.

In managerial terms, an intervention is effective when the result coincides
with the outcome targeted for that particular intervention. It is cost-effective if it
will do so at the lowest possible cost.

References

1. Senaratne MPL, Irwin ME, Shaben S et al (1999) Feasibility of direct discharge from the
   coronary/intermediate care unit after acute myocardial infarction. J Am Coll Cardiol 33:
   1040-1046
2. Keenan SP, Massel D, Inman KJ et al (1998) A systematic review of the cost-effectiveness of
   noncardiac transitional care units. Chest 113:172-177
3. Raoof S, Chowdhrey N, Raoof S et al (1999) Effects of combined kinetic therapy and percussion therapy on the resolution of atelectasis in critically ill patients. Chest 115:1658-1666
4. Barba CA, Angood PB, Kauder DR et al (1995) Bronchoscopic guidance makes percutaneous
   tracheostomy a safe, cost-effective, and easy-to-teach procedure. Surgery 118:879-883
5. Kollef MH, Shapiro SD, Boyd V et al (1998) A randomized clinical trial comparing an ex-
   tended-use hygroscopic condenser humidifier with heated-water humidification in mechanically ventilated patients. Chest 113:759-767
6. Ceelen W, Sonneville T, Randon C et al (1999) Cost-benefit analysis of endovascular versus
   open abdominal aortic aneurysm treatment. Acta Chir Belg 99:64-67
7. Hitchins DK (1992) Putting systems to work. J Wiley and Sons, New York, Brisbane
8. Reis Miranda D, Gyldmark M (1996) Evaluation and understanding of costs in the intensive
   care unit. In: Ryan DW (ed) Current practice in critical illness. Chapman & Hall, pp 129-149
9. Jegers M, Reis Miranda D (1999) Resource management in the intensive care unit. In: Oxford
   Textbook of Critical Care, pp 1013-1017
10. Reis Miranda D, Moreno R (1997) Intensive care models and their role in management and
    utilization programs. Curr Opin Crit Care 3:183-187
11. Broome J (1993) QALYs. J Publ Econ 50:149-167
12. Johannesson M (1995) QALYs: a comment. J Publ Econ 56:327-328
13. Mark DB, Hlatky MA, Califf RM et al (1995) Cost-effectiveness of thrombolytic therapy
    with tissue plasminogen activator as compared with streptokinase for acute myocardial infarc-
    tion. N Engl J Med 332:1418-1424

INDEX

4-aminopyridine 229
abbreviated injury score 411
abdominal surgery 211
abruptio placentae 266
acute
   - lung 109
   - phase proteins 469
   - renal failure 477, 499, 501, 502, 507
   - respiratory distress syndrome 79, 102,
     109, 116, 525, 527
   - respiratory failure 121, 141
adrenalin/epinephrine 538
advanced cardiac life support 536
airflow limitation 139
airway
   - obstruction 139, 144
   - resistance 162
   end-expiratory - occlusion 149
Alzheimer's disease 377
amino acids 477
amniotic fluid embolism 266, 268
amrinone 260
amyotrophic lateral sclerosis 377
anaesthesia 192, 201, 225, 265
   spinal - 268
   fast-track - 201, 206, 219
anaesthetic agents 191
analgesia 205, 333
   epidural - 269
anaesthesiologist 215
anaesthetic care 214
angiography 256
anticoagulation 508
apnea 149
apolipoprotein E 377
apoptosis 370
apparatus deadspace 57
aprotinin 306
arrhythmia
   supraventricular - 286, 287
   ventricular - 286
arterial
   - dissection 303
   - gas embolism 303
arthroscopy 219
asthma 89
   bronchial - 140

astrocytes 362
atherosclerosis 401
atracurium 186, 519
atrio-ventricular septal defect 251
atropine sulphate 181
basic life support 535
beta blockers 311
bethanechol 183
bicarbonate 538
biochemistry 191
body plethysmograph 135
bone morphogenetic protein 349
bradykinin 304
brain 369
breathing
   - retraining 163
   - technique 163
bronchoalveolar lavage 80
bronchopulmonary dysplasia 276
bubble oxygenators 302
bupivacaine 217
caesarean section 265
calpain 370
cardiac
   - arrest 543
   - surgery 201, 301, 303
cardiopulmonary
   - bypass 251, 252, 301
   - resuscitation 535, 543
caspases 371
central anticholinergic syndrome 180, 226
central nervous system 350
   - muscarinic receptors 180
   - transmitters 180
central respiratory drive 162
cerebral edema 230
chain-of-survival 543
cholecystectomy 216
chronic
   - heart failure 142, 288
   - lung disease 275
   - obstructive pulmonary disease (COPD)
     133, 140, 161
circulatory arrest 255
cisatracurium 185
cobalamin 173

colonic ileus 212

coma 225

compliance 25

conduction disorders 287

congenital cardiopathies 252

consciousness 225

continuous renal replacement therapy 477

coronary
- care unit 573
- circulation 281

corticosteroids 523

cost-effectiveness 573

cuprophane 500

cycloergometer 144

cytokines 304, 503

death 225, 567

defibrillation 535, 538

dendritogenesis 378, 380

deoxythymidine 174

deoxyuridine 174

dexamethasone 525

diethylether 194

disease
Alzheimer's - 377
chronic lung - 275
chronic obstructive pulmonary - 133, 140, 161
Gaucher's - 379
Huntington's - 372
neuromuscular - 161
Niemann-Pick type C - 377, 379
Parkinson's - 183
restrictive pulmonary - 165

dobutamine 258

dopamine 258

Doppler echocardiography 256

dyspnea 133, 168

elastic
- recoil pressure 162
- workload 166

embolism
amniotic fluid - 266, 268
arterial gas - 303

emergency cardiac care 543

end-expiratory
- airway occlusion 149
- lung volume 140

endotracheal tube 272

endurance 165

enflurane 192, 194

epidural analgesia 269

epinephrine 259, 273

esmolol 312

ethanol 194

etomidate 205

expiratory
- flow limitation 133, 139
- reserve volume 142

extracellular matrix 362

extracorporeal circulation 301, 302

face mask 272

failure
acute renal - 477, 499, 501, 502, 507
acute respiratory - 121, 141
chronic heart - 142, 288
multiple organ - 477
neonatal respiratory - 271
organ system - 511

fast-track
- anaesthesia 201, 206, 219
- surgical procedures 216

fatigue 162

femur 221

fentanyl 217

flow
- limitation 133, 162
- volume 133

flumazenil 229

folinic acid 175

forced expiratory vital capacity 133

functional residual capacity (FRC) 163

GABA-receptor 173

γ-aminobutyric acid 194

gas exchange 162

Gaucher's disease 379

gene therapy 383

Glasgow Coma Scale 412

glossopharyngeal method 166

glucocorticoids 306

glutamate 370
- receptors 194

glutamine 444

glutathione 440

glycopyrronium 181

glycosyl-phosphatidyl-inositol 362

Hageman factor 304

halothane 194

head injury 452

health care 574

heart 317

heat and moisture exchangers (HMEs) 57

hemodilution 253

hemofilters 500

hemofiltration 307, 499, 507
    continuous arterio-venous - 509
    continuous veno-venous - 509
    high-volume - 503

hemodiafiltration
    continuous - 509

hemoglobin 447

hemoperfusion 503

Hensen's node 349

heparin 220, 307

hepatic
    - arteries 442
    - failure 473

hepatocytes 441

hernia 217

homeostasis 469

Huntington's disease 372

hydrocortisone 526

hyperglycaemia 230

hyperinflation 162
    dynamic - 140, 147
    pulmonary - 133

hyperkalemia 317

hypertension 220, 266
    pulmonary - 65, 126

hypokalemia 317

hyponatriaemia 231

hypothermia 220, 230, 252, 307

hypoxia 369

ICU 517

infection 525

inflation 117

injury severity score 411

inspiratory
    - capacity 143
    - resistance 57
    - work 133

integrins 304

inter-atrial communication 251

intercellular adhesion molecule 304

intermediate care unit 573

inter-ventricular communication 251

ion-channels 192

ipratropium 183

ischemia 369
    - reperfusion syndrome 472
    myocardial - 283
    penumbra - 370

isocapnic hyperventilation 164

isoflurane 194

isoleucine 444

isoproterenol 259

kallikrein system 304

kidney 471

kininogen 304

Kuppfer cells 441

lactate 255

laudanosine 520

leucine 444

lidocaine 217

liver 439
    - transplantation 471, 473

lung
    - mechanics 162
    acute - 109
    end-expiratory - volume 140

lysosomal 378

maximal
    - inspiratory pressure (Pimax) 162
    - oxygen consumption 143
    - tidal volume 143

membrane oxygenators 301

methionine 444

methyl-atropine 181

methylprednisolone 525, 527

microglia 379

midazolam 205

milrinone 260

mivacurium 185

monitoring 291

monocytes 304

multiple organ failure 477
- syndrome 471

muscarinic receptors 181

muscle
- function 133
- proteolysis 469
- relaxants 185, 517
non-depolarizing - relaxants 520
- weakness 162

myoglobin 500

naloxon 229, 273, 274

neonatal
- intensive care units 271
- respiratory failure 271

neonates 271, 509

nerve growth factor 362

neural inducer 349

neuroepithelium 350

neuromuscular diseases 161

neutrophils 304

nicotine 180

nicotinic receptors 180

Niemann-Pick disease type C 377, 379

nitric oxide 66, 125, 261, 305

nitroglycerin 66, 261

nitroprusside 66

nitrous oxide 173, 194, 215

non invasive positive pressure ventilation
(NIPPV) 164

non-cardiac surgery 281

norepinephrine 259

nutrition 477

nutritional status 472, 474

obstetric emergencies 265

oesophageal pressure 26

organ
- system failure 511
- transplantation 470

orthopaedic surgery 219

oxidative catabolism 469

oxygen 66

pancreas 471

pancuronium 186, 519
- bromide 521

paralytic ileus 211

Parkinson's disease 183

peak expiratory flow 139

perinatal asphyxia 271

pernicious anaemia 176

phenylalanine 444

phosphodiesterase 260
- inhibitors 260

physostigmine 229

placenta praevia 266

plastoelastic model 30

plateau pressures 149

polyacrylonitrile 500

polycarbonate 500

polymethylmethacrylate 500

polysulphone 500

portal vein 442

positive end expiratory pressure (PEEP) 65,
116, 163
intrinsic - 57, 147, 162
extrinsic - 149
static intrinsic - 149
dynamic intrinsic - 149

positive pressure ventilation 272

postoperative
- care 201, 215, 219, 254
- ileus 211
- pain 333

pregnancy 266

pressure
elastic recoil - 162
maximal inspiratory - 162
positive end expiratory - 163
intrinsic positive end expiratory - 57,
147, 162
extrinsic positive end expiratory - 149
negative expiratory - 135
oesophageal - 26
plateau - 149

propofol 195, 205, 217

prostacyclin 66, 67

prostaglandin E1 66

pulmonary
- artery catheter 291

- hyperinflation 133
- hypertension 65, 126
- rehabilitation 161
restrictive - disease 165
- surfactant 89

pulseless electrical activity 538

quality of life 165

quality-adjusted life year 577

rapacuronium 185

rapid shallow breathing 162

recruitment 117

relaxation volume 140

resistance 25

respiratory
- acidosis 538
- care unit 573
- muscle weakness 167
- muscles 162
- system 27
- system compliance 166

rocuronium 185

scopolamine hydrobromide 181

score
abbreviated injury - 411
injury severity - 411
revised trauma - 412
trauma - 412

scoring system 411

selective decontamination of the digestive tract 577

sepsis 66, 271, 502, 525

septic shock 499, 525

severity characterisation of trauma 413

sodium
- bicarbonate 273
- nitroprusside 260

Spenmann's organizer 349

spinal cord 350

step-down unit 573

stroke 227, 401

sudden cardiac death 543

surfactant 80, 85, 102, 276
pulmonary - 89

surgeon 338

surgical care 214, 215

survival 165, 167

syndrome
acute respiratory distress - 79, 102, 109, 116, 525, 527
central anticholinergic - 180, 226
ischemia-reperfusion - 472
multiple organ failure - 471

Tay-Sachs 377, 378

tetrahydrofolate 173

tetralogy of Fallot 251

thrombin 307

thyroid hormones 362

tibia 221

tidal expiratory flow-volume 133

tourniquet 221

tracheal
- intubation 203, 205
- tubes 25

transesophageal echocardiography 294

trauma score 412

troponine 255

tryptophan 444

tumor necrosis factor 304

tyrosine 444

VA/Q mismatching 162

valine 444

vecuronium 186, 519

ventilation
assisted mechanical - 164
mechanical - 57, 102, 110, 121, 205
non invasive positive pressure - 164
positive pressure - 272

ventilator 25

ventricular
- fibrillation 535, 544
- tachycardia 544

Venturi device 135

viscoelastic 29

vitamin K 446

volume
- closure capacity 163
maximal tidal - 143
end-expiratory lung - 140
expiratory reserve - 142
relaxation - 140
tidal expiratory flow - 133

work of breathing 162

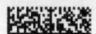